Medical Immunology

Medical Immunology

Edited by **Jim Wang**

hayle
medical

New York

Published by Hayle Medical,
30 West, 37th Street, Suite 612,
New York, NY 10018, USA
www.haylemedical.com

Medical Immunology
Edited by Jim Wang

International Standard Book Number: 978-1-63241-391-8 (Hardback)

Contents

Preface

Immune system is responsible for defending the body against disease causing agents whether internal or external. It generates antibodies to counter possible infections. Immunology is a rapidly progressing discipline playing a vital role in diverse fields of medical science such as oncology, parasitology, organ transplantation, etc. This book aims to shed light on some of the unexplored aspects and recent researches in this field. Different approaches, evaluations, methodologies and advanced studies have been included in this book. Scientists and students actively engaged in this area will find this book full of crucial and unexplored concepts.

This book is a comprehensive compilation of works of different researchers from varied parts of the world. It includes valuable experiences of the researchers with the sole objective of providing the readers (learners) with a proper knowledge of the concerned field. This book will be beneficial in evoking inspiration and enhancing the knowledge of the interested readers.

In the end, I would like to extend my heartiest thanks to the authors who worked with great determination on their chapters. I also appreciate the publisher's support in the course of the book. I would also like to deeply acknowledge my family who stood by me as a source of inspiration during the project.

Editor

fMLP-Induced IL-8 Release Is Dependent on NADPH Oxidase in Human Neutrophils

María A. Hidalgo,[1] María D. Carretta,[1] Stefanie E. Teuber,[1] Cristian Zárate,[1] Leonardo Cárcamo,[1] Ilona I. Concha,[2] and Rafael A. Burgos[1]

[1]*Laboratory of Molecular Pharmacology, Institute of Pharmacology and Morphophysiology, Faculty of Veterinary Sciences, Universidad Austral de Chile, Independencia 631, 5110566 Valdivia, Chile*

[2]*Institute of Biochemistry and Microbiology, Faculty of Sciences, Universidad Austral de Chile, Independencia 631, 5110566 Valdivia, Chile*

Correspondence should be addressed to María A. Hidalgo; mahidalgo@uach.cl and Rafael A. Burgos; rburgos1@uach.cl

Academic Editor: Carlos Rosales

N-Formyl-methionyl-leucyl-phenylalanine (fMLP) and platelet-activating factor (PAF) induce similar intracellular signalling profiles; but only fMLP induces interleukin-8 (IL-8) release and nicotinamide adenine dinucleotide phosphate reduced (NADPH) oxidase activity in neutrophils. Because the role of ROS on IL-8 release in neutrophils is until now controversial, we assessed if NADPH oxidase is involved in the IL-8 secretions and PI3K/Akt, MAPK, and NF-κB pathways activity induced by fMLP. Neutrophils were obtained from healthy volunteers. IL-8 was measured by ELISA, IL-8 mRNA by qPCR, and ROS production by luminol-amplified chemiluminescence, reduction of ferricytochrome c, and FACS. Intracellular pH changes were detected by spectrofluorescence. ERK1/2, p38 MAPK, and Akt phosphorylation were analysed by immunoblotting and NF-κB was analysed by immunocytochemistry. Hydroxy-3-methoxyaceto-phenone (HMAP), diphenyleneiodonium (DPI), and siRNA Nox2 reduced the ROS and IL-8 release in neutrophils treated with fMLP. HMAP, DPI, and amiloride (a Na^+/H^+ exchanger inhibitor) inhibited the Akt phosphorylation and did not affect the p38 MAPK and ERK1/2 activity. DPI and HMAP reduced NF-κB translocation induced by fMLP. We showed that IL-8 release induced by fMLP is dependent on NADPH oxidase, and ROS could play a redundant role in cell signalling, ultimately activating the PI3K/Akt and NF-κB pathways in neutrophils.

1. Introduction

Polymorphonuclear neutrophils (PMNs) are the first line of defence against microorganisms and are the main cellular component in the acute inflammatory response.

Neutrophils are primarily activated by chemotactic factors such as fMLP [1] and PAF [2].

Both compounds bind to the neutrophil cell surface via specific seven transmembrane domain G-protein coupled receptors [3, 4] and induce the activation of MAPK, PI3K, and NF-κB pathways in neutrophils [5, 6]. Notably, only fMLP has been described as a potent inducer of IL-8 in human neutrophils [7]. IL-8 is a member of the CXC chemokine family, relevant to the pathogenesis of several acute inflammatory processes and to the tissue damage associated with neutrophils [8]. Because PAF alone is not able

to induce IL-8 production [9], the existence of differential mechanisms of cell signalling, essential for neutrophil IL-8 release induced by fMLP, seems likely. It is widely known that fMLP induces a significant increase in superoxide production via NADPH oxidase; in contrast, basal levels of superoxide are unaltered in PAF activated neutrophils [9, 10]. In fact, neutrophils produce a strong respiratory burst, resulting in the release of a diversity of radical oxygen species (ROS), during phagocytosis or following stimulation with a wide variety of agents [11]. ROS originate from the activation of NADPH oxidase, which is assembled at the plasma membrane. This reaction produces two superoxide anions (O_2^-) and $2H^+$. The H^+ accumulation induces a transient intracellular acidification that activates several compensatory mechanisms such as Na^+/H^+ exchanger (NHE), H^+ channels, and V-ATPase [12], which promote intracellular alkalinisation [5]. ROS have been proposed as signalling molecules that regulate diverse responses in neutrophils, including cytokine expression [13–15]. It has been described that the superoxide anion induces NF-κB activation (IκBα degradation and p65 NF-κB translocation) and increases the expression of TNFα and macrophage inflammatory protein-2 in neutrophils [16]. However the role of ROS in cytokine expression is until now controversial in neutrophils. Human neutrophils from chronic granulomatous disease (CGD) that have genetic mutations in any of the components of the NADPH oxidase enzyme show an increase of IL-8 production induced by fMLP, suggesting that ROS reduce the IL-8 production in neutrophils [17]. Moreover, exposure of bone marrow-derived neutrophils to extracellular H_2O_2 diminished LPS induced activation of NF-B and expression of NF-B-dependent proinflammatory cytokines [18, 19].

In the present work, we present evidence that supports the role of NADPH oxidase in IL-8 release, the PI3K/Akt pathway, and NF-κB activity in human neutrophils treated with fMLP.

2. Materials and Methods

2.1. Reagents. Platelet-activating factor (C-16), fMLP, actinomycin D, SN50, UO126, LY294002, and SB203580 were obtained from Calbiochem (La Jolla, CA, USA). Histochoice, andrographolide, 4-hydroxy-3-methoxyaceto-phenone (HMAP), diphenyleneiodonium (DPI), and mon-oclonal antibody against β-actin were purchased from Sigma-Aldrich (St. Louis, MO, USA). The Akt inhibitor (sc-394003) 1L-6-hydroxymethyl-chiro-inositol-2-[(R)-2-O-methyl-3-O-octadecylcarbonate] was purchased from Santa Cruz Biotechnology (Dallas, TX, USA). Hank's balanced salt solution (HBSS), Iscove's Modified Dulbecco's medium (IMDM) Penicillin-streptomycin, certified foetal bovine serum, hydroethidine (HE), BCECF-AM, and nitrocellulose membrane were purchased from Invitrogen (Grand Island, NY, USA). Monoclonal antibodies against phospho-ERK1/2, phospho-p38, phospho-Akt (ser473), Akt, p38, rabbit IgG-HRP, and mouse IgG-HRP were purchased from Cell Signalling (Beverly, MA, USA). Polyclonal antibodies against ERK1 (sc-94), p65 NF-κB, Nox2 (sc-5827), gp91-phox siRNA, nonsilencing control siRNA, siRNA Transfection Reagent (sc-29528), and siRNA Transfection Medium (sc-36868) were purchased from Santa Cruz Biotechnology (Santa Cruz, CA, USA). Human IL-8 CytoSet Kit was purchased from Biosource International (Camarillo, CA, USA) and PE Mouse Anti-Human IL-8 (#554720) was purchased from BD Pharmingen. Proteases inhibitors were purchased from Roche Diagnostics (Indianapolis, IN, USA). Affinity Script Reverse Transcriptase and Brilliant II SYBR Green QPCR master mix were purchased from Stratagene (USA). SV Total RNA Isolation System was obtained from Promega (Madison, WI, USA). All other reagents and chemicals were purchased from Merck (Darmstadt, Germany).

2.2. Isolation of Neutrophils. Neutrophils were obtained from the fresh blood of healthy adult human volunteers in accordance with guidelines set by and with the approval

of the Bioethical and Bio-Safety Committee of Universidad Austral de Chile. Blood was collected in ACD vacutainer tubes, and neutrophils were purified by discontinuous Percoll gradient centrifugation. Neutrophils were suspended in Hank's Balanced Salt Solution (HBSS) (5.33 mM KCl, 0.441 mM KH_2PO_4, 138 mM NaCl, 0.34 mM Na_2HPO_4, and 5.56 mM D-glucose). Purity and viability were greater than 95% as determined by May-Grünwald Giemsa staining and trypan blue exclusion, respectively.

2.3. Cell Viability. Neutrophils (5×10^4/well) suspended in 100 μL HBSS were incubated with 500 μM HMAP, 10 μM DPI, 100 and 500 μM amiloride, 1 μM UO126, 10 μM LY294002, 10 μM SB203580, 10 μM AKT inhibitor, or vehicle (0.2% DMSO) for 30 min and stimulated with fMLP 100 nM for 4 h at 37°C. After that, we used the CellTiter-Glo Luminescent Cell Viability Assay according the manufacturer instruction (Promega, Madison, WI, USA).

2.4. Determination of IL-8 Release by ELISA. Neutrophils (2×10^6) were incubated with HMAP, DPI, amiloride, UO126, LY294002, SB203580, or vehicle for 30 min and stimulated with PAF or fMLP for 4 h. Supernatants were collected, and IL-8 was determined according the manufacturer's instructions (IL-8 Kit, Biosource).

2.5. Determination of Intracellular IL-8 by Flow Cytometer. Neutrophils (1×10^6) in HBSS were incubated with 500 μM HMAP, 10 μM DPI, 500 μM amiloride, 1 μM UO126, 10 μM LY294002, 10 μM Akt inhibitor, 10 μM SB203580, or vehicle (0.2% DMSO) for 30 min and stimulated with fMLP for 4 h at 37°C. Afterward neutrophils were centrifuged (300 ×g) for 6 min. The cells were fixed using paraformaldehyde 4% in PBS by 10 minutes at room temperature. Then the cells were washed twice using 500 μL of PBS. Afterward, the cells were permeabilized using 0.5% triton X-100 in PBS for 15 min and afterward washed twice with PBS. Then, neutrophils were incubated overnight at 4°C in 1% BSA-PBST (PBS-Tween 0.1%) containing PE Mouse Anti-Human IL-8 (1:100) or 0.25 μg mouse isotype antibody (5415 from Cell Signaling). A sample lacking the primary antibody was included as a control. Cells incubated with isotype antibody were incubated with 1% BSA-PBST with 1:1000 PE goat anti-mouse Ig (#550589) from BD Pharmingen (CA, USA) for 2 h at room temperature in the dark. Finally, the cells were washed with PBS and suspended in 300 μL of PBS, and they were assessed by flow cytometry FACSCanto II (BD, CA, USA) flow cytometer and analysed using FlowJo 7.6 software (FlowJo, OR, USA).

2.6. Real Time PCR of IL-8. Neutrophils (4×10^6) were incubated with fMLP for 1 h, and then 10 μM actinomycin D, 500 μM HMAP, 10 μM DPI, or vehicle was added for 1 or 3 h and total RNA was isolated. The RNA was treated with DNase and cDNA synthesis was made using 200 ng of total RNA. Real time PCR was performed using SYBR Green and primers of IL-8 and β-actin in MX3000P QPCR (Stratagene, USA) according to the conditions described elsewhere [20].

2.7. ROS Production. Luminol-amplified chemilumines-cence: neutrophils (1×10^6) were suspended in HBSS (250 μL/well) with 50 μM luminol in the presence or absence of inhibitors (HMAP, DPI, amiloride, UO126, LY294002, or SB203580) for 10 min. Cells were subsequently stimulated by the addition of different concentrations (1 nM–10 μM) of PAF or fMLP, or 100 nM PAF or fMLP, and the emission of light was recorded by a luminometer at 37°C for 30 min.

Superoxide production: O_2^- release was monitored spec-trophotometrically at 37°C by measuring O_2^- dismutase-inhibitable reduction of ferricytochrome c at 550 nm. Assays were performed in 96-well microtiter plates [21]. Control wells contained all components of the assay mixture plus O_2^- dismutase (20 U/mL) to correct for ferricytochrome c reduction by agents other than O_2^-. Cells (3×10^5) were suspended in HBSS (200 μL/well), incubated with inhibitors for 10 min, and stimulated by the addition of 100 nM PAF or fMLP. Absorbance (optical density) at 550 nm was recorded by a microplate reader (Tecan, Sunrise). O_2^- release was measured under conditions of linearity with respect to time and cell number, and O_2^- release was expressed as nmol $O_2^-/3 \times 10^5$ PMNs [21]. Additionally, superoxide production was assessed by flow cytometry using the fluorescent probe hydroethidine (HE). HL-60/neutrophils cells were loaded with 10 μM HE for 5 min at 37°C; then vehicle or fMLP was added and the superoxide production was measured at 10 min in FACSCanto II (BD, CA, USA) flow cytometer, with excitation at 488 nm and emission using a 610 nm absorbance long pass filter.

2.8. RNA Interference Assay. Small interfering RNA (siRNA) targeting human gp91-phox (Nox2) and a nonsilencing con-trol RNA were used. HL-60 cells were differentiated to neutrophils using 1.3% DMSO in IMDM medium for 5 days. Differentiated HL-60 cells were transiently transfected with each siRNA in siRNA Transfection Medium according to the manufacturer's protocol. Approximately 48 h posttrans-fection total proteins were isolated and gp91-phox levels were detected by immunoblot. Also, cells were stimulated with fMLP and assessed for superoxide production by flow cytometry and IL-8 production by ELISA, according to the protocols described above.

2.9. Neutrophil Intracellular pH. PMNs (2×10^7 cells/mL) were suspended in a pH 7.2 buffer (140 mM NaCl, 10 mM glucose, 1 mM KCl, 1 mM CaCl$_2$, 1 mM MgCl$_2$, and 20 mM HEPES) and incubated with BCECF-AM (2.5 μM; Molecular Probes, Oregon, USA) for 30 min at 37°C. The cells were then washed twice and suspended at 4×10^6 cells/mL. The 8×10^6 BCECF-loaded neutrophils were incubated with either vehicle, HMAP, DPI, amiloride, UO126, LY294002, or SB203580 for 10 min, followed by exposure to fMLP or PAF. Fluorescence was measured in a thermoregulated spectrofluorometer (LS55 Perkin-Elmer) at 490 and 440 nm of excitation and 535 nm of emission. The solution was continuously stirred. Fluorescence was converted to pH units using nigericin methods of calibration [5].

2.10. Immunoblotting. Neutrophils (5×10^6) were incubated with HMAP, DPI, amiloride, or vehicle for 30 min and then incubated with fMLP or PAF (100 nM) for 2 min. For ERK1/2, p38 MAPK, and Akt phosphorylation determinations, total protein extracts were prepared and resolved (50 μg) by 12% SDS/PAGE. Immunoblotting was performed using mono-clonal antibodies against phospho-ERK1/2 and total ERK1/2, phospho-p38 and total p38, and phospho-Akt (ser473) and total Akt [5]. Blots were developed with ECL. The primary antibodies were stripped, and each membrane was reprobed with an antibody recognising total nonphosphorylated pro-tein. Reprobed signal was detected as described above.

2.11. Immunocytochemistry. Neutrophils were incubated with UO126, LY294002, SB203580, HMAP, DPI, SN50, or vehicle for 30 min and stimulated with fMLP for 30 min. Cytospin was performed, and cells were fixed with Histochoice for 10 min and washed three times with PBS. Cells were sub-sequently permeabilized with 0.3% Triton X-100 in PBS for 15 min and washed three times with PBS. Each cytospin spot was then incubated with blocking buffer (1% BSA, 5% nonfat milk, and PBS) for 1 hour followed by incubation with an antibody directed against p65 NF-κB in blocking buffer overnight at room temperature. Cells were then washed three times with PBS and incubated with Alexa Fluor 488-conjugated goat anti-rabbit antibody (1 : 200) for 2 hours in the dark; nuclei were counterstained with propidium iodide. Cells were then washed with PBS, mounted with fluorescence medium, and examined by confocal microscopy (Fluoview 1000, Olympus). The Image ProPlus software 4.5.1 (Media Cybernetic, MD, USA) was used to measure nuclear or cytoplasm localization of p65 NF-κB.

2.12. Statistical Analysis. Results are expressed as fold increase compared to control, percentage, or area under the curve (AUC) and reported as mean $\pm$ SE. An ANOVA was performed and Dunnett's multiple comparison test was applied using GRAPH PAD V 2.0. The level of significance used was 5%.

3. Results

3.1. fMLP Produces High Levels of IL-8 and ROS and Increases the Intracellular pH. We determined the effects of fMLP and PAF on IL-8 release and ROS production as well as intracellular pH. The concentration of IL-8 was assessed by ELISA in supernatants of cells treated with each chemotactic factor for 4 hours. Only fMLP 1 induced an increase in IL-8 release compared to the basal control; IL-8 release induced by PAF was similar to the basal control (Figure 1(a)). Production of ROS was assessed by luminol-amplified chemi-luminescence and reduction of ferricytochrome c, to measure total ROS and extracellular superoxide release, respectively. A rapid and significant increase in ROS and superoxide production was observed in fMLP treated neutrophils with maximum peak at 112 s (Figure 1(b)). Following this peak, ROS release decreased rapidly and a second peak of smaller intensity in some volunteers was observed. This minor peak was distinctive and unique for each individual volunteer.

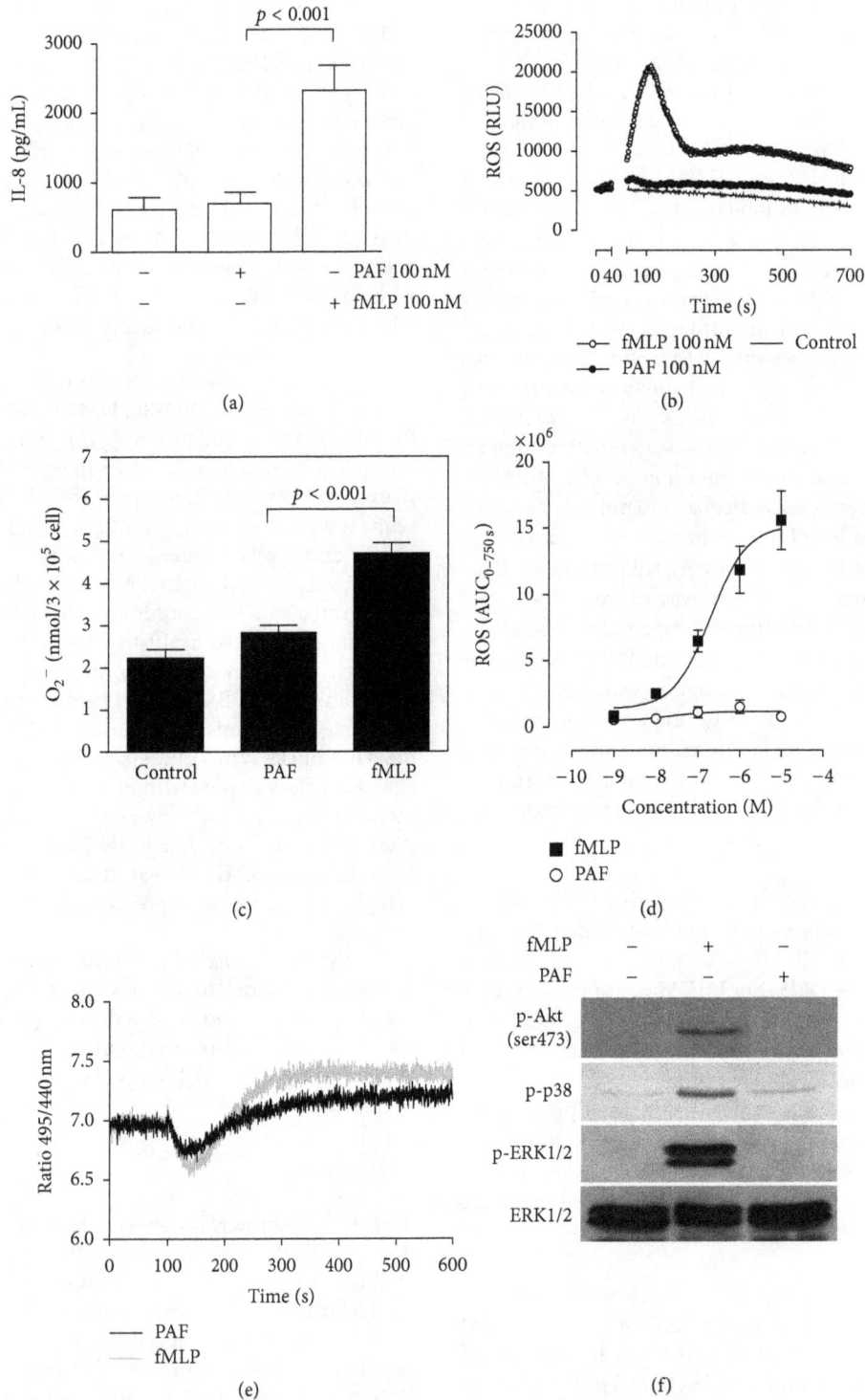

(a)

(b)

(c)

(d)

(e)

(f)

FIGURE 1: fMLP increases IL-8 release, ROS production, intracellular pH, and ERK1/2, p38 MAPK, and Akt phosphorylation. Human neutrophils were incubated with 100 nM fMLP or PAF for 4 h, and the IL-8 concentration in the supernatants was measured by ELISA (a). Neutrophils were incubated for 5 min at 37°C before fMLP or PAF was added. ROS production was monitored for 1200 s using a luminescence assay. RLU: relative luminescence unit (b), and superoxide production was measured following 30 min of incubation by a cytochrome c reduction assay (c). Curve dose response of ROS production in neutrophils stimulated with fMLP or PAF. AUC: area under curve for 700 s (AUC_{700}) (d). BCECF-AM-loaded neutrophils were incubated for 5 min at 37°C, fMLP or PAF was added, and the signal was measured for 600 s in a spectrofluorometer (e). Neutrophils were incubated with fMLP or PAF for 2 min, and total protein was analysed by immunoblot with specific antibodies against the phosphorylated form of Akt, p38 MAPK, and ERK1/2. In this case the same membrane was used after stripping procedure for reprobed and total ERK1/2 antibody was used as a charge control (f). Mean ± SE, $n = 3$.

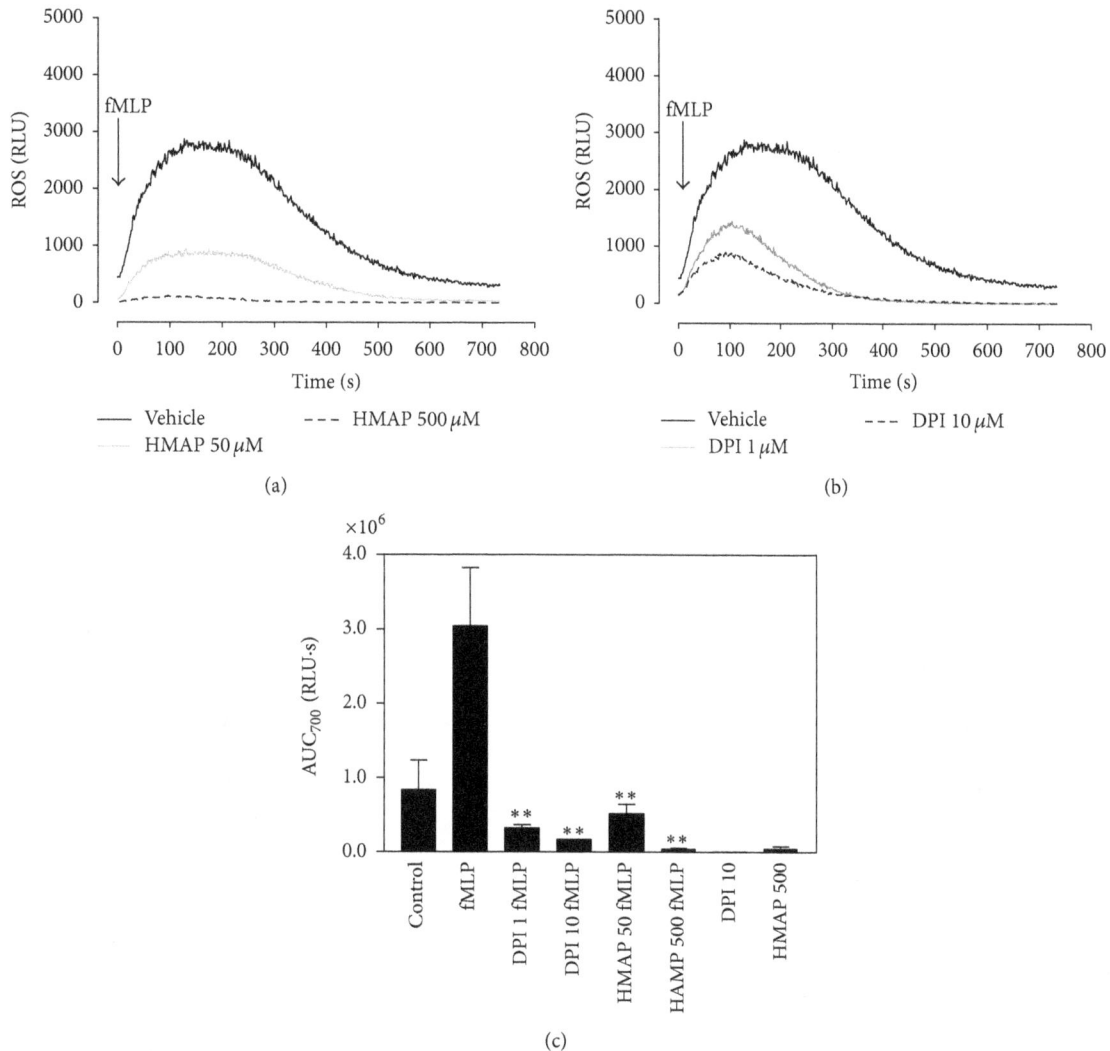

FIGURE 2: NADPH oxidase inhibition reduces ROS production. Neutrophils incubated with 50 or 500 μM HMAP (a), 1 or 10 μM DPI (b), or vehicle for 10 min were stimulated with 100 nM fMLP, and ROS production was detected by luminescence assay. In (c), the effect of NADPH oxidase inhibitors on AUC for 700 seconds (AUC_{700}) of ROS production is shown. Mean $\pm$ SE; $^{**}p < 0.01$ compared to fMLP; $n = 3$.

After 2 min of incubation, fMLP but not PAF stimulated an increase in superoxide release (Figure 1(c)). Only fMLP, in a dose-dependent manner, increased the ROS production (Figure 1(d)). NADPH oxidase activation also induces H^+ release in the intracellular space, contributing to slight and transient neutrophil acidification [12]. This lower pH is spontaneously restored to normal by activation of the Na^+/H^+ exchanger, producing an increase of intracellular pH [5]. We assessed the changes in intracellular pH in fMLP or PAF treated neutrophils using a fluorescent BCECF-AM probe. We found that fMLP and PAF induce a similar intracellular acidification in neutrophils; however, fMLP triggered a large rebound increase in intracellular pH following the period of acidification (Figure 1(e)).

Previously, it had been demonstrated that MAPK and Akt phosphorylation are induced by fMLP and PAF in neutrophils [6, 22, 23]. Here we show that ERK1/2, p38 MAPK, and Akt phosphorylation are more intense when induced by fMLP compared to PAF (Figure 1(f)).

3.2. NADPH Oxidase Inhibition Reduces IL-8 Release by Neutrophils Treated with fMLP.
ROS have been described as second messengers for the induction of cytokines [13]; however in neutrophils the role of ROS in the IL-8 release induced by fMLP is until now controversial. We assessed the role of ROS in IL-8 release by using DPI and HMAP, two known NADPH oxidase inhibitors. We observed that 1 and 10 μM DPI as well as 50 and 500 μM HMAP reduce, in a dose-dependent manner, the ROS production induced by fMLP in neutrophils as measured by luminol-amplified chemiluminescence (Figures 2(a)–2(c)).

Subsequently, IL-8 release was measured in neutrophils treated with DPI or HMAP for 30 min and stimulated with fMLP for 4 hr. We observed that IL-8 release was reduced following treatment with 500 μM HMAP and 10 μM of DPI (Figure 3(a)). Additionally, we assessed the effect of HMAP or DPI on stability of IL-8 mRNA. Neutrophils were stimulated with fMLP for 1 h and then actinomycin D plus HMAP, DPI, or vehicle for 1 or 3 h was added. The total RNA was used

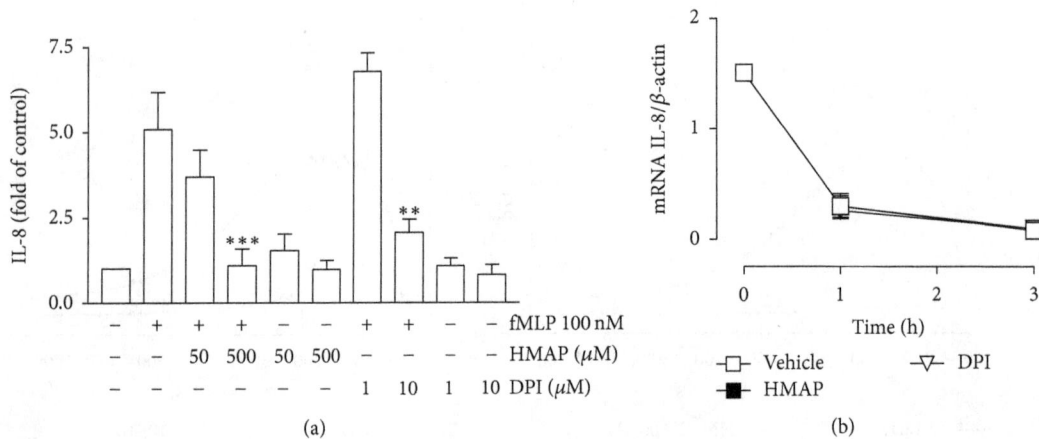

FIGURE 3: NADPH oxidase inhibition reduces IL-8 production. Neutrophils were treated with HMAP, DPI, or vehicle for 30 min and stimulated with fMLP for 4 h. IL-8 was measured in the supernatants by ELISA (a). Neutrophils were incubated with fMLP for 1 h, and then 10 μM actinomycin D and 500 μM HMAP, 10 μM DPI, or vehicle were added and incubated for 1 or 3 h. Total RNA was isolated and cDNA synthesis and qPCR of IL-8 and β-actin were done (b). Mean ± SE; $^{**}p < 0.01$; $^{***}p < 0.001$ compared to fMLP; $n = 3$.

for cDNA synthesis and real time PCR of IL-8 and β-actin. Figure 3(b) shows that the treatments with HMAP or DPI did not modify the slope of IL-8/β-actin compared to the vehicle, indicating that NADPHox inhibitors did not affect the mRNA stability, suggesting an effect on IL-8 at transcriptional level. siRNA assay targeting human Nox2 was used to verify the effect of NADPHox inhibition on IL-8 release. HL-60 cells differentiated to neutrophils were used for transfection assay.

Untransfected or transfected with siRNA Nox2 or siControl HL-60/neutrophils were used to determine Nox2 level, superoxide production, and IL-8 release. The transfection of siRNA Nox2 decreased the level of Nox2 compared to untransfected and siControl group (Figure 4(a)).

Also, a reduction of the superoxide production induced by fMLP in HL-60/neutrophils transfected with siRNA Nox2 compared to the untransfected or siControl group was observed (Figure 4(b)). Finally, we observed that the IL-8 release induced by fMLP was significantly reduced in HL-60/neutrophils transfected with siRNA Nox2 compared to untransfected or siControl transfected cells (Figure 4(c)).

3.3. HMAP and DPI Interfere with Intracellular pH Changes Induced by fMLP.

Intracellular pH changes induced during fMLP activation could be associated with the respiratory burst [24]. The intracellular pH drop induced by chemoattractants is transient (Figure 5(a)); the recovery of intracellular pH is NHE dependent [5]. To assess the impact of NADPH oxidase inhibitors on intracellular pH changes, we assessed the effects of HMAP and DPI on intracellular pH changes induced by fMLP. We observed that HMAP partially and DPI completely inhibited intracellular acidification. In addition, HMAP, but not DPI, partially interfered with the intracellular alkalinisation induced by fMLP (Figures 5(b) and 5(c)). We observed that amiloride, a NHE inhibitor, strongly reduced the intracellular alkalinisation induced by fMLP (Figure 5(d)).

3.4. Amiloride Reduces Release of IL-8 and ROS Production in Neutrophils Treated with fMLP.

It has been proposed that NHE is involved in IL-8 release [25]. To assess the role of NHE on ROS production and IL-8 release, we evaluated the effects of amiloride on human neutrophils treated with fMLP. Neutrophils were incubated with amiloride (an NHE inhibitor) for 30 min and stimulated with fMLP for 4 hr; IL-8 release was measured by ELISA. Amiloride (100 and 500 μM) reduced IL-8 release in neutrophils stimulated by fMLP, which suggests a role for NHE in the release of this chemokine (Figure 6(a)). However, it appears that amiloride interferes with ROS production, and the reduction of IL-8 release is secondary (Figure 6(b)). This was evident when we measured the AUC of ROS production over 25 min (Figure 6(c)), supporting that amiloride also affects the ROS production in neutrophils activated by fMLP.

3.5. fMLP Induces IL-8 Release via MAPK, PI3K/Akt, and NF-κB.

We analysed the signalling pathways that control IL-8 release. Neutrophils were pretreated with UO126 (MEK1/2 inhibitor), SB203580 (p38 MAPK inhibitor), or LY294002 (PI3K inhibitor) or with a specific Akt inhibitor for 30 min and stimulated with fMLP for 4 hr. A reduction in fMLP-induced IL-8 release was observed with all inhibitors analysed (Figure 7(a)). Furthermore, we demonstrated that andrographolide, a well-known NF-κB inhibitor [26–28], reduces the IL-8 release induced by fMLP. Neutrophils were incubated with the vehicle or inhibitors (UO126, LY294002, or SB203580) for 30 min and stimulated with fMLP for 2 min before ERK1/2, p38 MAPK, or Akt phosphorylation were analysed by immunoblotting (Figure 7(b)). fMLP induced an increase in ERK1/2 phosphorylation, a response that was completely inhibited by UO126. The p38 MAPK phosphorylation induced by fMLP was inhibited by SB203580. Furthermore, the increase in Akt phosphorylation induced by fMLP was inhibited by LY294002. Notably, Akt phosphorylation was also reduced by SB203580, suggesting that p38 MAPK could be upstream of Akt; this observation is consistent with previous reports in other cells which have indicated a possible role for p38 MAPK in regulating Akt phosphorylation [29].

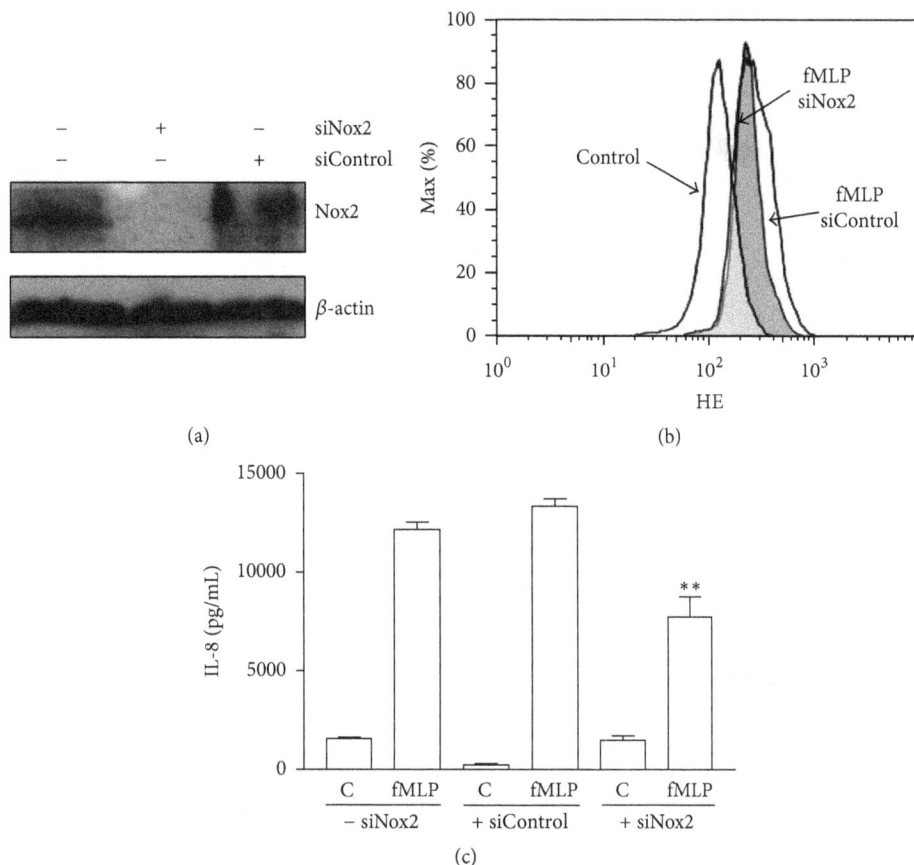

(a)

(b)

(c)

FIGURE 4: Nox2 siRNA interferes with ROS and IL-8 production in HL-60-derived neutrophilic cells. HL-60 cells were differentiated to neutrophils and transfected with Nox2 siRNA or control siRNA. (a) A representative immunoblot of Nox2 from cells untreated with siRNA or treated with unspecific siRNA (siControl) or specific siRNA (siNox2) is shown. As control β-actin was used. (b) HL-60/neutrophils transfected with siRNA siControl or Nox2 were loaded with HE and treated with vehicle (Control) or fMLP. The superoxide production was measured by flow cytometry. (c) HL-60/neutrophils untreated or treated with siRNA siControl or siNox2 were incubated with vehicle or fMLP for 4 h and IL-8 production in the supernatants by ELISA was analysed. Mean ± SE, **$p < 0.01$ compared to the siControl cells treated with fMLP, $n = 3$.

3.6. NADPH Oxidase, NHE, MAPK, and PI3K/Akt Inhibitors Increase the Intracellular IL-8 Level in fMLP Treated Cells. Because an interference of fMLP-induced IL-8 release was observed with the use of NADPH oxidase, NHE, MAPK, and PI3K/Akt inhibitors, a possible increase at intracellular level could be involved. To test this assumption we performed FACS experiments to assess the intracellular content of IL-8. We observed that DPI and HMAP increased the intracellular content of IL-8 in neutrophils stimulated with 100 nM fMLP. In a lesser extent, the inhibition of NHE or interference of PI3K/Akt, p38 MAPK, and ERK1/2 pathway also increased the intracellular level of this chemokine (Figure 8). Moreover, we discard a cytotoxic effect because none of these inhibitors affect the cellular viability (Supplemental Figure in Supplementary Material available online at http://dx.doi.org/10.1155/2015/120348).

3.7. NADPH Oxidase Inhibition Reduces Akt Phosphorylation. Because MAPK and PI3K/Akt participate in IL-8 release, we investigated whether NADPH oxidase activity has a role in ERK1/2, p38 MAPK, and Akt phosphorylation. Neutrophils were pretreated with DPI or HMAP for 30 min and subsequently stimulated with fMLP for 2 min; ERK1/2, p38 MAPK, and Akt phosphorylation were detected by immunoblotting. It was demonstrated that DPI and HMAP, in a dose-dependent manner, reduced Akt phosphorylation but did not affect ERK1/2 and p38 MAPK phosphorylation (Figure 9(a)). Also, we investigated the role of NHE in regulating MAPK and Akt phosphorylation. Amiloride strongly inhibited Akt phosphorylation but did not affect ERK1/2 or p38 MAPK phosphorylation, a pattern similar to that observed with NADPH oxidase inhibitors (Figure 9(b)).

3.8. fMLP Induces NF-κB Activation via MAPK, PI3K/Akt, and NADPH Oxidase. We evaluated NF-κB activation using confocal microscopy to analyse the p65 NF-κB translocation, a strongly expressed isoform in neutrophils [30]. In control cells, p65 NF-κB preferentially showed a cytoplasmic distribution. However, when the cells were activated by fMLP, p65 NF-κB was mainly localised in the nucleus (arrows in Figure 10); this localization was also visualised with the nuclear stain propidium iodide in merged images (Figure 10). UO126 markedly inhibited the nuclear translocation of p65

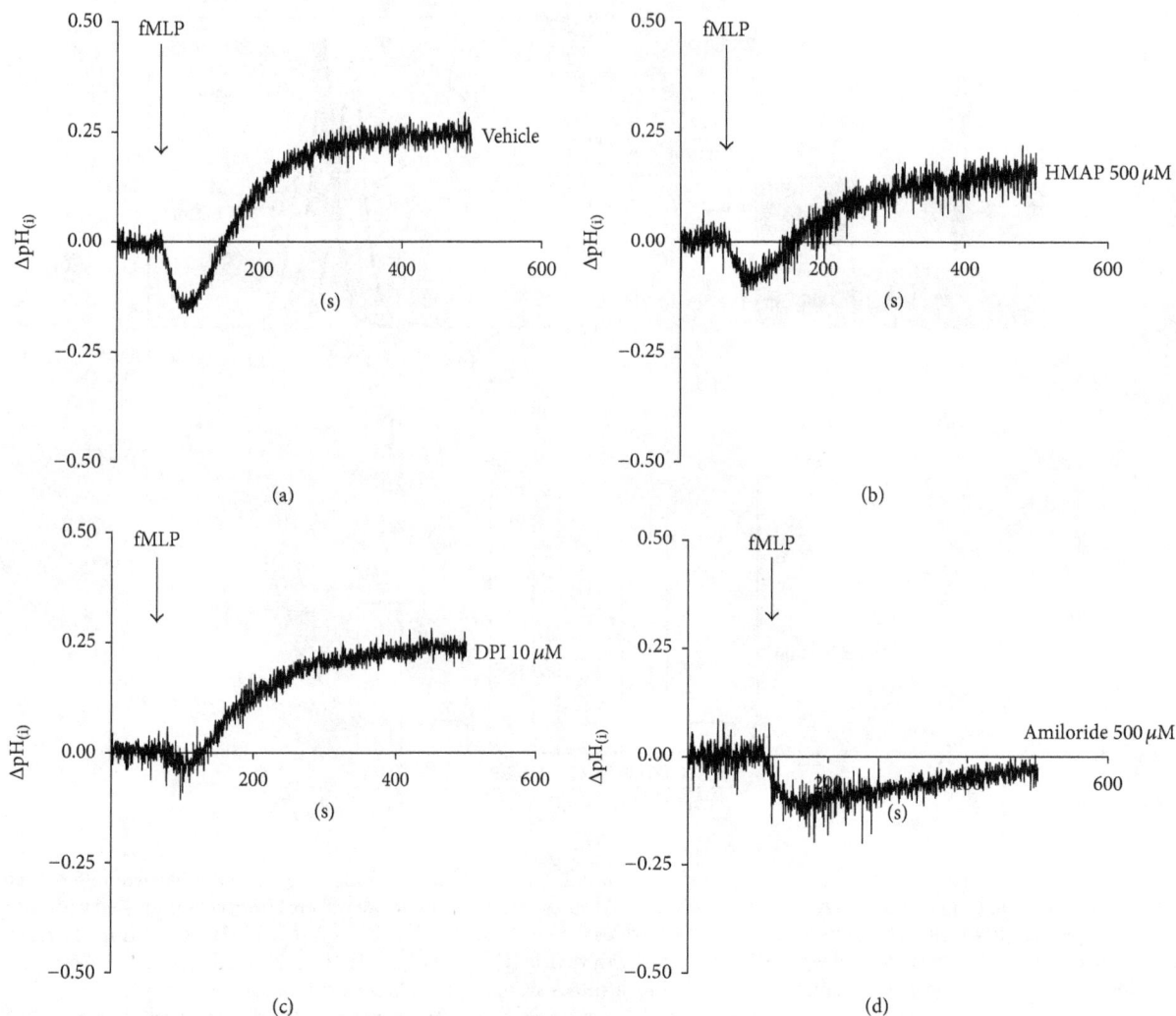

FIGURE 5: NADPH oxidase inhibition interferes with intracellular pH changes. BCECF-AM-loaded neutrophils were incubated with vehicle (a), 500 μM HMAP (b), 10 μM DPI (c), or 500 μM amiloride (d) for 10 min. A basal level was measured before 100 nM fMLP was added, and the intracellular pH was recorded for 500 s.

NF-κB in PAF activated cells, confirming participation of the ERK1/2 pathway in NF-κB activation. In cells activated with fMLP, preincubation with UO126, LY294002, and SB203580 significantly inhibited the p65 NF-κB translocation, resulting in a distribution similar to that of the control cells (Figure 10). These results demonstrate the importance of the ERK1/2, PI3K, and p38 MAPK pathways in NF-κB activation induced by fMLP. Additionally, we pretreated neutrophils with HMAP and DPI before stimulating the cells with fMLP. We observed that DPI and HMAP significantly interfered with NF-κB translocation, suggesting that NADPH oxidase is involved in the activation of this pathway. SN50, a cell-permeable peptide carrying a functional domain, nuclear localization sequence, that inhibits nuclear translocation of NF-κB/Rel complexes in intact cells, was used as control. SN50 significantly reduced the nuclear localization of p65 NF-κB induced by fMLP (p < 0.01). This result was in concordance with an inhibition of p65 NF-κB translocation from cytoplasmatic compartment.

4. Discussion

It has been reported that fMLP [7], but not PAF [9], is a potent inducer of IL-8 in human neutrophils. In fact, we demonstrated that fMLP, but not PAF, increases IL-8 release by neutrophils. Both chemoattractants induce a similar pattern of intracellular signaling pathways [5, 6, 31]. However, using two different approaches (luminol-chemiluminescence and reduction of cytochrome c) a clear difference between ROS production induced by fMLP and that induced by PAF in neutrophils was observed. It is widely known that PAF does not induce respiratory bursts and is considered mainly a priming stimulus in neutrophils [9]. There exist controversial antecedents in the role of ROS in neutrophils cytokine production. We hypothesised that fMLP induces IL-8 release via NADPH oxidase activity in neutrophils. We tested two NADPH oxidase inhibitors: HMAP, which reduces NADPH oxidase activity by competing with NADPH for the oxidase binding site [32], and DPI, which blocks flavin adenine dinucleotide binding to the oxidase [33]. HMAP and DPI,

(a)

(b)

(c)

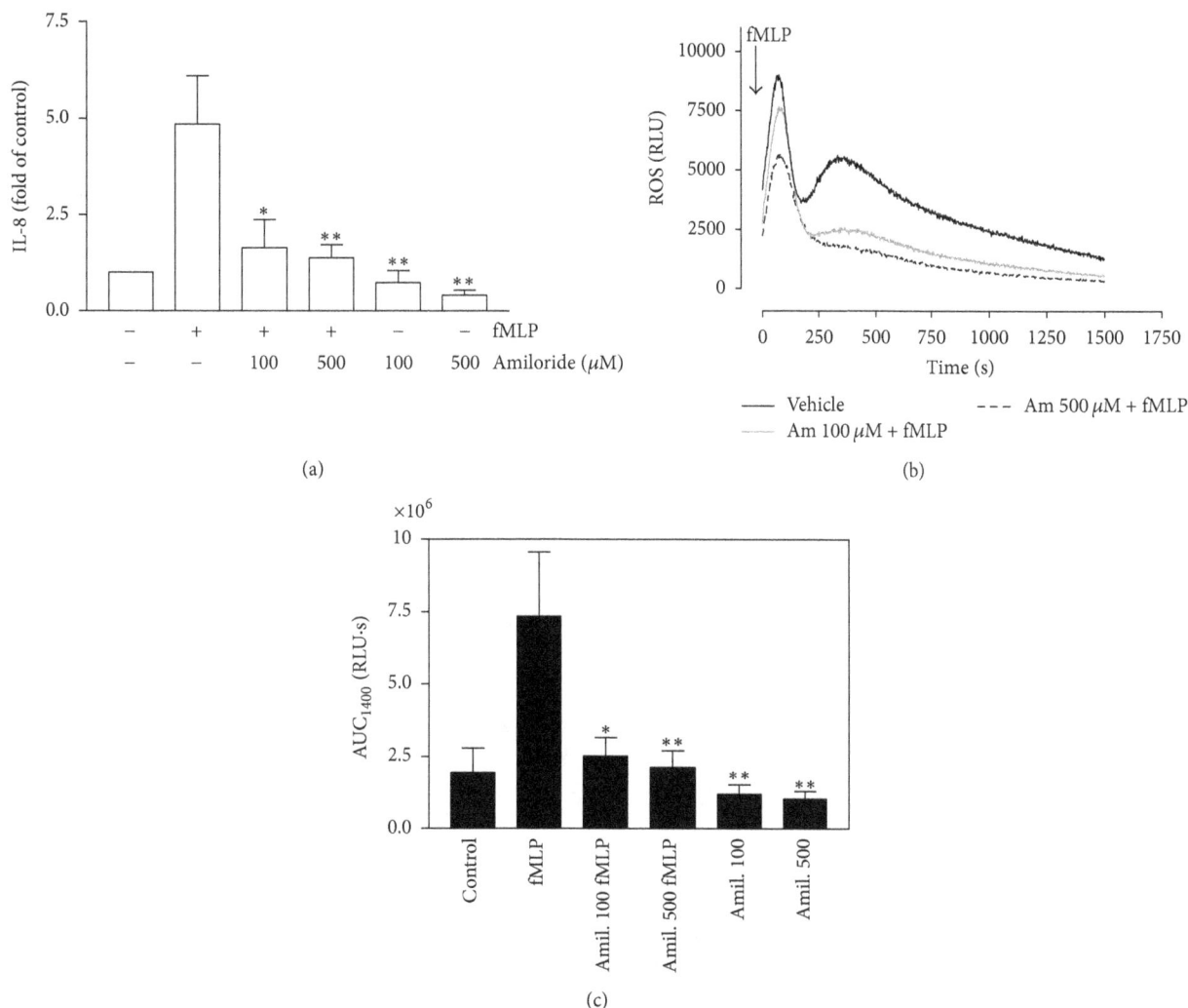

FIGURE 6: Amiloride reduces IL-8 and ROS production induced by fMLP. Neutrophils were incubated with vehicle or amiloride (100 or 500 μM) for 30 min and stimulated with fMLP for 4 h. IL-8 production was analysed in the supernatants by ELISA (a). Neutrophils were incubated with vehicle or amiloride (100 or 500 μM) for 10 min and then stimulated with 100 nM fMLP and the ROS production was detected by luminescence assay (b). In (c), the effect of amiloride on AUC for 1400 seconds (AUC$_{1400}$) of ROS production is shown. Mean $\pm$ SE; $^{*}p < 0.05$; $^{**}p < 0.01$ compared to fMLP; $n = 3$.

to a lesser extent, inhibited ROS production in neutrophils treated with fMLP. The observation that these compounds inhibit IL-8 release suggests that NADPH oxidase is involved in the secretion of this chemokine. We corroborate the role of NADPHox on IL-8 release induced by fMLP by using siRNA of Nox2 in HL-60/neutrophils. By the contrary, in neutrophils from chronic granulomatous disease that have genetic mutations in any of four components of the NADPH oxidase, fMLP increase the IL-8 neutrophil content [17]. These results could be explained by the different experimental conditions used. Because we measured the secretion of IL-8 but not total protein content, we propose that NADPH oxidase inhibition could be interfering with the release of IL-8, reducing the mobilization of a IL-8-containing organelle to the plasma membrane [34]. In fact, we observed that NADPH oxidase inhibitors increased the IL-8 at intracellular level in neutrophils treated with fMLP, suggesting interference in the release of this chemokine. In neutrophils, it has been

observed that ROS are involved in IgE-induced IL-8 release [35]. Moreover, in neutrophils treated with LPS the IL-8 release was inhibited using OH radical scavenger [36].

Because NADPH oxidase activity is involved in intracellular acidification in neutrophils [24], we assessed the effects of the NADPH oxidase inhibitors on intracellular pH changes induced by fMLP. fMLP induced biphasic pH changes characterised by transient intracellular acidification followed by intracellular alkalinisation. HMAP partially affected the intracellular acidification and alkalinisation, and DPI only affected the intracellular acidification. Sustained intracellular acidification has been demonstrated to increase H_2O_2 but not O_2^-, which is explained by an increased rate of dismutation of O_2^- at acidic intracellular pH [24]. Our results suggest that transient acidification alone is insufficient to increase IL-8; furthermore, PAF produced a similar intracellular pH pattern but did not induce IL-8 release in neutrophils. To assess the impact of intracellular acidification on IL-8 product,

(a)

(b)

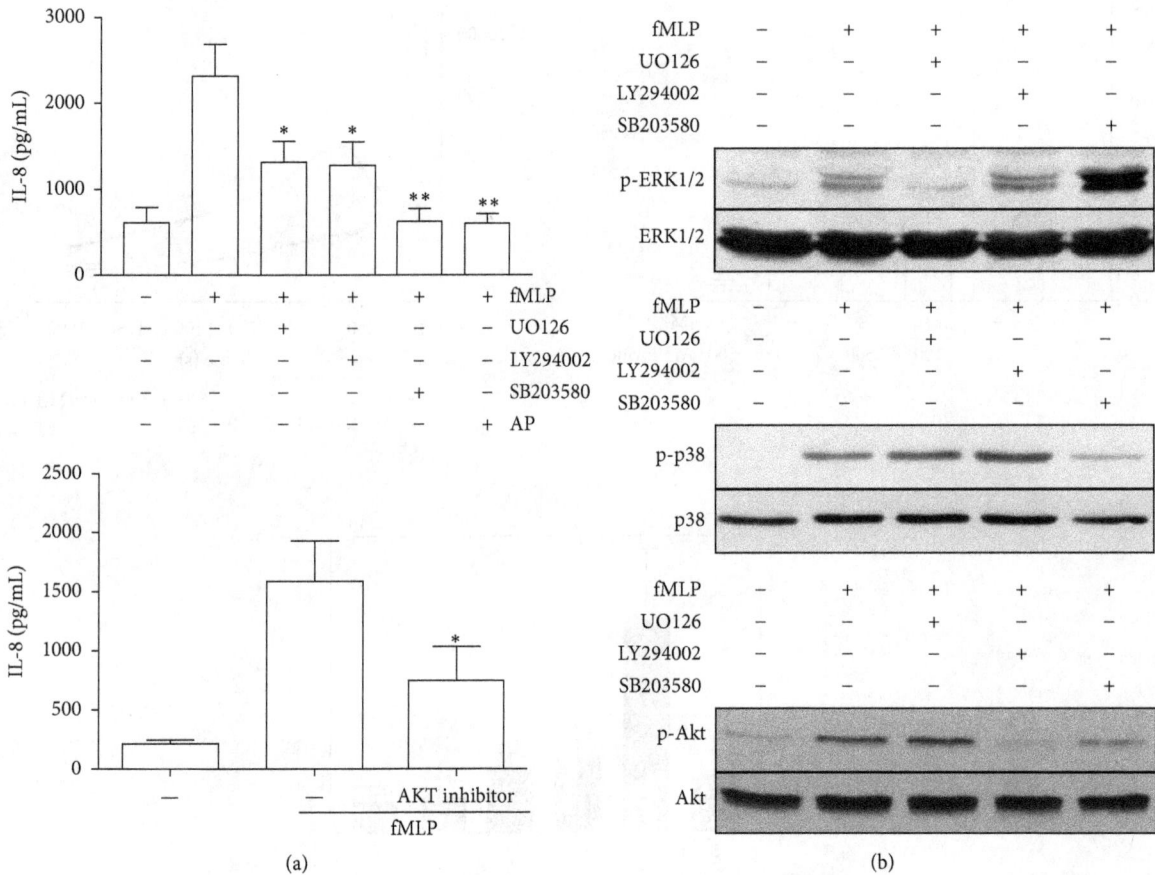

FIGURE 7: Effects of UO126, LY294002, Akt inhibitor, and SB203580 on IL-8 production and MAPK and Akt phosphorylation induced by fMLP. Neutrophils were incubated with vehicle, UO126 ($1\,\mu M$), LY294002 ($10\,\mu M$), SB203580 ($10\,\mu M$), andrographolide (AP) ($50\,\mu M$), or Akt inhibitor ($10\,\mu M$) for 30 min and stimulated with fMLP for 4 h. IL-8 production was analysed in the supernatants by ELISA (a). Neutrophils were incubated with vehicle, UO126 ($1\,\mu M$), LY294002 ($10\,\mu M$), or SB203580 ($10\,\mu M$) (b) for 30 min, stimulated with fMLP for 2 min, and analysed by immunoblot for ERK1/2, p38 MAPK, or Akt (Ser 473) phosphorylation. The blots were stripped and stained antibody specific to the unphosphorylated protein. Data presented are representative of three independent experiments. Mean ± SE; $^{*}p < 0.05$; $^{**}p < 0.01$ compared to fMLP; $n = 3$.

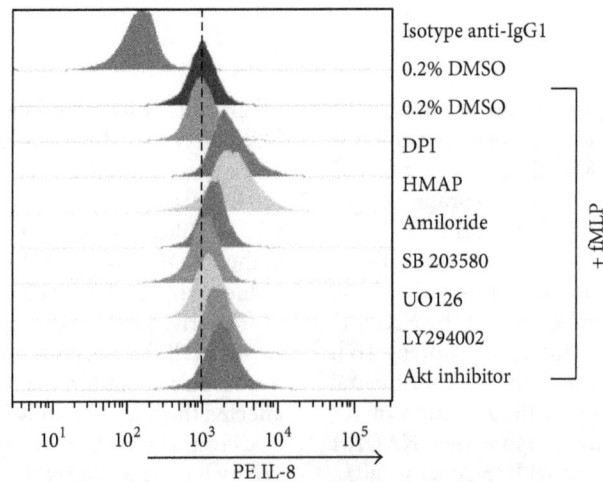

FIGURE 8: NAPDH oxidase, NHE, MAPK, and PI3K/Akt inhibitors increase the intracellular IL-8 level in fMLP treated cells. Neutrophils were incubated with vehicle, DPI ($10\,\mu M$), HMAP ($500\,\mu M$), amiloride ($500\,\mu M$), SB203580 ($10\,\mu M$), UO126 ($1\,\mu M$), LY294002 ($10\,\mu M$), or Akt inhibitor ($10\,\mu M$) for 30 min and stimulated with fMLP (100 nM) for 4 h. IL-8 intracellular content was measured by FACS. Data presented are representative of three independent experiments.

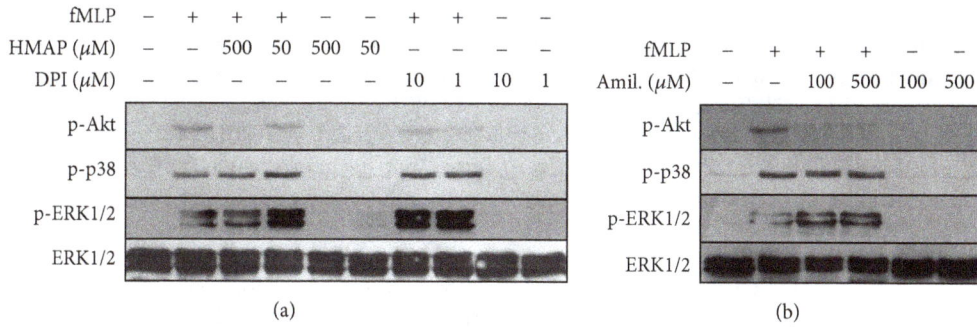

FIGURE 9: Effect of HMAP, DPI, and amiloride on MAPK and Akt phosphorylation induced by fMLP. Neutrophils were incubated with vehicle, HMAP, DPI (a), or amiloride (b) for 30 min, stimulated with fMLP for 2 min, and analysed by immunoblot for ERK1/2, p38 MAPK, or Akt (Ser 473) phosphorylation. The blots were stripped and stained antibody specific to the unphosphorylated protein. Data presented are representative of three independent experiments.

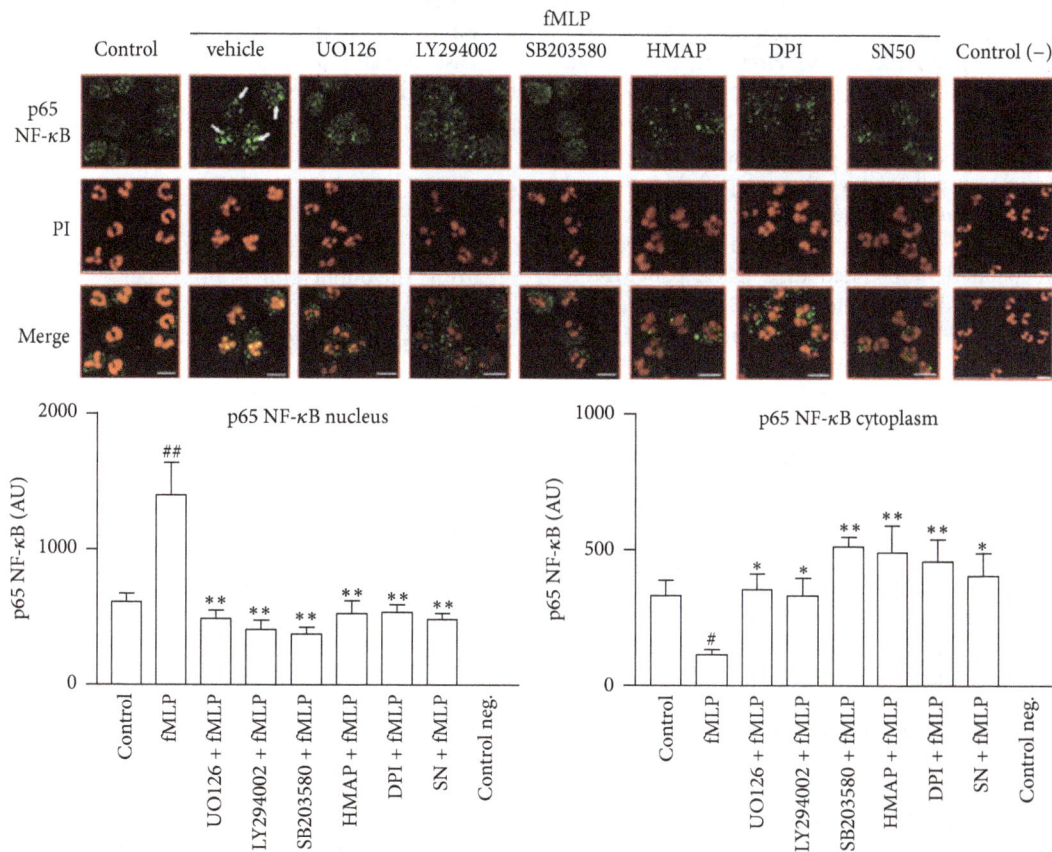

FIGURE 10: ERK1/2, PI3K, p38 MAPK, and NADPH inhibition reduce p65 NF-κB translocation induced by fMLP. Neutrophils were incubated with vehicle, UO126 (1 μM), LY294002 (10 μM), SB203580 (10 μM), HMAP (500 μM), DPI (10 μM), or SN50 (100 μg/mL) for 30 min and then stimulated with fMLP for 30 min. The cells were fixed and analysed by immunocytochemistry with an antibody targeted against p65 NF-κB. The nucleus was stained with propidium iodide (PI). The arrow shows the presence of p65 NF-κB in nucleus. The negative control was prepared without anti-p65 NF-κB. Bar: 10 μm. Figure is representative of three independent experiments. Each bar represents mean ± SE of arbitrary units (AU) of fluorescence intensity of p65 NF-κB, n = at least 5; $^{*}p < 0.05$; $^{**}p < 0.01$ compared to fMLP.

we subjected neutrophils to different concentrations of HCl. We found that intracellular acidification did not interfere with fMLP-induced chemokine secretion (data not shown). Additionally, we assess if intracellular alkalinisation via NHE could also be involved in IL-8 release. In monocytes and macrophages, LPS and IFN-γ via NHE promote the release of cytokines [25]. We found that amiloride inhibits fMLP-stimulated IL-8 secretion by neutrophils. However, amiloride also inhibited ROS production in neutrophils treated with fMLP, suggesting that NADPH oxidase could be involved in this IL-8 release. Moreover, PAF also activates NHE in neutrophils [5] but does not modify IL-8 basal levels or ROS production. Recently, it has been described that NHE inhibitors directly reduce mitochondrial function, thus preventing ROS production in cat myocardium induced by angiotensin II and endothelin-1 [37]. Therefore, we suggest that the effects of NHE inhibitors on neutrophils could be in part attributed to inhibition of ROS production.

The ROS could contribute to chemokine expression by acting as an intracellular second messenger, either directly or indirectly influencing the signalling pathways activated by chemoattractants such as fMLP. Our results show that NADPH oxidase inhibitors and amiloride reduced only the phosphorylation of Akt in neutrophils treated with fMLP, which indicate that MAPK pathways are not directly regulated by NADPH oxidase, suggesting the existence of a redundant effect of NADPH oxidase on PI3K/Akt pathways in neutrophils treated with fMLP, effect that could be cell and ligand specific. In support of this, LPS in macrophages, via NADPH oxidase, contribute to the phosphorylation of Akt but not p38 MAPK or ERK1/2 [38, 39]. However, angiotensin II potently induces phosphorylation of p38 MAPK and ERK1/2 in neutrophils, which is inhibited by NADPH oxidase inhibitors (e.g., DPI) and ROS scavengers [40]. In addition, HMAP reduces phosphorylation of p38 MAPK and ERK1/2 induced by α-IgE in neutrophils from sensitised allergic patients [41]; moreover, nonlethal concentrations of H_2O_2 have been demonstrated to activate p38 MAPK and ERK1/2 [42]. We demonstrated that SB203580, but not UO126, reduced Akt phosphorylation induced by fMLP in neutrophils. Therefore, our result supports that NADPH oxidase could contribute directly to the activation of PI3K in neutrophils stimulated by fMLP and would be necessary for IL-8 release [43]. In support of this, the inhibition of PI3K or Akt reduced the release of IL-8 induced by fMLP and increased the intracellular concentration of this chemokine. Our proposal suggests that NADPH oxidase participates in the activation of the PI3K pathway in neutrophils treated with fMLP. In fact, it recently has been described that Akt phosphorylation can be induced by ROS. Elevation of ROS can activate the PI3K/Akt pathway in TonB.210 cells with Bcr-Abl activated [44].

MAPK and PI3K/Akt pathways simultaneously play crucial roles in NF-κB activation [45]; therefore, the contribution of NADPH oxidase on NF-κB could be relevant in the IL-8 production induced with fMLP. HMAP and DPI reduced the p65 NF-κB translocation in neutrophils. In addition, NF-κB inhibition using andrographolide [27, 28, 45] reduced the IL-8 release in neutrophils treated with fMLP. In concordance with our results other reports show that NF-κB controls the expression and release of IL-8 in LPS- or TNF-α-stimulated neutrophils [46].

In the present study, we additionally showed that fMLP induces p65 NF-κB translocation in neutrophils and is upstream mediated by ERK1/2, PI3K, and p38 MAPK pathways. It has been suggested that there is a link between ERK1/2 and NF-κB in neutrophils activated with group IB secretory phospholipase A2 [47]. Previously, other authors have indirectly suggested that ERK1/2 MAPK could participate in NF-κB activation in human neutrophils, mainly because ERK1/2 is activated by TNF-α, a potent NF-κB

activator [48, 49]. A study showed that PI3K is upstream from NF-κB activation in neutrophils activated with type 1 IFN and exerts an antiapoptotic effect [50]. The role of p38 MAPK in the regulation of NF-κB activation in neutrophils is controversial. A report [46] concluded that p38 MAPK does not participate in NF-κB binding in LPS-stimulated neutrophils; however, in the present study we demonstrate a role for p38 MAPK in activating this transcription factor following fMLP stimulation. Our results agree with those of other authors who described the contribution of p38 MAPK to NF-κB activation in LPS-stimulated neutrophils [45]. The proteins downstream of p38 MAPK that control NF-κB are unknown in neutrophils; however, we did not exclude Akt as a possible candidate since inhibition of PI3K and p38 MAPK reduces Akt phosphorylation induced by fMLP. A similar cross talk between p38 and PI3K/Akt has been previously suggested in different cells [29].

Based on these results, we conclude that fMLP can increase NADPH oxidase activity and ROS production, favouring the activation of PI3K/Akt and NF-κB transduction pathways involved in the IL-8 release in neutrophils.

Conflict of Interests

The authors declare that there is no conflict of interests regarding the publication of this paper.

Acknowledgments

This work was supported by the following grants: FONDE-CYT 1090401 and DID-UACH S-200804. María A. Hidalgo was a Ph.D. student supported by CONICYT AT-4040024.

References

[1] M. A. Panaro and V. Mitolo, "Cellular responses to FMLP challenging: a mini-review," *Immunopharmacology and Immunotoxicology*, vol. 21, no. 3, pp. 397–419, 1999.

[2] W. G. Zhou, M. A. Javors, and M. S. Olson, "Impaired surface expression of PAF receptors on human neutrophils is dependent upon cell activation," *Archives of Biochemistry and Biophysics*, vol. 308, no. 2, pp. 439–445, 1994.

[3] F. Boulay, M. Tardif, L. Brouchon, and P. Vignais, "The human N-formylpeptide receptor. Characterization of two cDNA isolates and evidence for a new subfamily of G-protein-coupled receptors," *Biochemistry*, vol. 29, no. 50, pp. 11123–11133, 1990.

[4] M. Nakamura, Z.-I. Honda, T. Izumi et al., "Molecular cloning and expression of platelet-activating factor receptor from human leukocytes," *The Journal of Biological Chemistry*, vol. 266, no. 30, pp. 20400–20405, 1991.

[5] M. A. Hidalgo, F. Ojeda, P. Eyre et al., "Platelet-activating factor increases pH$_{(i)}$ in bovine neutrophils through the PI3K–ERK1/2 pathway," *British Journal of Pharmacology*, vol. 141, no. 2, pp. 311–321, 2004.

[6] J. A. Nick, N. J. Avdi, S. K. Young et al., "Common and distinct intracellular signaling pathways in human neutrophils utilized by platelet activating factor and FMLP," *The Journal of Clinical Investigation*, vol. 99, no. 5, pp. 975–986, 1997.

[7] T. Kimura, M. Iwase, G. Kondo et al., "Suppressive effect of selective cyclooxygenase-2 inhibitor on cytokine release in

human neutrophils," *International Immunopharmacology*, vol. 3, no. 10-11, pp. 1519–1528, 2003.

[8] A. Harada, N. Mukaida, and K. Matsushima, "Interleukin 8 as a novel target for intervention therapy in acute inflammatory diseases," *Molecular Medicine Today*, vol. 2, no. 11, pp. 482–489, 1996.

[9] S. Arbabi, M. R. Rosengart, I. Garcia, S. Jelacic, and R. V. Maier, "Priming interleukin 8 production: role of platelet-activating factor and p38," *Archives of Surgery*, vol. 134, no. 12, pp. 1348–1353, 1999.

[10] H. C. Steel and R. Anderson, "Dissociation of the PAF-receptor from NADPH oxidase and adenylate cyclase in human neutrophils results in accelerated influx and delayed clearance of cytosolic calcium," *British Journal of Pharmacology*, vol. 136, no. 1, pp. 81–89, 2002.

[11] J. M. Robinson, "Phagocytic leukocytes and reactive oxygen species," *Histochemistry and Cell Biology*, vol. 131, no. 4, pp. 465–469, 2009.

[12] R. J. Coakley, C. Taggart, N. G. McElvaney, and S. J. O'Neill, "Cytosolic pH and the inflammatory microenvironment modulate cell death in human neutrophils after phagocytosis," *Blood*, vol. 100, no. 9, pp. 3383–3391, 2002.

[13] L. Fialkow, Y. C. Wang, and G. P. Downey, "Reactive oxygen and nitrogen species as signaling molecules regulating neutrophil function," *Free Radical Biology and Medicine*, vol. 42, no. 2, pp. 153–164, 2007.

[14] T. Finkel, "Oxygen radicals and signaling," *Current Opinion in Cell Biology*, vol. 10, no. 2, pp. 248–253, 1998.

[15] H. J. Forman and M. Torres, "Reactive oxygen species and cell signaling—respiratory burst in macrophage signaling," *American Journal of Respiratory and Critical Care Medicine*, vol. 166, no. 12, part 2, pp. S4–S8, 2002.

[16] S. Mitra and E. Abraham, "Participation of superoxide in neutrophil activation and cytokine production," *Biochimica et Biophysica Acta—Molecular Basis of Disease*, vol. 1762, no. 8, pp. 732–741, 2006.

[17] J. A. Lekstrom-Himes, D. B. Kuhns, W. G. Alvord, and J. I. Gallin, "Inhibition of human neutrophil IL-8 production by hydrogen peroxide and dysregulation in chronic granulomatous disease," *Journal of Immunology*, vol. 174, no. 1, pp. 411–417, 2005.

[18] D. Strassheim, K. Asehnoune, J.-S. Park et al., "Modulation of bone marrow-derived neutrophil signaling by H_2O_2: disparate effects on kinases, NF-κB, and cytokine expression," *American Journal of Physiology—Cell Physiology*, vol. 286, no. 3, pp. C683–C692, 2004.

[19] J. W. Zmijewski, X. Zhao, Z. Xu, and E. Abraham, "Exposure to hydrogen peroxide diminishes NF-κB activation, IκB-α degradation, and proteasome activity in neutrophils," *American Journal of Physiology: Cell Physiology*, vol. 293, no. 1, pp. C255–C266, 2007.

[20] R. Natarajan, B. J. Fisher, and A. A. Fowler III, "Hypoxia inducible factor-1 modulates hemin-induced IL-8 secretion in microvascular endothelium," *Microvascular Research*, vol. 73, no. 3, pp. 163–172, 2007.

[21] E. Pick, "Microassays for superoxide and hydrogen peroxide production and nitroblue tetrazolium reduction using an enzyme immunoassay microplate reader," *Methods in Enzymology*, vol. 132, pp. 407–421, 1986.

[22] L.-W. Chen, M.-W. Lin, and C.-M. Hsu, "Different pathways leading to activation of extracellular signal-regulated kinase and p38 MAP kinase by formyl-methionyl-leucyl-phenylalanine or platelet activating factor in human neutrophils," *Journal of Biomedical Science*, vol. 12, no. 2, pp. 311–319, 2005.

[23] T. Khreiss, L. József, J. S. D. Chan, and J. G. Filep, "Activation of extracellular signal-regulated kinase couples platelet-activating factor-induced adhesion and delayed apoptosis of human neutrophils," *Cellular Signalling*, vol. 16, no. 7, pp. 801–810, 2004.

[24] A. S. Trevani, G. Andonegui, M. Giordano et al., "Extracellular acidification induces human neutrophil activation," *Journal of Immunology*, vol. 162, no. 8, pp. 4849–4857, 1999.

[25] P. De Vito, "The sodium/hydrogen exchanger: a possible mediator of immunity," *Cellular Immunology*, vol. 240, no. 2, pp. 69–85, 2006.

[26] Z. Bao, S. Guan, C. Cheng et al., "A novel antiinflammatory role for andrographolide in asthma via inhibition of the nuclear factor-κB pathway," *American Journal of Respiratory and Critical Care Medicine*, vol. 179, no. 8, pp. 657–665, 2009.

[27] M. A. Hidalgo, A. Romero, J. Figueroa et al., "Andrographolide interferes with binding of nuclear factor-κB to DNA in HL-60-derived neutrophilic cells," *British Journal of Pharmacology*, vol. 144, no. 5, pp. 680–686, 2005.

[28] Y.-F. Xia, B.-Q. Ye, Y.-D. Li et al., "Andrographolide attenuates inflammation by inhibition of NF-κB activation through covalent modification of reduced cysteine 62 of p50," *Journal of Immunology*, vol. 173, no. 6, pp. 4207–4217, 2004.

[29] M. J. Rane, P. Y. Coxon, D. W. Powell et al., "p38 kinase-dependent MAPKAPK-2 activation functions as 3-phosphoinositide-dependent kinase-2 for Akt in human neutrophils," *The Journal of Biological Chemistry*, vol. 276, no. 5, pp. 3517–3523, 2001.

[30] P. P. McDonald, A. Bald, and M. A. Cassatella, "Activation of the NF-kappaB pathway by inflammatory stimuli in human neutrophils," *Blood*, vol. 89, no. 9, pp. 3421–3433, 1997.

[31] E. Krump, J. S. Sanghera, S. L. Pelech, W. Furuya, and S. Grinstein, "Chemotactic peptide N-formyl-Met-Leu-Phe activation of p38 mitogen-activated protein kinase (MAPK) and MAPK-activated protein kinase-2 in human neutrophils," *Journal of Biological Chemistry*, vol. 272, no. 2, pp. 937–944, 1997.

[32] E. Van den Worm, C. J. Beukelman, A. J. J. Van den Berg, B. H. Kroes, R. P. Labadie, and H. Van Dijk, "Effects of methoxylation of apocynin and analogs on the inhibition of reactive oxygen species production by stimulated human neutrophils," *European Journal of Pharmacology*, vol. 433, no. 2-3, pp. 225–230, 2001.

[33] V. B. O'Donnell, D. G. Tew, O. T. G. Jones, and P. J. England, "Studies on the inhibitory mechanism of iodonium compounds with special reference to neutrophil NADPH oxidase," *Biochemical Journal*, vol. 290, no. 1, pp. 41–49, 1993.

[34] S. Pellmé, M. Mörgelin, H. Tapper, U.-H. Mellqvist, C. Dahlgren, and A. Karlsson, "Localization of human neutrophil interleukin-8 (CXCL-8) to organelle(s) distinct from the classical granules and secretory vesicles," *Journal of Leukocyte Biology*, vol. 79, no. 3, pp. 564–573, 2006.

[35] J. Monteseirín, P. Chacón, A. Vega et al., "Human neutrophils synthesize IL-8 in an IgE-mediated activation," *Journal of Leukocyte Biology*, vol. 76, no. 3, pp. 692–700, 2004.

[36] L. E. DeForge, A. M. Preston, E. Takeuchi, J. Kenney, L. A. Boxer, and D. G. Remick, "Regulation of interleukin 8 gene expression by oxidant stress," *The Journal of Biological Chemistry*, vol. 268, no. 34, pp. 25568–25576, 1993.

[37] C. D. Garciarena, C. I. Caldiz, M. V. Correa et al., "Na$^+$/H$^+$ exchanger-1 inhibitors decrease myocardial superoxide production via direct mitochondrial action," *Journal of Applied Physiology*, vol. 105, no. 6, pp. 1706–1713, 2008.

[38] J.-H. Kim, G. Lee, Y.-L. Cho et al., "Desmethylanhydroicaritin inhibits NF-κB-regulated inflammatory gene expression by modulating the redox-sensitive PI3K/PTEN/Akt pathway," *European Journal of Pharmacology*, vol. 602, no. 2-3, pp. 422–431, 2009.

[39] J.-H. Kim, H.-J. Na, C.-K. Kim et al., "The non-provitamin A carotenoid, lutein, inhibits NF-κB-dependent gene expression through redox-based regulation of the phosphatidylinositol 3-kinase/PTEN/Akt and NF-κB-inducing kinase pathways: role of H$_2$O$_2$ in NF-κB activation," *Free Radical Biology and Medicine*, vol. 45, no. 6, pp. 885–896, 2008.

[40] R. El Bekay, M. Álvarez, J. Monteseirín et al., "Oxidative stress is a critical mediator of the angiotensin II signal in human neutrophils: involvement of mitogen-activated protein kinase, calcineurin, and the transcription factor NF-κB," *Blood*, vol. 102, no. 2, pp. 662–671, 2003.

[41] A. Vega, P. Chacón, G. Alba, R. El Bekay, J. Martín-Nieto, and F. Sobrino, "Modulation of IgE-dependent COX-2 gene expression by reactive oxygen species in human neutrophils," *Journal of Leukocyte Biology*, vol. 80, no. 1, pp. 152–163, 2006.

[42] K. Z. Guyton, Y. Liu, M. Gorospe, Q. Xu, and N. J. Holbrook, "Activation of mitogen activated protein kinase by H$_2$O$_2$: role in cell survival following oxidant injury," *The Journal of Biological Chemistry*, vol. 271, no. 8, pp. 4138–4142, 1996.

[43] D. C. Newcomb, U. Sajjan, S. Nanua et al., "Phosphatidylinositol 3-kinase is required for rhinovirus-induced airway epithelial cell interleukin-8 expression," *Journal of Biological Chemistry*, vol. 280, no. 44, pp. 36952–36961, 2005.

[44] R. Naughton, C. Quiney, S. D. Turner, and T. G. Cotter, "Bcr-Abl-mediated redox regulation of the PI3K/AKT pathway," *Leukemia*, vol. 23, no. 8, pp. 1432–1440, 2009.

[45] J. A. Nick, N. J. Avdi, S. K. Young et al., "Selective activation and functional significance of p38α mitogen-activated protein kinase in lipopolysaccharide-stimulated neutrophils," *The Journal of Clinical Investigation*, vol. 103, no. 6, pp. 851–858, 1999.

[46] A. Cloutier, T. Ear, E. Blais-Charron, C. M. Dubois, and P. P. McDonald, "Differential involvement of NF-kappaB and MAP kinase pathways in the generation of inflammatory cytokines by human neutrophils," *Journal of Leukocyte Biology*, vol. 81, no. 2, pp. 567–577, 2007.

[47] E. J. Jo, H.-Y. Lee, Y.-N. Lee et al., "Group IB secretory phospholipase A2 stimulates CXC chemokine ligand 8 production via ERK and NF-kappa B in human neutrophils," *The Journal of Immunology*, vol. 173, no. 10, pp. 6433–6439, 2004.

[48] P. J. Barnes and M. Karin, "Nuclear factor-κB: a pivotal transcription factor in chronic inflammatory diseases," *The New England Journal of Medicine*, vol. 336, no. 15, pp. 1066–1071, 1997.

[49] K. R. McLeish, C. Knall, R. A. Ward et al., "Activation of mitogen-activated protein kinase cascades during priming of human neutrophils by TNF-alpha and GM-CSF," *Journal of Leukocyte Biology*, vol. 64, no. 4, pp. 537–545, 1998.

[50] K. Q. Wang, D. Scheel-Toellner, S. H. Wong et al., "Inhibition of neutrophil apoptosis by type 1 IFN depends on cross-talk between phosphoinositol 3-kinase, protein kinase C-δ, and NF-κB signaling pathways," *Journal of Immunology*, vol. 171, no. 2, pp. 1035–1041, 2003.

2

Reconciling the IPC and Two-Hit Models: Dissecting the Underlying Cellular and Molecular Mechanisms of Two Seemingly Opposing Frameworks

Carlos F. M. Morris,[1] Muhammad Tahir,[1] Samina Arshid,[1,2] Mariana S. Castro,[1] and Wagner Fontes[1]

[1]*Laboratory of Biochemistry and Protein Chemistry, Department of Cell Biology, Institute of Biology, University of Brasilia, 70910-900 Brasilia, DF, Brazil*
[2]*Laboratory of Surgical Physiopathology (LIM-62), Faculty of Medicine, University of Sao Paulo, 01246-904 Sao Paulo, SP, Brazil*

Correspondence should be addressed to Wagner Fontes; wagnerf@unb.br

Academic Editor: Carlos Rosales

Inflammatory cascades and mechanisms are ubiquitous during host responses to various types of insult. Biological models and interventional strategies have been devised as an effort to better understand and modulate inflammation-driven injuries. Amongst those the two-hit model stands as a plausible and intuitive framework that explains some of the most frequent clinical outcomes seen in injuries like trauma and sepsis. This model states that a first hit serves as a priming event upon which sequential insults can build on, culminating on maladaptive inflammatory responses. On a different front, ischemic preconditioning (IPC) has risen to light as a readily applicable tool for modulating the inflammatory response to ischemia and reperfusion. The idea is that mild ischemic insults, either remote or local, can cause organs and tissues to be more resilient to further ischemic insults. This seemingly contradictory role that the two models attribute to a first inflammatory hit, as priming in the former and protective in the latter, has set these two theories on opposing corners of the literature. The present review tries to reconcile both models by showing that, rather than debunking each other, each framework offers unique insights in understanding and modulating inflammation-related injuries.

1. Introduction

Many models have been put forward as an attempt to explain and counteract the real-life outcomes of several different inflammatory events in which neutrophil leukocytes play an outstanding role. Trauma, infection, hemorrhage, the response to both elective and emergency surgical interventions, and other pathological processes are incredibly prevalent in the human population. Such conditions are often complicated by nefarious immune responses that arise from these events that are, at least partially, mediated by neutrophils [1–4], since these are cells known for their central role in the mechanisms of inflammation in mammals [5, 6].

Logically, there is an ongoing effort to explain the inflammatory dynamics arising from these types of insults, as a first step in the direction of modulating and perhaps coordinating such responses in order to improve outcomes, reduce hospitalization times, and even prevent death.

The two-hit or multiple-hit hypothesis is a model that explains how sequential insults can synergically contribute to an inappropriate immune response [7] in which MODS/MOF (multiple organ dysfunction syndrome/multiple organ failure) is often the endpoint. As a broad definition, the two-hit model hypothesizes that an initial inflammation-triggering event, such as pancreatitis, trauma, burns, excessive bleeding, or elective surgery, can set in motion a priming condition for the immune system that can cause limited expression of SIRS (systemic inflammatory response syndrome) or other mild effects if left alone. Additional hits or insults (e.g., second-look laparotomy, infection, further blood loss, or ischemic injury during the process of aneurysm repair) are capable of causing an extraordinary and exaggerated immune response [8] that can evolve to MODS/MOF and death.

Ischemic preconditioning or IPC, on the other hand, does not represent an actual attempt to explain the inflammatory processes involved in SIRS/sepsis and its continuum of MODS/MOF. Rather, it is a collection of techniques that make use of the dynamics of the inflammatory response to generate a modulatory effect over these events. IPC is a demonstrable, observable, reproducible phenomenon in which a nonlethal, mild, and often cyclic ischemic event has the capacity to protect organs and tissues from a secondary, prolonged, and otherwise deleterious ischemic event [9], mitigating the response to ischemia and the ischemia-reperfusion injury (IRI).

Incidentally, the predominance of information in the literature about both models has a marked timeline difference. Throughout the late 1980s and early 1990s the two-hit model was considered a good standard as an intuitive and empirical explanation for some real-life chronologically based events seen in trauma and septic patients. Conversely, while the manipulation of the inflammatory response through exposure to controlled ischemic scenarios was already underway in the late 1980s [10], it was not until recently that IPC was shown to have clinical and surgical applications that far surpass those initially conceived and has, not without merit, been increasingly present in the literature.

The shift in the literature and the seemingly obvious difference as to how the two models treat a first inflammatory event, on one hand as a first/priming hit, and on the other hand as a protective/beneficial insult, have led to the notion that one model is capable of debunking the previous theory. In the following pages, we shed some light on some of the paradoxes regarding the coexistence of both models and try to reconcile both theories as simultaneously valid answers to some very different questions.

2. Two-Hit Model: An Intuitive Explanation for Empirical, Readily Observable Conditions

Sometime by the late 1990s the two-hit model soared to a unique position as a theory that successfully explained and accounted for many of the bedside events that accompanied trauma patients, which by the nature of their injuries were often exposed to sequential insults [11]. Another relevant well-known real-life example of the application of the two-hit model is the correction of ruptured aortic aneurysms [12], which requires imposing a second long-duration dry ischemic event for the actual repair of the initial naturally occurring hemorrhagic injury [13]. A host of experimental models has also been developed to mimic the events of multiple or sequential hits in order to further understand the processes involved in the augmentation of the inflammatory response. One example of those models is from the researchers that in 1998 demonstrated that neutrophil recruitment to the lung was increased when hemorrhagic shock (first hit) was followed by inoculation of LPS (second hit) if compared to a single-hit process [14]. Another group, on

the following year, demonstrated the same marked increase in PMN recruitment to the lung when subjects were exposed to a second hit with direct lung injury from LPS and immune complexes after a septic event that served as the first hit [15]. Nevertheless, examples of multiple-hit models that failed to induce the anticipated augmented immunological response can also be found in the literature. For instance, an American study from 2000 in which subjects were exposed to intratracheal injection of acid with or without previous induction of sepsis by CLP (cecal ligation and puncture) could not demonstrate a synergistic or even additive effect on the inflammatory response. Such study compared a two-hit insult versus a single-hit murine model, although their evaluation was limited to the number of PMN and the concentration of albumin present after BAL (bronchoalveolar lavage) [16]. This goes to show that the type and dynamics of the insult are to be considered when experimental models are designed to reproduce the inflammatory effects of multiple-hit insults.

As a rule, patients can be exposed to a variety of first-hit events, such as trauma itself or any number of hemorrhagic, ischemic, or infectious insults. During their hospital stay, patients are exposed to second, third, or further sequential events (e.g., laparotomy, fluid replacement therapy, blood transfusions, fracture repair surgeries, infection via catheter, or other sources). The mechanics behind it is that the first hit serves as a priming event that sets the patient towards the establishment of SIRS (systemic inflammatory syndrome). SIRS in itself is a fairly straightforward diagnosis, consisting in the identification of two or more of the following criteria [11]: (a) body temperature below $36°C$ or above $38°C$; (b) heart rate higher than 90 bpm; (c) respiratory rate in excess of 20 mpm or $PaCO_2$ lower than 32 mmHg; and (d) total white blood cell count above $12.000 \, mm^3$ or below $4.000 \, mm^3$ or the presence of over 10% band forms. If the first insult is by any chance infectious in nature, SIRS is loosely termed sepsis [17].

After the establishment of SIRS, a secondary, seemingly trivial, insult can jumpstart a detrimental organic response that can culminate in potentially lethal conditions such as MODS/MOF [14]. Depending on the type of sequential hits, the path following SIRS (which in this text is generally considered being end result of the first hit) is somewhat dualistic in nature. A first, anti-inflammatory state can ensue, which is called CARS (compensatory anti-inflammatory response syndrome) that, in and of itself, can be dangerous since it predisposes the body to infection that can in turn serve as one of the following hits. During CARS, immunosuppression occurs via impairment of T-cell function that can deteriorate the pathophysiological cascade and lead to infection, sepsis, MODS/MOF, and death [18–24]. A second proinflammatory state is triggered depending on the nature of the sequential events (additional hits). Major surgery, IR-like injury by fluid reperfusion in a previously hypovolemic patient, and infection by loss of gut barrier are some of the events that can serve as second or sequential hits. Cytokines and other molecular markers for both the anti- and proinflammatory states can be simultaneously found in patients facing hospitalization from several causes of SIRS/sepsis/MODS/MOF. This observation implies that these two biological conditions are not so clearly separated in real-life biological conditions but rather serve as a dynamic modulatory system that ideally keeps both the suppression and augmentation of the inflammatory response in check throughout the clinical evolution of the patient. Additional hits tend to throw this system out of balance, causing the inflammatory response and clinical presentation to escalate. Regardless of the type of insult, the two-hit model postulates that the inflammatory response to the additional challenges is generally exaggerated, since the body has already been primed by the first event, or hit. The complex molecular cascades and the serious remote injuries triggered by this proinflammatory state are responsible for the potentially fatal state of MODS/MOF [17]. The two-hit model clearly shows that severely injured or ill patients are commonly more easily susceptible to the sequential insults, which singly or cumulatively lead to their unfavorable outcomes, observation which indeed can be easily correlated to common clinical outcomes.

The molecular pathways that explain the two-hit model are incredibly complex and, to this date, there has not been a definitive flow of events identified. One can easily understand why this is the case, since the variable nature of the first and subsequent events imposes a humongous challenge to the definition of the underlying inflammatory biochemistry behind the two-hit model theory. For that reason, any discussion of the events occurring during the progression of the multiple inflammatory hits has to take into account the specifics of every single type of insult. Below we discuss some general molecular and physiological aspects underlying the two-hit or multiple-hit inflammatory events.

2.1. Cellular Responses. After an initial insult the immune system is affected at a cellular level as the inflammatory cells become easily susceptible and primed to any sequential stimulus/insult and are therefore further activated by a minor sequential exposure, allowing mildly injurious stimuli to synergistically set off the inflammatory machinery and cause tissue damage [25–28] both locally and remotely. The immune response induced by the first hit can be traumatic in nature and may be limited locally as in monotrauma or it may be a massive systemic immune activation as in polytrauma [18, 21, 29–31]. Different trauma-related inflammatory actors have been recently characterized among which the complement system stands out as a key mediator [20, 21, 24, 32–37]. When the complement system is activated by any of its three pathways, it plays a pivotal role in eliminating foreign pathogens by opsonization/phagocytosis (C3b, C4b) and chemotaxic attraction of leukocytes (C3a, C5a) and also directly lysing the pathogens through the membrane attack complex (MAC, C5b-9) [35, 38–40]. The anaphylatoxins like C3a and C5a recruit phagocytes and polymorphonuclear leukocytes (PMN) to the site of injury as these anaphylatoxins are strong chemoattractants for phagocytes [41] and also induce the degranulation of mast cells, basophils, and eosinophils [35, 39, 40]. It is clear from clinical and experimental studies that after trauma the complement system gets activated both locally and at the injury site, as well as systemically [42–47]. Tissue damage and cell injury cause the release of alarmins, which are non-pathogen-derived danger signals

capable of activating the innate immune responses. These include annexins, heat-shock proteins (HSPs), defensins, and classical markers of tissue injury like S100 protein and high mobility group box-1 (HMGB1) nuclear protein [48, 49]. Alarmins correlate with the heterogenic innate immune inflammatory molecules and pathogen-associated molecular patterns (PAMPs), which are recognized by the immune system as foreign molecules because of their characteristic molecular pattern [50, 51]. Together, alarmins and PAMPs form a large family of damage-associated molecular patterns (DAMPs) and are recognized by immune cells that express multiligand receptors, such as Toll-like receptors (TLRs), on their surfaces. Therefore DAMPs are capable of activating innate immune responses after trauma either when the traumatic injury is a standalone event or when the traumatic event is further complicated by infection [24, 48]. It is reasonable to assume that similar triggers are present when the first and sequential hits are not traumatic in nature.

2.2. Molecular Responses. Whatever the cause of the insult, it is generally accepted that cytokinemia or cytokine storm is of major importance during the biological responses inside the two-hit model [12]. Cytokines are molecules of low molecular weight that are secreted by immune cells and serve as mediators for the communication between leukocytes, interlinking innate and adaptive immune responses. Traumatic tissue injuries induce the expression of proinflammatory cytokines, such as tumor necrosis factor (TNF) and interleukin- (IL-) 1β, IL-6, IL-8, IL-12, IL-15, and IL-18 [52–54]. In addition to other biological roles, cytokines also activate neutrophils which are key players in the early inflammatory response to trauma or other first-hit insults [55]. Neutrophils are pulled away from the circulation to the site of injury by chemotactic molecules, such as complement anaphylatoxins and chemotactic cytokines, called chemokines, most notably IL-8 [39, 56]. Several studies have tracked cytokine production during inflammatory conditions, demonstrating their primary role in tissue damage by cellular priming/activation and also in the pathophysiology of SIRS. In particular, tumor necrosis factor-α (TNF-α), IL-1β, IL-6, and IL-8 have been consistently present during these observations. Nevertheless inconsistent results in terms of levels of TNF-α, IL-1β, and IL-6 have prevented a definitive association between high concentration of these agents and the risk for development of MODS/MOF [57, 58]. In an ideally regulated immune response, neutrophils play an important role in the defense and repair of injured tissues. PMN priming for cytotoxicity covers a wide range of physiologic responses, like degranulation of enzymes, superoxide anion generation, lipid mediator (LTB4) and cytokine (IL-8) production, decreased selectin expression (L-selectin), enhanced integrin expression (CD11b/CD18), cellular elongation, reduced deformability, and delayed apoptosis [59–63] in addition to other cellular events such as adhesion, rolling, and ultimately diapedesis [20, 64, 65]. Neutrophil priming results from the preexposure of the cell to priming molecules like platelet activating factor (PAF), anaphylatoxin C5a, granulocyte macrophage-colony stimulating factor (GM-CSF), LTB4, substance P, IL-8, interferon, TNF-α, LPS, L-selectin cross-linking, and

CD18 cross-linking [20, 66–68], which could arise from exposure to first-hit events [66, 69]. Some investigators have suggested that circulating monocytes and tissue macrophages also become primed after severe injury [70–72]. Despite the beneficial effects of neutrophils in host defense, a dysfunction in priming and subsequent cellular activation may result in an overwhelming inflammatory response. Such response leads to tissue injury of previously healthy sites via the local release of toxic metabolites and enzymes that may lead to acute respiratory distress syndrome (ARDS), MODS/MOF, secondary blood-brain barrier dysfunction, and brain edema after traumatic brain injury [21, 68, 73–79].

2.3. *Vascular Responses.* Aside from circulating cytokines and signaling molecules, the response of the endothelium and its relationship with immune cells are central in understanding the process through which sequential insults can cause tissue injury. Endothelial cells are obviously present in virtually every single organ and are in constant contact with immune molecular and cellular mediators. Therefore, rather than simply being a passive pipe-like structure, the endothelium serves as an important and complex immune agent and its dysfunction is closely associated with increased morbidity in SIRS and its complications via an increase of uncontrolled vascular permeability [80]. In addition, microvascular changes caused by a first hit such as hemorrhagic shock have been implicated as one of the mechanisms through which a second hit such as infection is able to cause an exaggerated systemic inflammatory response [7] that is more likely to trigger MODS/MOF.

Central to the role of the endothelium in immune responses is the glycocalyx, a thin and complex structure of proteoglycans, glycosaminoglycans, glycoproteins, and other soluble molecules, which serves as a dynamic interface through which the vascular bed communicates with the flowing blood through continuous shedding and synthesis of this layer [81, 82]. Functions of the glycocalyx vary widely, from conferring the outer surface of the endothelium an overall negative charge to regulating vascular permeability and fluidic balance, all the way to preventing erroneous and inadvertent adhesion of leukocytes and platelets to the vascular wall by mechanically shielding molecules such as intercellular adhesion molecule 1, vascular cell adhesion molecule 1, and selectins [81, 83]. The binding of cytokines in the glycocalyx also plays an important role in enclosing and effectively hiding these molecules from circulating leukocytes cell surface receptors. Loss of glycocalyx function has been observed under many inflammatory processes such as diabetes, atherosclerosis, sepsis, and IR injury due to, amongst other things, changes in the interaction of the exposed vascular bed and circulating leukocytes and increased vascular permeability [81, 82].

Endothelial cells express innate immune receptors, such as Toll-like receptors, which can trigger intracellular inflammatory responses through mediators such as MAPK and NF-κB that can ultimately modulate vascular permeability and coagulation [84]. It is even conceivable that thrombi inside the microvasculature may have a role in mechanically preventing infectious agents from spreading. Albeit never actually dormant, the overt activation of the endothelium can be triggered as a natural and physiological response to the stimulation of the innate immune response via reactive oxygen signaling dominance due to an uncoupled state of the endothelial nitric oxide synthase (eNOS) or as a pivotal part of many different disease processes involved mainly in cardiovascular illnesses [85].

In healthy and undisturbed endothelium, cell junctions are constantly regulated to preserve overall vascular barrier integrity while allowing for the passage of small molecules and immune cells that are responsible for tissue surveillance [86, 87]. Activated neutrophils and their interaction with the endothelium, involving neutrophil adhesion and subsequent transendothelial migration, play a crucial role in SIRS pathophysiology and are closely related to endothelial dysfunction, associated with loss of functional intracellular contact sites. This loss of integrity of cell-to-cell contact results in tissue edema and impairment of microcirculation and ultimately leads to organ dysfunction [88–90]. Microvascular endothelium also has an integral role in postinjury priming of the innate inflammatory response. Neutrophil priming agents such as LPS and TNF cause endothelial activation by stimulating the expression of adhesion molecules (e.g., ICAM and VCAM) on the vascular bed that can account for tissue damage-driven cell migration [91–93].

The process of neutrophil activation involves complement dependent and complement independent mechanisms. When the blood comes in contact with the activated endothelium it strongly activates the complement and clotting cascades which in turn causes neutrophil activation via the anaphylatoxins C3a, C5a, and C5b9 [94], as previously discussed. Neutrophil adhesion to the endothelium is carried out by cytokines such as IL-1 and PAF but also by adenosine, prostacyclin, and cAMP. Endothelial activation causes the high expression of adhesion molecules or activation of constitutively expressed molecules like ICAM-1, leukocyte function-associated antigen-1 (LFA-1), or E-selectin [95, 96]. The endothelial activation by cytokines leads to the upregulation of adhesion molecules and can be accompanied by the expression of anaphylatoxins C3a and C5b, PAF, and LTB4. TNF-α and IL-1 result in neutrophil degranulation and further activation of endothelial cells. For example, neutrophil degranulation induced by TNF-α leads to vascular endothelium architecture destruction by proteolytic enzymes such as elastase, gelatinase, and collagenase and subsequently to the disruption of vascular wall integrity as elastase degrades the endothelial homodimeric cadherin-cadherin binding [97]. The overall result of this process is augmented permeability, adhesion, and migration of PMN and other leukocytes to locally or remotely affected tissues and organs, causing tissue damage, organ dysfunction, and ultimately MODS/MOF [91–93].

The combination of these cellular, molecular, and vascular phenomena needs to be constantly and ever so delicately balanced and regulated. The sheer simplicity of the reasoning behind the two-hit argument is that sequential and superimposed insults tend to challenge this fragile environment and are capable of synergistically rerouting the inflammatory response to a tissue injury-driven path that can be ultimately recognized through the progression of the complex SIRS/sepsis/ARDS/MODS/MOF continuum, and possibly death.

3. IPC: An Elegant and Ingenious Solution for Modulating the Inflammatory Response to Ischemia

As early as 1986, researches were already noticing the protective effects that short-term nonlethal ischemic cycles could have over the heart if it were to be later exposed to a prolonged, potentially fatal ischemic event [10] and in 1990 a similar phenomenon had already been identified in the brain of gerbils [98]. This basic mechanism itself can be established in a variety of different organs and systems, and the initial protection-inducing ischemia can be of varying types and profiles. IPC or ischemic preconditioning is the general term that describes such phenomena. Some aspects of preconditioning through ischemia can even be naturally occurring as it is seen in patients that suffer from cerebral transient ischemic attacks (TIAs) and do not incur in structural damage to neurons but rather are actually protected from subsequent major episodes [99] demonstrating that IPC-like mechanisms can be adaptive in nature.

In general terms, IPC can be achieved by relatively gentle and often cyclic ischemic events. A tissue that undergoes an ischemic event is more likely to survive a subsequent prolonged deprivation of oxygen. Ideal duration and proportion of these initial insults of preconditioning are species- and tissue-specific. For example IPC can be achieved in rats during one to three cycles of IR [100, 101], while in rabbits a single 5 min cycle of IR is sufficient [102] and in dogs a 2.5 min single event of IR has been proven to be effective [103].

Processes involved during reperfusion of severe ischemic injuries are a consequence of a complex sequence of events leading to changes in capillary permeability, neutrophil recruitment, complement activation, and generation of reactive oxygen species [104], similar to other inflammation-driven insults. Preconditioned systems tend to attenuate these responses to IR and ultimately ameliorate IR injury. Two distinct phases of IPC can be observed [102, 105]. An early or classic stage of protection, independent of protein syntheses, begins almost immediately after the mild ischemic insult and can be sustained for up to 3 hours [106]. A second or delayed phase lasts for up to 24 hours after the first preconditioning hit and is based on synthesis of new proteins and altered gene expression [106].

Aside from local protection of tissues close to the preconditioned area, remote or distant protection of organs (RIPC, or remote ischemic preconditioning) can also occur. In broader terms, this notion means that exposing various tissues or organs (such as limbs) to mild preconditioning ischemic events can cause other distant organs and tissues to be more resilient to following ischemic insults, even though the latter were not directly preconditioned in the first place. This had already been demonstrated in 1993 when McClanahan and colleagues showed in a preliminary report that myocardial infarct size was reduced if rabbits were previously exposed to a brief transient occlusion of the renal artery [107].

In 1996 Gho et al. proved that brief occlusion of adjacent coronary arteries, left renal artery, and anterior mesenteric artery protected the myocardium from a subsequent prolonged ischemic event [108]. A murine model subject to two hours of ischemia of the hind limb showed significant protection against local (leg skeletal muscle) and distant (intestinal injury and lung infiltrates) organ injury by a subsequent severe ischemic event [109]. IPC also caused a marked mortality decrease up to one week after ischemia [109]. Due to its effect on decreasing neutrophil infiltrates in the lung [109–111] and because of the systemic attenuation of subsequent inflammatory responses, IPC could be a tool for modulating systemic inflammation and for preventing local and distant organ injury or even SIRS/sepsis or ARDS. Another clinical application of remote or distant IPC is the protection that it delivers against acute kidney injury following major cardiac surgery, demonstrated by the reduced rate in which patients subject to the procedure demand renal replacement therapy [112]. The possibility of remotely achieving IPC is pivotal in a number of conditions. During heart surgery, for instance, the repetitive clamping and declamping of major blood vessels to induce local IPC on the heart can cause the formation of emboli in addition to the risk that short repetitive ischemic episodes can be traumatic in nature to the organ itself [106]. Therefore, the possibility of triggering remote systemic protection against ischemia in organs such as the heart is invaluable [113, 114].

The molecular mechanisms through which IPC or RIPC protection occurs are still unclear and not a single definite pathway has been established. It seems that the protective state of IPC is achieved through a combination of humoral, neural, and systemic components [106, 115]. Principle mediators are adenosine, reactive oxygen species (ROS), NF-κB, bradykinin, opioids, angiotensin, endocannabinoids, and nitric oxide (NO) that alter cellular metabolism via ATP-sensitive K^+ ion channels and receptors that direct transcription of survival proteins and activation of intracellular kinases that ultimately protect against oxidative stress [105, 115–123]. The role of the endothelium seems to be central during the development of ischemic resistance through IPC. Local and systemic endothelial function was proven to be greatly enhanced when human subjects were exposed to daily short-term limb ischemia for a period of 7 days, with measurable improvements in resting skin microcirculation and brachial artery function assessed by FMD (flow-mediated dilation), effect which lingered after the late phase of ischemic protection was over [25]. Another study has shown that IPC is capable of protecting tight junctions both functionally and structurally on hearts that would otherwise suffer from cell-to-cell collapse and edema when exposed to severe IR injury [26]. Moreover, the role of endothelial nitric oxide synthase (eNOS) and its NO output has been implicated as relevant for the ischemic preconditioning both in early and late IPC [27, 124, 125].

The reasoning behind the triggering mechanisms of IPC is that short preconditioning insults generate enough tissue damage upon reperfusion as to cause the release of adenosine (from the breaking of ATP molecules), bradykinin, and ROS [105, 126]. These substances trigger a molecular cascade that begins in the translocation and activation of protein kinase C and culminates in the phosphorylation of HSP27 via p38 MAPK and the opening of ATP-sensitive K^+ channels [126]. The role of organelles such as mitochondria and their function in regulating intracellular Ca^{2+}/K^+ exchange has also been implicated in the mechanisms of IPC protection in neuronal tissues [127], since the artificial opening of ATP-sensitive K^+ channels can mimic some of the effects of IPC [128]. Many molecular mechanisms of IPC have the inhibition of mPTP (mitochondrial permeability transition pore) channels as their endpoint, which, if opened, mediate cell death by ATP depletion and mitochondrial swelling [115, 129]. Activation of PKC measured by its intracellular translocation and the role of several kinases such as PI3, ERK/MAPK, and JAK/STAT are pivotal in conferring the state of protection during IPC [115, 121, 129].

Furthermore, IPC can attenuate or eliminate O_2^- production and its effects by suppressing endothelin-1 (ET-1) secretion via the opening of these mitochondrial KATP channels prior to subsequent ischemic events, since ET-1 generation is related to increased production of superoxide anion and endothelial dysfunction with increased P-selectin expression and neutrophil adhesion [130].

Nevertheless, due to the complexity of these mechanisms, results generally lack consistency when it comes to defining pathways through which IPC occurs. For example, in two separate knockout models, NO produced by an increased expression of NF-κB has been shown to be relevant in the ischemic protection of the heart [131], while the same role could not be demonstrated in the protection of the intestines and brain tissue [132].

The suppression of TNF-α and Bax (both involved in apoptotic stimulation) and the stimulation of cellular survival mechanisms such as phosphorylation of ERK-1/2 and Akt simultaneous to the upregulation of Bcl-2 have been identified in IPC of the myocardium [133] as mechanisms through which cell survival surpasses the rate of apoptosis after IR injury. Once again, results concerning the role of TNF-α in IPC are inconsistent. Some studies have suggested a protective self-regulatory effect that the secretion of TNF-α could have on the stimulation of NF-κB and on the suppression of proinflammatory proteins during subsequent ischemic injury [133].

Other recently unveiled novel molecular mediators of IPC have risen to the stage as possible targets in the investigation of the protective cascades of preconditioning. A study from 2013 showed that concentrations of HIF1-α and procaspase-3 were higher in patients receiving RIPC by upper limb ischemia before cardiopulmonary bypass. These same patients had higher right atrial tissue and systemic concentrations of IL-1β, IL-8, and TNF-α, indicating the direct influence of RIPC in the modulation of apoptosis and inflammation [134]. The role of Cx43 (connexin 43) has also been established in both local and remote IPC, which attenuates the ischemia-induced dephosphorylation of Cx43 that would otherwise cause the mechanical, chemical, and electrical instabilities in cardiomyocytes gap junctions by opening of the Cx43 hemichannels [135, 136]. This stabilization of Cx43

might be related to its association with PKC and p38MAPK [135]. A relevant role of microRNA 144 has also recently been revealed. Levels of mRNA 144 were found to be increased after RIPC and the exogenous intravenous administration of mRNA 144 was capable of mimicking the protective effect of RIPC in rescuing tissue from IR injury. Furthermore, increased activation of Akt and p44/42MAPK and decreased levels of mTOR were observed after the administration of mRNA 144, suggesting that the molecule could serve as a biomarker for the efficacy of a conditioning procedure [115, 137].

IPC as a technique has very practical applications. It can potentially be used as therapeutic preparation for surgical procedures that require some kind of ischemic episode, like in organ transplants. Another very important application of the model for real-life pathologies is the identification of novel molecular targets that are involved in IR injury and in the protection against said injuries. The modulation of some of these molecular targets and pathways can serve as treatment for naturally occurring ischemic insults seen in strokes, in thromboembolic injuries, and in acute myocardial infarction, to name a few.

4. Conclusion

As stated before, neither IPC nor the multiple-hit hypotheses are particularly new ideas, but it was not until the beginning of the century that more and more research has focused on one of the two models. During this paradigm shift, the idea that the two-hit model can satisfactorily account for many real-life pathological processes has been somewhat pushed aside.

It is logical to assume that, because of its nature, IPC is a mechanism that can be spontaneously found in the body and its artificial mimicking consists of a way to tap into the underlying responses of the immune system upon inflammatory insults and can serve as a tool for modulating these responses. Therefore, the two-hit model and IPC are not competing models in principle. While the former serves as a tool to explain the intricate processes that can be brought about via multiple sequential inflammatory insults which occur during a host of disease processes, such as trauma, hemorrhagic shock, and sepsis, the latter is an active investigation of techniques and strategies that can modulate the inflammatory response to a number of ischemic insults.

Nevertheless, there is an obvious paradox surrounding the subject: how can an inflammatory, ischemic insult drive the triggering of a protective mechanism to a subsequent ischemic insult, while the two-hit model states that a priming insult, including ischemia, should prepare the body to an exaggerated response to a second hit or insult, which incidentally can also be ischemic in nature. To our knowledge, there are no definitive answers to this conundrum. That the initial preconditioning ischemic event should not be harsh enough to cause serious tissue injury while maintaining enough potency to trigger the molecular mechanisms relevant to preconditioning seems reasonable and intuitive, but, other than that, no clear differentiation has been established concerning the nature of the first event in each model. Researchers have already mapped protocols to ensure that certain ischemic events are limited in intensity and duration so that they would not serve as priming insults for the host while still holding their beneficial effects [100–103], but aside from this intuitive distinction little is known concerning what makes an insult behave in either a priming or protective manner.

During this review many pathways, examples, and applications of both the two-hit and IPC models were explored, and little juxtaposition was found. The goal behind this text was exactly that of reconciling both models and demonstrating that each of the seemingly contradictory perspectives has a lot to offer as platforms to better understand and intervene in some very real and relevant medical situations, while maintaining the fact that both theories are not mutually exclusive.

Conflict of Interests

The authors declare that there is no conflict of interests regarding the publication of this paper.

Authors' Contribution

Carlos F. M. Morris and Muhammad Tahir contributed equally to this work.

Acknowledgments

The authors acknowledge TWAS, CNPq, CAPES, FAPESP, and FUB-UnB for financial support.

References

[1] T. A. Mare, D. F. Treacher, M. Shankar-Hari et al., "The diagnostic and prognostic significance of monitoring blood levels of immature neutrophils in patients with systemic inflammation," *Critical Care*, vol. 19, no. 1, article 57, 2015.

[2] D. Stubljar and M. Skvarc, "Effective strategies for diagnosis of Systemic Inflammatory Response Syndrome (SIRS) due to bacterial infection in surgical patients," *Infectious Disorders: Drug Targets*, vol. 15, no. 1, pp. 53–56, 2015.

[3] M. Bhatia, R. L. Zemans, and S. Jeyaseelan, "Role of chemokines in the pathogenesis of acute lung injury," *American Journal of Respiratory Cell and Molecular Biology*, vol. 46, no. 5, pp. 566–572, 2012.

[4] B. Fontes, W. Fontes, E. M. Utiyama, and D. Birolini, "The efficacy of loop colostomy for complete fecal diversion," *Diseases of the Colon & Rectum*, vol. 31, no. 4, pp. 298–302, 1988.

[5] C. F. M. Morris, M. S. Castro, and W. Fontes, "Neutrophil proteome: lessons from different standpoints," *Protein and Peptide Letters*, vol. 15, no. 9, pp. 995–1001, 2008.

[6] M. de Souza Castro, N. M. de Sá, R. P. Gadelha et al., "Proteome analysis of resting human neutrophils," *Protein and Peptide Letters*, vol. 13, no. 5, pp. 481–487, 2006.

[7] R. N. Garrison, D. A. Spain, M. A. Wilson, P. A. Keelen, and P. D. Harris, "Microvascular changes explain the "two-hit" theory of multiple organ failure," *Annals of Surgery*, vol. 227, no. 6, pp. 851–860, 1998.

[8] N. Matsuda and Y. Hattori, "Systemic inflammatory response syndrome (SIRS): molecular pathophysiology and gene therapy," *Journal of Pharmacological Sciences*, vol. 101, no. 3, pp. 189–198, 2006.

[9] S. Okubo, L. Xi, N. L. Bernardo, K.-I. Yoshida, and R. C. Kukreja, "Myocardial preconditioning: basic concepts and potential mechanisms," *Molecular and Cellular Biochemistry*, vol. 196, no. 1-2, pp. 3–12, 1999.

[10] C. E. Murry, R. B. Jennings, and K. A. Reimer, "Preconditioning with ischemia: a delay of lethal cell injury in ischemic myocardium," *Circulation*, vol. 74, no. 5, pp. 1124–1136, 1986.

[11] A. Lenz, G. A. Franklin, and W. G. Cheadle, "Systemic inflammation after trauma," *Injury*, vol. 38, no. 12, pp. 1336–1345, 2007.

[12] M. J. Bown, M. L. Nicholson, P. R. F. Bell, and R. D. Sayers, "Cytokines and inflammatory pathways in the pathogenesis of multiple organ failure following abdominal aortic aneurysm repair," *European Journal of Vascular and Endovascular Surgery*, vol. 22, no. 6, pp. 485–495, 2001.

[13] M. J. Bown, M. L. Nicholson, P. R. F. Bell, and R. D. Sayers, "The systemic inflammatory response syndrome, organ failure, and mortality after abdominal aortic aneurysm repair," *Journal of Vascular Surgery*, vol. 37, no. 3, pp. 600–606, 2003.

[14] J. Fan, J. C. Marshall, M. Jimenez, P. N. Shek, J. Zagorski, and O. D. Rotstein, "Hemorrhagic shock primes for increased expression of cytokine-induced neutrophil chemoattractant in the lung: role in pulmonary inflammation following lipopolysaccharide," *The Journal of Immunology*, vol. 161, no. 1, pp. 440–447, 1998.

[15] B. J. Czermak, M. Breckwoldt, Z. B. Ravage et al., "Mechanisms of enhanced lung injury during sepsis," *American Journal of Pathology*, vol. 154, no. 4, pp. 1057–1065, 1999.

[16] J. A. Nemzek, D. R. Call, S. J. Ebong, D. E. Newcomb, G. L. Bolgos, and D. G. Remick, "Immunopathology of a two-hit murine model of acid aspiration lung injury," *The American Journal of Physiology—Lung Cellular and Molecular Physiology*, vol. 278, no. 3, pp. L512–L520, 2000.

[17] M. Van Griensven, M. Kuzu, M. Breddin et al., "Polymicrobial sepsis induces organ changes due to granulocyte adhesion in a murine two hit model of trauma," *Experimental and Toxicologic Pathology*, vol. 54, no. 3, pp. 203–209, 2002.

[18] A. E. Baue, R. Durham, and E. Faist, "Systemic Inflammatory Response Syndrome (SIRS), multiple organ dysfunction syndrome (MODS), multiple organ failure (MOF): are we winning the battle?" *Shock*, vol. 10, no. 2, pp. 79–89, 1998.

[19] C. J. Hauser, P. Joshi, Q. Jones, X. Zhou, D. H. Livingston, and R. F. Lavery, "Suppression of natural killer cell activity in patients with fracture/soft tissue injury," *Archives of Surgery*, vol. 132, no. 12, pp. 1326–1330, 1997.

[20] F. Hietbrink, L. Koenderman, G. T. Rijkers, and L. P. H. Leenen, "Trauma: the role of the innate immune system," *World Journal of Emergency Surgery*, vol. 1, article 15, 2006.

[21] M. Keel and O. Trentz, "Pathophysiology of polytrauma," *Injury*, vol. 36, no. 6, pp. 691–709, 2005.

[22] D. H. Livingston, S. H. Appel, S. R. Wellhausen, G. Sonnenfeld, and H. C. Polk Jr., "Depressed interferon gamma production and monocyte HLA-DR expression after severe injury," *Archives of Surgery*, vol. 123, no. 11, pp. 1309–1312, 1988.

[23] M. F. Osuchowski, K. Welch, J. Siddiqui, and D. G. Remick, "Circulating cytokine/inhibitor profiles reshape the understanding of the SIRS/CARS continuum in sepsis and predict mortality," *The Journal of Immunology*, vol. 177, no. 3, pp. 1967–1974, 2006.

[24] S. Zedler and E. Faist, "The impact of endogenous triggers on trauma-associated inflammation," *Current Opinion in Critical Care*, vol. 12, no. 6, pp. 595–601, 2006.

[25] H. Jones, N. Hopkins, T. G. Bailey, D. J. Green, N. T. Cable, and D. H. J. Thijssen, "Seven-day remote ischemic preconditioning improves local and systemic endothelial function and microcirculation in healthy humans," *American Journal of Hypertension*, vol. 27, no. 7, pp. 918–925, 2014.

[26] Z. Li and Z.-Q. Jin, "Ischemic preconditioning enhances integrity of coronary endothelial tight junctions," *Biochemical and Biophysical Research Communications*, vol. 425, no. 3, pp. 630–635, 2012.

[27] C. Yang, M. A. H. Talukder, S. Varadharaj, M. Velayutham, and J. L. Zweier, "Early ischaemic preconditioning requires Akt- and PKA-mediated activation of eNOS via serine1176 phosphorylation," *Cardiovascular Research*, vol. 97, no. 1, pp. 33–43, 2013.

[28] J. Brom and W. Konig, "Cytokine-induced (interleukins-3, -6 and -8 and tumour necrosis factor-beta) activation and deactivation of human neutrophils," *Immunology*, vol. 75, no. 2, pp. 281–285, 1992.

[29] W. Ertel, M. Keel, D. Marty et al., "Significance of systemic inflammation in 1,278 trauma patients]," *Unfallchirurg*, vol. 101, no. 7, pp. 520–526, 1998.

[30] G. Schlag, H. Redl, and S. Bahrami, "SIRS (systemic inflammatory response syndrome) following trauma and during sepsis," *Anästhesiologie, Intensivmedizin, Notfallmedizin, Schmerztherapie*, vol. 29, no. 1, pp. 37–41, 1994.

[31] L. M. Teles, E. N. Aquino, A. C. Neves et al., "Comparison of the neutrophil proteome in trauma patients and normal controls," *Protein and Peptide Ltters*, vol. 19, no. 6, pp. 663–672, 2012.

[32] M. C. Carroll and V. M. Holers, "Innate autoimmunity," *Advances in Immunology*, vol. 86, pp. 137–157, 2005.

[33] S. D. Fleming and G. C. Tsokos, "Complement, natural antibodies, autoantibodies and tissue injury," *Autoimmunity Reviews*, vol. 5, no. 2, pp. 89–92, 2006.

[34] D. Mastellos and J. D. Lambris, "Complement: more than a 'guard' against invading pathogens?" *Trends in Immunology*, vol. 23, no. 10, pp. 485–491, 2002.

[35] B. P. Morgan, K. J. Marchbank, M. P. Longhi, C. L. Harris, and A. M. Gallimore, "Complement: central to innate immunity and bridging to adaptive responses," *Immunology Letters*, vol. 97, no. 2, pp. 171–179, 2005.

[36] G. Schlag and H. Redl, "Mediators of injury and inflammation," *World Journal of Surgery*, vol. 20, no. 4, pp. 406–410, 1996.

[37] O. I. Schmidt, C. E. Heyde, W. Ertel, and P. F. Stahel, "Closed head injury—an inflammatory disease?" *Brain Research Reviews*, vol. 48, no. 2, pp. 388–399, 2005.

[38] B. J. Czermak, A. B. Lentsch, N. M. Bless, H. Schmal, H. P. Friedl, and P. A. Ward, "Synergistic enhancement of chemokine generation and lung injury by C5a or the membrane attack complex of complement," *The American Journal of Pathology*, vol. 154, no. 5, pp. 1513–1524, 1999.

[39] J. A. Ember and T. E. Hugli, "Complement factors and their receptors," *Immunopharmacology*, vol. 38, no. 1-2, pp. 3–15, 1997.

[40] D. Mastellos, D. Morikis, S. N. Isaacs, M. C. Holland, C. W. Strey, and J. D. Lambris, "Complement: structure, functions, evolution, and viral molecular mimicry," *Immunologic Research*, vol. 27, no. 2-3, pp. 367–386, 2003.

[41] R.-F. Guo and P. A. Ward, "Role of C5a in inflammatory responses," *Annual Review of Immunology*, vol. 23, pp. 821–852, 2005.

[42] B.-M. Bellander, S. K. Singhrao, M. Ohlsson, P. Mattsson, and M. Svensson, "Complement activation in the human brain after traumatic head injury," *Journal of Neurotrauma*, vol. 18, no. 12, pp. 1295–1311, 2001.

[43] R. Gallinaro, W. G. Cheadle, K. Applegate, and H. C. Polk Jr., "The role of the complement system in trauma and infection," *Surgery Gynecology and Obstetrics*, vol. 174, no. 5, pp. 435–440, 1992.

[44] M. Heideman, "The role of complement in trauma," *Acta Chirurgica Scandinavica, Supplement*, vol. 522, pp. 233–244, 1985.

[45] M. Heideman and L.-E. Gelin, "The general and local response to injury related to complement activation," *Acta Chirurgica Scandinavica. Supplementum*, vol. 145, no. 489, pp. 215–223, 1979.

[46] P. F. Stahel, M. C. Morganti-Kossmann, and T. Kossmann, "The role of the complement system in traumatic brain injury," *Brain Research Reviews*, vol. 27, no. 3, pp. 243–256, 1998.

[47] P. F. Stahel, M. C. Morganti-Kossmann, D. Perez et al., "Intrathecal levels of complement-derived soluble membrane attack complex (sC5b-9) correlate with blood-brain barrier dysfunction in patients with traumatic brain injury," *Journal of Neurotrauma*, vol. 18, no. 8, pp. 773–781, 2001.

[48] M. E. Bianchi, "DAMPs, PAMPs and alarmins: all we need to know about danger," *Journal of Leukocyte Biology*, vol. 81, no. 1, pp. 1–5, 2007.

[49] L. O. Carvalho, E. N. Aquino, A. C. Neves, and W. Fontes, "The neutrophil nucleus and its role in neutrophilic function," *Journal of Cellular Biochemistry*, vol. 116, no. 9, pp. 1831–1836, 2015.

[50] D. Foell, H. Wittkowski, T. Vogl, and J. Roth, "S100 proteins expressed in phagocytes: a novel group of damage-associated molecular pattern molecules," *Journal of Leukocyte Biology*, vol. 81, no. 1, pp. 28–37, 2007.

[51] C. A. Janeway Jr. and R. Medzhitov, "Innate immune recognition," *Annual Review of Immunology*, vol. 20, pp. 197–216, 2002.

[52] U. Felderhoff-Mueser, O. I. Schmidt, A. Oberholzer, C. Bührer, and P. F. Stahel, "IL-18: a key player in neuroinflammation and neurodegeneration?" *Trends in Neurosciences*, vol. 28, no. 9, pp. 487–493, 2005.

[53] F. Y. Liew and I. B. McInnes, "The role of innate mediators in inflammatory response," *Molecular Immunology*, vol. 38, no. 12-13, pp. 887–890, 2002.

[54] I. B. McInnes and J. A. Gracie, "Interleukin-15: a new cytokine target for the treatment of inflammatory diseases," *Current Opinion in Pharmacology*, vol. 4, no. 4, pp. 392–397, 2004.

[55] M. Perl, C. Hohmann, S. Denk et al., "Role of activated neutrophils in chest trauma-induced septic acute lung injury," *Shock*, vol. 38, no. 1, pp. 98–106, 2012.

[56] I. F. Charo and R. M. Ransohoff, "The many roles of chemokines and chemokine receptors in inflammation," *The New England Journal of Medicine*, vol. 354, no. 6, pp. 610–621, 2006.

[57] T. S. Blackwell and J. W. Christman, "Sepsis and cytokines: current status," *British Journal of Anaesthesia*, vol. 77, no. 1, pp. 110–117, 1996.

[58] W. L. Biffl, E. E. Moore, F. A. Moore, and V. M. Peterson, "Interleukin-6 in the injured patient: marker of injury or mediator of inflammation?" *Annals of Surgery*, vol. 224, no. 5, pp. 647–664, 1996.

[59] A. M. Condliffe, E. Kitchen, and E. R. Chilvers, "Neutrophil priming: pathophysiological consequences and underlying mechanisms," *Clinical Science*, vol. 94, no. 5, pp. 461–471, 1998.

[60] W. L. Biffl, E. E. Moore, G. Zallen et al., "Neutrophils are primed for cytotoxicity and resist apoptosis in injured patients at risk for multiple organ failure," *Surgery*, vol. 126, no. 2, pp. 198–202, 1999.

[61] G. Zallen, E. E. Moore, J. L. Johnson et al., "Circulating postinjury neutrophils are primed for the release of proinflammatory cytokines," *The Journal of Trauma*, vol. 46, no. 1, pp. 42–48, 1999.

[62] M. S. Libério, G. A. Joanitti, R. B. Azevedo et al., "Anti-proliferative and cytotoxic activity of pentadactylin isolated from *Leptodactylus labyrinthicus* on melanoma cells," *Amino Acids*, vol. 40, no. 1, pp. 51–59, 2011.

[63] A. Nascimento, A. Chapeaurouge, J. Perales et al., "Purification, characterization and homology analysis of ocellatin 4, a cytolytic peptide from the skin secretion of the frog *Leptodactylus ocellatus*," *Toxicon*, vol. 50, no. 8, pp. 1095–1104, 2007.

[64] M. M. Kapur, P. Jain, and M. Gidh, "The effect of trauma on serum C3 activation and its correlation with injury severity score in man," *The Journal of Trauma*, vol. 26, no. 5, pp. 464–466, 1986.

[65] H. Redl, H. Gasser, G. Schlag, and I. Marzi, "Involvement of oxygen radicals in shock related cell injury," *British Medical Bulletin*, vol. 49, no. 3, pp. 556–565, 1993.

[66] W. L. Biffl, E. E. Moore, F. A. Moore, V. S. Carl, F. J. Kim, and R. J. Franciose, "Interleukin-6 potentiates neutrophil priming with platelet-activating factor," *Archives of Surgery*, vol. 129, no. 11, pp. 1131–1139, 1994.

[67] R. S. Friese, T. F. Rehring, M. Wollmering et al., "Trauma primes cells," *Shock*, vol. 1, no. 5, pp. 388–394, 1994.

[68] D. A. Partrick, F. A. Moore, E. E. Moore, C. C. Barnett Jr., and C. C. Silliman, "Neutrophil priming and activation in the pathogenesis of postinjury multiple organ failure," *New Horizons*, vol. 4, no. 2, pp. 194–210, 1996.

[69] A. J. Botha, F. A. Moore, E. E. Moore, A. Sauaia, A. Banerjee, and V. M. Peterson, "Early neutrophil sequestration after injury: a pathogenic mechanism for multiple organ failure," *Journal of Trauma—Injury, Infection and Critical Care*, vol. 39, no. 3, pp. 411–417, 1995.

[70] H.-C. Pape, D. Remmers, M. Grotz et al., "Reticuloendothelial system activity and organ failure in patients with multiple injuries," *Archives of Surgery*, vol. 134, no. 4, pp. 421–427, 1999.

[71] M. R. Rosengart, A. B. Nathens, S. Arbabi et al., "Mitogen-activated protein kinases in the intensive care unit: prognostic potential," *Annals of Surgery*, vol. 237, no. 1, pp. 94–100, 2003.

[72] C. Waydhas, D. Nast-Kolb, A. Trupka et al., "Posttraumatic inflammatory response, secondary operations, and late multiple organ failure," *Journal of Trauma*, vol. 40, no. 4, pp. 624–630, 1996.

[73] A. J. Botha, F. A. Moore, E. E. Moore, F. J. Kim, A. Banerjee, and V. M. Peterson, "Postinjury neutrophil priming and activation: an early vulnerable window," *Surgery*, vol. 118, no. 2, pp. 358–365, 1995.

[74] D. J. Ciesla, E. E. Moore, J. L. Johnson, J. M. Burch, C. C. Cothren, and A. Sauaia, "The role of the lung in postinjury multiple organ failure," *Surgery*, vol. 138, no. 4, pp. 749–758, 2005.

[75] M. C. Morganti-Kossmann, M. Rancan, V. I. Otto, P. F. Stahel, and T. Kossmann, "Role of cerebral inflammation after traumatic brain injury: a revisited concept," *Shock*, vol. 16, no. 3, pp. 165–177, 2001.

[76] D. A. Partrick, E. E. Moore, F. A. Moore, W. L. Biffl, and C. C. Barnett Jr., "Release of anti-inflammatory mediators after major torso trauma correlates with the development of postinjury multiple organ failure," *The American Journal of Surgery*, vol. 178, no. 6, pp. 564–569, 1999.

[77] R. J. Schoettle, P. M. Kochanek, M. J. Magargee, M. W. Uhl, and E. M. Nemoto, "Early polymorphonuclear leukocyte accumulation correlates with the development of posttraumatic cerebral edema in rats," *Journal of Neurotrauma*, vol. 7, no. 4, pp. 207–217, 1990.

[78] M. Scholz, J. Cinatl, M. Schädel-Höpfner, and J. Windolf, "Neutrophils and the blood-brain barrier dysfunction after trauma," *Medicinal Research Reviews*, vol. 27, no. 3, pp. 401–416, 2007.

[79] A. W. Unterberg, J. Stover, B. Kress, and K. L. Kiening, "Edema and brain trauma," *Neuroscience*, vol. 129, no. 4, pp. 1021–1029, 2004.

[80] E. Rahbar, J. C. Cardenas, G. Baimukanova et al., "Endothelial glycocalyx shedding and vascular permeability in severely injured trauma patients," *Journal of Translational Medicine*, vol. 13, no. 1, article 117, 2015.

[81] H. Kolářová, B. Ambrůzová, L. Švihálková Šindlerová, A. Klinke, and L. Kubala, "Modulation of endothelial glycocalyx structure under inflammatory conditions," *Mediators of Inflammation*, vol. 2014, Article ID 694312, 17 pages, 2014.

[82] S. Reitsma, D. W. Slaaf, H. Vink, M. A. M. J. Van Zandvoort, and M. G. A. Oude Egbrink, "The endothelial glycocalyx: composition, functions, and visualization," *Pflügers Archiv*, vol. 454, no. 3, pp. 345–359, 2007.

[83] H. H. Lipowsky, "The endothelial glycocalyx as a barrier to leukocyte adhesion and its mediation by extracellular proteases," *Annals of Biomedical Engineering*, vol. 40, no. 4, pp. 840–848, 2012.

[84] S. Khakpour, K. Wilhelmsen, and J. Hellman, "Vascular endothelial cell Toll-like receptor pathways in sepsis," *Innate Immunity*, vol. 21, no. 8, pp. 827–846, 2015.

[85] U. K. Sampson, M. M. Engelgau, E. K. Peprah, and G. A. Mensah, "Endothelial dysfunction: a unifying hypothesis for the burden of cardiovascular diseases in sub-Saharan Africa," *Cardiovascular Journal of Africa*, vol. 26, no. 2, supplement 1, pp. S56–S60, 2015.

[86] S. Sukriti, M. Tauseef, P. Yazbeck, and D. Mehta, "Mechanisms regulating endothelial permeability," *Pulmonary Circulation*, vol. 4, no. 4, pp. 535–551, 2014.

[87] D. Mehta and A. B. Malik, "Signaling mechanisms regulating endothelial permeability," *Physiological Reviews*, vol. 86, no. 1, pp. 279–367, 2006.

[88] G. Asimakopoulos and K. M. Taylor, "Effects of cardiopulmonary bypass on leukocyte and endothelial adhesion molecules," *Annals of Thoracic Surgery*, vol. 66, no. 6, pp. 2135–2144, 1998.

[89] G. Matheis, M. Scholz, A. Simon, O. Dzemali, and A. Mortiz, "Leukocyte filtration in cardiac surgery: a review," *Perfusion*, vol. 16, no. 5, pp. 361–370, 2001.

[90] D. Vestweber, "Molecular mechanisms that control endothelial cell contacts," *Journal of Pathology*, vol. 190, no. 3, pp. 281–291, 2000.

[91] T. M. Carlos and J. M. Harlan, "Leukocyte-endothelial adhesion molecules," *Blood*, vol. 84, no. 7, pp. 2068–2101, 1994.

[92] W. F. Westlin and M. A. Gimbrone Jr., "Neutrophil-mediated damage to human vascular endothelium. Role of cytokine activation," *The American Journal of Pathology*, vol. 142, no. 1, pp. 117–128, 1993.

[93] J. Varani and P. A. Ward, "Mechanisms of endothelial cell injury in acute inflammation," *Shock*, vol. 2, no. 5, pp. 311–319, 1994.

[94] W. van Oeveren, C. R. H. Wildevuur, and M. D. Kazatchkine, "Biocompatibility of extracorporeal circuits in heart surgery," *Transfusion Science*, vol. 11, no. 1, pp. 5–31, 1990.

[95] S. D. Marlin and T. A. Springer, "Purified intercellular adhesion molecule-1 (ICAM-1) is a ligand for lymphocyte function-associated antigen 1 (LFA-1)," *Cell*, vol. 51, no. 5, pp. 813–819, 1987.

[96] W. Fontes, R. B. Cunha, M. V. Sousa, and L. Morhy, "Improving the recovery of lysine in automated protein sequencing," *Analytical Biochemistry*, vol. 258, no. 2, pp. 259–267, 1998.

[97] S. J. Weiss, "Tissue destruction by neutrophils," *The New England Journal of Medicine*, vol. 320, no. 6, pp. 365–376, 1989.

[98] K. Kitagawa, M. Matsumoto, M. Tagaya et al., "'Ischemic tolerance' phenomenon found in the brain," *Brain Research*, vol. 528, no. 1, pp. 21–24, 1990.

[99] J. Moncayo, G. R. de Freitas, J. Bogousslavsky, M. Altieri, and G. Van Melle, "Do transient ischemic attacks have a neuroprotective effect?" *Neurology*, vol. 54, no. 11, pp. 2089–2094, 2000.

[100] Y. W. Li, P. Whittaker, and R. A. Kloner, "The transient nature of the effect of ischemic preconditioning on myocardial infarct size and ventricular arrhythmia," *American Heart Journal*, vol. 123, no. 2, pp. 346–353, 1992.

[101] Y.-Z. Qian, J. E. Levasseur, K.-I. Yoshida, and R. C. Kukreja, "KATP channels in rat heart: blockade of ischemic and acetylcholine-mediated preconditioning by glibenclamide," *The American Journal of Physiology—Heart and Circulatory Physiology*, vol. 271, no. 1, part 2, pp. H23–H28, 1996.

[102] M. S. Marber, D. S. Latchman, J. M. Walker, and D. M. Yellon, "Cardiac stress protein elevation 24 hours after brief ischemia or heat stress is associated with resistance to myocardial infarction," *Circulation*, vol. 88, no. 3, pp. 1264–1272, 1993.

[103] M. Ovize, K. Przyklenk, S. L. Hale, and R. A. Kloner, "Preconditioning does not attenuate myocardial stunning," *Circulation*, vol. 85, no. 6, pp. 2247–2254, 1992.

[104] I. Laskowski, J. Pratschke, M. J. Wilhelm, M. Gasser, and N. L. Tilney, "Molecular and cellular events associated with ischemia/reperfusion injury," *Annals of Transplantation*, vol. 5, no. 4, pp. 29–35, 2000.

[105] I. E. Konstantinov, S. Arab, R. K. Kharbanda et al., "The remote ischemic preconditioning stimulus modifies inflammatory gene expression in humans," *Physiological Genomics*, vol. 19, no. 1, pp. 143–150, 2004.

[106] N. Tapuria, Y. Kumar, M. M. Habib, M. A. Amara, A. M. Seifalian, and B. R. Davidson, "Remote ischemic preconditioning: a novel protective method from ischemia reperfusion injury—a review," *Journal of Surgical Research*, vol. 150, no. 2, pp. 304–330, 2008.

[107] T. B. McClanahan, B. S. Nao, L. J. Wolke, B. J. Martin, T. E. Mertz, and K. P. Gallagher, "Brief renal occlusion and reperfusion reduces myocardial infarct size in rabbits," *The FASEB Journal*, vol. 7, no. A118, pp. 682–683, 1993.

[108] B. C. G. Gho, R. G. Schoemaker, M. A. Van den Doel, D. J. Duncker, and P. D. Verdouw, "Myocardial protection by brief ischemia in noncardiac tissue," *Circulation*, vol. 94, no. 9, pp. 2193–2200, 1996.

[109] K. R. Eberlin, M. C. McCormack, J. T. Nguyen, H. S. Tatlidede, M. A. Randolph, and W. G. Austen Jr., "Ischemic preconditioning of skeletal muscle mitigates remote injury and mortality," *Journal of Surgical Research*, vol. 148, no. 1, pp. 24–30, 2008.

[110] D. W. Harkin, A. A. B. D'Sa Barros, K. McCallion, M. Hoper, and F. C. Campbell, "Ischemic preconditioning before lower limb ischemia—reperfusion protects against acute lung injury," *Journal of Vascular Surgery*, vol. 35, no. 6, pp. 1264–1273, 2002.

[111] M. Tahir, S. Arshid, A. M. C. Heimbecker et al., "Evaluation of the effects of ischemic preconditioning on the hematological parameters of rats subjected to intestinal ischemia and reperfusion," *Clinics*, vol. 70, no. 1, pp. 61–68, 2015.

[112] A. Zuk and J. V. Bonventre, "Acute kidney injury: can remote ischaemic preconditioning prevent AKI?" *Nature Reviews Nephrology*, vol. 11, no. 9, pp. 512–513, 2015.

[113] K. Przyklenk, B. Bauer, M. Ovize, R. A. Kloner, and P. Whittaker, "Regional ischemic 'preconditioning' protects remote virgin myocardium from subsequent sustained coronary occlusion," *Circulation*, vol. 87, no. 3, pp. 893–899, 1993.

[114] D. J. Hausenloy, E. Boston-Griffiths, and D. M. Yellon, "Cardioprotection during cardiac surgery," *Cardiovascular Research*, vol. 94, no. 2, pp. 253–265, 2012.

[115] R. Gill, R. Kuriakose, Z. M. Gertz, F. N. Salloum, L. Xi, and R. C. Kukreja, "Remote ischemic preconditioning for myocardial protection: update on mechanisms and clinical relevance," *Molecular and Cellular Biochemistry*, vol. 402, no. 1-2, pp. 41–49, 2015.

[116] P. J. Sullivan, K. J. Sweeney, K. M. Hirpara, C. B. Malone, W. Curtin, and M. J. Kerin, "Cyclical ischaemic preconditioning modulates the adaptive immune response in human limb ischaemia-reperfusion injury," *British Journal of Surgery*, vol. 96, no. 4, pp. 381–390, 2009.

[117] T. J. Pell, G. F. Baxter, D. M. Yellon, and G. M. Drew, "Renal ischemia preconditions myocardium: role of adenosine receptors and ATP-sensitive potassium channels," *American Journal of Physiology—Heart and Circulatory Physiology*, vol. 275, part 2, no. 5, pp. H1542–H1547, 1998.

[118] R. G. Schoemaker and C. L. van Heijningen, "Bradykinin mediates cardiac preconditioning at a distance," *American Journal of Physiology—Heart and Circulatory Physiology*, vol. 278, no. 5, pp. H1571–H1576, 2000.

[119] H. H. Patel, J. Moore, A. K. Hsu, and G. J. Gross, "Cardioprotection at a distance: mesenteric artery occlusion protects the myocardium via an opioid sensitive mechanism," *Journal of Molecular and Cellular Cardiology*, vol. 34, no. 10, pp. 1317–1323, 2002.

[120] A. R. Hajrasouliha, S. Tavakoli, M. Ghasemi et al., "Endogenous cannabinoids contribute to remote ischemic preconditioning via cannabinoid CB2 receptors in the rat heart," *European Journal of Pharmacology*, vol. 579, no. 1–3, pp. 246–252, 2008.

[121] S. Wolfrum, K. Schneider, M. Heidbreder, J. Nienstedt, P. Dominiak, and A. Dendorfer, "Remote preconditioning protects the heart by activating myocardial PKCε-isoform," *Cardiovascular Research*, vol. 55, no. 3, pp. 583–589, 2002.

[122] D. Singh and K. Chopra, "Evidence of the role of angiotensin AT1 receptors in remote renal preconditioning of myocardium," *Methods and Findings in Experimental and Clinical Pharmacology*, vol. 26, no. 2, pp. 117–122, 2004.

[123] C. Weinbrenner, M. Nelles, N. Herzog, L. Sárváry, and R. H. Strasser, "Remote preconditioning by infrarenal occlusion of the aorta protects the heart from infarction: a newly identified non-neuronal but PKC-dependent pathway," *Cardiovascular Research*, vol. 55, no. 3, pp. 590–601, 2002.

[124] R. Bolli, S. Manchikalapudi, X.-L. Tang et al., "The protective effect of late preconditioning against myocardial stunning in

conscious rabbits is mediated by nitric oxide synthase: evidence that nitric oxide acts both as a trigger and as a mediator of the late phase of ischemic preconditioning," *Circulation Research*, vol. 81, no. 6, pp. 1094–1107, 1997.

[125] M. A. H. Talukder, F. Yang, H. Shimokawa, and J. L. Zweier, "eNOS is required for acute in vivo ischemic preconditioning of the heart: effects of ischemic duration and sex," *The American Journal of Physiology—Heart and Circulatory Physiology*, vol. 299, no. 2, pp. H437–H445, 2010.

[126] M. V. Cohen, C. P. Baines, and J. M. Downey, "Ischemic pre-conditioning: from adenosine receptor to K_{ATP} channel," *Annual Review of Physiology*, vol. 62, pp. 79–109, 2000.

[127] M. J. Sisalli, L. Annunziato, and A. Scorziello, "Novel cellular mechanisms for neuroprotection in ischemic preconditioning: a view from inside organelles," *Frontiers in Neurology*, vol. 6, p. 115, 2015.

[128] A. P. Wojtovich, W. R. Urciuoli, S. Chatterjee, A. B. Fisher, K. Nehrke, and P. S. Brookes, "Kir6.2 is not the mitochondrial KATP channel but is required for cardioprotection by ischemic preconditioning," *The American Journal of Physiology—Heart and Circulatory Physiology*, vol. 304, no. 11, pp. H1439–H1445, 2013.

[129] D. J. Hausenloy, "Cardioprotection techniques: precondition-ing, postconditioning and remote conditioning (basic science)," *Current Pharmaceutical Design*, vol. 19, no. 25, pp. 4544–4563, 2013.

[130] M. Duda, E. Czarnowska, M. Kurzelewski, A. Konior, and A. Beresewicz, "Ischemic preconditioning prevents endothelial dysfunction, P-selectin expression, and neutrophil adhesion by preventing endothelin and O_2- generation in the post-ischemic guinea-pig heart," *Journal of Physiology and Pharmacology*, vol. 57, no. 4, pp. 553–569, 2006.

[131] G. Li, F. Labruto, A. Sirsjö, F. Chen, J. Vaage, and G. Valen, "Myocardial protection by remote preconditioning: the role of nuclear factor κ-B p105 and inducible nitric oxide synthase," *European Journal of Cardio-thoracic Surgery*, vol. 26, no. 5, pp. 968–973, 2004.

[132] N. N. Petrishchev, T. D. Vlasov, V. G. Sipovsky, D. I. Kurapeev, and M. M. Galagudza, "Does nitric oxide generation contribute to the mechanism of remote ischemic preconditioning?" *Patho-physiology*, vol. 7, no. 4, pp. 271–274, 2001.

[133] C. C. Lai, C. Y. Tang, S. C. Chiang, K. W. Tseng, and C. H. Huang, "Ischemic preconditioning activates prosurvival kin-ases and reduces myocardial apoptosis," *Journal of the Chinese Medical Association*, vol. 78, no. 8, pp. 460–468, 2015.

[134] M. Albrecht, K. Zitta, B. Bein et al., "Remote ischemic precondi-tioning regulates HIF-1alpha levels, apoptosis and inflammation in heart tissue of cardiosurgical patients: a pilot experimental study," *Basic Research in Cardiology*, vol. 108, no. 1, article 314, 2013.

[135] T. Brandenburger, R. Huhn, A. Galas et al., "Remote ischemic preconditioning preserves Connexin 43 phosphorylation in the rat heart in vivo," *Journal of Translational Medicine*, vol. 12, p. 228, 2014.

[136] S. K. Jain, R. B. Schuessler, and J. E. Saffitz, "Mechanisms of delayed electrical uncoupling induced by ischemic precondi-tioning," *Circulation Research*, vol. 92, no. 10, pp. 1138–1144, 2003.

[137] J. Li, S. Rohailla, N. Gelber et al., "MicroRNA-144 is a circulating effector of remote ischemic preconditioning," *Basic Research in Cardiology*, vol. 109, no. 5, article 423, 2014.

3

Clinical Options in Relapsed or Refractory Hodgkin Lymphoma: An Updated Review

Roberta Fedele,[1] Massimo Martino,[1] Anna Grazia Recchia,[2] Giuseppe Irrera,[1] Massimo Gentile,[3] and Fortunato Morabito[2,3]

[1]Hematology and Stem Cell Transplant Unit, Azienda Ospedaliera BMM, 89100 Reggio Calabria, Italy
[2]Biotechnology Research Unit, Azienda Sanitaria Provinciale di Cosenza, 87051 Aprigliano, Italy
[3]Hematology Unit, Azienda Ospedaliera di Cosenza, 87100 Cosenza, Italy

Correspondence should be addressed to Roberta Fedele; r.fedele@yahoo.it

Academic Editor: Daniel Olive

Hodgkin lymphoma (HL) is a potentially curable lymphoma, and modern therapy is expected to successfully cure more than 80% of the patients. Second-line salvage high-dose chemotherapy and autologous stem cell transplantation (auto-SCT) have an established role in the management of refractory and relapsed HL, leading to long-lasting responses in approximately 50% of relapsed patients and a minority of refractory patients. Patients progressing after intensive treatments, such as auto-SCT, have a very poor outcome. Allogeneic SCT represents the only strategy with a curative potential for these patients; however, its role is controversial. Based on recent knowledge of HL pathology, biology, and immunology, antibody-drug conjugates targeting CD30, small molecule inhibitors of cell signaling, and antibodies that inhibit immune checkpoints are currently explored. This review will discuss the clinical results regarding auto-SCT and allo-SCT as well as the current role of emerging new treatment strategies.

1. Introduction

Hodgkin lymphoma (HL) is a potentially curable lymphoma with distinct histology, biological behavior, and clinical characteristics. Thomas Hodgkin first described the disorder in 1832. In the 20th century, with the realization that the disease consisted of a lymphoid malignancy, it was renamed HL. It is a relatively rare disease and accounts for approximately 10% of all malignant lymphomas, with about 9,200 estimated new cases and 1,200 estimated deaths per year in the United States [1]. The treatment of HL has evolved over the past three decades, and modern therapy is expected to successfully cure over 80% of patients [2]. Second-line salvage high-dose chemotherapy (HDC) and autologous stem cell transplantation (auto-SCT) have become the standard care for refractory/relapsed HL, leading to long-lasting responses in approximately 50% of relapsed patients and in a minority of refractory patients [3]. Disease recurrence or progression after auto-SCT is associated with very poor prognosis [4] and patients have an estimated average survival of less than 3

years [5]. However, because HL is a rare cancer that is highly curable, the development of new drugs for the treatment of HL has been very slow [6]. With growing knowledge of HL pathology, biology, and immunology, several therapeutic targets have been identified and are currently under preclinical and clinical investigation [7]. The aim of drug development in HL is not only to cure patients, but also to go further and decrease the toxic effects of therapy.

In this review, we summarize the most recent updates on the management of patients with relapsed or refractory HL and the role of novel therapeutic approaches. We also discuss the role of consolidation strategies such as HDC and auto-SCT and reduced-intensity (RIC) allogeneic stem cell transplantation (allo-SCT).

2. Autologous Stem Cell Transplantation

According to retrospective and prospective as well as randomized studies, HDC followed by auto-SCT can rescue 30% to 80% of relapsed/refractory HL patients [8–14].

In the BNLI trial [12], relapsed patients were treated with conventional dose mini-BEAM (carmustine, etoposide, cytarabine, and melphalan) or high-dose BEAM with auto-SCT. Both event-free survival (EFS) and progression-free survival (PFS) showed significant differences in favor of BEAM plus transplant ($p = 0.025$ and $p = 0.005$, resp.). In the GHSG trial [13], patients who relapsed after chemotherapy were randomly given four courses of mini-BEAM+dexamethasone (dexa-mini-BEAM) or two courses of dexa-mini-BEAM followed by BEAM and auto-SCT. Freedom from treatment failure (FFTF) in 3 years was significantly better for patients given BEAM and auto-SCT (55%) than for those on dexa-mini-BEAM (34%; $p = 0.019$). Overall survival (OS) of patients given either treatment did not differ significantly. Recently, the GHSG group [14] evaluated the impact of sequential HDC before myeloablative therapy. Patients with histologically confirmed, relapsed HL were treated with two cycles of dexamethasone, cytarabine, and cisplatin, and those without disease progression were then randomly divided between standard and experimental treatment arms. In the standard arm, patients received myeloablative therapy with BEAM followed by auto-SCT. In the experimental arm, patients received sequential cyclophosphamide, methotrexate, and etoposide in high doses before BEAM. Mortality was similar in both arms (20% and 18%). With a median observation time of 42 months, there was no significant difference in terms of FFTF ($p = 0.56$) and OS ($p = 0.82$) between arms. FFTF in 3 years was 62% and OS was 80%. Results demonstrated that sequential HDC did not improve outcome and was associated with more adverse events and toxicity. Based on the data presented, the authors concluded that two cycles of intensified conventional chemotherapy (DHAP) followed by HDC (BEAM) and auto-SCT are an effective and safe treatment strategy for patients with relapsed HL.

On the basis of this study, BEAM is considered the gold standard conditioning regimen for auto-SCT. However, due to drug constraints of carmustine, this drug is often replaced by a variety of agents, including fotemustine [15], bendamustine [16], and thiotepa [17].

Sweetenham et al. [18] published a retrospective analysis of 175 patients with HL who did not undergo remission after induction therapy and results were reported to the European Group for Bone Marrow Transplantation (EBMT). The 5-year actuarial OS and PFS rates were 36% and 32%, respectively, and results were very similar to those reported from single-institution series and from the Autologous Blood and Marrow Transplant Registry (ABMTR) [19]. The ABMTR series includes 122 patients with HL who have never achieved remission. The definition of failure to achieve remission differs from that in the EBMT series, in that it includes only those patients who had a documented disease progression or tissue confirmation of persistent disease in residual radiographic abnormalities. With a median follow-up of 28 months from the date of auto-SCT, the 3-year actuarial PFS and OS rates in this series were 38% and 50%, respectively. The GELTAMO Cooperative Group [20] presented the results of 62 patients treated with an auto-SCT for refractory HL. One-year transplant-related mortality (TRM) was 14%. The

response rate in 3 months after auto-SCT was 52%. Actuarial 5-year time to treatment failure (TTF) and OS were 15% and 26%, respectively. The presence of B symptoms at auto-SCT was the only adverse prognostic factor significantly influencing TTF. The presence of B symptoms at diagnosis, MOPP-like regimens as first-line therapy, bulky disease at auto-SCT, and two or more lines of therapy before auto-SCT adversely influenced OS.

Tandem auto-SCT for HL has been evaluated in a small number of studies [21–24] and in the most recent guidelines from the American Society for Blood and Marrow Transplantation it is not recommended, although further studies may be warranted in high-risk patients [25].

3. Allogeneic Stem Cell Transplantation

Although there is relatively limited accessible data regarding the best approach for patients who relapse after an auto-SCT, the available information supports the benefit of allo-SCT versus standard therapy [25–28]. Evidence of a graft versus HL (GVHL) effect comes from the demonstration that the development of graft versus host disease (GVHD) after allo-SCT is associated with a lower relapse rate [29, 30]. Moreover, the most direct evidence for a graft versus malignancy effect comes from the disease responses to donor lymphocyte infusions (DLIs). Peggs et al. [31] assessed the impact of DLI on relapse incidence when administered for mixed chimerism and the utility of DLI as salvage therapy when given for relapse in 76 consecutive patients with multiple relapsed or refractory HL, who underwent allo-SCT that incorporated in vivo T-cell depletion. The results demonstrated the potential for allogeneic immunotherapy with DLIs both to reduce relapse risk and to induce durable antitumor responses.

Despite early data showing promisingly low relapse rates after allo-SCT, the transplantation community was not very enthusiastic about considering allo-SCT for HL patients, because of the exceedingly high nonrelapse mortality (NRM). Registry data [32, 33] has shown that allo-SCT after myeloablative conditioning results in lower relapse rates but significantly higher toxicity than auto-SCT. Although the poor results after myeloablative conditioning can be explained by the very poor risk features of heavily pretreated patients included in these early trials, high TRM has been associated with high incidence of GVHD and infections after transplantation. Results of allo-SCT can be reasonably optimized with a better patient selection and the use of targeted and less toxic therapies to achieve an adequate response for patients.

In the last years, the use of RIC has reduced NRM and improved OS [34] and the percentage of patients with refractory and relapsed HL treated using this approach has been growing steadily in Europe [35]. Robinson et al. [36] conducted a retrospective analysis of 285 patients with HL who underwent a RIC allo-SCT in order to identify prognostic factors of outcome. Eighty percent of patients had undergone a prior auto-SCT and 25% had refractory disease at transplant. NRM was associated with chemorefractory disease, poor performance status, age > 45, and transplantation before 2002. For patients with no risk factors, the 3-year

NRM rate was 12.5% compared to 46.2% for patients with two or more risk factors. The use of an unrelated donor had no adverse effects on the NRM. The development of chronic GVHD was associated with a lower relapse rate. The disease progression rate in 1 and 5 years was 41% and 58.7%, respectively, and was associated with chemorefractory disease and extent of prior therapy. PFS and OS were both associated with performance status and disease status at transplant. Patients with neither risk factor had a 3-year PFS and OS of 42% and 56%, respectively, compared to 8% and 25% for patients with one or more risk factors. Relapse within 6 months of a prior auto-SCT was associated with a higher relapse rate and a lower PFS.

In the analysis by Robinson et al., the authors also identified important clinical parameters predicting transplant outcomes. RIC allo-SCT may be an effective salvage strategy for the minority of patients with good risk features who relapse after an auto-SCT, with similar outcomes for both sibling and matched unrelated donor (MUD) transplants. On the other hand, for patients with chemorefractory disease or a poor performance status, the overall outcome is poor and it is difficult to recommend RIC allo-SCT for these patients.

Burroughs et al. [37] evaluated the outcome of RIC allo-SCT for patients with relapsed or refractory HL based on different donor cell sources. Ninety patients with HL were treated with nonmyeloablative conditioning followed by allo-SCT from HLA-matched related, unrelated, or HLA-haploidentical related donors. The nonmyeloablative preparative regimen consisted in either 2-Gy total body irradiation (TBI) or combination with fludarabine 30 mg/m2/day followed by postgrafting immunosuppression with mycophenolate mofetil or cyclosporine/tacrolimus. Patients were heavily pretreated with a median of five regimens and most patients had failed auto-SCT and local radiation therapy. With a median follow-up of 25 months, the 2-year OS, the PFS, and incidence of relapsed/progressive disease were 53%, 23%, and 56% (HLA-matched related); 58%, 29%, and 63% (unrelated); and 58%, 51%, and 40% (HLA-haploidentical related), respectively. NRM was significantly lower for HLA-haploidentical related ($p = 0.02$) recipients compared to HLA-matched related recipients. There were promising results with significantly decreased risks of relapse for HLA-haploidentical related recipients compared to HLA-matched related ($p = 0.01$) and unrelated ($p = 0.03$) recipients. The incidence of acute GVHD grade III/IV and extensive chronic GVHD was 16%/50% (HLA-matched related), 8%/63% (unrelated), and 11%/35% (HLA-haploidentical related), respectively.

Raiola et al. [38] confirmed in 26 advanced HL patients the results published by the Baltimore/Seattle group [39], using haplo-mismatched marrow grafts and posttransplantation cyclophosphamide. The procedure was feasible, with a low rate of GVHD and NRM, and was associated with a durable remission in a high proportion of patients. The 4-year OS and EFS were 77% and 63%, respectively. EFS was statistically different when patients were stratified according to disease phase: 1-year PFS was 100%, 67%, and 37% for patients in complete remission (CR) ($n = 9$), partial remission (PR) ($n = 9$), or resistant disease ($n = 8$), respectively ($p = 0.02$). Actuarial survival was not statistically different in the three

groups ($p = 0.1$). The cumulative incidence of NRM was 4%. The 100-day cumulative incidence of grade I and grade II–IV acute GVHD was 4% and 24%, respectively; the cumulative 3-year incidence of moderate chronic GVHD was 9%.

The Lymphoma Working Party (LWP) of the EBMT, together with the GEL/TAMO [40], undertook the largest multicenter phase II prospective clinical trial presented up to now with the objective of analyzing the NRM and other major outcome parameters after allo-SCT in relapsed/refractory HL. In this study, 92 patients with an HLA-identical sibling, a MUD, or a one antigen mismatched, unrelated donor were treated with salvage chemotherapy followed by RIC allo-SCT. Fludarabine (150 mg/m2 intravenously) and melphalan (140 mg/m2 intravenously) were used as the conditioning regimen. The addition of antithymocyte globulin was used as GVHD prophylaxis for recipients of grafts from unrelated donors. The NRM rate was 8% in 100 days and 15% in 1 year. Relapse was the major cause of failure. The PFS rate was 48% in 1 year and 24% in 4 years. The OS rate was 71% in 1 year and 43% in 4 years. The results of this study emphasize the role of RIC allo-SCT in patients with relapsed/refractory HL after auto-SCT. The plateau phase in the survival curve of the subset of patients allografted in CR indicates the existence of a clinically beneficial GVHL effect. Chronic GVHD was associated with a significantly lower relapse incidence after transplantation and consequently a significant improvement of PFS.

Recently, the LWP of the EBMT has reported [41] the results on the outcome of the second allo-SCT (allo-SCT-2) performed in one hundred and forty patients with lymphoma, of which 31% were affected by HL. Three-year PFS, OS, relapse incidence, and NRM were 19%, 29%, 58%, and 23%, respectively. PFS and OS were significantly affected by refractory disease at allo-SCT-2 and by a short interval between allo-SCT-1 and allo-SCT-2. Long-term PFS was observed in particular in patients with HL, T-cell lymphoma, and indolent lymphoma where a GVHL effect was assumed [42]. In fact, considering that, in many patients, chronic GVHD was absent after allo-SCT-1 but not after allo-SCT-2, it is possible to conclude that the second allotransplant might induce an effective allo-response in patients in which GVHD failed to appear after the first transplant. Allo-SCT-2 can result in long-term disease control in patients with lymphoma recurrence after allo-SCT-1, in particular if relapse occurs late and is chemosensitive.

4. Brentuximab Vedotin

The expression of CD30 by Reed-Sternberg cells (RSc) coupled with its highly restricted expression makes it an obvious target for monoclonal antibody therapy [43, 44]. Results from two clinical studies using first-generation naked anti-CD30 monoclonal antibodies in patients with relapsed HL have been disappointing, perhaps reflecting their poor antigen binding and/or effector cell activation properties [45, 46]. In an alternate strategy, the anti-CD30 antibody cAC10 was conjugated to a synthetic antimicrotubule agent, monomethyl auristatin E (MMAE), resulting in the novel immunotoxin conjugate brentuximab vedotin [47]. In a phase I dose escalation trial that enrolled 45 patients with relapsed or refractory CD30+ hematologic malignancies [48], objective responses, including 11 CRs, were observed in 17 patients and tumor regression was observed in 86% of evaluable patients. Seventy-three percent of patients in that trial had undergone auto-SCT. Brentuximab vedotin (1.8 mg/kg intravenously every 3 weeks) was subsequently evaluated in a pivotal phase 2 study of 102 patients with relapsed/refractory CD30+ HL after auto-SCT [49]. Objective responses were documented in 75% of patients, with CRs observed in 34% of patients, as determined by an independent radiology review facility. The estimated 12-month survival rate was 89% and the median PFS was 5.6 months. Adverse events associated with brentuximab vedotin were typically of grade I/II and were treated through standard supportive care. Cumulative peripheral neuropathy, the most meaningful clinical adverse effect, improved or resolved completely in 80% of patients during the study.

Median OS and PFS were estimated in 40.5 months and 9.3 months, respectively. Improved outcomes were observed in patients who achieved a CR on brentuximab vedotin, with estimated 3-year OS and PFS rates of 73% and 58%, respectively, in this group of patients [50]. Of the 34 patients who obtained CR, 16 (47%) remain progression-free after a median of 53.3 months (range, 29.0 to 56.2 months); 12 patients remain progression-free without a consolidative allo-SCT. Younger age, good performance status, and lower disease burden at baseline were characteristic of patients who achieved a CR and were favorable prognostic factors for OS.

On the basis of these studies, brentuximab vedotin has been approved for the treatment of adult patients with relapsed or refractory CD30+ HL following auto-SCT or following at least two prior therapies with auto-SCT or multiagent chemotherapy.

The randomized, double-blind, placebo-controlled, phase 3 AETHERA study [51] demonstrated that brentuximab vedotin improves PFS when given as early consolidation after auto-SCT in patients with HL with risk factors for relapse or progression after transplantation. The high risk of progression after auto-SCT is defined by the presence of primary refractory HL (failure to achieve CR), relapsed HL with an initial remission duration of less than 12 months, or extranodal involvement at the start of pretransplantation salvage chemotherapy. Compared with historical survival data for high-risk patients with HL undergoing auto-SCT, the 3-year OS rate exceeding 80% in this study is remarkable.

A recent SIE, SIES, GITMO position paper declares that there is now evidence for recommending brentuximab vedotin also in HL patients refractory to salvage chemotherapy who are auto-SCT candidates and as a consolidation strategy after auto-SCT. The use of brentuximab vedotin in HL after relapse from allo-SCT or as first-line therapy is at present only experimental [52]. The Expert Panel recommends that, in the approved indications of brentuximab vedotin treatment for HL, treatment evaluation must be performed after 4 courses, and the subsequent treatment should be determined according to the response. In patients with HL attaining a CR, either an early consolidation program including allo-SCT or brentuximab vedotin therapy continued up to 16 cycles is the

approved indications. It is necessary to perform clinical trials to clarify which one of the two strategies is more appropriate. Early allo-SCT should strongly be considered in patients with HL attaining a PR. Patients not eligible for transplant should be treated with brentuximab vedotin up to a maximum of 16 cycles. In patients with HL and a stable disease, the decision to continue brentuximab vedotin should rely on a patient-centered balance between clinical benefits and risks. In patients with HL and a progressive disease, brentuximab vedotin therapy should be discontinued and patients must be enrolled in clinical trials.

5. Bendamustine

Bendamustine is a bifunctional alkylating agent with only partial cross-resistance to other alkylating drugs, making it an attractive agent for use in the relapsed setting [53]. Although it was developed in the 1960s and used in Germany for both HL and non-HL, it has been approved for treatment of chronic lymphatic leukemia and indolent B-cell non-HL [54] and limited data exist regarding its activity in HL patients. Moskowitz et al. [55] performed a phase II study evaluating the efficacy and toxicity of bendamustine in relapsed and refractory HL. Thirty-six patients were enrolled, and 25 patients were potentially eligible for allo-SCT. Bendamustine 120 mg/m2 was administered on days 1 and 2 of each 28-day cycle for a total of six cycles of treatment. The dose of bendamustine was reduced to 100 mg/m2 for treatment delays >5 days because of neutropenia or thrombocytopenia. The dose was further reduced to 70 mg/m2 for subsequent delays of >5 days for neutropenia or thrombocytopenia. The most common nonhematologic toxicities were fatigue (primarily grade I) and nausea (primarily grade I). Thrombocytopenia was the most common hematologic toxicity, with 20% of patients experiencing grade III or IV thrombocytopenia. The overall response rate (ORR) for the 36 patients was 53%, demonstrating that bendamustine is a good option for heavily treated patients with relapsed and refractory HL who could proceed to consolidative SCT. Zinzani et al. [56] reported two cases of patients relapsed/refractory after brentuximab vedotin were successfully treated with bendamustine indicating that patients with HL relapsed/refractory to brentuximab vedotin therapy may be chemosensitive and may obtain a good response to subsequent bendamustine treatment. Zinzani et al. [57], after these case reports, performed a retrospective study on 27 heavily pretreated patients with relapsed or refractory HL, who had all received brentuximab vedotin as their last treatment and who showed disease progression, refractory disease, or early relapse, when retreated with bendamustine. The ORR was 55.5%, with 10 of 27 patients (37.0%) obtaining a CR. In comparison, the ORR previously observed with brentuximab vedotin in the same subset of patients was much lower (18.5%).

Considering the promising results of brentuximab vedotin and bendamustine as single drugs on patients with relapsed/refractory HL and their independent mechanisms of action with manageable safety profiles, a phase I-II study was performed evaluating the safety and efficacy of brentuximab vedotin in combination with bendamustine for the treatment of patients with HL first relapse [58]. Brentuximab vedotin 1.8 mg/kg on day 1 in combination with bendamustine 90 mg/m2 on days 1 and 2 of 3-week-cycles for up to 6 cycles had a manageable safety profile with premedication. The CR rate of the combination was 82% and ORR 94%. The majority of CRs (24/28 patients) were documented after 2 cycles of combination therapy and, in these patients, stem cell mobilization and collection were performed with success. These data indicate a promising approach for maximizing responses prior SCT in relapsed/refractory HL patients after frontline therapy. Promising data were reported by O'Connor and colleagues [59] on the combination of brentuximab vedotin and bendamustine in relapsed/refractory HL and anaplastic large T-cell lymphoma.

6. Panobinostat and Mocetinostat

Agents that target acetylases may regulate several oncogenic pathways including cell cycle progression, cell survival, angiogenesis, and antitumor immunity. Panobinostat and mocetinostat target histone deacetylase (HDAC) and these agents may be effective in patients with HL by modulating serum cytokine levels and the expression of PD-1 on intratumoral T-cells.

Based on promising results from a phase I study that included 13 patients with relapsed HL [60], a large pivotal international phase II study was initiated. Oral panobinostat was administered at a dose of 40 mg three times per week, every week, in 21-day cycles. Dose delays and modifications for management of adverse events were permitted, but the lowest dose allowed on study was 20 mg. Efficacy was evaluated every 2 cycles by imaging studies. Surprisingly, patients were enrolled in less than one year. The median age was 32 years (range, 18–75), and the median number of prior chemotherapeutic regimens was 4 (range, 1–7). Importantly, the median time to relapse after the first auto-SCT was only 8 months, which represents a poor prognostic indicator. Moreover, 37% of the patients did not respond to their last prior therapy. Twelve patients also received prior allo-SCT.

In a phase II study, 129 patients with relapsed and refractory HL received 40 mg of panobinostat orally three times per week [61]. Treatment with panobinostat was effective as tumor reductions were seen in 74% of patients, and ORs were achieved by 35 patients (27%). Thirty patients (23%) had partial responses to treatment and five patients (4%) had CRs. The median duration of response was 6.9 months, and the median PFS was 6.1 months. The treatment was reasonably well tolerated with common drug-related grade I/II adverse effects as diarrhea, nausea, fatigue, vomiting, and anorexia. Common drug-related grade III/IV adverse events were thrombocytopenia, anemia, and neutropenia. The thrombocytopenia was manageable and reversible with dose hold and modification.

Considering the synergistic activity of HDAC inhibitors with other therapies [62, 63], association studies of HDAC inhibitors combined with chemotherapy, monoclonal antibodies, and small molecule inhibitors will be evaluated. A phase I study of panobinostat combined with lenalidomide in relapsed HL is ongoing [64].

The safety and efficacy of mocetinostat were recently evaluated in a phase II study in 51 patients with relapsed classical HL [65]. Mocetinostat was given orally 3 times per week (85 mg to 110 mg starting doses) for 1 year in the absence of disease progression or prohibitive toxicity. Initially, 23 patients were enrolled in the 110 mg cohort. Subsequently, because toxicity-related dose reductions were necessary in the 110 mg cohort, 28 additional patients were treated with a dose of 85 mg. The disease control rate was 35% (eight of 23 patients) in the 110 mg group and 25% (seven of 28) in the 85 mg group. Three of the 10 (30%) patients in the 85 mg group achieved partial remissions. Furthermore, grade III and IV toxicity (mainly fatigue, with no significant hematologic toxicity) was reduced to 20%. Overall, 80% of the 30 evaluable patients had some decrease in their tumor sizes. These data demonstrate that mocetinostat has a promising single-agent clinical activity with manageable toxicity in patients with relapsed classical HL.

7. Everolimus

The phosphatidylinositol 3-kinase/mammalian target of rapamycin (PI3K/mTOR) signaling pathway is one of the most aberrantly activated survival pathways in cancer, making it an important target for drug development [66]. Everolimus is an oral antineoplastic agent that targets this pathway, specifically the mTORcomplex1 (mTORC1) that has been shown to be activated in patients with HL. Everolimus not only may target the signaling pathways within the RSc but may also suppress signaling within the immune infiltrate and production of cytokines present in the tumor microenvironment [67]. Nineteen evaluable patients with relapsed HL were treated with daily doses of 10 mg everolimus, the ORR rate was 47%, and 8 patients achieved PR and 1 CR [68]. The median time to disease progression was 7.2 months. The majority of patients had received multiple previous lines of therapy and 84% of the patients had undergone a previous auto-SCT. Grade III adverse events included thrombocytopenia and anemia. Considering that several signal transduction pathways are critical for the proliferation and survival of neoplastic Hodgkin RSc, including NF-κB, JAK-STAT, PI3K-AkT, and ERK [69], a combination of therapeutic approaches capable of targeting RSc along with reactive cells of the microenvironment might prolong the response duration of mTOR inhibitors to overcome chemorefractoriness.

8. JAK Inhibitors

The Janus kinase (JAK) and signal transducer and activator of transcription (STAT) pathway is an active mediator of cytokine signaling in the pathogenesis of solid and hematologic malignancies. The seven-member STAT family is composed of latent cytoplasmic transcription factors that are activated by phosphorylation intertwined in a network with activation that ultimately leads to cell proliferation. Aberrant activation of the JAK-STAT pathway has been demonstrated in patients with large granular lymphocytic leukemia, aplastic anemia, myelodysplastic syndrome, myeloproliferative disorders, and HL [70]. Pacritinib is an inhibitor of JAK2 kinase with preclinical activity in a variety of hematological malignancies [71]. This JAK inhibitor has been used in a phase I clinical trial in patients with relapsed or refractory Hodgkin or non-Hodgkin lymphoma of any type except Burkitt or central nervous system lymphoma [72]. Doses of 100 to 600 mg/day were tested, and treatment was well tolerated, with mostly grade I/II toxicities. Among the 34 patients' study, the ORR was 14%, including three partial remissions. In the group of patients with HL, however, none of the 14 patients had a partial remission or better. However, at least five of the patients with HL did benefit from the treatment, with a decrease in the sites of active disease.

9. Rituximab

Rituximab has shown activity in nodular lymphocyte pre-dominant HL. It is active in relapsed/refractory classical HL regardless of subtype or degree of CD20 expression on RS cells. Rationale of using rituximab in classic HL includes elimination of CD20+ reactive B-cells supporting RS cells, hence depriving malignant cells of survival signals and potentially increasing host immune responses [73]. In a pilot study [74], 22 patients with recurrent, classic HL who had received a minimum of two prior treatment regimens, regardless of whether H/RS cells expressed CD20, were treated with 6 weekly doses of 375 mg/m2 rituximab to selectively deplete infiltrating benign B-cells. Five patients (22%) achieved partial or complete remission that lasted for a median of 7.8 months (range, 3.3–14.9 months). Remissions were observed in patients only at lymph node and splenic sites, but not at extranodal sites, and were irrespective of CD20 expression by H/RS cells. Furthermore, systemic (B) symptoms resolved in six of seven patients after therapy. These data need to be confirmed in clinical trial.

10. Lenalidomide

Lenalidomide is an immunomodulatory agent with several mechanisms of action, including direct induction of apopto-sis in tumor cells, antiangiogenic effects, and the modulation of immune cells, such as natural killer cells and T-cells [75]. Limited data suggest that lenalidomide has clinical activity in relapsed/refractory HL. Fehniger et al. [76] evaluated 38 relapsed HL patients with 25 mg/day of lenalidomide on days 1–21 of 28-day cycles; 33 of 38 patients had prior SCTs. The ORR to lenalidomide in the 35 evaluable patients was 17%, with one CR. Additional six patients had stable disease (SD) lasting >6 months, resulting in an overall cytostatic response rate (CR + PR + SD > 6 months) of 34%. Treatment continued until progressive disease or an unacceptable adverse event. Kuruvilla et al. [77] evaluated lenalidomide in 14 patients with relapsed or refractory HL. Two patients achieved a PR (14%), with additional seven patients having SD (50%). The median time to progression in that study was only 3.2 months, with a median OS time of 9.1 months. Böll and colleagues used lenalidomide in 42 patients [78]. Preliminary results involving the first 24 patients have been reported. Twelve patients (50%) had an objective response (11 with a PR and one with a CR), with additional eight patients achieving SD.

Further studies must be made to evaluate the actual efficacy and long-lasting effect of lenalidomide.

Lenalidomide was further evaluated in HL by the GHSG in a first-line phase I combination trial for older patients [79]. The GHSG aimed to improve the ABVD regimen by replacing bleomycin with lenalidomide (AVD-Rev) to improve both efficacy and tolerability of the regimen. Patients received four to eight cycles of AVD-Rev (standard-dose AVD on days 1 and 15 of a 28-day cycle and lenalidomide daily from days 1 to 21) followed by radiotherapy. The daily lenalidomide dose for the first patient was 5 mg; maximum dose in this dose escalation trial was 25 mg. Twenty-five patients with a median age of 67 were enrolled. Sixty-eight had advanced stage disease, and 80% had B symptoms at diagnosis. After dose-limiting toxicity evaluation of 20 patients, a prespecified stopping criterion was reached and the recommended dose for a phase II trial was 25 mg. At least one grade III/IV toxicity occurred in all 22 patients who were treated at dose levels 20 and 25 mg, and 16 of those patients had a grade IV toxicity. The 1-year estimates for PFS and OS were 69 and 91%, respectively. In summary, AVD-Rev displayed high efficacy and a manageable toxicity profile in older patients with HL and should be further evaluated in phase II/III trials. In addition, a phase II trial combining lenalidomide and panobinostat in patients with relapsed or refractory HL is currently recruiting.

11. Anti-PD-1 Antibodies

The concept that the immune system plays a critical role in controlling and eradicating cancer and that the immune response, driven by T-lymphocytes, is closely regulated through a complicated and delicate balance of inhibitory checkpoints and activating signals is well established [80, 81]. Programmed death-1 (PD-1) is one of the main immune checkpoint receptors that, when binding its programmed death-ligand-1 (PD-L1), determines the downregulation of the T-cell effector functions, thus contributing to the main-tenance of the tolerance to tumor cells. The blockade of this pathway by anti-PD-1 and anti-PD-L1 antibodies may prevent this downregulation and allows T-cells to maintain their antitumor property and ability to mediate the tumor cell death [82–84]. The genes encoding the PD-1 ligands, PD-L1 and PD-L2, are key targets of chromosome 9p24.1 amplification, a recurrent genetic abnormality in the nodular sclerosis type of HL. The 9p24.1 amplicon also includes JAK2, and gene dose-dependent JAK-STAT activity further induces PD-1 ligand transcription [85]. The complementary mechanisms of PD-1 ligand overexpression in HL suggest that this disease may have genetically determined vulnerability to PD-1 blockade. For these reasons, in a phase I study, 23 extensively pretreated patients with relapsed or refractory HL were given every 2 weeks 3 mg/kg nivolumab, a fully human monoclonal IgG4 antibody directed against PD-1 [86]. The majority of these patients had previously received an auto-SCT, and most had received previous brentuximab vedotin. Drug-related adverse events of any grade were reported in 18 (78%) of 23 patients, and grade III drug-related adverse events were reported in five (22%) patients. Of 23 patients,

TABLE 1: Novel agents evaluated in relapsed/refractory HL patients after auto-SCT.

Author	Therapeutic agent(s), study design	Pts. $N1$	Pts. $N2$	Response rate	Median duration of response
Younes et al., 2010 [48]	Brentuximab vedotin, phase I	42	33	ORR = 38% CR = 24%	9.7 months
Younes et al., 2012 [49]	Brentuximab vedotin, phase II	102	102	ORR = 75% CR = 34%	20.5 months for patients in CR
Moskowitz et al., 2013 [55]	Bendamustine, phase II	35	27	ORR = 53% CR = 33%	5 months
Zinzani et al., 2015 [57]	Bendamustine, retrospective	27	27	ORR = 55.5% CR = 37%	8 months
LaCasce et al., 2014 [58]	Bendamustine + brentuximab, phases I-II	45	—	ORR = 94% CR = 82%	NR
Younes et al., 2012 [61]	Panobinostat, phase II	129	129	ORR = 27% CR = 4%	6.9 months
Younes et al., 2011 [65]	Mocetinostat, phase II	51	43	ORR = 33%	NR
Johnston et al., 2010 [68]	Everolimus, phase II	19	16	ORR = 47% CR = 5%	7.2 months
Younes et al., 2012 [72]	Pacritinib, phase I	34	14	ORR = 14%	130 days
Younes et al., 2003 [74]	Rituximab, phase II	22	18	ORR = 22%	7.8 months
Fehniger et al., 2011 [76]	Lenalidomide, phase II	38	33	ORR = 17%	15 months
Kuruvilla et al., 2008 [77]	Lenalidomide, phase II	14	10	PR = 14% SD = 50%	Median OS was 9.1 months
Böll et al., 2010 [78]	Lenalidomide phase II	42	NR	ORR = 50%	NR
Ansell et al., 2015 [86]	Nivolumab, phase I	23	18	ORR = 87% SD = 13%	PFS in 24 weeks was 86%
Moskowitz et al. 2014 [87]	Pembrolizumab, phase I	15	15	ORR = 53% CR = 20%	NR

Pts. $N1$: total number of patients; Pts. $N2$: patients who received prior auto-SCT; ORR: overall response rate; CR: complete remission; PR: partial remission; SD: stable disease; OS: overall survival; PFS: progression-free survival; NR: not reported.

four (17%) had a CR, 16 (70%) had a PR, and three (13%) had SD. In 24 weeks, the rate of PFS was 86% resulting in a very high proportion of patients achieving an overall response and clinical benefit. The study shows promising results; however, larger trials are needed before introducing nivolumab in HL treatment.

A multicenter, open-label, phase Ib clinical trial is ongoing evaluating the use of the humanized IgG4 monoclonal antibody pembrolizumab (formerly MK-3475), targeting the PD-1 receptor, in relapsed or refractory HL patients who failed brentuximab vedotin treatment, with adequate performance status and organ function [87]. Pembrolizumab 10 mg/kg was administered in 15 patients intravenously every 2 weeks until confirmed tumor progression, excessive toxicity, or completion of 2 years of therapy. The drug was well tolerated with no serious adverse events, and only one patient experienced grade III pain and grade III joint swelling. The most common drug-related adverse events were grade I/II respiratory events (20%) and thyroid disorders (20%). Three patients (20%) had a CR in 12 weeks. Five additional patients (33%) had a PR as the best overall response, for an ORR of 53%. Four patients (27%) experienced progressive disease, although all 4 experienced a decrease in their overall tumor burden. In conclusion, pembrolizumab therapy appears to be safe, tolerable, and associated with clinical benefit in patients with heavily pretreated HL.

12. Conclusions

Auto-SCT is the standard of care for refractory/relapsed HL, leading to long-lasting responses in approximately 50% of relapsed patients and in a minority of refractory patients. Patients progressing after intensive treatments, such as auto-SCT, have a very poor outcome.

In the recent past, particularly effective novel therapies have been identified to treat these patients (Table 1). These agents have all been tested as single drugs acting on different pathways implicated in the pathogenesis of HL (Table 2), and therefore an important future approach will be to combine them with each other and with standard chemotherapies.

Up to now, brentuximab vedotin is the only FDA approved drug for the treatment of relapsed HL. There have been attempts to combine brentuximab vedotin in a pretransplant setting, either in sequential mode, that is, brentuximab vedotin as a single agent, followed by HDC, or concurrently (i.e., with bendamustine). Either way, there is an improvement in the overall response rate and complete response rate with these treatment strategies, and this may evolve with time to include brentuximab vedotin as part of the induction in pretransplant regimens.

PD1-targeted therapies, pembrolizumab and nivolumab, are becoming very good potential drugs, and most likely both will be approved in the near future.

TABLE 2: Competitive environment.

Agent	Indication	Development stage	Mechanism of action
Brentuximab vedotin	HL, NHL	Approved for HL and NHL	Anti-CD30 antibody-drug conjugate
Bendamustine	NHL, MM	Approved for NHL	Bifunctional alkylating agent
Panobinostat	AML, CML, breast cancer, prostate cancer, MM, idiopathic myelofibrosis, HL, NHL	Approved for MM	HDAC inhibitor
Mocetinostat	AML, solid tumors, CLL, MDS, NHL, HL	Phase II	HDAC inhibitor
Everolimus	Solid tumors, transplant rejection, HL, NHL	Approved for solid tumors and transplant rejection	mTOR inhibitor
Pacritinib	AML, myeloproliferative disorders, HL, NHL	Phase III	JAK2-inhibitor
Rituximab	NHL, CLL, rheumatoid arthritis, HL, granulomatosis, multiple sclerosis, MM	Approved for NHL, rheumatoid arthritis, granulomatosis, CLL	Anti-CD20 antibody
Lenalidomide	MDS, MM, NHL, HL, CLL	Approved for MDS, MM	Immunomodulator
Nivolumab	Melanoma, lung cancer, renal cancer, HL	Phase I	Anti-PD1 antibody
Pembrolizumab	Melanoma, lung cancer, renal cancer, HL	Phase I	Anti-PD1 antibody

HL: Hodgkin lymphoma; NHL: non-Hodgkin lymphoma; MM: multiple myeloma; AML: acute myeloid leukemia; CML: chronic myeloid leukemia; MDS: myelodysplastic syndrome; CLL: chronic lymphatic leukemia.

Although these new therapies have clearly demonstrated efficacy in HL, a molecularly targeted drug achieving long-term responses with good tolerability is still lacking. Moreover, the majority of patients are young, and in this scenario we believe that allo-SCT can play an important role in selected patients.

Conflict of Interests

The authors report no conflict of interests or funding sources.

Authors' Contribution

Quality control of data and algorithms has been done by Roberta Fedele, Massimo Martino, Anna Grazia Recchia, Massimo Gentile, and Fortunato Morabito. Paper preparation has been done by Roberta Fedele and Massimo Martino. Paper editing has been done by Roberta Fedele, Massimo Martino, and Anna Grazia Recchia. Paper review has been done by Roberta Fedele, Massimo Martino, Anna Grazia Recchia, and Fortunato Morabito. Approval of the submitted and final versions has been done by Roberta Fedele, Massimo Martino, Anna Grazia Recchia, Massimo Gentile, and Fortunato Morabito. Giuseppe Irrera contributed to paper review and the approval of the submitted and final versions.

References

[1] R. Siegel, J. Ma, Z. Zou, and A. Jemal, "Cancer statistics, 2014," *CA: A Cancer Journal for Clinicians*, vol. 64, no. 1, pp. 9–29, 2014.

[2] T. Chisesi, M. Bellei, S. Luminari et al., "Long-term follow-up analysis of HD9601 trial comparing ABVD versus Stanford V versus MOPP/EBV/CAD in patients with newly diagnosed advanced-stage Hodgkin's lymphoma: a study from the Intergruppo Italiano Linfomi," *Journal of Clinical Oncology*, vol. 29, no. 32, pp. 4227–4233, 2011.

[3] T. Moscato, R. Fedele, G. Messina, G. Irrera, G. Console, and M. Martino, "Hematopoietic progenitor cells transplantation for recurrent or refractory Hodgkin's lymphoma," *Expert Opinion on Biological Therapy*, vol. 13, no. 7, pp. 1013–1027, 2013.

[4] F. Montanari and C. Diefenbach, "Relapsed Hodgkin lymphoma: management strategies," *Current Hematologic Malignancy Reports*, vol. 9, no. 3, pp. 284–293, 2014.

[5] S. Horning and M. S. Fanale, "Defining a population of Hodgkin lymphoma patients for novel therapeutics: an international effort," *Annals of Oncology*, vol. 20, article 118, 2008.

[6] D. Buglio, G. Georgakis, and A. Younes, "Novel small-molecule therapy of Hodgkin lymphoma," *Expert Review of Anticancer Therapy*, vol. 7, no. 5, pp. 735–740, 2007.

[7] R. Küppers, "The biology of Hodgkin's lymphoma," *Nature Reviews Cancer*, vol. 9, no. 1, pp. 15–27, 2008.

[8] D. E. Reece, M. J. Barnett, J. M. Connors et al., "Intensive chemotherapy with cyclophosphamide, carmustine, and etoposide followed by autologous bone marrow transplantation for relapsed Hodgkin's disease," *The Journal of Clinical Oncology*, vol. 9, no. 10, pp. 1870–1879, 1991.

[9] R. Chopra, A. K. McMillan, D. C. Linch et al., "The place of high-dose BEAM therapy and autologous bone marrow transplantation in poor-risk Hodgkin's disease. A single-center eight-year study of 155 patients," *Blood*, vol. 81, no. 5, pp. 1137–1145, 1993.

[10] A. Sureda, R. Arranz, A. Iriondo et al., "Autologous stem-cell transplantation for Hodgkin's disease: results and prognostic factors in 494 patients from the Grupo Español de Linfomas/Transplante Autólogo de Médula Ósea Spanish Cooperative Group," *Journal of Clinical Oncology*, vol. 19, no. 5, pp. 1395–1404, 2001.

[11] M. D. Caballero, V. Rubio, J. Rifon et al., "BEAM chemotherapy followed by autologous stem cell support in lymphoma patients: analysis of efficacy, toxicity and prognostic factors," *Bone Marrow Transplantation*, vol. 20, no. 6, pp. 451–458, 1997.

[12] D. C. Linch, D. Winfield, A. H. Goldstone et al., "Dose intensification with autologous bone-marrow transplantation in relapsed and resistant Hodgkin's disease: results of a BNLI randomised trial," *The Lancet*, vol. 341, no. 8852, pp. 1051–1054, 1993.

[13] N. Schmitz, B. Pfistner, M. Sextro et al., "Aggressive conventional chemotherapy compared with high-dose chemotherapy with autologous haemopoietic stem-cell transplantation for relapsed chemosensitive Hodgkin's disease: a randomised trial," *The Lancet*, vol. 359, no. 9323, pp. 2065–2071, 2002.

[14] A. Josting, H. Müller, P. Borchmann et al., "Dose intensity of chemotherapy in patients with relapsed Hodgkin's lymphoma," *Journal of Clinical Oncology*, vol. 28, no. 34, pp. 5074–5080, 2010.

[15] M. Musso, R. Scalone, G. Marcacci et al., "Fotemustine plus etoposide, cytarabine and melphalan (FEAM) as a new conditioning regimen for lymphoma patients undergoing auto-SCT: a multicenter feasibility study," *Bone Marrow Transplantation*, vol. 45, no. 7, pp. 1147–1153, 2010.

[16] G. Visani, L. Malerba, P. M. Stefani et al., "BeEAM (bendamustine, etoposide, cytarabine, melphalan) before autologous stem cell transplantation is safe and effective for resistant/relapsed lymphoma patients," *Blood*, vol. 118, no. 12, pp. 3419–3425, 2011.

[17] R. L. Tombleson, M. R. Green, and K. M. Fancher, "Putting caution in TEAM: high-dose chemotherapy with autologous HSCT for primary central nervous system lymphoma," *Bone Marrow Transplantation*, vol. 47, no. 10, pp. 1383–1384, 2012.

[18] J. W. Sweetenham, A. M. Carella, G. Taghipour et al., "High-dose therapy and autologous stem-cell transplantation for adult patients with Hodgkin's disease who do not enter remission after induction chemotherapy: results in 175 patients reported to the European group for blood and marrow transplantation," *Journal of Clinical Oncology*, vol. 17, no. 10, pp. 3101–3109, 1999.

[19] H. M. Lazarus, P. A. Rowlings, M.-J. Zhang et al., "Autotransplants for Hodgkin's disease in patients never achieving remission: a report from the autologous blood and marrow transplant registry," *Journal of Clinical Oncology*, vol. 17, no. 2, pp. 534–545, 1999.

[20] M. Constans, A. Sureda, M. J. Terol et al., "Autologous stem cell transplantation for primary refractory Hodgkin's disease: results and clinical variables affecting outcome," *Annals of Oncology*, vol. 14, no. 5, pp. 745–751, 2003.

[21] T. Ahmed, K. Rashid, F. Waheed et al., "Long-term survival of patients with resistant lymphoma treated with tandem stem cell transplant," *Leukemia and Lymphoma*, vol. 46, no. 3, pp. 405–414, 2005.

[22] H. C. Fung, P. Stiff, J. Schriber et al., "Tandem autologous stem cell transplantation for patients with primary refractory or poor risk recurrent Hodgkin lymphoma," *Biology of Blood and Marrow Transplantation*, vol. 13, no. 5, pp. 594–600, 2007.

[23] L. Castagna, M. Magagnoli, M. Balzarotti et al., "Tandem high-dose chemotherapy and autologous stem cell transplantation in refractory/relapsed Hodgkin's lymphoma: a monocenter prospective study," *American Journal of Hematology*, vol. 82, no. 2, pp. 122–127, 2007.

[24] F. Morschhauser, P. Brice, C. Fermé et al., "Risk-adapted salvage treatment with single or tandem autologous stem-cell transplantation for first relapse/refractory Hodgkin's lymphoma: results of the prospective multicenter H96 trial by the GELA/SFGM study group," *Journal of Clinical Oncology*, vol. 26, no. 36, pp. 5980–5987, 2008.

[25] M. A. Perales, I. Ceberio, P. Armand et al., "Role of cytotoxic therapy with hematopoietic cell transplantation in the treatment of Hodgkin lymphoma: guidelines from the American Society for Blood and Marrow Transplantation," *Biology of Blood and Marrow Transplantation*, vol. 21, no. 6, pp. 971–983, 2015.

[26] K. J. Thomson, K. S. Peggs, P. Smith et al., "Superiority of reduced-intensity allogeneic transplantation over conventional treatment for relapse of Hodgkin's lymphoma following autologous stem cell transplantation," *Bone Marrow Transplantation*, vol. 41, no. 9, pp. 765–770, 2008.

[27] L. Castagna, B. Sarina, E. Todisco et al., "Allogeneic stem cell transplantation compared with chemotherapy for poor-risk Hodgkin lymphoma," *Biology of Blood and Marrow Transplantation*, vol. 15, no. 4, pp. 432–438, 2009.

[28] B. Sarina, L. Castagna, L. Farina et al., "Allogeneic transplantation improves the overall and progression-free survival of Hodgkin lymphoma patients relapsing after autologous transplantation: a retrospective study based on the time of HLA typing and donor availability," *Blood*, vol. 115, no. 18, pp. 3671–3677, 2010.

[29] J. L. Gajewski, G. L. Phillips, K. A. Sobocinski et al., "Bone marrow transplants from HLA-identical siblings in advanced Hodgkin's disease," *Journal of Clinical Oncology*, vol. 14, no. 2, pp. 572–578, 1996.

[30] A. Claviez, C. Canals, D. Dierickx et al., "Allogeneic hematopoietic stem cell transplantation in children and adolescents with recurrent and refractory Hodgkin lymphoma: an analysis of the European Group for Blood and Marrow Transplantation," *Blood*, vol. 114, no. 10, pp. 2060–2067, 2009.

[31] K. S. Peggs, I. Kayani, N. Edwards et al., "Donor lymphocyte infusions modulate relapse risk in mixed chimeras and induce durable salvage in relapsed patients after T-cell-depleted allogeneic transplantation for Hodgkin's lymphoma," *Journal of Clinical Oncology*, vol. 29, no. 8, pp. 971–978, 2011.

[32] N. Milpied, A. K. Fielding, R. M. Pearce, P. Ernst, and A. H. Goldstone, "Allogeneic bone marrow transplant is not better than autologous transplant for patients with relapsed Hodgkin's disease," *Journal of Clinical Oncology*, vol. 14, no. 4, pp. 1291–1296, 1996.

[33] J. E. Anderson, M. R. Litzow, F. R. Appelbaum et al., "Allogeneic, syngeneic, and autologous marrow transplantation for Hodgkin's disease: the 21-year seattle experience," *Journal of Clinical Oncology*, vol. 11, no. 12, pp. 2342–2350, 1993.

[34] A. Sureda, S. Robinson, C. Canals et al., "Reduced-intensity conditioning compared with conventional allogeneic stem-cell transplantation in relapsed or refractory Hodgkin's lymphoma: an analysis from the lymphoma working party of the European Group for Blood and Marrow Transplantation," *Journal of Clinical Oncology*, vol. 26, no. 3, pp. 455–462, 2008.

[35] J. R. Passweg, H. Baldomero, A. Gratwohl et al., "The EBMT activity survey: 1990–2010," *Bone Marrow Transplantation*, vol. 47, no. 7, pp. 906–923, 2012.

[36] S. P. Robinson, A. Sureda, C. Canals et al., "Reduced intensity conditioning allogeneic stem cell transplantation for Hodgkin's lymphoma: identification of prognostic factors predicting outcome," *Haematologica*, vol. 94, no. 2, pp. 230–238, 2009.

[37] L. M. Burroughs, P. V. O'Donnell, B. M. Sandmaier et al., "Comparison of outcomes of HLA-matched related, unrelated, or HLA-haploidentical related hematopoietic cell transplantation following nonmyeloablative conditioning for relapsed or refractory Hodgkin lymphoma," *Biology of Blood and Marrow Transplantation*, vol. 14, no. 11, pp. 1279–1287, 2008.

[38] A. Raiola, A. Dominietto, R. Varaldo et al., "Unmanipulated haploidentical BMT following non-myeloablative conditioning and post-transplantation CY for advanced Hodgkin's lymphoma," *Bone Marrow Transplantation*, vol. 49, no. 2, pp. 190–194, 2014.

[39] L. Luznik, P. V. O'Donnell, H. J. Symons et al., "HLA-haploidentical bone marrow transplantation for hematologic malignancies using nonmyeloablative conditioning and high-dose, posttransplantation cyclophosphamide," *Biology of Blood and Marrow Transplantation*, vol. 14, no. 6, pp. 641–650, 2008.

[40] A. Sureda, C. Canals, R. Arranz et al., "Allogeneic stem cell transplantation after reduced intensity conditioning in patients with relapsed or refractory Hodgkin's lymphoma. Results of the HDR-ALLO study—a prospective clinical trial by the Grupo Español de Linfomas/Trasplante de Médula Osea (GEL/TAMO) and the Lymphoma Working Party of the European Group for Blood and Marrow Transplantation," *Haematologica*, vol. 97, no. 2, pp. 310–317, 2012.

[41] K. Horstmann, A. Boumendil, J. Finke et al., "Second allo-SCT in patients with lymphoma relapse after a first allogeneic transplantation. A retrospective study of the EBMT Lymphoma Working Party," *Bone Marrow Transplantation*, vol. 50, no. 6, pp. 790–794, 2015.

[42] C. Kahl, B. E. Storer, B. M. Sandmaier et al., "Relapse risk in patients with malignant diseases given allogeneic hematopoietic cell transplantation after nonmyeloablative conditioning," *Blood*, vol. 110, no. 7, pp. 2744–2748, 2007.

[43] A. Younes and A. Carbone, "CD30/CD30 ligand and CD40/CD40 ligand in malignant lymphoid disorders," *The International Journal of Biological Markers*, vol. 14, no. 3, pp. 135–143, 1999.

[44] A. Younes and B. B. Aggarwall, "Clinical implications of the tumor necrosis factor family in benign and malignant hematologic disorders," *Cancer*, vol. 98, no. 3, pp. 458–467, 2003.

[45] S. M. Ansell, S. M. Horwitz, A. Engert et al., "Phase I/II study of an anti-CD30 monoclonal antibody (MDX-060) in Hodgkin's lymphoma and anaplastic large-cell lymphoma," *Journal of Clinical Oncology*, vol. 25, no. 19, pp. 2764–2769, 2007.

[46] A. Forero-Torres, J. P. Leonard, A. Younes et al., "A Phase II study of SGN-30 (anti-CD30 mAb) in Hodgkin lymphoma or systemic anaplastic large cell lymphoma," *British Journal of Haematology*, vol. 146, no. 2, pp. 171–179, 2009.

[47] E. Oflazoglu, K. M. Kissler, E. L. Sievers, I. S. Grewal, and H.-P. Gerber, "Combination of the anti-CD30-auristatin-E antibody-drug conjugate (SGN-35) with chemotherapy improves anti-tumour activity in Hodgkin lymphoma," *British Journal of Haematology*, vol. 142, no. 1, pp. 69–73, 2008.

[48] A. Younes, N. L. Bartlett, J. P. Leonard et al., "Brentuximab vedotin (SGN-35) for relapsed CD30-positive lymphomas," *The New England Journal of Medicine*, vol. 363, no. 19, pp. 1812–1821, 2010.

[49] A. Younes, A. K. Gopal, S. E. Smith et al., "Results of a pivotal phase II study of brentuximab vedotin for patients with relapsed or refractory Hodgkin's lymphoma," *Journal of Clinical Oncology*, vol. 30, no. 18, pp. 2183–2189, 2012.

[50] A. K. Gopal, R. Chen, S. E. Smith et al., "Durable remissions in a pivotal phase 2 study of brentuximab vedotin in relapsed or refractory Hodgkin lymphoma," *Blood*, vol. 125, no. 8, pp. 1236–1243, 2015.

[51] C. H. Moskowitz, A. Nademanee, T. Masszi et al., "Brentuximab vedotin as consolidation therapy after autologous stem-cell transplantation in patients with Hodgkin's lymphoma at risk of relapse or progression (AETHERA): a randomised, double-blind, placebo-controlled, phase 3 trial," *The Lancet*, vol. 385, no. 9980, pp. 1853–1862, 2015.

[52] P. L. Zinzani, P. Corradini, A. M. Gianni et al., "Brentuximab vedotin in CD30-positive lymphomas. A SIE, SIES, GITMO position paper," *Clinical Lymphoma, Myeloma & Leukemia*, vol. 15, no. 9, pp. 507–513, 2015.

[53] V. Gandhi, "Metabolism and mechanisms of action of bendamustine: rationales for combination therapies," *Seminars in Oncology*, vol. 4, supplement 13, pp. 4–11, 2002.

[54] M. M. Goldenberg, "Pharmaceutical approval update," *P&T*, vol. 33, no. 5, pp. 299–302, 2008.

[55] A. J. Moskowitz, P. A. Hamlin Jr., M.-A. Perales et al., "Phase II study of bendamustine in relapsed and refractory Hodgkin lymphoma," *Journal of Clinical Oncology*, vol. 31, no. 4, pp. 456–460, 2013.

[56] P. L. Zinzani, E. Derenzini, C. Pellegrini, M. Celli, A. Broccoli, and L. Argnani, "Bendamustine efficacy in Hodgkin lymphoma patients relapsed/refractory to brentuximab vedotin," *British Journal of Haematology*, vol. 163, no. 5, pp. 681–683, 2013.

[57] P. L. Zinzani, U. Vitolo, S. Viviani et al., "Safety and efficacy of single-agent bendamustine after failure of brentuximab vedotin in patients with relapsed or refractory Hodgkin's lymphoma: experience with 27 patients," *Clinical Lymphoma, Myeloma and Leukemia*, vol. 15, no. 7, pp. 404–408, 2015.

[58] A. LaCasce, R. G. Bociek, J. Matous et al., "Brentuximab vedotin in combination with bendamustine for patients with Hodgkin lymphoma who are relapsed or refractory after frontline therapy," *Blood*, vol. 124, no. 21, p. 293, 2014.

[59] O. A. O'Connor, J. Kuruvilla, A. Sawas et al., "A Phase 1-2 study of brentuximab vedotin (Bv) and bendamustine (B) in patients with relapsed or refractory hodgkin lymphoma (HL) and anaplastic large T-cell lymphoma (ALCL)," *Blood*, vol. 124, no. 21, p. 3084, 2014.

[60] M. Dickinson, D. Ritchie, D. J. Deangelo et al., "Preliminary evidence of disease response to the pan deacetylase inhibitor panobinostat (LBH589) in refractory Hodgkin Lymphoma," *British Journal of Haematology*, vol. 147, no. 1, pp. 97–101, 2009.

[61] A. Younes, A. Sureda, D. Ben-Yehuda et al., "Panobinostat in patients with relapsed/refractory Hodgkin's lymphoma after autologous stem-cell transplantation: results of a phase II study," *Journal of Clinical Oncology*, vol. 30, no. 18, pp. 2197–2203, 2012.

[62] P. Atadja, "Development of the pan-DAC inhibitor panobinostat (LBH589): successes and challenges," *Cancer Letters*, vol. 280, no. 2, pp. 233–241, 2009.

[63] M. Lemoine, E. Derenzini, D. Buglio et al., "The pandeacetylase inhibitor panobinostat induces cell death and synergizes with everolimus in Hodgkin lymphoma cell lines," *Blood*, vol. 119, no. 17, pp. 4017–4025, 2012.

[64] B. Christian, A. Kopko, T. A. Fehniger, N. L. Bartlett, and K. A. A. Blum, "Phase I. Trial of the histone deacetylase (HDAC)

inhibitor, panobinostat, in combination with lenalidomide in patients with relapsed/refractory Hodgkin's lymphoma (HL)," *Blood*, vol. 120, no. 21, p. 1644, 2012.

[65] A. Younes, Y. Oki, R. G. Bociek et al., "Mocetinostat for relapsed classical Hodgkin's lymphoma: an open-label, single-arm, phase 2 trial," *The Lancet Oncology*, vol. 12, no. 13, pp. 1222–1228, 2011.

[66] N. T. Ihle and G. Powis, "Take your PIK: phosphatidylinositol 3-kinase inhibitors race through the clinic and toward cancer therapy," *Molecular Cancer Therapeutics*, vol. 8, no. 1, pp. 1–9, 2009.

[67] A. Guarini, C. Minoia, M. Giannoccaro et al., "mTOR as a target of everolimus in refractory/relapsed Hodgkin Lymphoma," *Current Medicinal Chemistry*, vol. 19, no. 7, pp. 945–954, 2012.

[68] P. B. Johnston, D. J. Inwards, J. P. Colgan et al., "A phase II trial of the oral mTOR inhibitor everolimus in relapsed Hodgkin lymphoma," *American Journal of Hematology*, vol. 85, no. 5, pp. 320–324, 2010.

[69] A. Carbone, A. Gloghini, L. Castagna, A. Santoro, and C. Carlo-Stella, "Primary refractory and early-relapsed Hodgkin's lymphoma: strategies for therapeutic targeting based on the tumour microenvironment," *The Journal of Pathology*, vol. 237, no. 1, pp. 4–13, 2015.

[70] J. Munoz, N. Dhillon, F. Janku, S. S. Watowich, and D. S. Hong, "STAT3 inhibitors: finding a home in lymphoma and leukemia," *The Oncologist*, vol. 19, no. 5, pp. 536–544, 2014.

[71] L. M. Scott and M. K. Gandhi, "Deregulated JAK/STAT signalling in lymphomagenesis, and its implications for the development of new targeted therapies," *Blood Reviews*, 2015.

[72] A. Younes, J. Romaguera, M. Fanale et al., "Phase I study of a novel oral Janus kinase 2 inhibitor, SB1518, in patients with relapsed lymphoma: evidence of clinical and biologic activity in multiple lymphoma subtypes," *Journal of Clinical Oncology*, vol. 30, no. 33, pp. 4161–4167, 2012.

[73] R. J. Jones, C. D. Gocke, Y. L. Kasamon et al., "Circulating clonotypic B cells in classic Hodgkin lymphoma," *Blood*, vol. 113, no. 23, pp. 5920–5926, 2009.

[74] A. Younes, J. Romaguera, F. Hagemeister et al., "A pilot study of rituximab in patients with recurrent, classic Hodgkin disease," *Cancer*, vol. 98, no. 2, pp. 310–314, 2003.

[75] R. Ramchandren, "Advances in the treatment of relapsed or refractory Hodgkin's lymphoma," *The Oncologist*, vol. 17, no. 3, pp. 367–376, 2012.

[76] T. A. Fehniger, S. Larson, K. Trinkaus et al., "A phase 2 multicenter study of lenalidomide in relapsed or refractory classical Hodgkin lymphoma," *Blood*, vol. 118, no. 19, pp. 5119–5125, 2011.

[77] J. Kuruvilla, D. Taylor, L. Wang, C. Blattler, A. Keating, and M. Crump, "Phase II trial of Lenalidomide in patients with relapsed or refractory Hodgkin lymphoma," *Blood*, vol. 112, no. 11, p. 3052, 2008.

[78] B. Böll, M. Fuchs, K. S. Reiners et al., "Lenalidomide in patients with relapsed or refractory Hodgkin lymphoma," *Blood*, vol. 116, no. 21, p. 2828, 2010.

[79] B. Böll, A. Plutschow, M. Fuchs et al., "German hodgkin study group phase I trial of doxorubicin, vinblastine, dacarbazine, and lenalidomide (AVD-Rev) for older Hodgkin lymphoma patients," *Blood*, vol. 122, no. 21, p. 3054, 2013.

[80] D. M. Pardoll, "The blockade of immune checkpoints in cancer immunotherapy," *Nature Reviews Cancer*, vol. 12, no. 4, pp. 252–264, 2012.

[81] S. Topalian, C. Drake, and D. Pardoll, "Immune checkpoint blockade: a common denominator approach to cancer therapy," *Cancer Cell*, vol. 27, no. 4, pp. 450–461, 2015.

[82] A. Ribas, "Tumor immunotherapy directed at PD-1," *The New England Journal of Medicine*, vol. 366, no. 26, pp. 2517–2519, 2012.

[83] S. L. Topalian, F. S. Hodi, J. R. Brahmer et al., "Safety, activity, and immune correlates of anti-PD-1 antibody in cancer," *The New England Journal of Medicine*, vol. 366, no. 26, pp. 2443–2454, 2012.

[84] M. A. Postow, M. K. Callahan, and J. D. Wolchok, "Immune checkpoint blockade in cancer therapy," *Journal of Clinical Oncology*, vol. 33, no. 17, pp. 1974–1982, 2015.

[85] M. R. Green, S. Monti, S. J. Rodig et al., "Integrative analysis reveals selective 9p24.1 amplification, increased PD-1 ligand expression, and further induction via JAK2 in nodular sclerosing Hodgkin lymphoma and primary mediastinal large B-cell lymphoma," *Blood*, vol. 116, no. 17, pp. 3268–3277, 2010.

[86] S. M. Ansell, A. M. Lesokhin, I. Borrello et al., "PD-1 blockade with nivolumab in relapsed or refractory Hodgkin's lymphoma," *The New England Journal of Medicine*, vol. 372, no. 4, pp. 311–319, 2015.

[87] C. H. Moskowitz, V. Ribrag, J. M. Michot et al., "PD-1 Blockade with the monoclonal antibody Pembrolizumab (MK-3475) in patients with classical Hodgkin lymphoma after brentuximab vedotin failure: preliminary results from a Phase 1B study (KEYNOTE-013)," *Blood*, vol. 124, no. 21, p. 290, 2014.

4

Autoimmune Hepatitis in Brazilian Children: IgE and Genetic Polymorphisms in Associated Genes

Léa Campos de Oliveira,[1] Anna Carla Goldberg,[2,3] Maria Lucia Carnevale Marin,[4,5] Karina Rosa Schneidwind,[6] Amanda Farage Frade,[7] Jorge Kalil,[3,4,5,7] Irene Kasue Miura,[6] Renata Pereira Sustovich Pugliese,[6] Vera Lucia Baggio Danesi,[6] and Gilda Porta[6]

[1]*Laboratório de Medicina Laboratorial (LIM03), Hospital das Clínicas, Faculdade de Medicina, Universidade de São Paulo, 05403-000 São Paulo, SP, Brazil*

[2]*Hospital Israelita Albert Einstein, 05652-900 São Paulo, SP, Brazil*

[3]*Instituto de Investigação em Imunologia, Instituto Nacional de Ciência e Tecnologia, 05403-000 São Paulo, SP, Brazil*

[4]*Laboratório de Imunologia, Instituto do Coração (InCor), Hospital das Clínicas, Faculdade de Medicina, Universidade de São Paulo, 05403-000 São Paulo, SP, Brazil*

[5]*Laboratório de Histocompatibilidade e Imunidade Celular (LIM19), Hospital das Clínicas, Faculdade de Medicina, Universidade de São Paulo, 05403-000 São Paulo, SP, Brazil*

[6]*Departamento de Hepatologia, Instituto da Criança, Hospital das Clínicas, Faculdade de Medicina, Universidade de São Paulo, 05403-000 São Paulo, SP, Brazil*

[7]*Divisão de Alergia e Imunologia Clínica, Faculdade de Medicina, Universidade de São Paulo, 05403-000 São Paulo, SP, Brazil*

Correspondence should be addressed to Anna Carla Goldberg; goldberg@einstein.br

Academic Editor: Fulvia Ceccarelli

Pediatric autoimmune hepatitis (AIH) patients present hypergammaglobulinemia, periportal CD8$^+$ cytotoxic T cell infiltration, and cirrhosis. Autoantibody profile defines AIH types 1 and 2 in addition to strong association with HLA-DRB1. We previously detected increased IgE serum levels and sought to compare clinical and histological features according to IgE levels in AIH ($n = 74$, ages 1–14 years) patients. Additionally, we typed 117 patients and 227 controls for functional polymorphisms of IL4, IL13, IL5, and IL4RA genes involved in IgE switching and eosinophil maturation that might contribute to overall genetic susceptibility to AIH. Serum IgE levels were high in 55% of AIH-1, but only in 12% of AIH-2 ($P = 0.003$) patients. Liver IgE was present in 91.3% of AIH-1 patients. The A alleles at both IL13 rs20541 and IL4RA rs1805011 were associated with AIH-1 ($P = 0.024$, OR = 1.55 and $P < 0.0001$, OR = 2.15, resp.). Furthermore, individuals presenting homozygosis for the A allele at IL4RA rs1805011 and HLA-DRB1*03 and/or *13 allele had sixfold greater risk to develop the disease (OR = 14.00, $P < 0.001$). The novel association suggests an additional role for IgE-linked immune response genes in the pathogenesis of AIH.

1. Introduction

Autoimmune hepatitis (AIH) is a chronic inflammatory disease characterized by progressive destruction of the hepatic parenchyma [1]. The disease displays female predominance and is considered rare in childhood, although it may occur in very young children [2]. The hallmark of the disease is the presence of circulating autoantibodies, defining two major subtypes: type 1 (AIH-1) [3, 4] and type 2 (AIH-2) [5].

Equally striking is the strong genetic susceptibility identified by specific MHC class II molecules, especially HLA-DRB1, which discriminates between the two types of AIH. Brazilian AIH-1 patients carry HLA-DRB1*13 and/or HLA-DRB1*03 whereas AIH-2 patients present mainly carry HLA-DRB1*07 [6].

Hypergammaglobulinemia is a diagnostic feature of AIH but other immunoglobulins may be altered as well. Low IgA levels are particularly common in AIH-2 [7] and we have observed high IgE levels in children with AIH-1 [8]. Elevated serum IgE levels have been previously described in acute and chronic liver diseases usually linked to alcohol abuse or viral infection [9]. This phenomenon is traditionally linked to allergy, asthma, and atopy, but elevated IgE serum levels in specific autoimmune diseases have been increasingly acknowledged. To date, elevated IgE serum levels have been identified in Churg–Strauss vasculitis [10], sclerosing cholangitis [11], bullous pemphigus [12], autoimmune pancreatitis [13], and Grave's disease [14]. IgE seems also to play a role in the pathogenesis of rheumatoid arthritis contributing to the immune response against citrullinated proteins [15]. Atta et al. [16] also observed specific IgE antinuclear antibodies in systemic lupus erythematosus suggesting there is an important contribution to the pathogenesis of the disease. B lymphocyte switching to IgE is induced by IL4 and its neighbor gene IL13 [17], which form, together with IL5, a well-studied cytokine gene cluster (5q31.1) controlling TH2 type immune responses. IL4 is a pleiotropic cytokine essential for IgE synthesis by B cells and for T cell differentiation into a TH2 phenotype and upregulation of MHC class II expression. The functions of IL13 in immune surveillance and in TH2 type immune responses partially overlap with those of IL4. In addition to the classic TH2 pathway shared with IL4, IL13 has other important functions. IL13, together with IL5 [18], is a potent mediator of tissue fibrosis and tissue remodeling, as shown in experimental models of schistosomiasis [19]. A steadily increasing literature indicates that there is an important role for IL13 in the development of hepatic fibrosis, signaling through the IL13 receptor to induce collagen production by local fibroblasts [20] AIH-1 pediatric patients typically exhibit liver fibrosis, including most patients in our study. About 25% of AIH patients, despite treatment with corticosteroids, present progressive fibrosis, highlighting the importance of any gene which might be involved in this process [21]. In addition, both IL4 and IL13 genes harbor functionally relevant polymorphisms [22, 23].

Histological findings in AIH include typical piecemeal necrosis with infiltrating T lymphocytes. T cell-mediated cytotoxicity is believed to be the central mechanism responsible for hepatic damage, but other cells are involved. Typically, $CD4^+$ helper T and B cells gather around portal tracts, whereas $CD8^+$ cytotoxic T cells have a periportal distribution [24]. In addition to the abundant infiltrating mononuclear cells, plasma cells and eosinophils may also be present [1]. Interestingly, a previous study has highlighted the increased production of IL4 messenger RNA in AIH-1 liver biopsies in parallel with the expected increase in inflammatory interferon gamma and other proinflammatory cytokines [25]. These findings led us to try to identify additional factors involved in the autoimmune processes present in this liver disease, which might act either as prognostic disease markers or as novel targets for a therapeutic approach. To this end, we analyzed the major clinical manifestations and biopsies from Brazilian children grouped according to the AIH type and serum IgE levels. We also investigated, in the predominant AIH-1 group of patients, functional polymorphisms of the IL4, IL13, IL5, and IL4RA (IL4 receptor alpha chain) genes involved in IgE switching and eosinophil differentiation and

maturation that we believe might contribute to overall genetic susceptibility to AIH.

2. Patients and Methods

A total of 141 patients diagnosed as AIH, according to the International Autoimmune Hepatitis Group Report [26], were studied. Patients were followed at the Pediatric Hepatology Unit of the Children's Institute, General Hospital, Faculty of Medicine, University of São Paulo in São Paulo, Brazil. Clinical, biochemical, and histological features of 74 AIH patients (61 with AIH-1 and 24 with AIH-2) aged 1 to 14 years were evaluated.

To increase statistical power for analysis of gene polymorphisms, we included a further 43 children with AIH-1 (a total of 117). Non-HLA matched siblings of bone marrow recipients from the same hospital and with similar social and ethnic background, without any autoimmune and/or other severe disease, were enrolled as healthy controls (HC, $n = 227$). Written informed consents were obtained from all participants and/or legal guardians, and the Internal Review Board of the University of São Paulo approved the study.

Laboratory liver tests, including alanine aminotransferase (ALT), aspartate aminotransferase (AST), alkaline phosphatase, gamma glutamyl transpeptidase (γGT), albumin, γ-globulins, prothrombin, and total bilirubin, and autoantibody profiles were performed in all patients. Fecal samples collected in all patients were negative for parasitic infection. Radioallergosorbent test (RAST) for specific allergen against house dust, animal fur, food, and fungi was assayed by radioimmunoassay using Unicap100E (Pharmacia & Upjohn Company LLC, MI, USA) system. I. Immunoglobulins M, G, A, and E were assayed by nephelometry using a DADE Behring System Nephelometer BN 100 (Dade Behring Diagnostics Inc., Somerville, NJ). Serological tests for hepatitis A, B, and C were negative in all patients. Clinicians involved in this study ruled out other hepatic diseases such as alpha-1 antitrypsin deficiency and Wilson's disease.

Histological features of liver biopsies were graded semi-quantitatively using the Brazilian Consensus for Histopathology of Chronic Hepatitis [27]. Specific monoclonal antibodies for IgE, CD3, CD4, CD8, CD20, and CD16 (BD Biosciences, San Jose, CA, USA) were used for immunohistochemistry [28].

Genomic DNA was extracted using a dodecyl/hexadecyl-trimethylammonium bromide (DTAB/CTAB) method [29]. IL4 rs2243250, rs2070874, IL5 rs2069812, and IL13 rs20541 polymorphisms were typed by restriction fragment length polymorphism (RFLP). IL4 rs2070874 and IL13 rs20541 typing by RFLP is described elsewhere [30, 31]. The primers and restriction enzymes for IL4 rs2243250 and IL5 rs2069812 were 5′CCTAAACTTGGGGAGAACATGGT, 3′TCCTCC-TGGGGAAAGATAGA (AvaII) and 5′TTCCTGCTGCTC-ATGAACAGAATACGT, 3′CATTTTGATGGCTTCAGT-GACTCTTCC (RsaI), respectively. IL4 rs2227284 and IL4RA rs1805011 polymorphisms were typed by ASPCR (allele-specific polymerase chain reaction). Primers for IL4RA rs1805011 have been described [32] and primers used for IL4 rs2227284 were 5′TTGGGTGGACAAGTAGTTGGAGCG,

TABLE 1: Clinical and laboratory findings of children with type 1 and type 2 autoimmune hepatitis.

	AIH-1 $n = 117$	AIH-2 $n = 24$
Clinical features		
Age onset; median (min–max)	8.2 (1.6–15.2)	4.8 (11.1–9.0)
Sex; n (F/M)	78/39	21/3
Onset; n (acute/insidious)	98/19	20/4
Concurrent autoimmune disease[1]; n (%)	15 (12.8)	3 (12.5)
Autoimmune diseases in relatives[2]; n (%)	23 (19.6)	11 (45.8)
Laboratory findings		
AA: type 1, SMA/ANA/SMA + ANA; type 2, LKM (n)	64/7/46	24
Alanine aminotransferase IU/L (× upper normal limit); median (min–max)	18 (2–128)	28 (4–85)
Albumin g/dL; median (min-max)	3.3 (2.2–5.1)	3.5 (2.6–4.7)
Bilirubin mg/dL; median (min-max)	3.3 (0.3–27.2)	5.8 (0.6–35)
γ-globulin g/dL; median (min-max)	3.4 (0.9–6.3)	3.3 (0.9–4.8)
IgE IU/mL; median (min-max)	96 (11–2245)	65 (6–560)
Histological features		
Cirrhosis; n (yes/no)	64/41	10/10
Not done	12	4

F = female; M = male; AA = autoantibody; SMA = smooth muscle antibody; ANA = antinuclear antibody; LKM = Liver Kidney Microsomal; n = number of individuals.
Normal albumin = 3.5–5.0 g/dL; normal bilirubin ≤ 1.1 mg/dL; normal γ-globulin = 0.7–1.6 g/dL; normal IgE = 20–100 IU/mL.
[1]Vitiligo, thyroiditis, diabetes mellitus, psoriasis, or Behçet's disease.
[2]First degree relatives.

5′TTGGGTGGACAAGTAGTTGGAGCT and 3′ATGTCC-CATCCTGCCCAGGATAG.

2.1. Statistical Analysis. All statistical analyses were carried out using GraphPad Prism 5 or SPSS, v.13 Software. The clinical and laboratory parameters were analyzed using Student's t-test or Fisher's exact test, as well as the Mann-Whitney test where necessary. P values under 0.05 were considered as significant. The power was estimated for all studied SNPs and values ranged from 76 to 82%, indicating adequate sample size. In addition, all SNPs were in HWE and, as expected, Haploview analysis confirmed that the three studied IL4 SNPs were in linkage disequilibrium.

For the possible genetic associations, χ^2 or exact Fisher's test were applied. Unpaired t-test was used to evaluate associations between IgE and the genotypes of all studied SNPs. For regression analysis, variables presenting P value <0.100 in the univariate analysis were included. To identify possible gene-gene interactions, a binary logistic regression was performed considering changes in the OR.

3. Results

The majority of the AIH patients were classified as type 1 (85% versus 15% type 2). The median age of diagnosis was 8.2 and 4.8 years, respectively, for AIH-1 and AIH-2. In addition, 54% (13/24) of AIH-2 patients developed the disease before the age of 5 years, whereas this occurred only in 8/117 (7%) of AIH-1 patients ($P < 0.001$). Twenty-three (20%) AIH-1 and 11 (46%) AIH-2 patients ($P = 0.006$) had relatives presenting autoimmune diseases. In addition, median serum

alanine aminotransferase values were higher in the AIH-2 group (28 versus 18 × upper normal limit; see Table 1).

Serum IgG, IgA, and IgE levels were significantly higher in AIH-1 in comparison to the AIH-2 group of patients (Figure 1). High IgE levels were observed in 50/91 (55%) of patients with AIH-1, but only in 2/17 (12%) of those with AIH-2 ($P = 0.003$) (Table 1).

Histopathology showed presence of cirrhosis in the majority of AIH-1 patients (57 out of 60) analyzed, usually accompanied by necroinflammatory activity corresponding to a score 3 and a score 4 panacinar necrosis. Liver cell rosettes were also present in almost 90% of livers, accompanied by infiltrating eosinophils and/or plasma cells, independently of patients IgE serum levels (Table 2). Importantly, in contrast to increased IgE serum levels present in about half of the patients, liver IgE was absent in only 4 of the 46 AIH-1 patients. Finally, most patients exhibited CD8$^+$ cytotoxic T cell and NK infiltrating cells, in some cases without detectable CD4$^+$ helper T cells (Table 3). However, irrespective of serum IgE levels, in most patients, moderate to high infiltration levels of CD4$^+$ helper T cells usually accompanied by moderately elevated liver NK cells were in fact present. In conclusion and in spite of having analyzed only a subgroup (46/60) of patients, our results clearly show that the well-known infiltrating proinflammatory cell profile coexists side by side with IgE, eosinophils, and the plasma cells possibly involved in IgE production. The reason for this mixed cell profile is currently unknown.

Among the studied SNPs in AIH-1, two functionally relevant SNPs present, respectively, in the IL13 gene and in its receptor IL4RA disclosed statistically significant increases.

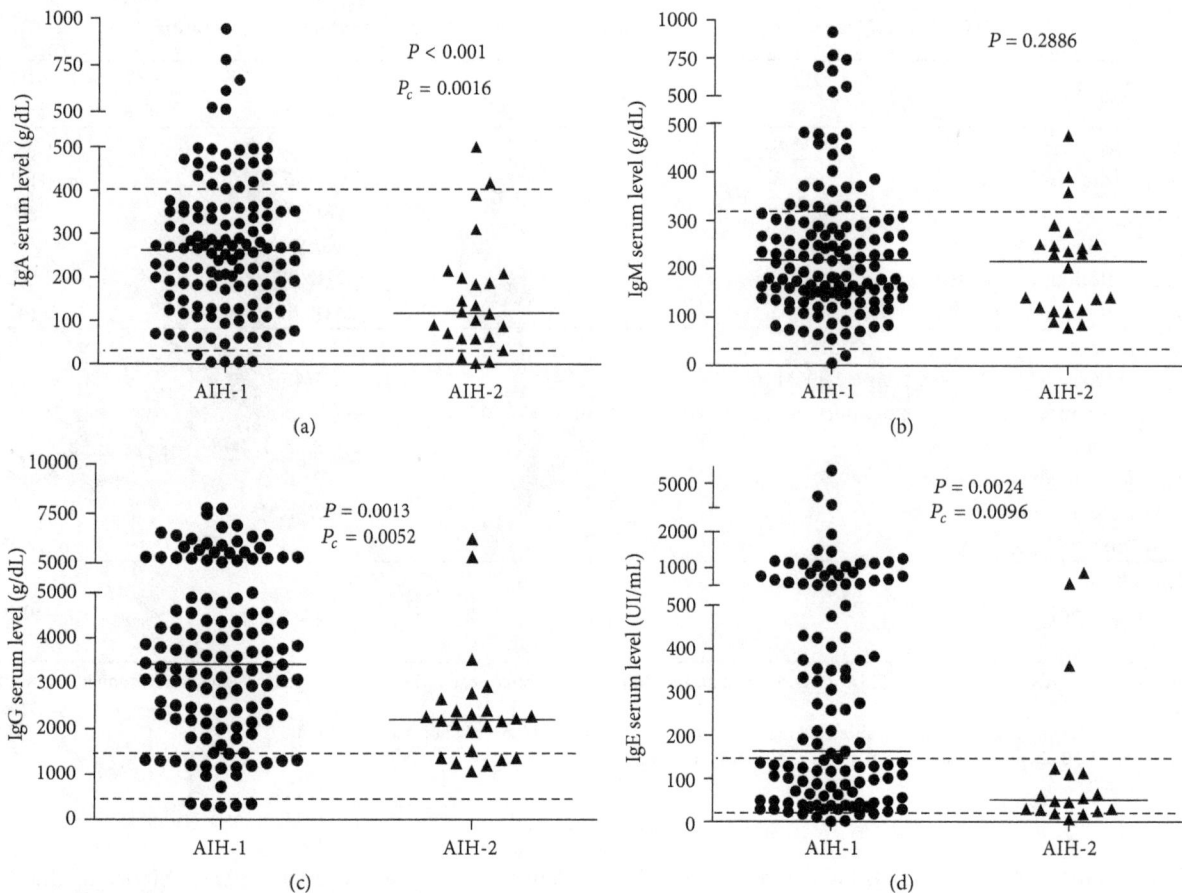

FIGURE 1: Immunoglobulins concentrations according to autoimmune hepatitis type. (a) IgA (g/dL); (b) IgM (g/dL); (c) IgG (g/dL), and (d) IgE (UI/mL). The immunoglobulins concentrations were assessed by nephelometry. Statistical analysis by Mann-Whitney nonparametric test (for medians).

The first SNP is IL13 rs20541 (31 versus 23% of HC; $P = 0.024$, OR = 1.55) and, moreover, homozygosis for the A allele at IL13 rs20541, known to impact upon receptor ligand affinity, was also significantly increased compared to healthy controls ($P < 0.001$, OR = 4.62). Increased frequencies were also found for A allele at IL4RA rs1805011 (68% versus 49%; $P < 0.0001$, OR = 2.15) and homozygosis for A (47% versus 19%; $P < 0.001$, OR = 3.75) (Table 4). The remaining polymorphisms did not show any relevant difference when AIH-1 and HC groups were compared (Supplementary Table 1 in Supplementary Material available online at http://dx.doi.org/10.1155/2015/679813).

Finally, we carried out analysis using a logistic regression model, which included allele carriage of the different SNPs as well as clinical and laboratory parameters. Three modes of analysis were tested. In the first mode (mode 1), presence of disease was considered as the dependent variable. The results confirmed the findings for both IL13 rs20541 (OR = 9.45 (95% 2.28–39.18) $P = 0.002$) and IL4RA rs1805011 (OR = 3.72 (95% 1.78–7.77) $P < 0.001$). To investigate a possible association of SNPs with pathogenesis of the disease, a second mode (mode 2) of analysis considered each SNP as the dependent variable. The T allele at IL5 rs2069812 showed association with treatment suspension (remission by

clinical and laboratory standards) ($P = 0.004$) but was a very rare outcome, present only in 7 patients (7/117, 6%) where 5 achieved regression of fibrosis after treatment (grades IV to II). IL5 is directly involved in eosinophil activation and is a key molecule in allergy and eosinophilic inflammation [33], expressed by CD4$^+$ helper T and B cells, mast cells, and eosinophils. It remains to be seen if an extended analysis confirms this indication. Finally, IgE was considered as the dependent variable in another analysis (mode 3). The presence of the T allele at IL4 rs2227284 showed association with high IgE levels (OR = 7.42 (95% CI 1.33 to 41.34), $P = 0.02$) (Table 5), an expected result.

The genes individually associated with susceptibility to the disease were examined for potential gene-gene interactions. Gene-gene interactions considered grouped genotypes for IL4RA rs1805011, IL4 rs2243250, IL4 rs2070874, rs2227284, IL13 rs20541, and IL5 rs2069812 and the presence of *03 and/or *13 alleles at the HLA-DRB1 locus. Individuals presenting homozygosis for the A allele at IL4RA rs1805011 and HLA-DRB1*03 and/or *13 allele were at six times greater risk to develop the disease (OR = 14.00, $P < 0.001$) compared to the risks conferred by the same alleles individually (HLA-DRB1*03 and/or *13, OR = 8.28; IL4RA rs1805011, OR = 3.72). Individuals homozygous for the A allele at IL13 rs20541,

TABLE 2: Semiquantitative assessment of the histopathological variables by serum IgE levels in AIH-1 and AIH-2 patients.

| Histopathological variables | Score | AIH-1 IgE | | AIH-2 IgE | |
		Normal $n = 27$ (%)	Increased $n = 33$ (%)	Normal $n = 11$ (%)	Increased $n = 2$ (%)
Structural changes	1-2	2 (7)	1 (3)	1 (9)	0 (0)
	3	2 (7)	2 (6)	1 (9)	1 (50)
	4	23 (86)	30 (91)	9 (82)	1 (50)
Portal inflammation	1-2	8 (30)	11 (33)	5 (45)	0 (0)
	3	15 (55)	11 (33)	4 (36)	1 (50)
	4	4 (15)	11 (33)	2 (18)	1 (50)
Periportal inflammation	1-2	6 (22)	7 (21)	3 (27)	0 (0)
	3	11 (41)	10 (30)	3 (27)	1 (50)
	4	10 (37)	19 (55)	5 (46)	1 (50)
Panacinar necrosis	Present	12 (44)	21 (64)	3 (27)	2 (100)
Plasmocytes	Present	20 (74)	27 (82)	8 (73)	1 (50)
Eosinophils	Present	16 (59)	19 (58)	7 (64)	1 (50)
Rosettes	Present	24 (89)	29 (88)	10 (91)	2 (100)

1 = minimal portal fibrosis; 2 = moderate portal fibrosis; 3 = bridging fibrosis; 4 = cirrhosis.

combined with HLA-DRB1*13 and/or *03 allele also showed a slightly greater risk to develop the disease (OR = 8.88, P = 0.04).

4. Discussion

The recurrent presence of plasmocytes and eosinophils in liver biopsies along with the unusual finding of increased circulating IgE antibodies in Brazilian pediatric patients with AIH was the basis for this retrospective study. To further understand if those cells might be disease markers for AIH-1, we investigated gene polymorphisms of cytokines involved in plasmocyte and eosinophil maturation and IgE production. Our hypothesis was that these SNPs might play an additional role in the development of AIH, a disease primarily caused by autoreactive T cells, acting as disease modifiers in synergy with the strongly associated MHC class II HLA-DRB1*13 and *03 alleles in the Brazilian admixed population [34]. Our cross-sectional analysis of laboratory and clinical parameters aimed to distinguish if the increased levels of circulating IgE are markers for the presence of an autoimmune process and therefore present in all patients irrespective of other markers or an indicator of a pathogenic role varying according to disease severity. It is also possible that IgE levels are simply an epiphenomenon caused by widespread inflammatory and immune activity.

The degree of portal inflammation and, especially, parenchymal lesions and interface necroinflammatory activity were remarkable in AIH-1 patients and occurred irrespective of IgE serum levels. A major feature in the present series of analysis was the finding of panacinar necrosis in about half of all patients, again regardless of IgE serum levels, eosinophil count, or other histology characteristics. In spite of liver-infiltrating eosinophils in about 60% of these patients, eosinophil count in peripheral blood of all patients was in the normal range (data not shown). This observation is in accordance with the observed lack of RAST reactivity in the patients. We concluded that despite the high IgE serum levels, the laboratory and clinical findings are not indicative of a concomitant allergy or atopy occurring in these children. In addition, eosinophils have a circulating half-life of only a few hours, with rapid removal of tissues by leukocyte extravasation [35]. In tissues, eosinophils live from 2 to 14 days, especially in liver and spleen. Eosinophils are not usually present in livers from healthy or CMV-infected patients, in contrast to liver transplanted patients, where eosinophil count correlates with degree of rejection [36]. In our patients, and arguably due to the widespread inflammation, not only were eosinophils present but also IgE was identified in most biopsies analyzed. In addition, plasma cells, T and B lymphocytes, and NK cells were also found in the liver of most patients, confirming the generalized inflammatory process. In AIH, T cell-mediated cytotoxicity is believed to be the central mechanism responsible for hepatic damage. In fact, the intriguingly mixed immune profile included also the clearly defined CD8[+] cytotoxic T cell periportal infiltration responsible for the piecemeal necrosis that is a hallmark of the disease whereas CD4[+] helper T cell and B cells gathered around portal tracts. Of note, in our group of patients, we observed a more modest score in the case of CD4[+] helper T cell infiltrating cells than described elsewhere [24].

Our data are similar to a recent study in adult AIH and drug-induced liver injury patients. Infiltrating liver cells were profiled and the presence of eosinophils was detected after standard staining in varying percentages in both groups of patients [37], but tissue IgE was not measured. Added to the unambiguous detection of eosinophils in the biopsies of our group of pediatric patients, we show that liver IgE is present in the vast majority of patients.

TABLE 3: Immunohistochemical analysis for tissue IgE, liver-infiltrating T and B lymphocytes, and NK cells in the liver of AIH-1 patients, grouped according to serum IgE levels.

Infiltrate	AIH-1 IgE serum levels	
	Normal $n = 26$ (%)	Increased $n = 20$ (%)
	IgE	
Negative	3 (12)	1 (5)
Low	11 (42)	11 (55)
Moderate/elevated	8 (31)	8 (40)
Not done	4 (15)	0
	CD3	
Negative	0	0
Low	6 (23)	6 (30)
Moderate/elevated	20 (77)	14 (70)
Not done	0	0
	CD8	
Negative	0	1 (5)
Low	14 (54)	9 (45)
Moderate/elevated	10 (38)	9 (45)
Not done	2 (8)	1 (5)
	CD4	
Negative	6 (23)	6 (30)
Low	9 (35)	7 (35)
Moderate/elevated	11 (42)	6 (30)
Not done	0	1 (5)
	CD20	
Negative	1 (4)	1 (5)
Low	11 (42)	10 (50)
Moderate/elevated	14 (54)	8 (40)
Not done	0	1 (5)
	CD16	
Negative	0	0
Low	13 (50)	11 (55)
Moderate/elevated	13 (50)	5 (25)
Not done	0	4 (20)

TABLE 4: Genotype and allele frequencies of *IL13* rs20541 and *IL4RA* rs1805011 in children with type 1 autoimmune hepatitis (AIH-1) and in healthy controls (HC).

	AIH-1 $n = 117$	HC $n = 160$	P	OR	95% CI
IL13 rs20541	n (%)	n (%)			
Genotype					
AA	18 (15)	6 (4)			
AG	37 (32)	60 (38)	0.003		
GG	62 (53)	94 (58)			
AA versus AG+GG			<0.001	4.62	1.77–12.04
Allele					
A	73 (31)	72 (23)	0.024	1.55	1.06–2.27
G	161 (69)	248 (77)			
IL4RA rs1805011	$n = 88$	$n = 212$			
Genotype					
AA	41 (47)	40 (19)			
AG	37 (42)	129 (61)	<0.001		
GG	10 (11)	43 (20)			
AA versus AG+GG			<0.001	3.75	2.18–6.45
Allele					
A	119 (68)	209 (49)	<0.001	2.15	1.49–3.11
G	57 (32)	215 (51)			

IL13 codon 110 (rs20541): A allele = Q (glutamic acid) and G allele = R (arginine); *IL4RA* codon 50 (rs1805011): A allele = I (isoleucine) and G allele = V (valine); n = number of individuals; OR = odds ratio; CI = confidence interval.

Taken together, beyond the characteristic portal and periportal inflammatory cell profile, the ubiquitous presence of IgE deposits, plasma cells, and eosinophils suggests a yet unidentified additional role in the pathogenesis of AIH. In rheumatoid arthritis, the involvement of eosinophils [38] has been linked to IL-5 and TGF-β1, profibrogenic cytokines that contribute to collagen accumulation in tissues [39]. It is possible that, likewise, the excess liver-infiltrating eosinophils take part in the development of the severe fibrosis typical of the disease in young children.

On the other hand, IL4 and IL13 are major cytokines involved in IgE synthesis by B cells [17] and exhibit overlapping functions due to the interaction with the type II receptor composed of the IL4Rα and IL13Rα1 expressed in nonhematopoietic cells and shared by both cytokines [40]. IL13 additionally impacts upon tissue eosinophilia, tissue remodeling, and fibrosis, especially in the liver [17]. We observed an association between presence of the IL13 codon 110 A allele (coding for glutamine) and susceptibility to AIH-1. This variant has been associated with increased IgE levels in both atopic and healthy children [41]. Association with the functional polymorphism coding for valine in the alpha chain of the IL4 receptor was also identified (see multivariate analysis, model 1). Chen et al. (2004) [42] have previously shown that the IL13 glutamine carrying variant displays increased activity compared to the wild type arginine variant. Furthermore, they showed that signal transduction by the variant was further enhanced when the IL4 receptor alpha chain carried valine in position 50. The results suggest that the joint presence of these two polymorphisms in AIH pediatric patients may indeed impact AIH pathology and contribute to disease severity. It is possible that the presence of higher circulating and liver IgE reflects an overall stimulus of the immune system that results in enhanced immunoglobulin levels, which could include target-driven autoantibodies. It remains to be seen if any specific autoantigen is recognized by these IgE antibodies, but without a defined target this analysis remains difficult to be achieved.

The IL4 rs2243250, rs2070874, and rs2227284 SNPs included in this study have been shown to impact IL4 transcriptional activity [43] and IL4 rs2227284 (G>T), which resides in a putative transcription factor binding site, may act independently to regulate IL4 transcription and IgE production. Furthermore, presence of the T allele at IL4

TABLE 5: Multivariate analysis of factors associated with AIH-1, using three different models.

	Dependent variable	P	OR	95% CI
	AIH-1			
Model 1				
*HLA-DRB1**	Different from 03 and/or 13	<0.001	8.28	3.46–19.82
	03 and/or 13			
IL13 rs20541	AG plus GG	0.002	9.45	2.28–39.18
	AA			
IL4RA rs1805011	AG plus GG	0.001	3.72	1.78–7.77
	AA			
	IL5 rs2069812			
Model 2				
Treatment suspension	Yes[a]	0.004	6.41	1.83–22.44
	No			
	IgE levels			
Model 3				
IL4 rs2227284	TT and GT	0.022	7.42	1.33–41.34
	GG			

Dependent variable in model 1: AIH-1 susceptibility.
Dependent variable in model 2: *IL5* rs2069812.
Dependent variable in model 3: IgE levels.
IL13 codon 110 (rs20541): A allele = Q (glutamic acid) and G allele = R (arginine); *IL4RA* codon 50 (rs1805011): A allele = I (isoleucine) and G allele = V (valine).
[a]Homozigosis for T allele.

rs2227284 has been associated with higher IgE levels in White, African-American, and Hispanic asthma patients [40]. In the multivariate analysis (see model 3), the same T allele was significantly associated with serum IgE levels strengthening our hypothesis of an additional role for the IL4, IL13 cytokine pathway in the pathogenesis of AIH.

5. Conclusion

In conclusion, in agreement with the recurrent observation of high serum IgE levels and presence of eosinophils, plasmocytes, and IgE in the liver of AIH-1 pediatric patients, we have identified novel associations with polymorphic variants of the IL13 gene and the functionally related IL4 receptor alpha chain which suggest IgE-linked immune responses may be involved in the overall susceptibility to AIH-1.

Abbreviations

AIH: Autoimmune hepatitis
MHC: Major Histocompatibility Complex
SNP: Single nucleotide polymorphism
TGF: Transforming growth factor
OR: Odds ratio
CI: Confidence interval
LD: Linkage disequilibrium
HWE: Hardy-Weinberg equilibrium.

Conflict of Interests

All authors declare no conflict of interests regarding the publication of this paper.

Authors' Contribution

Léa Campos de Oliveira designed the study, performed the analyses and interpreted the data, drafted the initial paper, and wrote the report. Anna Carla Goldberg and Gilda Porta designed and supervised the study and wrote the report. Maria Lucia Carnevale Marin performed the analyses and interpreted the data, drafted the initial paper, and wrote the report. Karina Rosa Schneidwind designed the study, performed the analyses, and drafted the initial paper. Amanda Farage Frade performed the analyses. Jorge Kalil supervised the study. Irene Kasue Miura, Renata Pereira Sustovich Pugliese, and Vera Lucia Baggio Danesi were in charge of patient follow-up and clinical data collection. All authors approved the decision to submit the final paper. Anna Carla Goldberg and Gilda Porta contributed equally to the study.

Acknowledgments

The authors thank Venâncio Avancini Ferreira Alves, M.D., Ph.D., and Evandro Sobroza de Mello, M.D., Ph.D., for histological and immunohistochemical analysis and thank Paulo Lisboa Bittencourt, M.D., Ph.D., for his review of the paper. Anna Carla Goldberg and Jorge Kalil are recipients of personal grants for scientific achievement from CNPq. All phases of this study were supported by the Brazilian National Council for Scientific and Technological Development (CNPq) and São Paulo State Research Foundation (FAPESP).

References

[1] E. L. Krawitt, "Autoimmune hepatitis," *The New England Journal of Medicine*, vol. 354, no. 1, pp. 54–66, 2006.

[2] G. V. Gregorio, B. Portmann, F. Reid et al., "Autoimmune hepatitis in childhood: a 20-year experience," *Hepatology*, vol. 25, no. 3, pp. 541–547, 1997.

[3] A. J. Czaja, F. Cassani, M. Cataleta, P. Valentini, and F. B. Bianchi, "Frequency and significance of antibodies to actin in type 1 autoimmune hepatitis," *Hepatology*, vol. 24, no. 5, pp. 1068–1073, 1996.

[4] G. F. Bottazzo, A. Florin-Christensen, A. Fairfax, G. Swana, D. Doniach, and U. Groeschel-Stewart, "Classification of smooth muscle autoantibodies detected by immunofluorescence," *Journal of Clinical Pathology*, vol. 29, no. 5, pp. 403–410, 1976.

[5] L. Bridoux-Henno, G. Maggiore, C. Johanet et al., "Features and outcome of autoimmune hepatitis type 2 presenting with isolated positivity for anti-liver cytosol antibody," *Clinical Gastroenterology and Hepatology*, vol. 2, no. 9, pp. 825–830, 2004.

[6] P. L. Bittencourt, A. C. Goldberg, E. L. R. Cançado et al., "Genetic heterogeneity in susceptibility to autoimmune hepatitis types 1 and 2," *American Journal of Gastroenterology*, vol. 94, no. 7, pp. 1906–1913, 1999.

[7] G. Porta, "Clinical and laboratory features of Brazilian children with autoimmune hepatitis types 1 and 2," *Journal of Pediatric Gastroenterology and Nutrition*, vol. 31, supplement 2, pp. S4–S19, 2000.

[8] G. Porta, K. Rosa, I. K. Miura et al., "Autoimmune hepatitis type 1 in children is associated with high IgE levels," *Journal of Pediatric Gastroenterology and Nutrition*, vol. 39, supplement 2, pp. S175–S176, 2004.

[9] E. Van Epps, G. Husby, R. C. Williams Jr., and R. G. Strickland, "Liver disease—a prominent cause of serum IgE elevation," *Clinical and Experimental Immunology*, vol. 23, no. 3, pp. 444–450, 1976.

[10] S. Ghosh, M. Bhattacharya, and S. Dhar, "Churg-strauss syndrome," *Indian Journal of Dermatology*, vol. 56, no. 6, pp. 718–721, 2011.

[11] I. Shimomura, Y. Takase, S. Matsumoto et al., "Primary sclerosing cholangitis associated with increased peripheral eosinophils and serum IgE," *Journal of Gastroenterology*, vol. 31, no. 5, pp. 737–741, 1996.

[12] J. A. Fairley, L. F. Chang, and G. J. Giudice, "Mapping the binding sites of anti-BP180 immunoglobulin E autoantibodies in bullous pemphigoid," *Journal of Investigative Dermatology*, vol.ernational Histocompatibility Workshop for typin 125, no. 3, pp. 467–472, 2005.

[13] K. Hirano, M. Tada, H. Isayama et al., "Clinical analysis of high serum IgE in autoimmune pancreatitis," *World Journal of Gastroenterology*, vol. 16, no. 41, pp. 5241–5246, 2010.

[14] K. Yabiku, M. Hayashi, I. Komiya et al., "Polymorphisms of interleukin (IL)-4 receptor alpha and signal transducer and activator of transcription-6 (Stat6) are associated with increased IL-4Ralpha-Stat6 signalling in lymphocytes and elevated serum IgE in patients with Graves' disease," *Clinical and Experimental Immunology*, vol. 148, no. 3, pp. 425–431, 2007.

[15] A. J. M. Schuerwegh, A. Ioan-Facsinay, A. L. Dorjée et al., "Evidence for a functional role of IgE anticitrullinated protein antibodies in rheumatoid arthritis," *Proceedings of the National Academy of Sciences of the United States of America*, vol. 107, no. 6, pp. 2586–2591, 2010.

[16] A. M. Atta, M. B. Santiago, F. G. Guerra, M. M. Pereira, and M. L. B. S. Atta, "Autoimmune response of IgE antibodies to cellular self-antigens in systemic lupus erythematosus," *International Archives of Allergy and Immunology*, vol. 152, no. 4, pp. 401–406, 2010.

[17] J. Punnonen, R. de Waal Malefyt, P. van Vlasselaer, J.-F. Gauchat, and J. E. de Vries, "IL-10 and viral IL-10 prevent IL-4-induced IgE synthesis by inhibiting the accessory cell function of monocytes," *Journal of Immunology*, vol. 151, no. 3, pp. 1280–1289, 1993.

[18] R. M. Reiman, R. W. Thompson, C. G. Feng et al., "Interleukin-5 (IL-5) augments the progression of liver fibrosis by regulating IL-13 activity," *Infection and Immunity*, vol. 74, no. 3, pp. 1471–1479, 2006.

[19] M. G. Chiaramonte, D. D. Donaldson, A. W. Cheever, and T. A. Wynn, "An IL-13 inhibitor blocks the development of hepatic fibrosis during a T-helper type 2-dominated inflammatory response," *The Journal of Clinical Investigation*, vol. 104, no. 6, pp. 777–785, 1999.

[20] T. A. Wynn, "IL-13 effector functions," *Annual Review of Immunology*, vol. 21, pp. 425–456, 2003.

[21] A. J. Czaja and H. A. Carpenter, "Progressive fibrosis during corticosteroid therapy of autoimmune hepatitis," *Hepatology*, vol. 39, no. 6, pp. 1631–1638, 2004.

[22] H. Mitsuyasu, Y. Yanagihara, X.-Q. Mao et al., "Cutting edge: dominant effect of Ile50Val variant of the human IL-4 receptor alpha-chain in IgE synthesis," *The Journal of Immunology*, vol. 162, no. 3, pp. 1227–1231, 1999.

[23] F. Alvarez, P. A. Berg, F. B. Bianchi et al., "International autoimmune hepatitis group report: review of criteria for diagnosis of autoimmune hepatitis," *Journal of Hepatology*, vol. 31, no. 5, pp. 929–938, 1999.

[24] M. B. De Biasio, N. Periolo, A. Avagnina et al., "Liver infiltrating mononuclear cells in children with type 1 autoimmune hepatitis," *Journal of Clinical Pathology*, vol. 59, no. 4, pp. 417–423, 2006.

[25] A. C. Cherñavsky, N. Paladino, A. E. Rubio et al., "Simultaneous expression of Th1 cytokines and IL-4 confers severe characteristics to type I autoimmune hepatitis in children," *Human Immunology*, vol. 65, no. 7, pp. 683–691, 2004.

[26] F. Alvarez, P. A. Berg, F. B. Bianchi et al., "International Autoimmune Hepatitis Group Report: review of criteria for diagnosis of autoimmune hepatitis," *Journal of Hepatology*, vol. 31, no. 5, pp. 929–938, 1999.

[27] L. C. C. Gayotto, V. A. F. Alves, and E. Strauss, *Doenças do Fígado e Vias Biliares*, Atheneu, Sao Paulo, Brazil, 1st edition, 2001.

[28] C. E. Bacchi and A. M. Gown, "Detection of cell proliferation in tissue sections," *Brazilian Journal of Medical and Biological Research*, vol. 26, no. 7, pp. 677–687, 1993.

[29] J. D. Bignon and M. A. Fernandes-Viña, "Protocols of the 12th International Histocompatibility Workshop for typing of HLA class II alleles by DNA amplification by polymerase chain reaction (PCR) and hybridization with sequence specific oligonucleotide probes (SSOP)," in *Genetic Diversity of HLA. Functional and Medical Implications*, D. Charron, Ed., p. 584, EDK, Paris, France, 1997.

[30] N. Shibata, T. Ohnuma, T. Takahashi et al., "The effect of IL4 +33C/T polymorphism on risk of Japanese sporadic Alzheimer's disease," *Neuroscience Letters*, vol. 323, no. 2, pp. 161–163, 2002.

[31] Y. Hiromatsu, T. Fukutani, M. Ichimura et al., "Interleukin-13 gene polymorphisms confer the susceptibility of Japanese populations to Graves' disease," *The Journal of Clinical Endocrinology and Metabolism*, vol. 90, no. 1, pp. 296–301, 2005.

[32] H. Mitsuyasu, Y. Yanagihara, X.-Q. Mao et al., "Cutting edge: dominant effect of Ile50Val variant of the human IL-4 receptor α-chain in IgE synthesis," *The Journal of Immunology*, vol. 162, no. 3, pp. 1227–1231, 1999.

[33] K. Takatsu, "Interleukin 5 and B cell differentiation," *Cytokine and Growth Factor Reviews*, vol. 9, no. 1, pp. 25–35, 1998.

[34] A. C. Goldberg, P. L. Bittencourt, B. Mougin et al., "Analysis of HLA haplotypes in autoimmune hepatitis type 1: identifying the major susceptibility locus," *Human Immunology*, vol. 62, no. 2, pp. 165–169, 2001.

[35] N. Farahi, N. R. Singh, S. Heard et al., "Use of 111-Indium-labeled autologous eosinophils to establish the in vivo kinetics of human eosinophils in healthy subjects," *Blood*, vol. 120, no. 19, pp. 4068–4071, 2012.

[36] Z. Ben-Ari Shpirer, J. D. Booth, S. D. Gupta, K. Rolles, A. P. Dhillon, and A. K. Burroughs, "Morphometric image analysis and eosinophil counts in human liver allografts," *Transplant International*, vol. 8, no. 5, pp. 346–352, 1995.

[37] A. Suzuki, E. M. Brunt, D. E. Kleiner et al., "The use of liver biopsy evaluation in discrimination of idiopathic autoimmune hepatitis versus drug-induced liver injury," *Hepatology*, vol. 54, no. 3, pp. 931–939, 2011.

[38] A. Kargili, N. Bavbek, A. Kaya, A. Koşar, and Y. Karaaslan, "Eosinophilia in rheumatologic diseases: a prospective study of 1000 cases," *Rheumatology International*, vol. 24, no. 6, pp. 321–324, 2004.

[39] A. J. Lucendo, Á. Arias, L. C. De Rezende et al., "Subepithelial collagen deposition, profibrogenic cytokine gene expression, and changes after prolonged fluticasone propionate treatment in adult eosinophilic esophagitis: a prospective study," *Journal of Allergy and Clinical Immunology*, vol. 128, no. 5, pp. 1037–1046, 2011.

[40] A. E. Kelly-Welch, E. M. Hanson, M. R. Boothby, and A. D. Keegan, "Interleukin-4 and interleukin-13 signaling connections maps," *Science*, vol. 300, no. 5625, pp. 1527–1528, 2003.

[41] P. E. Graves, M. Kabesch, M. Halonen et al., "A cluster of seven tightly linked polymorphisms in the IL-13 gene is associated with total serum IgE levels in three populations of white children," *Journal of Allergy and Clinical Immunology*, vol. 105, no. 3, pp. 506–513, 2000.

[42] W. Chen, M. B. Ericksen, L. S. Levin, and G. K. K. Hershey, "Functional effect of the R110Q IL13 genetic variant alone and in combination with IL4RA genetic variants," *Journal of Allergy and Clinical Immunology*, vol. 114, no. 3, pp. 553–560, 2004.

[43] M. J. Basehore, T. D. Howard, L. A. Lange et al., "A comprehensive evaluation of IL4 variants in ethnically diverse populations: association of total serum IgE levels and asthma in white subjects," *The Journal of Allergy and Clinical Immunology*, vol. 114, no. 1, pp. 80–87, 2004.

5

Immune Checkpoint Modulators: An Emerging Antiglioma Armamentarium

Eileen S. Kim,[1] Jennifer E. Kim,[1] Mira A. Patel,[1] Antonella Mangraviti,[1] Jacob Ruzevick,[1] and Michael Lim[1,2]

[1]*Department of Neurosurgery, Johns Hopkins University School of Medicine, Baltimore, MD 21205, USA*
[2]*Department of Oncology, Johns Hopkins University School of Medicine, Baltimore, MD 21205, USA*

Correspondence should be addressed to Michael Lim; mlim3@jhmi.edu

Academic Editor: Daniel Olive

Immune checkpoints have come to the forefront of cancer therapies as a powerful and promising strategy to stimulate antitumor T cell activity. Results from recent preclinical and clinical studies demonstrate how checkpoint inhibition can be utilized to prevent tumor immune evasion and both local and systemic immune suppression. This review encompasses the key immune checkpoints that have been found to play a role in tumorigenesis and, more specifically, gliomagenesis. The review will provide an overview of the existing preclinical and clinical data, antitumor efficacy, and clinical applications for each checkpoint with respect to GBM, as well as a summary of combination therapies with chemotherapy and radiation.

1. Introduction

Over the past five years, a series of landmark publications heralded the advances of checkpoint inhibitors as cancer immunotherapy [1–3]. Recent clinical trials have demonstrated significant response rates with anti-CTLA-4 and anti-PD-1 antibodies in patients with late stage melanoma and squamous cell lung cancer [1, 4]. These results, along with the recent FDA approval of ipilimumab (anti-CTLA-4) and nivolumab (anti-PD-1), continue to highlight checkpoint inhibitors' potential as powerful new additions to the modern anticancer armamentarium.

Preclinical and clinical studies have shown that immunotherapy can improve survival and generate a robust antitumor immune response to improve cancer therapy [5, 6]. Under normal physiologic conditions, immune homeostasis is regulated by a careful balance of activating and inhibitory signals. These "immune checkpoints" (Figure 1) play a critical role in regulating the cells of the immune system. Dysregulation of these checkpoints has been implicated in the pathologically up- or downregulated immune responses seen in chronic infection, autoimmunity, and cancer.

Tumor cells have developed several strategies to exploit these checkpoints and circumvent the host immune defenses.

Glioblastoma multiforme (GBM) is the most common central nervous system (CNS) tumor, which has been shown to evade host antitumor response by decreasing immune activation and antigen recognition through several mechanisms. These methods include inducing T cell anergy and lymphopenia, decreasing synthesis of antibodies, increasing immunosuppressive cytokines (i.e., IL10 and TGF-β), upregulating inhibitory molecules of T cells (i.e., Fas ligand [FasL] and programmed death ligand-1 [PDL-1]), and recruiting regulatory T cells (Tregs) and myeloid derived suppressor cells (MDSCs) to subdue immune response [7–13].

The recent discovery of lymphatic vessels in the brain has generated much excitement towards an immune approach to treatment of brain malignancies [14]. This finding provides anatomic evidence for immune communications between the periphery and CNS and may support the long-standing theory that activated, circulating T cells can cross the blood brain barrier after peripheral vaccination or checkpoint inhibition. At present, several studies have demonstrated a positive correlation between high lymphocytic infiltration of primary brain tumors and overall survival [15–21]. Targeted immunotherapy has, therefore, emerged as a promising new approach for treatment, based on the principle that augmenting tumor infiltrating lymphocytes (TILs) activity

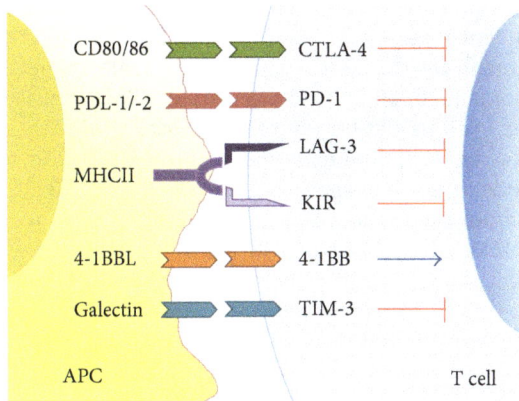

FIGURE 1: Negative and positive immune checkpoint receptors and ligands.

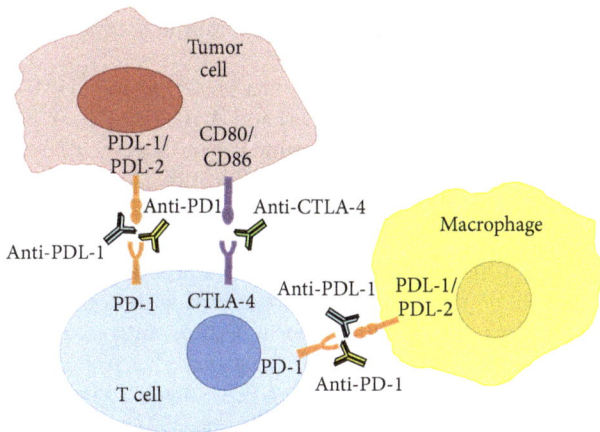

FIGURE 2: Anti-checkpoint antibodies and their targets.

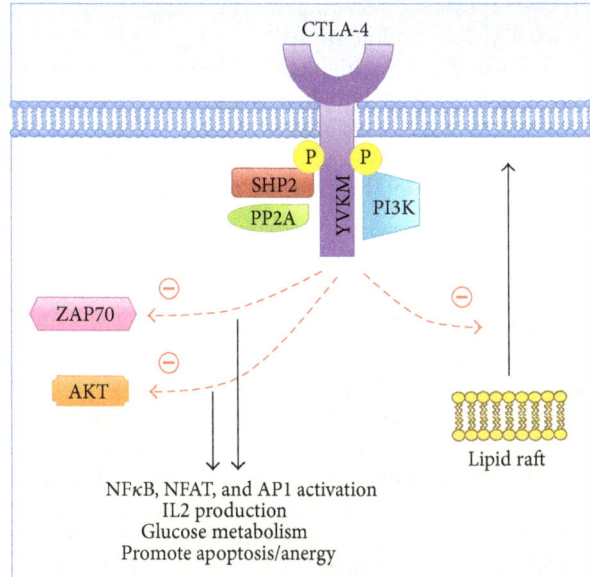

FIGURE 3: CTLA-4 signaling cascade.

in the tumor microenvironment could translate to tumor regression [22, 23]. Monoclonal antibodies as agonists or antagonists that target checkpoint inhibitors have emerged as potential strategies to restrict TIL inhibiting signals from the tumor and circulating monocytes, block negative signals and cytokines that inhibit T cell activity, and stimulate systemic immunity (Figure 2) [24].

In this review, we will discuss a series of immune checkpoints that have emerged as potential targets for therapeutic blockade, with an emphasis on those pertinent to the treatment of malignant gliomas. This discussion will touch upon cellular mechanisms, clinical relevance, and outcomes of both preclinical and clinical studies pertaining to each checkpoint. We will also address the topics of combination therapy with other checkpoints molecules as well as other modalities.

2. Immune Checkpoints

2.1. CTLA-4. Cytotoxic T lymphocyte antigen-4 (CTLA-4) is widely regarded as the archetypal T cell intrinsic inhibitory checkpoint. A member of the immune regulatory CD28-B7 immunoglobulin superfamily [25], CTLA-4, acts largely on

naïve and resting T lymphocytes to promote immunosuppression through both B7-dependent and B7-independent pathways. The B7-1 (CD80) and B7-2 (CD86) proteins found on the surface of antigen presenting cells (APCs) interact with CD28 receptors on T cells to provide the costimulatory "Signal 2" for T cell activation ("Signal 1" being the primary interaction of the T cell receptor [TCR] and Major Histocompatibility Complex [MHC]). Though the B7:CD28 pathway is one of the best-understood mechanisms for T cell costimulation, it is complicated by the addition of CTLA-4 (CD152), a lymphocyte surface protein with 30% homology to CD28 [26]. This transmembrane glycoprotein is a negative T cell regulator that also associates with B7, but with nearly 20 times greater affinity. CTLA-4:B7 engagement not only is quick and effective, but also segregates and prevents B7 from interacting with the activating CD28 [27–29].

B7-dependent immunosuppression occurs through direct engagement of CTLA-4, which may be expressed in a constitutive or rapidly inducible manner on CD4+, CD8+, and regulatory T cells (Tregs) [30]. Though the exact signaling mechanism for T cell inactivation has not yet been fully characterized, existing evidence suggests that upon phosphorylation, CTLA-4 binds to phosphoinositide 3-kinase (PI3K) via a Tyr-Val-Lys-Met (YVKM) motif and activates phosphatases SHP2 and PP2A. Downstream effects of the proposed signaling cascades (see Figure 3) may include inhibition of metabolism [31, 32], inactivation of transcription factors [33, 34], inhibition of CD28-mediated lipid raft formation, [35, 36], and loss of calcium mobilization required for cell proliferation [37].

As an effector molecule, CTLA-4 modulates the threshold for T cell activation [38]. Along with direct signal transduction, engagement with B7 has been shown to control rapid cell surface accumulation of CTLA-4 [39]. CTLA-4 may also actively capture and remove B7-1 (CD80) and B7-2 (CD86) proteins on the opposing APC through a process of transendocytosis, resulting in "signaling independent" negative T cell regulation [40, 41].

In vivo studies have highlighted the regulatory role that CTLA-4 may play in lymphoproliferation. Early lethality due to uncontrolled polyclonal CD4+ T cell expansion was demonstrated in CTLA-4-deficient mice, ostensibly resulting from dysregulated self-tolerance of peripheral autoantigens [42–44].

2.1.1. Preclinical Evidence. The role of CTLA-4 in glioma maintenance is complex and incompletely understood. While early characterizations of glioma tissue noted dramatic CD4+ lymphopenia and T cell anergy [45–47], the mechanisms by which gliomas achieved global immunocompromise were not yet known. Studies from the early 2000s implicated CTLA-4 in the development of Tregs, a population of immune suppressor cells that is often expanded in gastric [48, 49], pancreatic [50, 51], ovarian [52], and lung cancers [52]. In 2006, using flow cytometry on human GBM samples, El Andaloussi and Lesniak demonstrated that the number of FOXP3+ Tregs were significantly increased in TIL populations compared to controls and that CTLA-4 expression was also elevated within the glioma Treg population compared to those in the control samples [8]. That same year, Fecci et al. reported their findings that while absolute CD4+ cell counts (including CD4+ T helper cells and CD4+CD25+FoxP3+CD4RO+ Tregs) were lower in malignant glioma samples compared to controls, Tregs represented an increased fraction of the existing T cells, and though diminished in number, they were sufficient to significantly impair immune responsiveness [53]. These findings have helped implicate CTLA-4 in the maintenance of an immunosuppressive tumor microenvironment and highlight its potential as a target for immunotherapy in malignant gliomas.

In a follow-up study by Fecci et al, monoclonal anti-CTLA-4 antibody was administered in murine glioma-bearing mice to investigate the immune consequences of CTLA-4 checkpoint blockade. A long-term survival of 80% was reported in the treated group, as well as a restoration of CD4+ proliferation and antitumor capacity. Interestingly, the treatment effects seemed to be exclusive to the CD4+ helper T cell compartment, while Tregs remained functionally unaffected or unsuppressed [9]. Additional animal studies explored the effects of combining anti-CTLA-4 with other immunotherapies. Grauer et al. reported a 50% survival with anti-CTLA-4 alone, compared to 100% survival in mice treated with both anti-CTLA-4 and anti-CD25 (alpha chain of the IL-2 receptor) [54]. Agarwalla et al. found that while high dose anti-CTLA-4 alone was ineffective against large, well-established tumors, the addition of a whole tumor cell vaccination (Gvax) significantly improved long term survival in mice with murine intracranial gliomas [55]. Findings such as these have helped promote the development of clinical trials using anti-CTLA antibody for malignant gliomas.

2.1.2. Clinical Evidence. In light of promising results in animal models, clinical testing of two fully humanized anti-CTLA-4 antibodies, ipilimumab (Bristol Meyer-Squibb) and tremelimumab (Pfizer), began in 2000. The findings from subsequent studies culminated in the 2011 FDA approval of ipilimumab for the treatment of unresectable or metastatic melanoma [3, 6, 41, 56]. With regard to GBM, The National Cancer Institute has begun a Phase I trial to identify safety and dosage of ipilimumab and/or nivolumab with temozolomide in newly diagnosed glioblastoma (NCT02311920). In addition, a randomized, 2-arm, Phase II-III study of ipilimumab in combination with standard-of-care temozolomide for the treatment of newly diagnosed glioblastoma is also currently underway, helmed by the Radiation Therapy Oncology Group (RTOG 1125) [57].

2.2. PD-1/PDL-1. Like CTLA-4, programmed cell death protein 1 (PD-1, also known as CD279) is an inhibitory receptor that negatively regulates the immune system. However, while CTLA-4 mainly affects naïve T cells, PD-1 is more broadly expressed on immune cells and regulates mature T cell activity in peripheral tissues and in the tumor microenvironment [41].

The PD-1 receptor binds two ligands, PD ligand 1 (PDL-1, also known as B7-H1 or CD274) and PDL2 (B7-DC or 273) [58–61], each belonging to the same B7 family as the B7-1 and B7-2 proteins that interact with CD28 and CTLA-4. In the first paper detailing the discovery of the ligand, Dong et al. noted that ligation of PDL-1 not only decreased IFNγ, TNFα, and IL-2 production but also stimulated production of IL10, an anti-inflammatory cytokine associated with decreased T cell reactivity and proliferation as well as antigen-specific T cell anergy [58, 60, 61]. PDL2 ligation also results in T cell suppression, but where PDL-1-PD-1 interactions inhibits proliferation via cell cycle arrest in the G1/G2 phase [62], PDL2-PD-1 engagement has been shown to inhibit TCR-mediated signaling by blocking B7:CD28 signals at low antigen concentrations and reducing cytokine production at high antigen concentrations [59].

Though both CTLA-4 activity and PD-1 activity have immunosuppressive effects, PD-1 relies on different signaling pathways and mechanisms to suppress the T cell inflammatory response and limit autoimmunity (Figure 4).

Ligation of this 288-amino acid transmembrane receptor results in the dephosphorylation (and deactivation) of ZAP70 and the recruitment of SHP2. Upon binding PD-1, SHP-2 directly dephosphorylates PI3K, which inhibits downstream activation of Akt and thereby decreases production of inflammatory cytokine production and cell survival proteins (i.e., Bcl-xL) [63, 64]. Of note, PD-1 activity may be countered or overcome by strong TCR signaling or concomitant CD28 [65] or IL-2 [66] costimulation, allowing recovery of cytokine production and cell survival [61].

2.2.1. Preclinical Evidence. PDL-1 has been shown to be highly expressed on multiple malignant gliomas, as compared to normal brain or benign tumor tissues [67–70]. The mechanism for ligand upregulation has been elucidated in part by Parsa et al., who found that loss of the phosphatase and tensin homolog (PTEN) led to increased PDL-1 gene transcription; furthermore, gliomas with wild-type PTEN were more likely

TABLE 1: Immune checkpoint antibodies under clinical development.

Target	Biological function	Agent	Stage of clinical development
CTLA-4	Inhibitory receptor	Ipilimumab Tremelimumab	Phase I/II/III/IV Phase I/II/III
PD-1	Inhibitory receptor	Nivolumab (MDX1106, BMS-936558) Pembrolizumab (MK-3475) Pidilizumab (CT-011)	Phase I/II/III/IV Phase I/II/III Phase I/II
PD-L1	Ligand for PD-1	BMS935559 (MDX1105) MPDL3280A MEDI4736 MSB0010718C	Phase I Phase I Phase I Phase I
PD-1-positive T cells	PD-1 inhibitor	AMP-224	Phase I
LAG-3	Inhibitory protein	IMP321	Phase I/II (terminated)
KIR	Inhibitory receptor	Lirilumab (IPH2101, BMS)	Phase I/II
4-1BB	Stimulatory receptor	Urelumab (BMS-663513)	Phase I
GITR	Stimulatory receptor	TRX518	Phase I
TIM-3	Inhibitory receptor	Anti-TIM-3	Preclinical

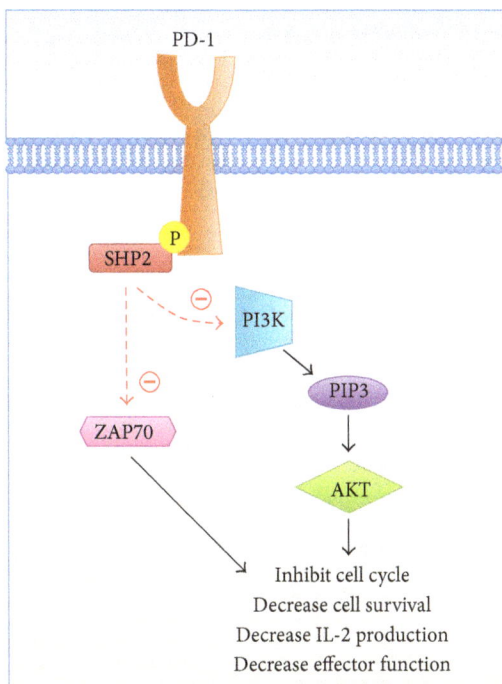

FIGURE 4: PD-1 signaling cascade.

to be lysed by tumor-specific T cells than gliomas with mutant or inactivated PTEN [68]. The presence of PDL-1 has been associated with potent inhibition of CD4+ and CD8+ T cell activation and cytokine release (IFNγ, IL2, and IL10) [67]. PDL-1 expression levels have also been shown to have significant correlation with tumor grade [71]. Using a mouse orthotopic glioblastoma model, Zeng et al. demonstrated that the combined used of anti-PD-1 and focal radiation therapy led to robust antitumor activity and immunologic memory, as demonstrated by significantly improved survival, increased tumor infiltration of CD8+ T cells, and decreased Tregs populations [5]. These findings have spurred interest in further testing of PD-1 blockade in the clinical trials setting.

2.2.2. *Clinical Evidence.* At present, several forms of monoclonal anti-PD-1 and anti-PDL-1 antibodies are undergoing clinical development, several of which have shown promising results in early Phase I and II trials (Table 1).

Therapeutic IgGs that target the PD-1 receptor include AMP-224 (Amplimmune), Pembrolizumab (Merck), Nivolumab (BMS), and Pidilizumab (CureTech). Human IgGs targeting the PDL-1 ligand include BMS-936559 (BMS), MEDI4736 (Medimmune), MPDL3280A (Genentech), and MSB0010718C (Merck); additionally, rHigM12B7 (Mayo Foundation) is a human IgM that targets the PDL2 ligand.

Recent results from a clinical trial examining the safety and efficacy of Nivolumab with and without ipilimumab have shown that monotherapy with Nivolumab had fewer treatment related adverse effects than combination therapy and that immune therapy seems to have biologic effects. This has led to Phase III of the trial comparing the safety and efficacy of Nivolumab versus Bevacizumab with or without ipilimumab (NCT02017717). There are several clinical trials recruiting patients to study the effects of anti-PD-1 in patients with GBM. These trials include a Phase I/II clinical trial (NCT01952769) to study the safety and efficacy of Pidilizumab in diffuse intrinsic pontine glioma and relapsed GBM, a Phase II trial of neoadjuvant Nivolumab in primary and recurrent GBM (NCT02550249), a Phase II trial of Pembrolizumab in recurrent GBM (NCT02337686), and several trials examining the effects of combination therapy of anti-PD-1 antibodies with Temozolomide with and without radiation therapy (NCT02311920, NCT02530502), INCB24360 (NCT02327078), FPA008 (NCT02526017), and dendritic cell vaccine (NCT02529072).

3. Additional Checkpoints

3.1. LAG-3. Lymphocyte-activation gene 3 (LAG-3, also known as CD223) is a CD4-related transmembrane protein that competitively binds MHC II and acts as a coinhibitory checkpoint for T cell activation [72, 73]. The mechanism by which LAG-3 negatively regulates the TCR-CD3 complex and inhibits T cell proliferation and cytokine production is not well understood, but several studies have suggested that the inhibitory function depends on a conserved KIEELE motif in the protein's cytoplasmic domain [72–74]. An additional domain binds LAP (LAG-3-associated protein), which may play a role in microtubule association after TCR engagement [75].

LAG-3 is expressed in vivo on the surface of activated CD4+, CD8+, and NK cells [75, 76] under inflammatory conditions. In vitro studies have shown that LAG-3 is upregulated by IL12 and promotes the production of IFNγ [77]. LAG-3 expression is required for maximal Treg function, and ectopic expression may be sufficient for inducing regulatory activity, with suppressive capacities comparable to ectopically expressed FOXP3 [78, 79]. LAG-3 may also play a role in regulating DC function; engagement with DC MHCII molecules has been shown to induce morphologic changes and upregulate IL12 and TNFα secretion [76]. In a study by Workman and Vignali, LAG-3(−/−) T cells exhibited the following characteristics as compared to LAG-3+ cells: (1) delayed cell cycle arrest after stimulation with a superantigen, (2) greater proliferation after in vivo stimulation, (3) and higher numbers of memory T cells after viral exposure [73]. These data suggested LAG-3 plays an important role in regulating T cell expansion, a hypothesis that was further supported by a study by Huang et al. Using LAG-3 knockout mice, the authors demonstrated that, compared to wild-type Tregs, more than double the number of LAG-3(−/−) Tregs were required to control CD4+ helper T cell proliferation at high antigen peptide concentrations; furthermore, the authors reported that administration of anti-LAG-3 antibodies resulted in a reversal of Treg-mediated immune suppression [78]. Grosso et al. also employed antibodies against LAG-3 to increase proliferation and effector function of tumor-specific CD8+ cytotoxic T cells and resulting in disrupted tumor architecture and growth inhibition [80]. A recent study by Woo et al. demonstrated the efficacy of combined checkpoint blockade using three distinct tumor types (B16 melanoma, MC38 colorectal adenocarcinoma, and SalN fibrosarcoma); in each of these tumors types, tolerized T cells were found to coexpress LAG-3 and PD-1. Whereas treatment with anti-LAG-3 alone or anti-PD-1 alone delayed tumor growth in a minority of treated mice (0–40%), dual therapy with anti-LAG-3 and anti-PD-1 resulted in complete tumor regression in 70 and 80% of mice with fibrosarcoma and colorectal tumors, respectively. Though no therapeutic effects were observed in the melanoma-inoculated mice, these findings provided compelling evidence for a synergistic benefit of combination checkpoint blockade [81]

3.2. TIM-3. T cell immunoglobulin mucin 3 (TIM-3) was discovered in 2002 as a marker of IFNγ producing CD4+ and CD8+ T cells in mice and humans [82, 83]. A type I glycoprotein receptor that binds to S-type lectin galectin-9 (Gal-9), TIM-3, is a widely expressed ligand on lymphocytes, liver, small intestine, thymus, kidney, spleen, lung, muscle, reticulocytes, and brain tissue [84]. Binding of Gal-9 by the TIM-3 receptor triggers downstream signaling to negatively regulate T cell survival and function. In vitro studies have shown that Gal-9 induced TIM-3 activation induced intracellular calcium influx, aggregation, and cell death (mixed apoptosis and necrosis) of CD4+ T cells; additionally, Gal-9 administration in vivo can cause rapid elimination of IFNγ-producing CD4+ T cells and suppress Th1-mediated autoimmunity [85].

TIM-3 is a marker of CD8+ T cell exhaustion in the setting of chronic viral infections and immunogenic tumor microenvironments [82, 86–90]. TIM-3+PD-1+ TILs have been identified in murine models of colon adenocarcinoma, breast adenocarcinoma, and melanoma; coexpression of these two T cell "exhaustion" markers has been shown to be the most functionally impaired group of CD8+ TIL populations as determined by lowest IL2, TNF and IFNγ production and progression through the cell cycle [90, 91]. In advanced AML tumor models where PD-1+TIM-3+ CD8+ cells have been correlated with disease progression, dual therapy with anti-PDL-1 and TIM-3Ig has been shown to significantly decrease tumor burden and improve survival [86].

Recent evidence suggests that TIM-3 may also play a role in myeloid-derived suppressor cell (MDSC) development. Composed of a heterogeneous group of CD11b+Gr1+ myeloid cells, MDSCs are powerful T cell suppressors that have been shown to proliferate under conditions of infection, autoimmunity, trauma, and malignancy, and their presence has been identified as negative predictive factor predictor for oncologic outcomes [10]. Both Gal-9 and transgenic TIM-3 overexpression have been shown to induce MDSC expansion, with subsequent T cell inhibition [92]; conversely, tumor growth was found to be significantly delayed in TIM-3(−/−) mice implanted with T1 mammary adenocarcinoma, as compared to TIM-3+ wild type mice [92].

3.3. KIR. Killer immunoglobulin-like receptors (KIRs) comprise a diverse repertoire of MHCI binding molecules that negatively regulate NK function to protect cells from NK-mediated cell lysis. KIRs are generally expressed on NK cells but have also been detected on tumor specific CTLs [93]. Members of the KIR family of molecules contain 2-3 Ig ectodomains and cytoplasmic tails of variable length [94]. While some "noninhibitory" KIRs have truncated cytoplasmic tails, others possess longer tails containing two immune receptor tyrosine-based inhibitory motifs (ITIMs) that mediate downstream signaling and confer anti-NK potential [95–98]. The KIR locus is most likely polymorphic and polygenic, with inhibitory KIR haplotypes remaining relatively specific for HLA-B and HLA-C ligands, while noninhibitory phenotypes display greater variability [99].

Unlike adaptive B and T cells, NK cells lack such meticulous antigen sensitivity and instead rely on several activating and inhibitory receptors to modulate and direct their killing capacity [100]. When expressed on the cell surface, KIRs may play a role in inducing NK tolerance through a process of "licensing," in which each inhibitory receptor recognizes a self HLA class I molecule and prevents NK activation against autoantigens and self-tissue [101, 102]. Knowledge of these germline-encoded receptors has provided valuable insight into the mechanisms of NK-tumor interactions [103, 104]. The phenomenon of NK-dependent rejection of syngeneic or human solid and hematopoietic tumor grafts [105, 106] is partially explained by the "missing" self-recognition phenomenon, where NK cells have been found to target aberrant cells that specifically lack self MHC I expression [107–109]. Though controversial, a few studies have also demonstrated that a lack of KIR ligands or KIR ligand incompatibility with foreign tissues is associated with improved survival and lower relapse rates [110–112] and suggest KIR inhibition as a viable means of enabling or augmenting NK cell-mediated antitumor lytic activity. This hypothesis has been borne out in adoptive transfer experiments of KIR-ligand mismatched or KIR-ligand nonexpressing NK cells which led to significantly increased cytotoxicity of multiple tumor cell lines [113, 114]. KIR blockade using anti-KIR antibodies has also been shown to prevent tolerogenicity and reconstitute NK-mediated cell lysis in both in vivo and in vitro hematopoietic cancer models [115–117].

3.4. 41BB.

A member of the tumor necrosis factor (TNF) receptor superfamily that includes the FAS receptor (apoptosis antigen), CD40 (T cell costimulatory receptor), CD27 (TNF receptor), and CD30 (tumor marker), and 4-1BB (CD137) is a Type II transmembrane glycoprotein [118] that is inducibly expressed on primed CD4+ and CD8+ T cells [119], activated NK cells, DCs, and neutrophils [120] and acts as a T cell costimulatory molecule when bound to the 4-1BB ligand (4-1BBL) found on activated macrophages, B cells, and DCs [121, 122]. Ligation of the 4-1BB receptor leads to activation of the NF-κB, c-Jun and p38 signaling pathways [123] and has been shown to promote survival of CD8+ T cells, specifically, by upregulating expression of the antiapoptotic genes BcL-x(L) and Bfl-1 [124]. In this manner, 4-1BB serves to boost or even salvage a suboptimal immune response [120]. Its expression may also be contingent on activation of the B7:CD28 pathway (see above section on *CTLA-4*), with 4-1BB producing its own feedforward loop to maintain T cell activity, and the B7-CD28 complex serving to temper the immune response and protect against inappropriate immune activation [21].

Unlike negative T cell regulators (i.e., CTLA-4, PD-1, LAG-3, and TIM-3), 4-1BB is an activating checkpoint that mediates prosurvival and proinflammatory signaling pathways. 4-1BB costimulation has been shown to profoundly enhance antigen-specific CD8 T cell survival and proliferation [125] and has therefore become a target of interest in tumor immunotherapy, especially against poorly immunogenic tumors for which the host antitumor immune response may prove inadequate. Monoclonal agonist antibodies are one promising method of harnessing the proinflammatory potential of this checkpoint molecule. Anti-4-1BB antibodies have been shown to cause tumor regression in animal models of sarcoma and mastocytoma [119], breast cancer [126], and

metastatic colon carcinoma [127] with concomitant increase in tumor selective cytotoxic T cell activity. Synergy with IL-12 gene therapy and anti-4-1BB antibody [127] or local 4-1BB gene [126] delivery has also been shown with significant tumor rejection and long-term immunity seen in metastatic breast and colon cancer models. In intracranial tumor models, anti-41BB has been shown to have moderate cure rates (2/5 mice with GL261 glioma and 4/5 with MCA205 sarcoma), but no effect against the poorly immunogenic B16/D5 melanoma model [128]. Adoptive transfer experiments have also been used to highlight 4-1BB's role in antitumor immunity. CD28 and 4-1BB costimulated T cells adoptively transferred into mice bearing poorly immunogenic melanoma have been shown to result in a 60% cure rate [129] and prolong survival in murine fibrosarcoma models [130]. Whole cell vaccines using tumor cells transfected with 4-1BBL cDNA have also been shown to induce vigorous antitumor CD8+ T cell activity and long term survival in various tumor models [131–134]. However, the technical difficulty and feasibility of culturing and administering lymphocyte or transfected tumor cells for either adoptive transfer or whole cell vaccination have limited their translation into clinical practice.

3.5. GITR.

Glucocorticoid-induced TNFR family related gene (GITR) is a member of the tumor necrosis factor receptor (TNFR) superfamily that is constitutively or conditionally expressed on Treg, CD4, and CD8 T cells [135, 136]. Initially described as a unique CD4+CD25+FoxP3+ Treg marker [137], subsequent studies demonstrated rapid upregulation of GITR on effector T cells following TCR ligation and activation [138–142]. The human GITR ligand (GITRL) is constitutively expressed on APCs in secondary lymphoid organs and has also been found on nonlymphoid tissues including vascular endothelial and various epithelial cells [135, 143]. The downstream effect of GITR:GITRL interaction is believed to be at least twofold, including (1) attenuation of Treg activity and (2) enhancement of CD4+ T cell activity [137–139, 141, 144, 145]. The net result is a reversal of Treg-mediated immunosuppression and increased immune stimulation [142, 146].

Like the 4-1BB costimulatory molecule, GITR is an activating checkpoint that enhances inflammatory pathways and host immune response. Overexpression or experimental GITR agonism is associated with autoimmunity [138, 140, 147] and pathologic inflammatory responses such as in asthma [148] and post-stroke states [149]. Preclinical studies have elucidated the differential effects of GITR upregulation on Tregs versus effector T lymphocytes, and its potential role in facilitating the antitumor immune response. Using anti-GITR monoclonal antibodies, Cohen et al. demonstrated that GITR agonism led to lower intratumoral Treg accumulation, loss of FoxP3 expression, decreased Treg suppressor function, and, ultimately, regression of B16 melanoma in mouse models [150]. While these findings were initially implicated Tregs as the primary substrate for GITR:GITRL interactions, subsequent studies have suggested that effector T cells, as opposed to Tregs, may be the principal mediators of the GITR signaling pathway [139–141]. Using GITR knockout mice that still retained functional Treg populations, Stephens et al. elegantly demonstrated that GITR engagement on CD4+CD25− T cells, and not CD25+ Treg cells, was required to abrogate Treg suppressive activity [151]. Conversely, antagonizing GITRL using blocking antibodies seemed to increase CD4+ T cell susceptibility to Treg-mediated suppression [151]. Additional studies that demonstrated the efficacy of anti-GITR agonist antibodies in inducing tumor regression and preventing regrowth upon secondary challenge have raised interest in GITR as a potential target of tumor immunotherapy [138, 152, 153].

3.5.1. Clinical Evidence. At present, there are no clinical trials for GBM involving IMP321 (a soluble LAG-3 chimeric IgG1 and MHCII agonist), anti-TIM-3 antibody, IPH2101 (anti-KIR), BMS-663513 (a fully humanized anti-4-1BB agonist antibody), or TRX518 (a first in class, humanized anti-GITR monoclonal antibody). However, these immune modulators have tremendous therapeutic potential for the treatment of CNS tumors.

4. Integrating Checkpoint Inhibitors into the Standard of Care

Despite aggressive treatment with chemotherapy and radiation, the refractory nature of high-grade gliomas has become strong motivation to seek novel treatment regimens. The clinical successes of immunomodulating antibodies in both CNS and non-CNS cancers have raised the possibility of adding checkpoint inhibitors to the current anticancer armamentarium as a complementary or even synergistic modality.

Unlike vaccine therapies or adoptive cell transfer, checkpoint inhibition is a nonspecific strategy that relies on generalized activation of the immune system. While T cells are the best-characterized targets of checkpoint inhibition at present, it is becoming clear that these therapies have wide-ranging effects on other immune players such as NK cells, monocytes, macrophages, and dendritic cells [78, 100, 154, 155] (Figure 2). Nonspecific checkpoint-based therapies may therefore benefit from concurrent therapies that either deplete immunosuppressive cells (i.e., chemotherapy) or increase access to tumor-specific antigens (i.e., ionizing radiation).

The following discussion will focus on the possible synergistic effects of concurrent chemoradiation therapy and the challenges of integrating checkpoint inhibitors into the current standard of care.

4.1. Checkpoint Inhibitors and Radiation Therapy. RT is a nonselective cytocidal treatment modality that targets rapidly dividing cells. T cells, which are the main effectors of cancer immunotherapy, are known to be exquisitely sensitive to its effects [156, 157]. Studies testing combined RT and TMZ [158] or RT and steroid [47] regimens have demonstrated significant, long-lasting drops in CD4 counts with concomitant systemic immune compromise. Though these findings could suggest an antagonistic interaction between RT and immunotherapy, the significant cellular and stromal

destruction caused by ionizing radiation has been shown to act as a powerful "danger," or activation, signal to the host immune system [159, 160]. Apoptotic tumor cells provide APCs with tumor-specific antigens that can be presented on MHC class I molecules to CD8+ cells, leading to enhanced, antitumor immune activation [161–163]. RT has also been shown to counteract MHC downregulation, a strategy used by GBM to escape immune detection [164, 165]; a study by Newcomb et al. reported a significant upregulation of the β2-microglobulin light chain subunit of the MHCI molecule in GL261 glioma cells following whole body radiation therapy [166].

Elucidating the pathways for radiation-induced immune stimulation provides a mechanism for the observed synergy between radiation and immunotherapy. Prolonged survival with the addition of anti-CTLA-4 to stereotactic radiosurgery has been reported in breast cancer-bearing mice, largely attributed to CD8+ T cell activity [167]. Although it has not been seen in GBM, combination therapy with ipilimumab (anti-CTLA-4 antibody) and local radiation has also been shown to cause tumor regression at both irradiated and nonirradiated sites—the latter known as the abscopal effect [168, 169]. Zeng et al. demonstrated that the addition of SRS to PD-1 blockade increased in vitro expression of proinflammatory molecules such as MHCI, CXCL16, and ICAM and correlated with a survival advantage in glioma-bearing mice [5]. The results of these preclinical studies indicate that RT can work synergistically with checkpoint inhibitors, and at present, a Phase I trial is underway testing the combined used of Pembrolizumab and radiation in GBM (NCT02530502). Results from these studies will help guide future strategies to integrate immunotherapy into the current standard of care therapeutic regimen.

4.2. Checkpoint Inhibitors and Chemotherapy. Approved by the FDA in 2001 for refractory anaplastic astrocytomas and in 2005 for newly diagnosed GBMs, TMZ is a second-generation DNA alkylating agent that is currently the chemotherapeutic standard for the treatment of malignant gliomas. Since its adoption as a first-line agent, population studies have demonstrated an increase in 2-year survival from 7% in cases that were diagnosed between 1993 and 1995 to 17% in those diagnosed between 2005 and 2007 [170]. Use of TMZ in combination with radiation has also been shown to increase two-year survival from 10.4% to 26.5%, as compared to radiation monotherapy [171].

Chemotherapy has been widely hypothesized to be antagonistic or counterproductive to immunotherapy due to its systemic immune toxic effects. Cytotoxic drugs such as TMZ have been associated with severe lymphopenia [172, 173]. In a prospective, multicenter study of patients with high-grade gliomas, Grossman et al. observed long-lasting, systemic CD4+ lymphodepletion with poor clinical outcomes in patients who underwent treatment with oral TMZ and radiation. In this study, median CD4 count was 664 cells/mm^3 before treatment, reached its lowest point at 255 cells/mm^3 two months after the start of TMZ + RT, and remained persistently low for the duration of observation (12 months) [158].

In theory, these effects—in combination with the locally immunosuppressive tumor microenvironment—could abrogate immunotherapy's efficacy by depleting the peripheral pool of effector T cells.

Contrary to these suppositions, numerous clinical studies combining chemotherapy with immunotherapy such as monoclonal antibodies, active specific immunotherapy, and adoptive lymphocyte immunotherapy have shown promising results, though larger studies are needed to verify and assess efficacy [174]. Heimberger et al. published a case study in 2008 demonstrating successful immune activation in a GBM patient following treatment with both TMZ and EGFRvIII vaccine [7]. Of note, the authors observed no significant decline in CD4+ and CD8+ T cell counts and concluded that as long as the cytotoxic chemotherapy was administered outside of the vaccine's therapeutic window, the two modalities could be used in a synergistic manner [7]. Furthermore, some authors have suggested the use of local or intratumoral TMZ as a less immunosuppressive alternative compared to oral TMZ. Using glioma-bearing mice, Brem et al. found that polymeric implants for local TMZ delivery were associated with improved survival, and that the addition of RT prolonged survival even further without additional toxicity [175]. Fritzell et al. later demonstrated that intratumoral TMZ may synergistically increase survival rates in immunized mice by sustained proliferation of CD8+ T cells and decreased intratumoral immunosuppressive cells such as myeloid-derived suppressor cells (MDSCs) [176].

With respect to checkpoint inhibitors, these findings imply that carefully timed, interdigitated or alternating chemotherapy would not only protect immunotherapy-activated effector T cells but also ablates immunosuppressive Tregs that could otherwise reduce the efficacy of immunomodulating antibodies [7, 177]. The use of intratumoral chemotherapy may also further protect the effector T cells and provide a survival advantage due to a more robust immune profile. At present, there are no published clinical trials data on the use of TMZ plus checkpoint inhibitors. Further preclinical and clinical studies will be required to examine the risks and benefits of this particular multimodal therapeutic strategy.

5. Summary

Immune checkpoint therapy has emerged as a welcome and potent addition to the current arsenal of anticancer treatment. While certain checkpoint blockades such as CTLA-4 and PD-1 have proven clinically successful, both alone and in conjunction with each other, there are several other targets that such as LAG-3, TIM-3, KIR, and GITR that have shown promise for passive immunotherapy. Anti-CTLA-4 and anti-PD-1 have had promising outcomes in preclinical studies for the treatment of malignant GBMs. Those studies have spurred further ongoing clinical trials that look to solidify immune therapy as a mainstay for treating primary and recurrent brain tumors. Checkpoint inhibitors may be effective not only as monotherapy, but also in combination with chemotherapy and/or radiation therapy. Synergy between the antibodies and either of the two conventional modalities could lead to significant improvements in tumor regression and overall survival. Further research on the mechanisms and therapeutic efficacy of specific antibodies, as well as their interactions with other treatment modalities, is needed to successfully incorporate checkpoint modulators into the current standard of care.

Conflict of Interests

The authors declare that there is no conflict of interests regarding the publication of this paper.

Authors' Contribution

Eileen S. Kim and Jennifer E. Kim contributed equally to this work.

References

[1] J. R. Brahmer, S. S. Tykodi, L. Q. M. Chow et al., "Safety and activity of anti-PD-L1 antibody in patients with advanced cancer," The New England Journal of Medicine, vol. 366, no. 26, pp. 2455–2465, 2012.

[2] D. T. Le, J. N. Uram, H. Wang et al., "PD-1 blockade in tumors with mismatch-repair deficiency," The New England Journal of Medicine, vol. 372, no. 26, pp. 2509–2520, 2015.

[3] F. S. Hodi, S. J. O'Day, D. F. McDermott et al., "Improved survival with ipilimumab in patients with metastatic melanoma," The New England Journal of Medicine, vol. 363, no. 8, pp. 711–723, 2010.

[4] J. D. Wolchok, H. Kluger, M. K. Callahan et al., "Nivolumab plus Ipilimumab in advanced melanoma," The New England Journal of Medicine, vol. 369, no. 2, pp. 122–133, 2013.

[5] J. Zeng, A. P. See, J. Phallen et al., "Anti-PD-1 blockade and stereotactic radiation produce long-term survival in mice with intracranial gliomas," International Journal of Radiation Oncology Biology Physics, vol. 86, no. 2, pp. 343–349, 2013.

[6] F. Aranda, E. Vacchelli, A. Eggermont et al., "Trial watch: immunostimulatory monoclonal antibodies in cancer therapy," Oncoimmunology, vol. 3, no. 1, Article ID e27297, 2014.

[7] A. B. Heimberger, W. Sun, S. F. Hussain et al., "Immunological responses in a patient with glioblastoma multiforme treated with sequential courses of temozolomide and immunotherapy: case study," Neuro-Oncology, vol. 10, no. 1, pp. 98–103, 2008.

[8] A. El Andaloussi and M. S. Lesniak, "An increase in CD4+CD25+FOXP3+ regulatory T cells in tumor-infiltrating lymphocytes of human glioblastoma multiforme," Neuro-Oncology, vol. 8, no. 3, pp. 234–243, 2006.

[9] P. E. Fecci, H. Ochiai, D. A. Mitchell et al., "Systemic CTLA-4 blockade ameliorates glioma-induced changes to the CD4+ T cell compartment without affecting regulatory T-cell function," Clinical Cancer Research, vol. 13, no. 7, pp. 2158–2167, 2007.

[10] D. I. Gabrilovich and S. Nagaraj, "Myeloid-derived suppressor cells as regulators of the immune system," Nature Reviews Immunology, vol. 9, no. 3, pp. 162–174, 2009.

[11] A. P. See, J. E. Han, J. Phallen et al., "The role of STAT3 activation in modulating the immune microenvironment of GBM," Journal of Neuro-Oncology, vol. 110, no. 3, pp. 359–368, 2012.

[12] C. Jackson, J. Ruzevick, A. G. Amin, and M. Lim, "Potential role for STAT3 inhibitors in glioblastoma," *Neurosurgery Clinics of North America*, vol. 23, no. 3, pp. 379–389, 2012.

[13] M. Kortylewski and H. Yu, "Stat3 as a potential target for cancer immunotherapy," *Journal of Immunotherapy*, vol. 30, no. 2, pp. 131–139, 2007.

[14] A. Louveau, I. Smirnov, T. J. Keyes et al., "Structural and functional features of central nervous system lymphatic vessels," *Nature*, vol. 523, no. 7560, pp. 337–341, 2015.

[15] R. I. von Hanwehr, F. M. Hofman, C. R. Taylor, and M. L. J. Apuzzo, "Mononuclear lymphoid populations infiltrating the microenvironment of primary CNS tumors. Characterization of cell subsets with monoclonal antibodies," *Journal of Neurosurgery*, vol. 60, no. 6, pp. 1138–1147, 1984.

[16] L. Palma, N. Di Lorenzo, and B. Guidetti, "Lymphocytic infiltrates in primary glioblastomas and recidivous gliomas. Incidence, fate, and relevance to prognosis in 228 operated cases," *Journal of Neurosurgery*, vol. 49, no. 6, pp. 854–861, 1978.

[17] W. H. Brooks, W. R. Markesbery, G. D. Gupta, and T. L. Roszman, "Relationship of lymphocyte invasion and survival of brain tumor patients," *Annals of Neurology*, vol. 4, no. 3, pp. 219–224, 1978.

[18] D. K. Boker, R. Kalff, F. Gullotta, S. Weekes-Seifert, and U. Möhrer, "Mononuclear infiltrates in human intracranial tumors as a prognostic factor. Influence of preoperative steroid treatment. I. Glioblastoma," *Clinical Neuropathology*, vol. 3, no. 4, pp. 143–147, 1984.

[19] D. Schiffer, D. Cavicchioli, M. T. Giordana, L. Palmucci, and A. Piazza, "Analysis of some factors effecting survival in malignant gliomas," *Tumori*, vol. 65, no. 1, pp. 119–125, 1979.

[20] Y.-F. Yang, J.-P. Zou, J. Mu et al., "Enhanced induction of antitumor T-cell responses by cytotoxic T lymphocyte-associated molecule-4 blockade: the effect is manifested only at the restricted tumor-bearing stages," *Cancer Research*, vol. 57, no. 18, pp. 4036–4041, 1997.

[21] Y.-J. Kim, S. H. Kim, P. Mantel, and B. S. Kwon, "Human 4-1BB regulates CD28 co-stimulation to promote Th1 cell responses," *European Journal of Immunology*, vol. 28, no. 3, pp. 881–890, 1998.

[22] G. P. Dunn, A. T. Bruce, H. Ikeda, L. J. Old, and R. D. Schreiber, "Cancer immunoediting: from immunosurveillance to tumor escape," *Nature Immunology*, vol. 3, no. 11, pp. 991–998, 2002.

[23] R. D. Schreiber, L. J. Old, and M. J. Smyth, "Cancer immunoediting: integrating immunity's roles in cancer suppression and promotion," *Science*, vol. 331, no. 6024, pp. 1565–1570, 2011.

[24] S. L. Topalian, C. G. Drake, and D. M. Pardoll, "Targeting the PD-1/B7-H1(PD-L1) pathway to activate anti-tumor immunity," *Current Opinion in Immunology*, vol. 245, no. 2, pp. 207–212, 2012.

[25] R. J. Greenwald, G. J. Freeman, and A. H. Sharpe, "The B7 family revisited," *Annual Review of Immunology*, vol. 23, pp. 515–548, 2005.

[26] M.-L. Alegre, K. A. Frauwirth, and C. B. Thompson, "T-cell regulation by CD28 and CTLA-4," *Nature Reviews Immunology*, vol. 1, no. 3, pp. 220–228, 2001.

[27] A. V. Collins, D. W. Brodie, R. J. C. Gilbert et al., "The interaction properties of costimulatory molecules revisited," *Immunity*, vol. 17, no. 2, pp. 201–210, 2002.

[28] P. S. Linsley, J. L. Greene, W. Brady, J. Bajorath, J. A. Ledbetter, and R. Peach, "Human B7-1 (CD80) and B7-2 (CD86) bind with similar avidities but distinct kinetics to CD28 and CTLA-4 receptors," *Immunity*, vol. 1, no. 9, pp. 793–801, 1994.

[29] R. J. Peach, J. Bajorath, W. Brady et al., "Complementary determining region 1 (CDR1)- and CDR3-analogous regions in CTLA-4 and CD28 determine the binding to B7-1," *The Journal of Experimental Medicine*, vol. 180, no. 6, pp. 2049–2058, 1994.

[30] T. Lindsten, K. P. Lee, E. S. Harris et al., "Characterization of CTLA-4 structure and expression on human T cells," *The Journal of Immunology*, vol. 151, no. 7, pp. 3489–3499, 1993.

[31] C. E. Rudd, A. Taylor, and H. Schneider, "CD28 and CTLA-4 coreceptor expression and signal transduction," *Immunological Reviews*, vol. 229, no. 1, pp. 12–26, 2009.

[32] E. Chuang, T. S. Fisher, R. W. Morgan et al., "The CD28 and CTLA-4 receptors associate with the serine/threonine phosphatase PP2A," *Immunity*, vol. 13, no. 3, pp. 313–322, 2000.

[33] J. H. Fraser, M. Rincón, K. D. McCoy, and G. L. Gros, "CTLA4 ligation attenuates AP-1, NFAT and NF-κB activity in activated T cells," *European Journal of Immunology*, vol. 29, no. 3, pp. 838–844, 1999.

[34] H. Bour-Jordan, J. H. Esensten, M. Martinez-Llordella, C. Penaranda, M. Stumpf, and J. A. Bluestone, "Intrinsic and extrinsic control of peripheral T-cell tolerance by costimulatory molecules of the CD28/B7 family," *Immunological Reviews*, vol. 241, no. 1, pp. 180–205, 2011.

[35] S. Chikuma, J. B. Imboden, and J. A. Bluestone, "Negative regulation of T cell receptor-lipid raft interaction by cytotoxic T lymphocyte-associated antigen 4," *The Journal of Experimental Medicine*, vol. 197, no. 1, pp. 129–135, 2003.

[36] M. Martin, H. Schneider, A. Azouz, and C. E. Rudd, "Cytotoxic T lymphocyte antigen 4 and CD28 modulate cell surface raft expression in their regulation of T cell function," *Journal of Experimental Medicine*, vol. 194, no. 11, pp. 1675–1681, 2001.

[37] H. Schneider, X. Smith, H. Liu, G. Bismuth, and C. E. Rudd, "CTLA-4 disrupts ZAP70 microcluster formation with reduced T cell/APC dwell times and calcium mobilization," *European Journal of Immunology*, vol. 38, no. 1, pp. 40–47, 2008.

[38] T. F. Gajewski, F. Fallarino, P. E. Fields, F. Rivas, and M.-L. Alegre, "Absence of CTLA-4 lowers the activation threshold of primed CD8$^+$ TCR-transgenic T cells: lack of correlation with Src homology domain 2-containing protein tyrosine phosphatase," *The Journal of Immunology*, vol. 166, no. 6, pp. 3900–3907, 2001.

[39] M.-L. Alegre, P. J. Noel, B. J. Eisfelder et al., "Regulation of surface and intracellular expression of CTLA4 on mouse T cells," *Journal of Immunology*, vol. 157, no. 11, pp. 4762–4770, 1996.

[40] O. S. Qureshi, Y. Zheng, K. Nakamura et al., "Trans-endocytosis of CD80 and CD86: a molecular basis for the cell-extrinsic function of CTLA-4," *Science*, vol. 332, no. 6029, pp. 600–603, 2011.

[41] D. M. Pardoll, "The blockade of immune checkpoints in cancer immunotherapy," *Nature Reviews Cancer*, vol. 12, no. 4, pp. 252–264, 2012.

[42] P. Waterhouse, J. M. Penninger, E. Timms et al., "Lymphoproliferative disorders with early lethality in mice deficient in Ctla-4," *Science*, vol. 270, no. 5238, pp. 985–988, 1995.

[43] C. A. Chambers, T. J. Sullivan, and J. P. Allison, "Lymphoproliferation in CTLA-4-deficient mice is mediated by costimulation-dependent activation of CD4$^+$ T cells," *Immunity*, vol. 7, no. 6, pp. 885–895, 1997.

[44] B. Salomon and J. A. Bluestone, "Complexities of CD28/B7: CTLA-4 costimulatory pathways in autoimmunity and transplantation," *Annual Review of Immunology*, vol. 19, pp. 225–252, 2001.

[45] L. A. Morford, L. H. Elliott, S. L. Carlson, W. H. Brooks, and T. L. Roszman, "T cell receptor-mediated signaling is defective in T cells obtained from patients with primary intracranial tumors," *Journal of Immunology*, vol. 159, no. 9, pp. 4415–4425, 1997.

[46] T. L. Roszman and W. H. Brooks, "Immunobiology of primary intracranial tumours. III. demonstration of a qualitative lymphocyte abnormality in patients with primary brain tumours," *Clinical & Experimental Immunology*, vol. 39, no. 2, pp. 395–402, 1980.

[47] M. A. Hughes, M. Parisi, S. Grossman, and L. Kleinberg, "Primary brain tumors treated with steroids and radiotherapy: low CD4 counts and risk of infection," *International Journal of Radiation Oncology Biology Physics*, vol. 62, no. 5, pp. 1423–1426, 2005.

[48] F. Ichihara, K. Kono, A. Takahashi, H. Kawaida, H. Sugai, and H. Fujii, "Increased populations of regulatory T cells in peripheral blood and tumor-infiltrating lymphocytes in patients with gastric and esophageal cancers," *Clinical Cancer Research*, vol. 9, no. 12, pp. 4404–4408, 2003.

[49] K. D. Lute, K. F. May Jr., P. Lu et al., "Human CTLA4 knock-in mice unravel the quantitative link between tumor immunity and autoimmunity induced by anti-CTLA-4 antibodies," *Blood*, vol. 106, no. 9, pp. 3127–3133, 2005.

[50] U. K. Liyanage, T. T. Moore, H.-G. Joo et al., "Prevalence of regulatory T cells is increased in peripheral blood and tumor microenvironment of patients with pancreas or breast adenocarcinoma," *The Journal of Immunology*, vol. 169, no. 5, pp. 2756–2761, 2002.

[51] T. Sasada, M. Kimura, Y. Yoshida, M. Kanai, and A. Takabayashi, "CD4$^+$CD25$^+$ regulatory T cells in patients with gastrointestinal malignancies: possible involvement of regulatory T cells in disease progression," *Cancer*, vol. 98, no. 5, pp. 1089–1099, 2003.

[52] E. Y. Woo, C. S. Chu, T. J. Goletz et al., "Regulatory CD4$^+$CD25$^+$ T cells in tumors from patients with early-stage non-small cell lung cancer and late-stage ovarian cancer," *Cancer Research*, vol. 61, no. 12, pp. 4766–4772, 2001.

[53] P. E. Fecci, D. A. Mitchell, J. F. Whitesides et al., "Increased regulatory T-cell fraction amidst a diminished CD4 compartment explains cellular immune defects in patients with malignant glioma," *Cancer Research*, vol. 66, no. 6, pp. 3294–3302, 2006.

[54] O. M. Grauer, S. Nierkens, E. Bennink et al., "CD4+FoxP3+ regulatory T cells gradually accumulate in gliomas during tumor growth and efficiently suppress antiglioma immune responses in vivo," *International Journal of Cancer*, vol. 121, no. 1, pp. 95–105, 2007.

[55] P. Agarwalla, Z. Barnard, P. Fecci, G. Dranoff, and W. T. Curry Jr., "Sequential immunotherapy by vaccination with GM-CSF-expressing glioma cells and CTLA-4 blockade effectively treats established murine intracranial tumors," *Journal of Immunotherapy*, vol. 35, no. 5, pp. 385–389, 2012.

[56] J. S. Weber, R. Dummer, V. de Pril, C. Lebbé, and F. S. Hodi, "Patterns of onset and resolution of immune-related adverse events of special interest with ipilimumab: detailed safety analysis from a phase 3 trial in patients with advanced melanoma," *Cancer*, vol. 119, no. 9, pp. 1675–1682, 2013.

[57] S. Tanaka, D. N. Louis, W. T. Curry, T. T. Batchelor, and J. Dietrich, "Diagnostic and therapeutic avenues for glioblastoma: no longer a dead end?" *Nature Reviews Clinical Oncology*, vol. 10, no. 1, pp. 14–26, 2013.

[58] H. Dong, G. Zhu, K. Tamada, and L. Chen, "B7-H1, a third member of the B7 family, co-stimulates T-cell proliferation and interleukin-10 secretion," *Nature Medicine*, vol. 5, no. 12, pp. 1365–1369, 1999.

[59] Y. Latchman, C. R. Wood, T. Chernova et al., "PD-L2 is a second ligand for PD-1 and inhibits T cell activation," *Nature Immunology*, vol. 2, no. 3, pp. 261–268, 2001.

[60] K. W. Moore, A. O'Garra, R. de Waal Malefyt, P. Vieira, and T. R. Mosmann, "Interleukin-10," *Annual Review of Immunology*, vol. 11, pp. 165–190, 1993.

[61] M. E. Keir, M. J. Butte, G. J. Freeman, and A. H. Sharpe, "PD-1 and its ligands in tolerance and immunity," *Annual Review of Immunology*, vol. 26, pp. 677–704, 2008.

[62] N. Patsoukis, J. Brown, V. Petkova, F. Liu, L. Li, and V. A. Boussiotis, "Selective effects of PD-1 on Akt and ras pathways regulate molecular components of the cell cycle and inhibit T cell proliferation," *Science Signaling*, vol. 5, no. 230, article ra46, 2012.

[63] M. E. Keir, S. C. Liang, I. Guleria et al., "Tissue expression of PD-L1 mediates peripheral T cell tolerance," *Journal of Experimental Medicine*, vol. 203, no. 4, pp. 883–895, 2006.

[64] R. V. Parry, J. M. Chemnitz, K. A. Frauwirth et al., "CTLA-4 and PD-1 receptors inhibit T-cell activation by distinct mechanisms," *Molecular and Cellular Biology*, vol. 25, no. 21, pp. 9543–9553, 2005.

[65] G. J. Freeman, A. J. Long, Y. Iwai et al., "Engagement of the PD-1 immunoinhibitory receptor by a novel B7 family member leads to negative regulation of lymphocyte activation," *The Journal of Experimental Medicine*, vol. 192, no. 7, pp. 1027–1034, 2000.

[66] L. Carter, L. A. Fouser, J. Jussif et al., "PD-1:PD-L inhibitory pathway affects both CD4$^+$ and CD8$^+$ T cells and is overcome by IL-2," *European Journal of Immunology*, vol. 32, no. 3, pp. 634–643, 2002.

[67] S. Wintterle, B. Schreiner, M. Mitsdoerffer et al., "Expression of the B7-related molecule B7-H1 by glioma cells: a potential mechanism of immune paralysis," *Cancer Research*, vol. 63, no. 21, pp. 7462–7467, 2003.

[68] A. T. Parsa, J. S. Waldron, A. Panner et al., "Loss of tumor suppressor PTEN function increases B7-H1 expression and immunoresistance in glioma," *Nature Medicine*, vol. 13, no. 1, pp. 84–88, 2007.

[69] T. Avril, S. Saikali, E. Vauleon et al., "Distinct effects of human glioblastoma immunoregulatory molecules programmed cell death ligand-1 (PDL-1) and indoleamine 2,3-dioxygenase (IDO) on tumour-specific T cell functions," *Journal of Neuroimmunology*, vol. 225, no. 1-2, pp. 22–33, 2010.

[70] J. F. M. Jacobs, A. J. Idema, K. F. Bol et al., "Regulatory T cells and the PD-L1/PD-1 pathway mediate immune suppression in malignant human brain tumors," *Neuro-Oncology*, vol. 11, no. 4, pp. 394–402, 2009.

[71] R. Wilmotte, K. Burkhardt, V. Kindler et al., "B7-homolog 1 expression by human glioma: a new mechanism of immune evasion," *Neuroreport*, vol. 16, no. 10, pp. 1081–1085, 2005.

[72] N. Li, C. J. Workman, S. M. Martin, and D. A. A. Vignali, "Biochemical analysis of the regulatory T cell protein lymphocyte activation gene-3 (LAG-3; CD223)," *The Journal of Immunology*, vol. 173, no. 11, pp. 6806–6812, 2004.

[73] C. J. Workman and D. A. A. Vignali, "The CD4-related molecule, LAG-3 (CD223), regulates the expansion of activated T cells," *European Journal of Immunology*, vol. 33, no. 4, pp. 970–979, 2003.

[74] S. Hannier, M. Tournier, G. Bismuth, and F. Triebel, "CD3/TCR complex-associated lymphocyte activation gene-3 molecules

inhibit CD3/TCR signaling," *The Journal of Immunology*, vol. 161, no. 8, pp. 4058–4065, 1998.

[75] F. Triebel, "LAG-3: a regulator of T-cell and DC responses and its use in therapeutic vaccination," *Trends in Immunology*, vol. 24, no. 12, pp. 619–622, 2003.

[76] S. Andreae, F. Piras, N. Burdin, and F. Triebel, "Maturation and activation of dendritic cells induced by lymphocyte activation gene-3 (CD223)," *The Journal of Immunology*, vol. 168, no. 8, pp. 3874–3880, 2002.

[77] F. Annunziato, R. Manetti, L. Tomasévic et al., "Expression and release of LAG-3-encoded protein by human CD4$^+$ T cells are associated with IFN-γ production," *The FASEB Journal*, vol. 10, no. 7, pp. 769–776, 1996.

[78] C.-T. Huang, C. J. Workman, D. Flies et al., "Role of LAG-3 in regulatory T cells," *Immunity*, vol. 21, no. 4, pp. 503–513, 2004.

[79] M. V. Goldberg and C. G. Drake, "LAG-3 in cancer immuno-therapy," *Current Topics in Microbiology and Immunology*, vol. 344, pp. 269–278, 2011.

[80] J. F. Grosso, C. C. Kelleher, T. J. Harris et al., "LAG-3 regulates CD8$^+$ T cell accumulation and effector function in murine self- and tumor-tolerance systems," *The Journal of Clinical Investigation*, vol. 117, no. 11, pp. 3383–3392, 2007.

[81] S.-R. Woo, M. E. Turnis, M. V. Goldberg et al., "Immune inhibitory molecules LAG-3 and PD-1 synergistically regulate T-cell function to promote tumoral immune escape," *Cancer Research*, vol. 72, no. 4, pp. 917–927, 2012.

[82] K. Sakuishi, P. Jayaraman, S. M. Behar, A. C. Anderson, and V. K. Kuchroo, "Emerging Tim-3 functions in antimicrobial and tumor immunity," *Trends in Immunology*, vol. 32, no. 8, pp. 345–349, 2011.

[83] C. Zhu, A. C. Anderson, and V. K. Kuchroo, "TIM-3 and its regulatory role in immune responses," *Current Topics in Microbiology and Immunology*, vol. 350, pp. 1–15, 2011.

[84] J. Wada and Y. S. Kanwar, "Identification and characterization of galectin-9, a novel β-galactoside-binding mammalian lectin," *The Journal of Biological Chemistry*, vol. 272, no. 9, pp. 6078–6086, 1997.

[85] C. Zhu, A. C. Anderson, A. Schubart et al., "The tim-3 ligand galectin-9 negatively regulates T helper type 1 immunity," *Nature Immunology*, vol. 6, no. 12, pp. 1245–1252, 2005.

[86] Q. Zhou, M. E. Munger, R. G. Veenstra et al., "Coexpression of Tim-3 and PD-1 identifies a CD8$^+$ T-cell exhaustion phenotype in mice with disseminated acute myelogenous leukemia," *Blood*, vol. 117, no. 17, pp. 4501–4510, 2011.

[87] L. Golden-Mason, B. E. Palmer, N. Kassam et al., "Negative immune regulator Tim-3 is overexpressed on T cells in hepatitis C virus infection and its blockade rescues dysfunctional CD4$^+$ and CD8$^+$ T cells," *Journal of Virology*, vol. 83, no. 18, pp. 9122–9130, 2009.

[88] R. H. McMahan, L. Golden-Mason, M. I. Nishimura et al., "Tim-3 expression on PD-1+ HCV-specific human CTLs is associated with viral persistence, and its blockade restores hepatocyte-directed in vitro cytotoxicity," *The Journal of Clinical Investigation*, vol. 120, no. 12, pp. 4546–4557, 2010.

[89] H.-T. Jin, A. C. Anderson, W. G. Tan et al., "Cooperation of Tim-3 and PD-1 in CD8 T-cell exhaustion during chronic viral infection," *Proceedings of the National Academy of Sciences of the United States of America*, vol. 107, no. 33, pp. 14733–14738, 2010.

[90] J. Fourcade, Z. Sun, M. Benallaoua et al., "Upregulation of Tim-3 and PD-1 expression is associated with tumor antigen-specific CD8$^+$ T cell dysfunction in melanoma patients," *Journal of Experimental Medicine*, vol. 207, no. 10, pp. 2175–2186, 2010.

[91] K. Sakuishi, L. Apetoh, J. M. Sullivan, B. R. Blazar, V. K. Kuchroo, and A. C. Anderson, "Targeting tim-3 and PD-1 pathways to reverse T cell exhaustion and restore anti-tumor immunity," *Journal of Experimental Medicine*, vol. 207, no. 10, pp. 2187–2194, 2010.

[92] V. Dardalhon, A. C. Anderson, J. Karman et al., "Tim-3/galectin-9 pathway: regulation of Th1 immunity through promotion of CD11b$^+$Ly-6G$^+$ myeloid cells," *The Journal of Immunology*, vol. 185, no. 3, pp. 1383–1392, 2010.

[93] D. E. Speiser, M. J. Pittet, D. Valmori et al., "In vivo expression of natural killer cell inhibitory receptors by human melanoma-specific cytolytic T lymphocytes," *The Journal of Experimental Medicine*, vol. 190, no. 6, pp. 775–782, 1999.

[94] E. O. Long, D. N. Burshtyn, W. P. Clark et al., "Killer cell inhibitory receptors: diversity, specificity, and function," *Immunological Reviews*, vol. 155, pp. 135–144, 1997.

[95] D. N. Burshtyn, A. M. Scharenberg, N. Wagtmann et al., "Recruitment of tyrosine phosphatase HCP by the killer cell inhibitory receptor," *Immunity*, vol. 4, no. 1, pp. 77–85, 1996.

[96] S. Lazetic, C. Chang, J. P. Houchins, L. L. Lanier, and J. H. Phillips, "Human natural killer cell receptors involved in MHC class I recognition are disulfide-linked heterodimers of CD94 and NKG2 subunits," *Journal of Immunology*, vol. 157, no. 11, pp. 4741–4745, 1996.

[97] R. Biassoni, C. Cantoni, M. Falco et al., "The human leukocyte antigen (HLA)-C-specific 'activatory' or 'inhibitory' natural killer cell receptors display highly homologous extracellular domains but differ in their transmembrane and intracytoplas-mic portions," *Journal of Experimental Medicine*, vol. 183, no. 2, pp. 645–650, 1996.

[98] N. Wagtmann, R. Biassoni, C. Cantoni et al., "Molecular clones of the p58 NK cell receptor reveal immunoglobulin-related molecules with diversity in both the extra- and intracellular domains," *Immunity*, vol. 2, no. 5, pp. 439–449, 1995.

[99] K. C. Hsu, S. Chida, D. E. Geraghty, and B. Dupont, "The killer cell immunoglobulin-like receptor (KIR) genomic region: gene-order, haplotypes and allelic polymorphism," *Immunological Reviews*, vol. 190, pp. 40–52, 2002.

[100] H. J. Pegram, D. M. Andrews, M. J. Smyth, P. K. Darcy, and M. H. Kershaw, "Activating and inhibitory receptors of natural killer cells," *Immunology and Cell Biology*, vol. 89, no. 2, pp. 216–224, 2011.

[101] S. Kim, J. B. Sunwoo, L. Yang et al., "HLA alleles determine differences in human natural killer cell responsiveness and potency," *Proceedings of the National Academy of Sciences of the United States of America*, vol. 105, no. 8, pp. 3053–3058, 2008.

[102] J. Yu, J. M. Venstrom, X.-R. Liu et al., "Breaking tolerance to self, circulating natural killer cells expressing inhibitory KIR for non-self HLA exhibit effector function after T cell-depleted allogeneic hematopoietic cell transplantation," *Blood*, vol. 113, no. 16, pp. 3875–3884, 2009.

[103] H.-G. Ljunggren and K.-J. Malmberg, "Prospects for the use of NK cells in immunotherapy of human cancer," *Nature Reviews Immunology*, vol. 7, no. 5, pp. 329–339, 2007.

[104] L. Moretta and A. Moretta, "Unravelling natural killer cell function: triggering and inhibitory human NK receptors," *The EMBO Journal*, vol. 23, no. 2, pp. 255–259, 2004.

[105] L. Ruggeri, A. Mancusi, E. Burchielli et al., "NK cell alloreac-tivity and allogeneic hematopoietic stem cell transplantation," *Blood Cells, Molecules, and Diseases*, vol. 40, no. 1, pp. 84–90, 2008.

[106] J. S. Miller, Y. Soignier, A. Panoskaltsis-Mortari et al., "Successful adoptive transfer and in vivo expansion of human haploidentical NK cells in patients with cancer," *Blood*, vol. 105, no. 8, pp. 3051–3057, 2005.

[107] H.-G. Ljunggren and K. Kärre, "In search of the 'missing self': MHC molecules and NK cell recognition," *Immunology Today*, vol. 11, no. 7, pp. 237–244, 1990.

[108] H.-G. Ljunggren and K. Karre, "Host resistance directed selectively against H-2-deficient lymphoma variants. Analysis of the mechanism," *The Journal of Experimental Medicine*, vol. 162, no. 6, pp. 1745–1759, 1985.

[109] K. Karre, H. G. Ljunggren, G. Piontek, and R. Kiessling, "Selective rejection of H-2-deficient lymphoma variants suggests alternative immune defence strategy," *Nature*, vol. 319, no. 6055, pp. 675–678, 1986.

[110] S. Giebel, F. Locatelli, T. Lamparelli et al., "Survival advantage with KIR ligand incompatibility in hematopoietic stem cell transplantation from unrelated donors," *Blood*, vol. 102, no. 3, pp. 814–819, 2003.

[111] D. W. Beelen, H. D. Ottinger, S. Ferencik et al., "Genotypic inhibitory killer immunoglobulin-like receptor ligand incompatibility enhances the long-term antileukemic effect of unmodified allogeneic hematopoietic stem cell transplantation in patients with myeloid leukemias," *Blood*, vol. 105, no. 6, pp. 2594–2600, 2005.

[112] J. S. Miller, S. Cooley, P. Parham et al., "Missing KIR ligands are associated with less relapse and increased graft-versus-host disease (GVHD) following unrelated donor allogeneic HCT," *Blood*, vol. 109, no. 11, pp. 5058–5061, 2007.

[113] Y. K. Tam, J. A. Martinson, K. Doligosa, and H.-G. Klingemann, "Ex vivo expansion of the highly cytotoxic human natural killer cell line NK-92 under current good manufacturing practice conditions for clinical adoptive cellular immunotherapy," *Cytotherapy*, vol. 5, no. 3, pp. 259–272, 2003.

[114] H.-G. Klingemann, "Natural killer cell-based immunotherapeutic strategies," *Cytotherapy*, vol. 7, no. 1, pp. 16–22, 2005.

[115] H. E. Kohrt, A. Thielens, A. Marabelle et al., "Anti-KIR antibody enhancement of anti-lymphoma activity of natural killer cells as monotherapy and in combination with anti-CD20 antibodies," *Blood*, vol. 123, no. 5, pp. 678–686, 2014.

[116] F. Romagné, P. André, P. Spee et al., "Preclinical characterization of 1-7F9, a novel human anti-KIR receptor therapeutic antibody that augments natural killer-mediated killing of tumor cells," *Blood*, vol. 114, no. 13, pp. 2667–2677, 2009.

[117] C. Y. Koh, B. R. Blazar, T. George et al., "Augmentation of antitumor effects by NK cell inhibitory receptor blockade in vitro and in vivo," *Blood*, vol. 97, no. 10, pp. 3132–3137, 2001.

[118] R. G. Goodwin, W. S. Din, T. Davis-Smith et al., "Molecular cloning of a ligand for the inducible T cell gene 4-1BB: a member of an emerging family of cytokines with homology to tumor necrosis factor," *European Journal of Immunology*, vol. 23, no. 10, pp. 2631–2641, 1993.

[119] I. Melero, W. W. Shuford, S. A. Newby et al., "Monoclonal antibodies against the 4-1BB T-cell activation molecule eradicate established tumors," *Nature Medicine*, vol. 3, no. 6, pp. 682–685, 1997.

[120] A. T. C. Cheuk, G. J. Mufti, and B.-A. Guinn, "Role of 4-1BB:4-1BB ligand in cancer immunotherapy," *Cancer Gene Therapy*, vol. 11, no. 3, pp. 215–226, 2004.

[121] T. H. Watts, "TNF/TNFR family members in costimulation of T cell responses," *Annual Review of Immunology*, vol. 23, pp. 23–68, 2005.

[122] D. S. Vinay, K. Cha, and B. S. Kwon, "Dual immunoregulatory pathways of 4-1BB signaling," *Journal of Molecular Medicine*, vol. 84, no. 9, pp. 726–736, 2006.

[123] J. L. Cannons, Y. Choi, and T. H. Watts, "Role of TNF receptor-associated factor 2 and p38 mitogen-activated protein kinase activation during 4-1BB-dependent immune response," *Journal of Immunology*, vol. 165, no. 11, pp. 6193–6204, 2000.

[124] H.-W. Lee, S.-J. Park, B. K. Choi, H. H. Kim, K.-O. Nam, and B. S. Kwon, "4-1BB promotes the survival of CD8$^+$ T lymphocytes by increasing expression of Bcl-^{x}L and Bfl-1," *The Journal of Immunology*, vol. 169, no. 9, pp. 4882–4888, 2002.

[125] L. Myers, C. Takahashi, R. S. Mittler, R. J. Rossi, and A. T. Vella, "Effector CD8 T cells possess suppressor function after 4-1BB and Toll-like receptor triggering," *Proceedings of the National Academy of Sciences of the United States of America*, vol. 100, no. 9, pp. 5348–5353, 2003.

[126] O. Martinet, C. M. Divino, Y. Zang et al., "T cell activation with systemic agonistic antibody versus local 4-1BB ligand gene delivery combined with interleukin-12 eradicate liver metastases of breast cancer," *Gene Therapy*, vol. 9, no. 12, pp. 786–792, 2002.

[127] S.-H. Chen, K. B. Pham-Nguyen, O. Martinet et al., "Rejection of disseminated metastases of colon carcinoma by synergism of IL-12 gene therapy and 4-1BB costimulation," *Molecular Therapy*, vol. 2, no. 1, pp. 39–46, 2000.

[128] J. A. Kim, B. J. Averbook, K. Chambers et al., "Divergent effects of 4-1BB antibodies on antitumor immunity and on tumor-reactive T-cell generation," *Cancer Research*, vol. 61, no. 5, pp. 2031–2037, 2001.

[129] S. E. Strome, B. Martin, D. Flies et al., "Enhanced therapeutic potential of adoptive immunotherapy by in vitro CD28/4-1BB costimulation of tumor-reactive T cells against a poorly immunogenic, major histocompatibility complex class I-negative A9P melanoma," *Journal of Immunotherapy*, vol. 23, no. 4, pp. 430–437, 2000.

[130] Q. Li, A. Carr, F. Ito, S. Teitz-Tennenbaum, and A. E. Chang, "Polarization effects of 4-1BB during CD28 costimulation in generating tumor-reactive T cells for cancer immunotherapy," *Cancer Research*, vol. 63, no. 10, pp. 2546–2552, 2003.

[131] I. Melero, N. Bach, K. E. Hellström, A. Aruffo, R. S. Mittler, and L. Chen, "Amplification of tumor immunity by gene transfer of the co-stimulatory 4-1BB ligand: synergy with the CD28 co-stimulatory pathway," *European Journal of Immunology*, vol. 28, no. 3, pp. 1116–1121, 1998.

[132] B.-A. Guinn, M. A. DeBenedette, T. H. Watts, and N. L. Berinstein, "4-IBBL cooperates with B7-1 and B7-2 in converting a B cell lymphoma cell line into a long-lasting antitumor vaccine," *The Journal of Immunology*, vol. 162, no. 8, pp. 5003–5010, 1999.

[133] S. Mogi, J. Sakurai, T. Kohsaka et al., "Tumour rejection by gene transfer of 4-1BB ligand into a CD80$^+$ murine squamous cell carcinoma and the requirements of co-stimulatory molecules on tumour and host cells," *Immunology*, vol. 101, no. 4, pp. 541–547, 2000.

[134] J. Xiang, "Expression of Co-stimulatory 4-1BB ligand induces significant tumor regression and protective immunity," *Cancer Biotherapy and Radiopharmaceuticals*, vol. 14, no. 5, pp. 353–361, 1999.

[135] A. L. Gurney, S. A. Marsters, A. Huang et al., "Identification of a new member of the tumor necrosis factor family and its receptor, a human ortholog of mouse GITR," *Current Biology*, vol. 9, no. 4, pp. 215–218, 1999.

[136] B. Kwon, K.-Y. Yu, J. Ni et al., "Identification of a novel activation-inducible protein of the tumor necrosis factor receptor superfamily and its ligand," *The Journal of Biological Chemistry*, vol. 274, no. 10, pp. 6056–6061, 1999.

[137] R. S. McHugh, M. J. Whitters, C. A. Piccirillo et al., "CD4$^+$CD25$^+$ immunoregulatory T cells: gene expression analysis reveals a functional role for the glucocorticoid-induced TNF receptor," *Immunity*, vol. 16, no. 2, pp. 311–323, 2002.

[138] J. Shimizu, S. Yamazaki, T. Takahashi, Y. Ishida, and S. Sakaguchi, "Stimulation of CD25$^+$CD4$^+$ regulatory T cells through GITR breaks immunological self-tolerance," *Nature Immunology*, vol. 3, no. 2, pp. 135–142, 2002.

[139] S. Ronchetti, O. Zollo, S. Bruscoli et al., "Frontline: GITR, a member of the TNF receptor superfamily, is costimulatory to mouse T lymphocyte subpopulations," *European Journal of Immunology*, vol. 34, no. 3, pp. 613–622, 2004.

[140] A. P. Kohm, J. S. Williams, and S. D. Miller, "Ligation of the glucocorticoid-induced TNF receptor enhances autoreactive CD4$^+$ T cell activation and experimental autoimmune encephalomyelitis," *The Journal of Immunology*, vol. 172, no. 8, pp. 4686–4690, 2004.

[141] F. Kanamaru, P. Youngnak, M. Hashiguchi et al., "Costimulation via glucocorticoid-induced TNF receptor in both conventional and CD25$^+$ regulatory CD4$^+$ T cells," *Journal of Immunology*, vol. 172, no. 12, pp. 7306–7314, 2004.

[142] G. Nocentini and C. Riccardi, "GITR: a multifaceted regulator of immunity belonging to the tumor necrosis factor receptor superfamily," *European Journal of Immunology*, vol. 35, no. 4, pp. 1016–1022, 2005.

[143] B. J. Kim, Z. Li, R. N. Fariss et al., "Constitutive and cytokine-induced GITR ligand expression on human retinal pigment epithelium and photoreceptors," *Investigative Ophthalmology and Visual Science*, vol. 45, no. 9, pp. 3170–3176, 2004.

[144] E. M. Shevach and G. L. Stephens, "The GITR-GITRL interaction: co-stimulation or contrasuppression of regulatory activity?" *Nature Reviews Immunology*, vol. 6, no. 8, pp. 613–618, 2006.

[145] D. A. Schaer, "GITR pathway activation abrogates tumor immune suppression through loss of regulatory T cell lineage stability," *Cancer Immunology Research*, vol. 1, no. 5, pp. 320–331, 2013.

[146] R.-R. Ji, S. D. Chasalow, L. Wang et al., "An immune-active tumor microenvironment favors clinical response to ipilimumab," *Cancer Immunology, Immunotherapy*, vol. 61, no. 7, pp. 1019–1031, 2012.

[147] S. Cuzzocrea, E. Ayroldi, R. Di Paola et al., "Role of glucocorticoid-induced TNF receptor family gene (GITR) in collagen-induced arthritis," *The FASEB Journal*, vol. 19, no. 10, pp. 1253–1265, 2005.

[148] M. Patel, D. Xu, P. Kewin et al., "Glucocorticoid-induced TNFR family-related protein (GITR) activation exacerbates murine asthma and collagen-induced arthritis," *European Journal of Immunology*, vol. 35, no. 12, pp. 3581–3590, 2005.

[149] M. Takata, T. Nakagomi, S. Kashiwamura et al., "Glucocorticoid-induced TNF receptor-triggered T cells are key modulators for survival/death of neural stem/progenitor cells induced by ischemic stroke," *Cell Death and Differentiation*, vol. 19, no. 5, pp. 756–767, 2012.

[150] A. D. Cohen, D. A. Schaer, C. Liu et al., "Agonist anti-GITR monoclonal antibody induces melanoma tumor immunity in mice by altering regulatory T cell stability and intra-tumor accumulation," *PLoS ONE*, vol. 5, no. 5, Article ID e10436, 2010.

[151] G. L. Stephens, R. S. McHugh, M. J. Whitters et al., "Engagement of glucocorticoid-induced TNFR family-related receptor on effector T cells by its ligand mediates resistance to suppression by CD4$^+$CD25$^+$ T cells," *The Journal of Immunology*, vol. 173, no. 8, pp. 5008–5020, 2004.

[152] M. J. Turk, J. A. Guevara-Patiño, G. A. Rizzuto, M. E. Engelhorn, and A. N. Houghton, "Concomitant tumor immunity to a poorly immunogenic melanoma is prevented by regulatory T cells," *The Journal of Experimental Medicine*, vol. 200, no. 6, pp. 771–782, 2004.

[153] D. A. Schaer, J. T. Murphy, and J. D. Wolchok, "Modulation of GITR for cancer immunotherapy," *Current Opinion in Immunology*, vol. 24, no. 2, pp. 217–224, 2012.

[154] D.-M. Kuang, Q. Zhao, C. Peng et al., "Activated monocytes in peritumoral stroma of hepatocellular carcinoma foster immune privilege and disease progression through PD-L1," *The Journal of Experimental Medicine*, vol. 206, no. 6, pp. 1327–1337, 2009.

[155] J. Krempski, L. Karyampudi, M. D. Behrens et al., "Tumor-infiltrating programmed death receptor-1$^+$ dendritic cells mediate immune suppression in ovarian cancer," *The Journal of Immunology*, vol. 186, no. 12, pp. 6905–6913, 2011.

[156] M. J. Gough and M. R. Crittenden, "Combination approaches to immunotherapy: the radiotherapy example," *Immunotherapy*, vol. 1, no. 6, pp. 1025–1037, 2009.

[157] E. M. Rosen, S. Fan, S. Rockwell, and I. D. Goldberg, "The molecular and cellular basis of radiosensitivity: implications for understanding how normal tissues and tumors respond to therapeutic radiation," *Cancer Investigation*, vol. 17, no. 1, pp. 56–72, 1999.

[158] S. A. Grossman, X. Ye, G. Lesser et al., "Immunosuppression in patients with high-grade gliomas treated with radiation and temozolomide," *Clinical Cancer Research*, vol. 17, no. 16, pp. 5473–5480, 2011.

[159] W. H. McBride, C.-S. Chiang, J. L. Olson et al., "A sense of danger from radiation," *Radiation Research*, vol. 162, no. 1, pp. 1–19, 2004.

[160] S. Demaria and S. C. Formenti, "Sensors of ionizing radiation effects on the immunological microenvironment of cancer," *International Journal of Radiation Biology*, vol. 83, no. 11-12, pp. 819–825, 2007.

[161] M. L. Albert, B. Sauter, and N. Bhardwaj, "Dendritic cells acquire antigen from apoptotic cells and induce class I-restricted CTLS," *Nature*, vol. 392, no. 6671, pp. 86–89, 1998.

[162] E. J. Friedman, "Immune modulation by ionizing radiation and its implications for cancer immunotherapy," *Current Pharmaceutical Design*, vol. 8, no. 19, pp. 1765–1780, 2002.

[163] B. Sauter, M. L. Albert, L. Francisco, M. Larsson, S. Somersan, and N. Bhardwaj, "Consequences of cell death: exposure to necrotic tumor cells, but not primary tissue cells or apoptotic cells, induces the maturation of immunostimulatory dendritic cells," *Journal of Experimental Medicine*, vol. 191, no. 3, pp. 423–433, 2000.

[164] D. Zagzag, K. Salnikow, L. Chiriboga et al., "Downregulation of major histocompatibility complex antigens in invading glioma cells: stealth invasion of the brain," *Laboratory Investigation*, vol. 85, no. 3, pp. 328–341, 2005.

[165] H. Wiendl, M. Mitsdoerffer, V. Hofmeister et al., "A functional role of HLA-G expression in human gliomas: an alternative strategy of immune escape," *The Journal of Immunology*, vol. 168, no. 9, pp. 4772–4780, 2002.

[166] E. W. Newcomb, S. Demaria, Y. Lukyanov et al., "The combination of ionizing radiation and peripheral vaccination produces

long-term survival of mice bearing established invasive GL261 gliomas," *Clinical Cancer Research*, vol. 12, no. 15, pp. 4730–4737, 2006.

[167] S. Demaria, N. Kawashima, A. M. Yang et al., "Immune-mediated inhibition of metastases after treatment with local radiation and CTLA-4 blockade in a mouse model of breast cancer," *Clinical Cancer Research*, vol. 11, no. 2, part 1, pp. 728–734, 2005.

[168] M. Z. Dewan, A. E. Galloway, N. Kawashima et al., "Fractionated but not single-dose radiotherapy induces an immune-mediated abscopal effect when combined with anti-CTLA-4 antibody," *Clinical Cancer Research*, vol. 15, no. 17, pp. 5379–5388, 2009.

[169] A. W. Silk, M. F. Bassetti, B. T. West, C. I. Tsien, and C. D. Lao, "Ipilimumab and radiation therapy for melanoma brain metastases," *Cancer Medicine*, vol. 2, no. 6, pp. 899–906, 2013.

[170] A. S. Darefsky, J. T. King Jr., and R. Dubrow, "Adult glioblastoma multiforme survival in the temozolomide era: a population-based analysis of surveillance, epidemiology, and end results registries," *Cancer*, vol. 118, no. 8, pp. 2163–2172, 2012.

[171] R. Stupp, M. E. Hegi, T. Gorlia et al., "Cilengitide combined with standard treatment for patients with newly diagnosed glioblastoma with methylated MGMT promoter (CENTRIC EORTC 26071-22072 study): a multicentre, randomised, open-label, phase 3 trial," *The Lancet Oncology*, vol. 15, no. 10, pp. 1100–1108, 2014.

[172] C. L. Mackall, T. A. Fleisher, M. R. Brown et al., "Lymphocyte depletion during treatment with intensive chemotherapy for cancer," *Blood*, vol. 84, no. 7, pp. 2221–2228, 1994.

[173] Y. B. Su, S. Sohn, S. E. Krown et al., "Selective CD4$^+$ lymphopenia in melanoma patients treated with temozolomide: a toxicity with therapeutic implications," *Journal of Clinical Oncology*, vol. 22, no. 4, pp. 610–616, 2004.

[174] J. L. Frazier, J. E. Han, M. Lim, and A. Olivi, "Immunotherapy combined with chemotherapy in the treatment of tumors," *Neurosurgery Clinics of North America*, vol. 21, no. 1, pp. 187–194, 2010.

[175] S. Brem, B. Tyler, K. Li et al., "Local delivery of temozolomide by biodegradable polymers is superior to oral administration in a rodent glioma model," *Cancer Chemotherapy and Pharmacology*, vol. 60, no. 5, pp. 643–650, 2007.

[176] S. Fritzell, E. Sandén, S. Eberstål, E. Visse, A. Darabi, and P. Siesjö, "Intratumoral temozolomide synergizes with immunotherapy in a T cell-dependent fashion," *Cancer Immunology, Immunotherapy*, vol. 62, no. 9, pp. 1463–1474, 2013.

[177] C. Banissi, F. Ghiringhelli, L. Chen, and A. F. Carpentier, "Treg depletion with a low-dose metronomic temozolomide regimen in a rat glioma model," *Cancer Immunology, Immunotherapy*, vol. 58, no. 10, pp. 1627–1634, 2009.

6

Dendritic Cells and *Leishmania* Infection: Adding Layers of Complexity to a Complex Disease

Daniel Feijó,[1] Rafael Tibúrcio,[1,2] Mariana Ampuero,[1,2] Cláudia Brodskyn,[1,2,3] and Natalia Tavares[1]

[1]*Centro de Pesquisas Gonçalo Moniz (CPqGM), 40296-710 Salvador, BA, Brazil*
[2]*Universidade Federal da Bahia (UFBA), 40170-115 Salvador, BA, Brazil*
[3]*Instituto de Investigação em Imunologia (iii), 01246-903 São Paulo, SP, Brazil*

Correspondence should be addressed to Daniel Feijó; danielffeijo@gmail.com and Natalia Tavares; natalia.tavares@bahia.fiocruz.br

Academic Editor: Alice O. Kamphorst

Leishmaniasis is a group of neglected diseases whose clinical manifestations depend on factors from the host and the pathogen. It is an important public health problem worldwide caused by the protozoan parasite from the *Leishmania* genus. Cutaneous Leishmaniasis (CL) is the most frequent form of this disease transmitted by the bite of an infected sandfly into the host skin. The parasites can be uptook and/or recognized by macrophages, neutrophils, and/or dendritic cells (DCs). Initially, DCs were described to play a protective role in activating the immune response against *Leishmania* parasites. However, several reports showed a dichotomic role of DCs in modulating the host immune response to susceptibility or resistance in CL. In this review, we discuss (1) the interactions between DCs and parasites from different species of *Leishmania* and (2) the crosstalk of DCs and other cells during CL infection. The complexity of these interactions profoundly affects the adaptive immune response and, consequently, the disease outcome, especially from *Leishmania* species of the New World.

1. Introduction

Leishmaniasis are a complex of vector-borne diseases caused by an intracellular protozoan parasite from *Leishmania* sp. (Kinetoplastida, Trypanosomatidae). Its clinical spectra depends largely on parasite species and host immune response. Although the disease has been known and studied for a long time, it is still considered as a neglected and public health problem worldwide. Such diseases affect approximately 12 million people in 88 countries, where 350 million inhabitants are exposed, mainly in remote rural areas and underserved urban areas [1]. The clinical forms range from asymptomatic infection to two main clinical syndromes: visceral leishmaniasis (VL) and cutaneous leishmaniasis (CL).

VL is a chronic infection, fatal if not treated. It is characterized by progressive fever, weight loss, splenomegaly, hepatomegaly, anemia, and spontaneous bleeding associated with marked inflammatory imbalance [2]. The hallmark of this disease is thought to be a lack of cellular immune response against the parasite and high systemic levels of IFN-g and IL-10 [3].

CL is the most frequent form of this disease. It is characterized by chronic evolution, which affects the skin and cartilaginous structures [4]. The main clinical forms of diseases associated with CL are the Localized Cutaneous Leishmaniasis (LCL), Mucocutaneous Leishmaniasis (ML), disseminated and diffuse Leishmaniasis [1].

LCL is mainly caused by the species *Leishmania tropica*, *L. aethiopica*, and *L. major* in the Old World. However, New World LCL is mainly caused by multiple species of both *Leishmania* subgenera *Leishmania* (*L. amazonensis*, *L. infantum*, *L. mexicana*, and *L. venezuelensis*) and *Viannia* subgenera (*L. braziliensis*, *L. guyanensis*, *L. panamensis*, and *L. peruviana*). The incubation period lasts on average from 2 weeks to 3 months with the appearance of papules or nodules and, sometimes, is preceded or accompanied by the swelling of underlying nodes. The hallmark of this illness is the development of single or multiple ulcerated dermal lesions. Over time, the lesion may evolve spontaneously to healing or develop into different frames of gravity in ulceration of the lesion with its expansion [4].

Some patients (a fraction of 3%) may develop the ML, caused by the infection with *L. braziliensis* and *L. guyanensis*. The symptoms are associated with the destruction of the nasal cavity and oropharyngeal tissues [4]. Genetic diversity of *Leishmania* species contributes to the difficulty of controlling the disease and to the increase in the number of cases that are resistant to conventional treatment [5]. Although both forms of CL are rarely fatal, they can cause nasty scars on the skin and severe problems in the oropharyngeal device [4].

Dendritic cells (DCs) are a family of professional antigen-presenting cells (APCs) that resides in all peripheral tissues in an immature state, capable of antigen uptake and processing. As such, they function as sentinel of the immune system. After contact with microorganisms or substances associated with infection or inflammation, DCs undergo a process of maturation and migrate to the T cell areas of lymphoid organs. There, they present antigens to naïve T cells and modulate their responses [6]. The maturation process consists of (1) increased expression of major histocompatibility complex (MHC) and costimulatory molecules, such as CD40, CD80, CD86, and CD54; (2) downregulation of antigen capture and phagocytic capacity; (3) enhanced cytokine secretion; (4) different patterns of chemokine receptor expression and chemokine production, enabling DC migration and recruitment of other cell types [7, 8].

DCs are able to take up antigens via different groups of receptor families, such as Fc receptors, C-type lectin receptors (CLRs), and pattern recognition receptors (PRRs), such as Toll-like receptors (TLRs) [9]. The engagement between ligand and its receptor enables DCs to recognize a wide range of microbial stimuli [10].

DCs are a heterogeneous population of cells that can be divided into 2 main categories: the plasmacytoid DCs (pDCs), experts in type I interferon synthesis, and the conventional DCs (cDCs), specialized in antigen capture, processing, and presentation for T cell priming. pDCs constitutively express MHC class II molecules and lineage markers, such as CD45RA/B220[+], Ly6C/GR-1[+], and siglec-H [11–13]. Two cDCs subsets can be distinguished based on functional specialization. cDC1s are particularly efficient in CD8[+] T cell activation and cross-presentation. cDC2s are most efficient for CD4[+] T helper polarization, especially Th2 or Th17 [14]. In mice, cDC1s express high levels of CD8α or CD103 [15, 16] and cDC2s express CD11b and CD172a (also known as SIRPα) [17]. In humans, DCs can be subdivided into two main populations: CD141[+] DCs (also referred to as BDCA3[+]) and CD1c[+] DCs (also known as BDCA1[+]). Based on gene expression profiles and functions similarities, human CD141[+] DCs and CD1c[+] DCs resemble those of mouse cDC1s and cDC2s, respectively [18–21]. Also, monocytes can adopt a DC morphology and antigen-presenting functions in inflammatory sites, leading to their designation as monocytes-derived DCs (MoDCs) [22, 23]. In mice, MoDCs derived from Ly6C[hi] monocytes can express CD11c and MHC class II, and, similarly to macrophages, F4/80 and CD64 [23, 24].

In humans, MoDCs derived from CD14[+] monocytes and can express CD1a [24]. Langerhans cells (LCs) present DC morphology and antigen-presenting functions in the skin [25, 26]. They constitutively express major histocompatibility complex (MHC) class II and high levels of the lectin Langerin [27]. The most current phenotypes described for each type of DC are summarized in Table 1.

Several reports show a central role for DCs in orchestrating immune responses in leishmaniasis [28–30]. In this review, we discuss the heterogeneity of the interaction between DCs and different species of *Leishmania* that causes CL.

2. Interaction of DC with Different *Leishmania* Species

Infection with *Leishmania* parasites leads to lifelong immunity against the same subspecies, after the infection is healed. Experimental models of CL infections are largely used to study the mechanism under this lifelong immunity. Most of these studies have been carried out by inoculation of *L. major*, a species present in the Old World. However, experimental studies with the New World *Leishmania* sp., such as *L. amazonensis* and *L. braziliensis*, are scarce. This reinforces the importance of studies about the immune response induced by specific species of *Leishmania*.

2.1. Interaction of DC Subtypes with Leishmania major. Current paradigms of the involvement of T helper subsets in infectious diseases are based, in large part, on the results of studies about resistance and susceptibility to *L. major* in inbred mice. In murine LCL, BALB/c mice respond to infection with production of Th2-type cytokines, in particular IL-4 and IL-10. These cytokines are associated with disease progression and susceptibility to *L. major*. In contrast, recovery from infection of resistant mice (e.g., C57BL/6) depends on the induction of a polarized Th1-type response, resulting in macrophage activation and killing of parasites.

Early studies demonstrated that epidermal LCs phagocyte *L. major in vivo* and migrate to draining lymph nodes (dLNs) for presentation to antigen-specific T cells [31]. However, later studies showed that DCs harboring parasites in dLNs are Langerin negative and express dermal DC markers [32]. Besides, mice deficient for MHC class II exclusively in LCs (but not in dermal DCs) control *L. major* infection, similar to wild type animals [33]. This finding suggests that LCs are dispensable for triggering T cell response during *Leishmania* infection. Moreover, a recent study showed that LCs might even play a pathogenic role during low dose infection via the induction and expansion of regulatory T cells [34]. Some studies showed that dermal DCs harboring parasites migrate out of the skin and transport antigens to the dLNs [32, 35]. Another study suggested that blood MoDCs might phagocyte parasites and transport them to the dLN, where they present parasite-derived antigen to T cells [29]. In this way, depending on the tissue and the subtype involved, DCs could have different biological response towards *Leishmania* interaction.

TABLE 1: Summary of current phenotypes described for different DC subsets.

DC type	Phenotype/markers	Function	Reference
Plasmacytoid DC (pDC)	MHC-II, CD45RA/B220, Ly6C/GR-1, Siglec-H	Type I-IFN synthesis	[11–13]
Conventional DC type 1 (cDC1)	CD8α, CD103 (mice); CD141/BDCA3 (humans)	Antigen cross-presentation, CD8α^+ T cell activation	[15, 16, 18, 19]
Conventional DC type 2 (cDC2)	CD11b, CD172/SIRPα (mice); CD1c/BDCA1 (humans)	CD4$^+$ T cell polarization	[17, 20, 21]
Monocyte-derived DC (MoDC)	CD11c, MHC-II, F4/80, CD64 (mice); CD1a (humans)	Antigen presentation at inflammatory sites	[23, 24]
Langerhans cell (LC)	MHC-II, Langerin	Antigen presentation in the skin	[25–27]

The production of IL-12 by APCs is critically important for the polarization of naïve T cells toward Th1 subset and subsequent IFN-γ production [30, 36]. Infection of DC with *L. major* results in functional IL-12p70 production [37]. Interestingly, DC subsets are differentially permissive to *Leishmania* parasites and this differential infectivity seems to be inversely correlated with the ability of infected cells to produce IL-12p70 [38, 39]. CD8α^+ DCs are less permissive to *L. major* amastigotes compared to CD8α^- DCs. However, CD8α^+ and CD103$^+$ DCs are the most powerful IL-12p70 producers in response to this infection [36, 38]. The mechanism(s) that control the induction of IL-12 from DCs and the functional differences between IL-12-producing DCs and nonproducers are still not known.

It has been speculated that different outcomes of *Leishmania* infection between resistant and susceptible mice may be related to differences in their DC functions, particularly in the differentiation of naïve TCD4$^+$ into effector cells [40, 41]. However, *L. major*-infected skin-derived DCs from BALB/c and C57BL/6 mice upregulated costimulatory molecules and produced comparable levels of proinflammatory cytokines [30]. In further contrast, LCs from BALB/c mice upregulate IL-4 receptor expression and downregulate IL-12p40 production in response to *L. major* infection [42]. These findings suggest that *L. major* is able to inhibit Th1 immune response through altering DCs functions, depending on the cell type involved. Baldwin et al. [43] found that *L. major*-infected BALB/c mice have an increased number of plasmacytoid DCs in their dLNs [43]. This was associated with increased pDC recruitment early after infection, compared to infected C57BL/6 mice.

Ashok and Acha-Orbea [44] proposed a model of infection based on DCs subtypes at the different time points after *L. major* infection. This model nicely explains many features and contradiction in the role of DCs subsets in cutaneous leishmaniasis: (1) dermal DCs and LCs play a role early in infection and (2) monocyte-derived dendritic cells and lymph node resident DCs are important to establish an efficient immune response at later time points [44]. However, this proposed model only focuses on DCs role in murine models based on *L. major* infection. It is not clear whether the differences observed in DCs from susceptible and resistant mice are relevant to the pathogenesis of the disease in humans. At present, there is still limited information on initial or late DC responses to other species of *Leishmania*

and their contribution to prime protective or pathogenic T cell responses in cutaneous leishmaniasis.

2.2. Role of DCs Interaction with Other Leishmania Species. Even though cutaneous leishmaniasis is caused by almost 20 species of *Leishmania*, most studies about the role of DCs are focused on experimental models of 4 species: *L. major*, *L. mexicana*, *L. amazonensis*, and *L. braziliensis*.

The role of Langerhans cells (LCs) was examined in patients with different forms of cutaneous leishmaniasis (CL) caused by the New World *Leishmania* sp. (*L. braziliensis*, *L. mexicana*, and *L. amazonensis*) [45, 46]. The analysis of LCs density among different clinical forms of CL showed a reduced LC density in *L. braziliensis* infection with a positive DTH response (delayed type IV hypersensibility). In comparison to nonreactive DTH from severe forms caused by *L. amazonensis*, an increase of LC density was observed [46]. These results indicate a species-specific negative correlation between LC density and DTH reaction among clinical forms of CL. This could lead to a suppression of T cell immune response. However, in CL caused by *L. mexicana*, the LCs density is similar between mild and severe clinical forms [45]. These findings indicate that *L. amazonensis* may use LCs to prime regulatory T cells, inhibiting the T cell responses, in a similar way to *L. major* infection [34].

Moreover, corroborating this clinical observation, experimental evidence confirms that early stages of *L. amazonensis* infection in BALB/c mice may impair multiple immune functions, leading to an antigen-specific T cell immune suppression [47]. Similar results were observed in murine and human DCs infected *in vitro* by *L. amazonensis* [48, 49]. However, for *L. braziliensis* murine infection, a full DC maturation process and activation were observed [50]. Together, these studies point out the specificity of strategies from different *Leishmania* species to modulate T cell immune response through DCs. Besides, there is a lack of information about the importance of other DC types for the development of different clinical forms caused by one species.

The dynamics of DCs migration to lymph nodes and to nonlymphoid tissues is also an important issue for the disease outcome. DCs progenitors and monocytes terminally differentiate into DCs subsets, depending on the nonlymphoid tissue they migrate, such as the skin. When activated, skin DCs upregulate CCR7 and migrate again to draining lymph node via afferent lymphatics in response to CCL19 and CCL21 [14, 51]. The migration of monocyte-derived DCs to the lymph nodes is driven by CCR2 and its ligands [52]. In VL, there is a lack of protective immune response, partially, due to an altered DC migration to the spleen and dLNs [53–56]. This is also observed in CL. During *L. major* infection, MoDCs are preferentially recruited to the infected skin and dLN. They are important to mediate a Th1 response and to control the infection [29]. Such enhanced recruitment of DCs to dLN leads to hypertrophy of the LN, which is associated with a protective response against *L. major* [57]. On the other hand, *L. mexicana* infection induces limited recruitment of MoDCs and decreased LN expansion, without affecting T cell proliferation [58, 59]. This diminished recruitment is independent of IL-10 and leads to disease progression, since treatment with neutralizing antibodies against IL-10 increases MoDCs migration and decreases parasite burden [59]. The modulation of DC recruitment to the infected skin and dLN could be used as a mechanism of immune evasion by different *Leishmania* sp. that causes CL.

3. Differences in Recognition of *Leishmania* Parasites by DCs

DCs express a wide variety of pattern recognition receptors (PRRs) that are important for initiating and directing subsequent adaptive immunity. The recognition of pathogen associated molecular patterns (PAMPs) can vary among species of *Leishmania*. de Veer et al. [60] found that MyD88 deficient (MyD88$^{-/-}$) C57BL/6 mice are more susceptible to *L. major* infection, suggesting a critical role of TLR signaling in initiating anti-*Leishmania* immunity [60]. They further demonstrated that LPG, the most abundant surface molecule of *Leishmania* and a TLR2 ligand, is responsible for the generation of protective immunity against leishmaniasis. Neutralization of TLR2 and TLR4 *in vivo* reduced the expression of costimulatory molecules on DCs infected with *L. major* [61]. However, the lack of TLR2 in mice infected with *L. braziliensis* resulted in an enhanced DC activation and increased IL-12 production. As such, *L. braziliensis*-infected DCs from TLR2$^{-/-}$ were more competent in priming naïve CD4$^+$ T cells *in vitro*. These findings correlated with an increased IFN-γ production *in vivo* and enhanced resistance to infection [62]. On the other hand, *L. braziliensis*-infected DCs from MyD88$^{-/-}$ exhibited less activation and decreased production of interleukin-12 [62].

Furthermore, it has been shown that TLR9 signaling is crucial to the release of IL-12 and type I IFN from DCs exposed *in vitro* to *L. major* and *L. braziliensis*. *In vivo* assays with *L. major* infection also confirmed the importance of TLR9 to IL-12 production from DCs [63, 64]. However, for *L. braziliensis* infection, *in vivo* experiments established that TLR9$^{-/-}$ mice could generate a Th1 response and activate DC, despite the diminished DC activation *in vitro* [65]. Together these data from TLR assays reinforce the importance to define *in vitro* and *in vivo* approaches to better characterize the modulation of DC induced by different *Leishmania* sp. on the immune response.

The recognition of pathogens could be optimized by the action of antibodies, a process called opsonization [66]. The uptake of *L. amazonensis* amastigotes by DC and LCs can be promoted by opsonization [67]. This process leads to IL-10 production from these DCs, as well as the consequent priming of IL-10-producing T CD4$^+$ and lesion progress in mice [67]. In contrast, the uptake of opsonized *L. major* by murine DCs leads to cell activation, IL-12 production, and protective immunity [68, 69]. In further contrast, *L. mexicana* and *L. braziliensis* are highly efficient in infecting DCs, even in the absence of antibodies [62, 70]. These findings point out that the profile of cytokine production from DC is differently induced in a species-specific way, despite the same pathway recognition of *Leishmania*.

4. Interaction of DC with Other Leukocytes

Dendritic cells are the most important APCs, making a link among innate and adaptive immunity. They can have direct and diverse functions on the immune response, leading to activation as well as tolerance and anergy. In the context of CL, the functions of DCs could be modulated by the interaction with other leukocytes, such as neutrophils and NK cells.

It has been shown that genomic DNA of *L. major* and *L. braziliensis* promastigotes activate cDCs and pDCs to produce IL-12 and IFN-α/β, respectively. After, they were cocultured with NK cells, leading to an increased IFN-γ release and NK cytotoxicity [63, 64]. Certain *Leishmania* species (*L. tropica*, *L. amazonensis*, and *L. mexicana*), in their amastigotes phase, are poor inducers of IL-12 by DC. This might account for the limited NK cell response during prolonged infections *in vivo* [71, 72]. Hernandez Sanabria et al. [73] demonstrated that infection of *L. amazonensis* amastigotes triggers minimal DC activation, but the interaction with activated NK cells could partially overcome the deficiencies in DC activation *in vitro* [73]. The injection of activated NK cells 24 hours after infection *in vivo* promoted IL-12 release and increased the expression of costimulatory molecules in infected DCs (CD40, CD83, and CD80) [73]. Regarding NK cells in this context, they showed increased expression of IFN-γ and CXCL10. Such interaction forms a positive loop, leading to the induction of a Th1 immune response to reduce parasite loads.

In a vaccination context against *L. major*, BALB/c depleted of NK cells and vaccinated with DCs pulsed with parasites lysates and, then, challenged with *L. major* showed a significant increase in footpad swelling and parasite load in the dLN [74]. In order to evaluate the mechanisms under this process, coculture of these cells was assessed. This resulted in upregulation of CD69 and IFN-γ on NK cells as well as CD86 and MHC-II on pulsed DCs. The interaction of DC and NK cells is a good example of a positive interaction that leads to cross activation and host immune protection, either, in the context of an infection or vaccination.

Neutrophils are also an important cell type which interact with DCs. The ingestion of *L. major* by neutrophils in parasite-inoculated mice increased cell apoptosis. This

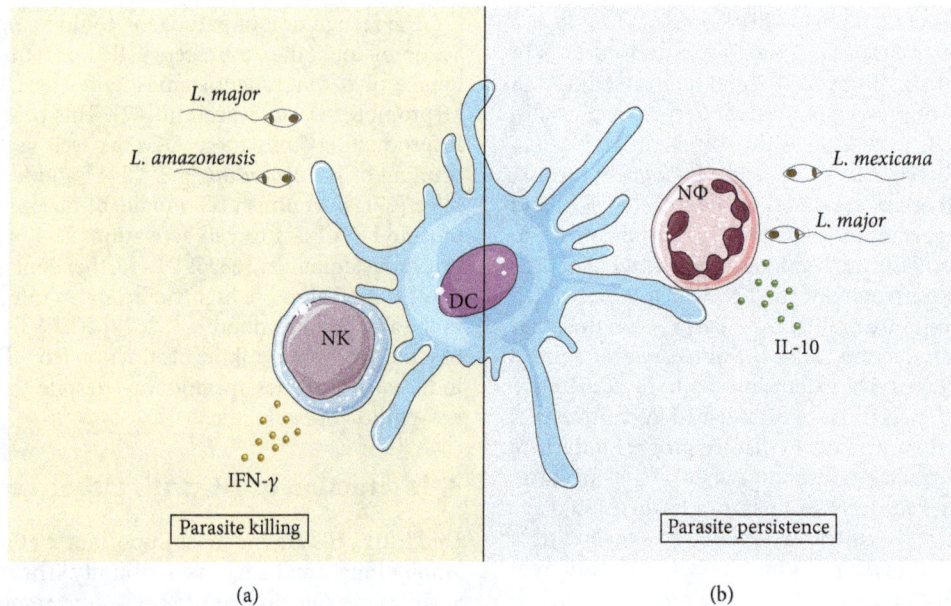

FIGURE 1: Interaction of DC with different leukocytes in the cutaneous leishmaniasis context. (a) shows the interaction among NK and infected DCs that leads to host immune protection and parasite killing through IFN-γ production during *L. amazonensis* [73] or *L. major* [74] infection. (b) shows the outcome induced by the increased production of IL-10 after the interaction between infected neutrophils (NΦ) with *L. major* [75] or *L. mexicana* [76] and DCs, leading to parasite persistence.

favored the capture of apoptotic neutrophils by DCs, preventing the activation of infected DCs in the skin [75]. In the case of *L. mexicana* infection, this effect was not observed, since the infection did not induce neutrophil apoptosis. Parasites sequestration by neutrophils impaired DC migration to the site of infection, through reduced CCL2, CCL3, and CCL5 release. Furthermore, the diminished DCs that migrate to the site of infection had a decreased motility and parasite uptake [76]. The interaction among DCs and neutrophils is a good example of negative regulation of the immune response, regardless of the *Leishmania* sp. Although the consequences of DCs and neutrophils interaction lead to immune suppression, the mechanisms of action could be diverse and *Leishmania* species-specific (summarized in Figure 1).

5. Systems Biology as a Tool to Develop Vaccines against CL Based on DCs

Recently, Matos et al. [77] showed the potential of targeting DC *in vivo* for induction of protective immune response against *L. major* in murine model of CL [77]. However, the role of DCs in CL is diverse and complex. Such role could explain some unique clinical manifestations, depending on the species of *Leishmania* that causes the disease. Because of that, the use of vaccines based on DCs is not yet a reality for CL. This is not only due to the complexity of the disease. Genomic and transcriptional profiles vary not only interspecifically in *Leishmania* parasites that causes CL [78–81], but also within parasites strains isolated from patients [82]. This variability leads to a difficult task to identify a universal antigen vaccine candidate to clinical trials.

Systems Biology could be a useful tool to overcome these difficulties. Systems Biology have a holistic approach to describe complex interactions between multiple components in a biological context [83]. Using high dimensional molecular approaches, Systems Biology identifies changes caused by perturbations, such as infection or vaccination, combined with computational analysis to model and predict responses [84]. The first studies of Systems Biology about the immune response predicted that certain signatures of CD8[+] T cells and B lymphocytes correlated with a protective immune response induced by a vaccine against Yellow Fever Virus [85, 86]. Since then, there is an increased interest about the research of immune responses based on Systems Biology approaches. These studies lead to the identification of interactions between pathogens and hosts and factors for parasite dissemination and disease progression, as well as to the selection of promising antigens as vaccine candidates [87–89]. For instance, hub genes with unknown functions were identified from *Plasmodium falciparum* parasites isolated from noncerebral clinical complications of malaria. The presence of these genes correlates parasite burden and survival with complicated clinical manifestations [90]. These findings revealed the crucial roles of these genes in parasite biology and their potential as candidates for intervention strategies.

Regarding leishmaniasis, Albergante et al. [91] have developed an *in silico* Petri net model that simulates hepatic granuloma development during the infection in experimental visceral context. This model identified an intergranuloma diversity of the antileishmanial activity and a dominant regulatory role of IL-10 produced by infected Kupffer cells at the core of the granuloma [91]. This approach raised new insights into how effector mechanisms may be regulated within the granuloma and revealed a useful tool to interpret how interventions may operate. For cutaneous leishmaniasis, the analysis of DNA sequence of *L. braziliensis* and *L. guyanensis* isolated from patients with different treatment outcomes identified polymorphisms related to drug resistance [92]. This study showed that genes related to drug resistance could be used to discriminate the two species of the subgenus *L. Viannia* and also could predict treatment failure.

Those studies mentioned above demonstrate the use of System Biology as a useful tool to better understand an infection, to identify unknown pathogen cell signaling pathways, potential biomarkers of disease susceptibility, and immunological alterations that aggravates the pathology. However, the studies employing this approach are few, but they will be very promising for the development of new technologies on the leishmaniasis field.

A successful application of the System Biology approach was modeled to study the function and the role of pDC during cytopathic virus infection to identify multiscale interactions involved in the protection against the virus [93]. The results obtained from this analysis identified and predicted that (1) one infected pDC secretes sufficient type I IFN to protect up to 10^4 macrophages from cytopathic viral infection; (2) pDC population in the spleen protects against virus variants which inhibit IFN production; and (3) antiviral therapy should primarily limit viral replication within peripheral organs. Together, these results demonstrate the importance of System Biology application to direct and optimize the use of different technologies based on DCs.

In this way, the application of System Biology could be a useful tool to design and develop promising vaccines candidates based on DCs pulsed with *Leishmania* antigens. Studies about DC signaling network based on Systems Biology approach are already published and they stand for the feasibility of this technique [94, 95]. However, the development of vaccines based on DCs through Systems Biology approach needs to be well designed to avoid undesired effects, such as the exacerbation of the CL through the increase of inflammation [96].

6. Conclusion and Future Directions

Given the fact that the disease pathology of CL is highly variable depending on the species of *Leishmania*, it is very hard to generalize specific modulatory mechanisms to all strains and in all hosts. This is important because most of the studies about the role of DCs during *Leishmania* infection were usually conducted with a single species of the parasite, which precludes multi-species/strain comparison. Not all *Leishmania* species and its interaction with DCs were studied. For instance, infection caused by *L. guyanensis* paradoxically induces a specific immune response via TLR3 early after infection that impairs killing of parasites [97]. A more comprehensive study would be very helpful for a better understanding about the role of these cells and the mechanisms that regulate their antigen presentation functions and also pathogen factors that could influence the antigen

presentation and subsequent activation of the adaptive immune system. Besides that, the development and use of computational immunology have been constantly increasing its value. Nowadays, different *in silico* approaches are available for identification of potential epitopes and antigens for vaccines, since experimental methods are difficult and time-consuming [98]. In addition, the DNA sequencing techniques became less expensive and, therefore, many parasite genome strains can be sequenced. Their predicted proteomes can be assessed considering their variability, an important feature of antigen candidates for vaccine development to one or all *Leishmania* species that cause CL. In this way, the use of DCs is promising for generation of potential alternatives therapies and vaccines protocols to improve the quality of life of patients infected by these protozoan parasites.

Conflict of Interests

The authors declare that they do not have a commercial association that might pose a conflict of interests.

Authors' Contribution

Cláudia Brodskyn and Natalia Tavares contributed equally to this review.

Acknowledgments

This review was supported by Conselho Nacional de Desenvolvimento Científico e Tecnológico (CNPq), Fundação de Amparo à Pesquisa do Estado da Bahia (FAPESB), and Instituto de Investigação em Imunologia-Instituto Nacional de Ciência e Tecnologia (iii-INCT), Brazil. Daniel Feijó receives fellowship from CNPq. Cláudia Brodskyn is a senior investigator at CNPq. Rafael Tibúrcio and Mariana Ampuero receive fellowships from FAPESB. The authors thank Drs. Leonardo Farias, Bruno Andrade, and Pablo Oliveira for suggestions and comments. They also thank Elaine Santos and Andrezza Souza for technical support.

References

[1] WHO/Leishmaniasis, "Leishmaniasis: Magnitude of the problem," 2014, http://www.who.int/leishmaniasis/burden/magnitude/burden_magnitude/en/index.html.

[2] S. Saha, S. Mondal, A. Banerjee, J. Ghose, S. Bhowmick, and N. Ali, "Immune responses in kala-azar," *The Indian Journal of Medical Research*, vol. 123, no. 3, pp. 245–266, 2006.

[3] A. Caldas, C. Favali, D. Aquino et al., "Balance of IL-10 and interferon-γ plasma levels in human visceral leishmaniasis: implications in the pathogenesis," *BMC Infectious Diseases*, vol. 5, article 113, 2005.

[4] H. Goto and J. A. L. Lindoso, "Current diagnosis and treatment of cutaneous and mucocutaneous leishmaniasis," *Expert Review of Anti-Infective Therapy*, vol. 8, no. 4, pp. 419–433, 2010.

[5] P. J. Guerin, P. Olliaro, S. Sundar et al., "Visceral leishmaniasis: current status of control, diagnosis, and treatment, and a proposed research and development agenda," *The Lancet Infectious Diseases*, vol. 2, no. 8, pp. 494–501, 2002.

[6] C. Reis e Sousa, "Activation of dendritic cells: translating innate into adaptive immunity," *Current Opinion in Immunology*, vol. 16, no. 1, pp. 21–25, 2004.

[7] H. Moll, "Dendritic cells and host resistance to infection," *Cellular Microbiology*, vol. 5, no. 8, pp. 493–500, 2003.

[8] M. Sundquist, A. Rydström, and M. J. Wick, "Immunity to *Salmonella* from a dendritic point of view," *Cellular Microbiology*, vol. 6, no. 1, pp. 1–11, 2004.

[9] T. B. H. Geijtenbeek, S. J. van Vliet, A. Engering, B. A. t Hart, and Y. van Kooyk, "Self- and nonself-recognition by C-type lectins on dendritic cells," *Annual Review of Immunology*, vol. 22, pp. 33–54, 2004.

[10] K. Takeda and S. Akira, "Microbial recognition by Toll-like receptors," *Journal of Dermatological Science*, vol. 34, no. 2, pp. 73–82, 2004.

[11] Y.-J. Liu, "IPC: professional type 1 interferon-producing cells and plasmacytoid dendritic cell precursors," *Annual Review of Immunology*, vol. 23, pp. 275–306, 2005.

[12] K. Shortman and Y.-J. Liu, "Mouse and human dendritic cell subtypes," *Nature Reviews Immunology*, vol. 2, no. 3, pp. 151–161, 2002.

[13] J. Zhang, A. Raper, N. Sugita et al., "Characterization of Siglec-H as a novel endocytic receptor expressed on murine plasmacytoid dendritic cell precursors," *Blood*, vol. 107, no. 9, pp. 3600–3608, 2006.

[14] M. Merad, P. Sathe, J. Helft, J. Miller, and A. Mortha, "The dendritic cell lineage: ontogeny and function of dendritic cells and their subsets in the steady state and the inflamed setting," *Annual Review of Immunology*, vol. 31, pp. 563–604, 2013.

[15] K. Crozat, R. Guiton, V. Contreras et al., "The XC chemokine receptor 1 is a conserved selective marker of mammalian cells homologous to mouse CD8α⁺ dendritic cells," *The Journal of Experimental Medicine*, vol. 207, no. 6, pp. 1283–1292, 2010.

[16] M. Guilliams, F. Ginhoux, C. Jakubzick et al., "Dendritic cells, monocytes and macrophages: a unified nomenclature based on ontogeny," *Nature Reviews Immunology*, vol. 14, no. 8, pp. 571–578, 2014.

[17] S. Gurka, E. Hartung, M. Becker, and R. A. Kroczek, "Mouse conventional dendritic cells can be universally classified based on the mutually exclusive expression of XCR1 and SIRPα," *Frontiers in Immunology*, vol. 6, article 35, 2015.

[18] M. Haniffa, A. Shin, V. Bigley et al., "Human tissues contain CD141^hi cross-presenting dendritic cells with functional homology to mouse CD103⁺ nonlymphoid dendritic cells," *Immunity*, vol. 37, no. 1, pp. 60–73, 2012.

[19] S. L. Jongbloed, A. J. Kassianos, K. J. McDonald et al., "Human CD141⁺ (BDCA-3)⁺ dendritic cells (DCs) represent a unique myeloid DC subset that cross-presents necrotic cell antigens," *The Journal of Experimental Medicine*, vol. 207, no. 6, pp. 1247–1260, 2010.

[20] S. H. Robbins, T. Walzer, D. Dembélé et al., "Novel insights into the relationships between dendritic cell subsets in human and mouse revealed by genome-wide expression profiling," *Genome Biology*, vol. 9, no. 1, article R17, 2008.

[21] A. Schlitzer, N. McGovern, P. Teo et al., "IRF4 transcription factor-dependent CD11b⁺ dendritic cells in human and mouse control mucosal IL-17 cytokine responses," *Immunity*, vol. 38, no. 5, pp. 970–983, 2013.

[22] C. Cheong, I. Matos, J.-H. Choi et al., "Microbial stimulation fully differentiates monocytes to DC-SIGN/CD209⁺ dendritic cells for immune T cell areas," *Cell*, vol. 143, no. 3, pp. 416–429, 2010.

[23] C. Langlet, S. Tamoutounour, S. Henri et al., "CD64 expression distinguishes monocyte-derived and conventional dendritic cells and reveals their distinct role during intramuscular immunization," *Journal of Immunology*, vol. 188, no. 4, pp. 1751–1760, 2012.

[24] S. Tamoutounour, M. Guilliams, F. M. Sanchis et al., "Origins and functional specialization of macrophages and of conventional and monocyte-derived dendritic cells in mouse skin," *Immunity*, vol. 39, no. 5, pp. 925–938, 2013.

[25] M. Greter, I. Lelios, P. Pelczar et al., "Stroma-derived interleukin-34 controls the development and maintenance of langerhans cells and the maintenance of microglia," *Immunity*, vol. 37, no. 6, pp. 1050–1060, 2012.

[26] J. C. Miller, B. D. Brown, T. Shay et al., "Deciphering the transcriptional network of the dendritic cell lineage," *Nature Immunology*, vol. 13, no. 9, pp. 888–899, 2012.

[27] M. Merad and M. G. Manz, "Dendritic cell homeostasis," *Blood*, vol. 113, no. 15, pp. 3418–3427, 2009.

[28] P. M. A. Gorak, C. R. Engwerda, and P. M. Kaye, "Dendritic cells, but not macrophages, produce IL-12 immediately following *Leishmania donovani* infection," *European Journal of Immunology*, vol. 28, no. 2, pp. 687–695, 1998.

[29] B. León, M. López-Bravo, and C. Ardavín, "Monocyte-derived dendritic cells formed at the infection site control the induction of protective T helper 1 responses against *Leishmania*," *Immunity*, vol. 26, no. 4, pp. 519–531, 2007.

[30] E. von Stebut, Y. Belkaid, T. Jakob, D. L. Sacks, and M. C. Udey, "Uptake of *Leishmania major* amastigotes results in activation and interleukin 12 release from murine skin-derived dendritic cells: implications for the initiation of anti-*Leishmania* immunity," *The Journal of Experimental Medicine*, vol. 188, no. 8, pp. 1547–1552, 1998.

[31] H. Moll, H. Fuchs, C. Blank, and M. Rollinghoff, "Langerhans cells transport *Leishmania* major from the infected skin to the draining lymph node for presentation to antigen-specific T cells," *European Journal of Immunology*, vol. 23, no. 7, pp. 1595–1601, 1993.

[32] U. Ritter, A. Meißner, C. Scheidig, and H. Körner, "CD8α- and Langerin-negative dendritic cells, but not Langerhans cells, act as principal antigen-presenting cells in leishmaniasis," *European Journal of Immunology*, vol. 34, no. 6, pp. 1542–1550, 2004.

[33] M. P. Lemos, F. Esquivel, P. Scott, and T. M. Laufer, "MHC class II expression restricted to CD8α⁺ and CD11b⁺ dendritic cells is sufficient for control of *Leishmania* major," *Journal of Experimental Medicine*, vol. 199, no. 5, pp. 725–730, 2004.

[34] K. Kautz-Neu, M. Noordegraaf, S. Dinges et al., "Langerhans cells are negative regulators of the anti-*Leishmania* response," *The Journal of Experimental Medicine*, vol. 208, no. 5, pp. 885–891, 2011.

[35] L. G. Ng, A. Hsu, M. A. Mandell et al., "Migratory dermal dendritic cells act as rapid sensors of protozoan parasites," *PLoS Pathogens*, vol. 4, no. 11, Article ID e1000222, 2008.

[36] M. Martínez-López, S. Iborra, R. Conde-Garrosa, and D. Sancho, "Batf3-dependent CD103⁺ dendritic cells are major producers of IL-12 that drive local Th1 immunity against *Leishmania major* infection in mice," *European Journal of Immunology*, vol. 45, no. 1, pp. 119–129, 2015.

[37] M. A. Marovich, M. A. McDowell, E. K. Thomas, and T. B. Nutman, "IL-12p70 production by Leishmania major-harboring human dendritic cells is a CD40/CD40 ligand-dependent process," *Journal of Immunology*, vol. 164, no. 11, pp. 5858–5865, 2000.

[38] S. Henri, J. Curtis, H. Hochrein, D. Vremec, K. Shortman, and E. Handman, "Hierarchy of susceptibility of dendritic cell subsets to infection by *Leishmania* major: inverse relationship to interleukin-12 production," *Infection and Immunity*, vol. 70, no. 7, pp. 3874–3880, 2002.

[39] M. Akbari, K. Honma, D. Kimura et al., "IRF4 in dendritic cells inhibits IL-12 production and controls TH1 immune responses against leishmania major," *Journal of Immunology*, vol. 192, no. 5, pp. 2271–2279, 2014.

[40] K. Suzue, S. Kobayashi, T. Takeuchi, M. Suzuki, and S. Koyasu, "Critical role of dendritic cells in determining the Th1/Th2 balance upon *Leishmania major* infection," *International Immunology*, vol. 20, no. 3, pp. 337–343, 2008.

[41] M. J. Girard-Madoux, K. Kautz-Neu, B. Lorenz, J. L. Ober-Blöbaum, E. von Stebut, and B. E. Clausen, "IL-10 signaling in dendritic cells attenuates anti-*Leishmania major* immunity without affecting protective memory responses," *Journal of Investigative Dermatology*, vol. 135, no. 11, pp. 2890–2894, 2015.

[42] H. Moll, A. Scharner, and E. Kämpgen, "Increased interleukin 4 (IL-4) receptor expression and IL-4-induced decrease in IL-12 production by langerhans cells infected with *Leishmania* major," *Infection and Immunity*, vol. 70, no. 3, pp. 1627–1630, 2002.

[43] T. M. Baldwin, C. Elso, J. Curtis, L. Buckingham, and E. Handman, "The site of *Leishmania* major infection determines disease severity and immune responses," *Infection and Immunity*, vol. 71, no. 12, pp. 6830–6834, 2003.

[44] D. Ashok and H. Acha-Orbea, "Timing is everything: dendritic cell subsets in murine *Leishmania* infection," *Trends in Parasitology*, vol. 30, no. 10, pp. 499–507, 2014.

[45] U. Ritter, H. Moll, T. Laskay et al., "Differential expression of chemokines in patients with localized and diffuse cutaneous American leishmaniasis," *The Journal of Infectious Diseases*, vol. 173, no. 3, pp. 699–709, 1996.

[46] M. B. Xavier, F. T. Silveira, S. Demachki, M. M. R. Ferreira, and J. L. M. do Nascimento, "American tegumentary leishmaniasis: a quantitative analysis of Langerhans cells presents important differences between *L. (L.) amazonensis* and *Viannia subgenus*," *Acta Tropica*, vol. 95, no. 1, pp. 67–73, 2005.

[47] J. Ji, J. Sun, and L. Soong, "Impaired expression of inflammatory cytokines and chemokines at early stages of infection with Leishmania amazonensis," *Infection and Immunity*, vol. 71, no. 8, pp. 4278–4288, 2003.

[48] C. Favali, N. Tavares, J. Clarêncio, A. Barral, M. Barral-Netto, and C. Brodskyn, "*Leishmania* amazonensis infection impairs differentiation and function of human dendritic cells," *Journal of Leukocyte Biology*, vol. 82, no. 6, pp. 1401–1406, 2007.

[49] L. Soong, "Modulation of dendritic cell function by leishmania parasites," *Journal of Immunology*, vol. 180, no. 7, pp. 4355–4360, 2008.

[50] A. K. Carvalho, F. T. Silveira, L. F. D. Passero, C. M. C. Gomes, C. E. P. Corbett, and M. D. Laurenti, "*Leishmania (V.) braziliensis* and *L. (L.) amazonensis* promote differential expression of dendritic cells and cellular immune response in murine model," *Parasite Immunology*, vol. 34, no. 8-9, pp. 395–403, 2012.

[51] L. Ohl, M. Mohaupt, N. Czeloth et al., "CCR7 governs skin dendritic cell migration under inflammatory and steady-state conditions," *Immunity*, vol. 21, no. 2, pp. 279–288, 2004.

[52] F. Geissmann, S. Gordon, D. A. Hume, A. M. Mowat, and G. J. Randolph, "Unravelling mononuclear phagocyte heterogeneity," *Nature Reviews Immunology*, vol. 10, no. 6, pp. 453–460, 2010.

[53] M. K. Ibrahim, J. L. Barnes, E. Y. Osorio et al., "Deficiency of lymph node-resident dendritic cells (DCs) and dysregulation of DC chemoattractants in a malnourished mouse model of *Leishmania donovani* infection," *Infection and Immunity*, vol. 82, no. 8, pp. 3098–3112, 2014.

[54] M. Ato, A. Maroof, S. Zubairi, H. Nakano, T. Kakiuchi, and P. M. Kaye, "Loss of dendritic cell migration and impaired resistance to *Leishmania donovani* infection in mice deficient in CCL19 and CCL21," *The Journal of Immunology*, vol. 176, no. 9, pp. 5486–5493, 2006.

[55] M. Ato, S. Stäger, C. R. Engwerda, and P. M. Kaye, "Defective CCR7 expression on dendritic cells contributes to the development of visceral leishmaniasis," *Nature Immunology*, vol. 3, no. 12, pp. 1185–1191, 2002.

[56] A. C. Stanley, J. E. Dalton, S. H. Rossotti et al., "VCAM-1 and VLA-4 modulate dendritic cell IL-12p40 production in experimental visceral leishmaniasis," *PLoS Pathogens*, vol. 4, no. 9, Article ID e1000158, 2008.

[57] L. P. Carvalho, P. M. Petritus, A. L. Trochtenberg et al., "Lymph node hypertrophy following *Leishmania major* infection is dependent on TLR9," *The Journal of Immunology*, vol. 188, no. 3, pp. 1394–1401, 2012.

[58] A. C. Hsu and P. Scott, "Leishmania mexicana infection induces impaired lymph node expansion and Th1 cell differentiation despite normal T cell proliferation," *The Journal of Immunology*, vol. 179, no. 12, pp. 8200–8207, 2007.

[59] P. M. Petritus, D. Manzoni-de-Almeida, C. Gimblet, C. Gonzalez Lombana, and P. Scott, "*Leishmania mexicana* mexicana induces limited recruitment and activation of monocytes and monocyte-derived dendritic cells early during infection," *PLoS Neglected Tropical Diseases*, vol. 6, no. 10, Article ID e1858, 2012.

[60] M. J. de Veer, J. M. Curtis, T. M. Baldwin et al., "MyD88 is essential for clearance of *Leishmania major*: possible role for lipophosphoglycan and Toll-like receptor 2 signaling," *European Journal of Immunology*, vol. 33, no. 10, pp. 2822–2831, 2003.

[61] M. Komai-Koma, D. Li, E. Wang, D. Vaughan, and D. Xu, "Anti-Toll-like receptor 2 and 4 antibodies suppress inflammatory response in mice," *Immunology*, vol. 143, no. 3, pp. 354–362, 2014.

[62] D. A. Vargas-Inchaustegui, W. Tai, L. Xin, A. E. Hogg, D. B. Corry, and L. Soong, "Distinct roles for MyD88 and toll-like receptor 2 during *Leishmania braziliensis* infection in mice," *Infection and Immunity*, vol. 77, no. 7, pp. 2948–2956, 2009.

[63] J. Liese, U. Schleicher, and C. Bogdan, "TLR9 signaling is essential for the innate NK cell response in murine cutaneous leishmaniasis," *European Journal of Immunology*, vol. 37, no. 12, pp. 3424–3434, 2007.

[64] U. Schleicher, J. Liese, I. Knippertz et al., "NK cell activation in visceral leishmaniasis requires TLR9, myeloid DCs, and IL-12, but is independent of plasmacytoid DCs," *The Journal of Experimental Medicine*, vol. 204, no. 4, pp. 893–906, 2007.

[65] T. Weinkopff, A. Mariotto, G. Simon et al., "Role of toll-like receptor 9 signaling in experimental *Leishmania braziliensis* infection," *Infection and Immunity*, vol. 81, no. 5, pp. 1575–1584, 2013.

[66] L. T. Vogelpoel, D. L. Baeten, E. C. de Jong, and J. den Dunnen, "Control of cytokine production by human fc gamma receptors: implications for pathogen defense and autoimmunity," *Frontiers in Immunology*, vol. 6, article 79, 2015.

[67] N. Wanasen, L. Xin, and L. Soong, "Pathogenic role of B cells and antibodies in murine *Leishmania amazonensis* infection,"

International Journal for Parasitology, vol. 38, no. 3-4, pp. 417–429, 2008.

[68] A. P. Nigg, S. Zahn, D. Rückerl et al., "Dendritic cell-derived IL-12p40 homodimer contributes to susceptibility in cutaneous leishmaniasis in BALB/c mice," *The Journal of Immunology*, vol. 178, no. 11, pp. 7251–7258, 2007.

[69] F. Woelbing, S. L. Kostka, K. Moelle et al., "Uptake of *Leishmania major* by dendritic cells is mediated by Fcγ receptors and facilitates acquisition of protective immunity," *The Journal of Experimental Medicine*, vol. 203, no. 1, pp. 177–188, 2006.

[70] E. Prina, S. Z. Abdi, M. Lebastard, E. Perret, N. Winter, and J.-C. Antoine, "Dendritic cells as host cells for the promastigote and amastigote stages of *Leishmania amazonensis*: the role of opsonins in parasite uptake and dendritic cell maturation," *Journal of Cell Science*, vol. 117, no. 2, pp. 315–325, 2004.

[71] C. L. Bennett, A. Misslitz, L. Colledge, T. Aebischer, and C. C. Blackburn, "Silent infection of bone marrow-derived dendritic cells by *Leishmania mexicana* amastigotes," *European Journal of Immunology*, vol. 31, no. 3, pp. 876–883, 2001.

[72] M. A. McDowell, M. Marovich, R. Lira, M. Braun, and D. Sacks, "Leishmania priming of human dendritic cells for CD40 ligand-induced interleukin-12p70 secretion is strain and species dependent," *Infection and Immunity*, vol. 70, no. 8, pp. 3994–4001, 2002.

[73] M. X. Hernandez Sanabria, D. A. Vargas-Inchaustegui, L. Xin, and L. Soong, "Role of natural killer cells in modulating dendritic cell responses to *Leishmania amazonensis* infection," *Infection and Immunity*, vol. 76, no. 11, pp. 5100–5109, 2008.

[74] K. A. Remer, B. Roeger, C. Hambrecht, and H. Moll, "Natural killer cells support the induction of protective immunity during dendritic cell-mediated vaccination against *Leishmania major*," *Immunology*, vol. 131, no. 4, pp. 570–582, 2010.

[75] F. L. Ribeiro-Gomes, N. C. Peters, A. Debrabant, and D. L. Sacks, "Efficient capture of infected neutrophils by dendritic cells in the skin inhibits the early anti-leishmania response," *PLoS Pathogens*, vol. 8, no. 2, Article ID e1002536, 2012.

[76] B. P. Hurrell, S. Schuster, E. Grün et al., "Rapid sequestration of *Leishmania mexicana* by neutrophils contributes to the development of chronic lesion," *PLoS Pathogens*, vol. 11, no. 5, Article ID e1004929, 2015.

[77] I. Matos, O. Mizenina, A. Lubkin, R. M. Steinman, and J. Idoyaga, "Targeting antigens to dendritic cells in vivo induces protective immunity," *PLoS ONE*, vol. 8, no. 6, Article ID e67453, 2013.

[78] L. A. Dillon, K. Okrah, V. K. Hughitt et al., "Transcriptomic profiling of gene expression and RNA processing during *Leishmania major* differentiation," *Nucleic Acids Research*, vol. 43, no. 14, pp. 6799–6813, 2015.

[79] M. Fiebig, S. Kelly, E. Gluenz, and P. J. Myler, "Comparative life cycle transcriptomics revises *Leishmania mexicana* genome annotation and links a chromosome duplication with parasitism of vertebrates," *PLoS Pathogens*, vol. 11, no. 10, Article ID e1005186, 2015.

[80] C. S. Peacock, K. Seeger, D. Harris et al., "Comparative genomic analysis of three *Leishmania* species that cause diverse human disease," *Nature Genetics*, vol. 39, no. 7, pp. 839–847, 2007.

[81] D. A. Tschoeke, G. L. Nunes, R. Jardim et al., "The comparative genomics and phylogenomics of *Leishmania amazonensis* parasite," *Evolutionary Bioinformatics*, vol. 10, pp. 131–153, 2014.

[82] E. V. Alves-Ferreira, J. S. Toledo, A. H. De Oliveira et al., "Differential gene expression and infection profiles of cutaneous and mucosal *Leishmania braziliensis* isolates from the same patient," *PLoS Neglected Tropical Diseases*, vol. 9, no. 9, Article ID e0004018, 2015.

[83] L. H. Hartwell, J. J. Hopfield, S. Leibler, and A. W. Murray, "From molecular to modular cell biology," *Nature*, vol. 402, no. 6761, supplement, pp. C47–C52, 1999.

[84] H. Kitano, "Systems biology: a brief overview," *Science*, vol. 295, no. 5560, pp. 1662–1664, 2002.

[85] D. Gaucher, R. Therrien, N. Kettaf et al., "Yellow fever vaccine induces integrated multilineage and polyfunctional immune responses," *The Journal of Experimental Medicine*, vol. 205, no. 13, pp. 3119–3131, 2008.

[86] T. D. Querec, R. S. Akondy, E. K. Lee et al., "Systems biology approach predicts immunogenicity of the yellow fever vaccine in humans," *Nature Immunology*, vol. 10, no. 1, pp. 116–125, 2009.

[87] C. J. Blohmke, D. O'Connor, and A. J. Pollard, "The use of systems biology and immunological big data to guide vaccine development," *Genome Medicine*, vol. 7, no. 1, article 114, 2015.

[88] J. B. Gutierrez, M. R. Galinski, S. Cantrell, and E. O. Voit, "From within host dynamics to the epidemiology of infectious disease: scientific overview and challenges," *Mathematical Biosciences B*, vol. 270, pp. 143–155, 2015.

[89] D. E. Zak and A. Aderem, "Systems integration of innate and adaptive immunity," *Vaccine*, vol. 33, no. 40, pp. 5241–5248, 2015.

[90] A. K. Subudhi, P. A. Boopathi, I. Pandey et al., "Disease specific modules and hub genes for intervention strategies: a co-expression network based approach for *Plasmodium falciparum* clinical isolates," *Infection, Genetics and Evolution*, vol. 35, pp. 96–108, 2015.

[91] L. Albergante, J. Timmis, L. Beattie, and P. M. Kaye, "A Petri net model of granulomatous inflammation: implications for IL-10 mediated control of *Leishmania donovani* infection," *PLoS Computational Biology*, vol. 9, no. 11, Article ID e1003334, 2013.

[92] D. C. Torres, M. Ribeiro-Alves, G. A. S. Romero, A. M. R. Dávila, and E. Cupolillo, "Assessment of drug resistance related genes as candidate markers for treatment outcome prediction of cutaneous leishmaniasis in Brazil," *Acta Tropica*, vol. 126, no. 2, pp. 132–141, 2013.

[93] G. Bocharov, R. Züst, L. Cervantes-Barragan et al., "A systems immunology approach to plasmacytoid dendritic cell function in cytopathic virus infections," *PLoS Pathogens*, vol. 6, no. 7, Article ID e1001017, pp. 1–15, 2010.

[94] D. Cavalieri, D. Rivero, L. Beltrame et al., "DC-ATLAS: a systems biology resource to dissect receptor specific signal transduction in dendritic cells," *Immunome Research*, vol. 6, no. 1, article 10, 2010.

[95] S. Patil, H. Pincas, J. Seto, G. Nudelman, I. Nudelman, and S. C. Sealfon, "Signaling network of dendritic cells in response to pathogens: a community-input supported knowledgebase," *BMC Systems Biology*, vol. 4, article 137, 2010.

[96] P. Tsagozis, E. Karagouni, and E. Dotsika, "Dendritic cells pulsed with peptides of gp63 induce differential protection against experimental cutaneous leishmaniasis," *International Journal of Immunopathology and Pharmacology*, vol. 17, no. 3, pp. 343–352, 2004.

[97] A. Ives, C. Ronet, F. Prevel et al., "Leishmania RNA virus controls the severity of mucocutaneous leishmaniasis," *Science*, vol. 331, no. 6018, pp. 775–778, 2011.

[98] D. R. Flower, I. K. Macdonald, K. Ramakrishnan, M. N. Davies, and I. A. Doytchinova, "Computer aided selection of candidate vaccine antigens," *Immunome Research*, vol. 6, supplement 2, article S1, 2010.

7

Neutrophil-Mediated Regulation of Innate and Adaptive Immunity: The Role of Myeloperoxidase

Dragana Odobasic,[1] **A. Richard Kitching,**[1,2] **and Stephen R. Holdsworth**[1,2]

[1]*Centre for Inflammatory Diseases, Monash University, Department of Medicine, Monash Medical Centre, Clayton, VIC 3168, Australia*
[2]*Department of Nephrology, Monash Health, Clayton, VIC 3168, Australia*

Correspondence should be addressed to Dragana Odobasic; dragana.odobasic@monash.edu

Academic Editor: Carlos Rosales

Neutrophils are no longer seen as leukocytes with a sole function of being the essential first responders in the removal of pathogens at sites of infection. Being armed with numerous pro- and anti-inflammatory mediators, these phagocytes can also contribute to the development of various autoimmune diseases and can positively or negatively regulate the generation of adaptive immune responses. In this review, we will discuss how myeloperoxidase, the most abundant neutrophil granule protein, plays a key role in the various functions of neutrophils in innate and adaptive immunity.

1. Neutrophils in Innate and Adaptive Immunity: The Role of MPO

Neutrophils are capable of affecting many aspects of both innate and adaptive immunity. They are well known to be the first leukocyte to arrive at sites of infection. There, they play a key role in the clearance of pathogens, both by phagocytosis and by subsequent intracellular killing, as well as the release of neutrophil extracellular traps (NETs) into the extracellular space [1]. However, through the release of various inflammatory mediators, neutrophils can also contribute to tissue injury and organ damage in inflammatory and autoimmune diseases. On the other hand, neutrophil proteins are targets in autoimmune anti-neutrophil cytoplasmic antibody- (ANCA-) associated vasculitis (AAV) [2]. In more recent years, evidence has been accumulating to show that not only do neutrophils act at sites of inflammation, but they also infiltrate secondary lymphoid organs where they regulate the development of adaptive immunity [3]. MPO, the major protein in neutrophil granules, has been shown to be one of the key players in the neutrophil functions described above. This paper will review the contribution of MPO to neutrophil-mediated intracellular microbial killing,

formation of NETs, and tissue damage, as well as the development of AAV. Particular attention will be given to the more recently described and less well known function of neutrophil MPO as a regulator of adaptive immunity.

2. Biosynthesis, Cellular Sources, Storage, and Release of MPO

MPO, which was originally named verdoperoxidase due to its intense green colour, is a highly cationic, heme-containing, glycosylated enzyme [4] which is found mainly in primary (azurophilic) granules of neutrophils, making up approximately 5% of the total dry cell weight [5]. Human neutrophils contain about 5–10-fold higher levels of MPO than murine neutrophils [6]. MPO is also found, to a lesser extent, in monocytes where it constitutes about 1% of total cell protein [7]. During monocyte-to-macrophage differentiation, MPO expression is generally lost [8]. However, MPO can be found in some macrophage subpopulations including resident tissue macrophages such as Kupffer cells [9], peritoneal macrophages [10], and microglia [11], as well as in organ infiltrating macrophages in various inflammatory diseases including atherosclerosis [12], multiple sclerosis (MS) [13],

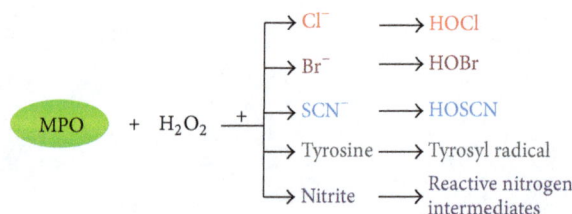

FIGURE 1: *Reactive intermediates formed by MPO*. In the presence of hydrogen peroxide and chloride, bromide, thiocyanate, tyrosine, or nitrite, MPO catalyses the formation of hypochlorous, hypobromous, and hypothiocyanous acids, tyrosyl radical, and reactive nitrogen intermediates. H_2O_2, hydrogen peroxide; Cl^-, chloride; Br^-, bromide; SCN^-, thiocyanate; HOCl, hypochlorous acid; HOBr, hypobromous acid; HOSCN, hypothiocyanous acid.

and AAV [14]. Macrophages can also acquire neutrophil-derived MPO by phagocytosis of apoptotic neutrophils or uptake of extracellular MPO through the mannose receptor [15].

Although it is possible for MPO transcription to be reinitiated in macrophages under certain conditions [16], MPO synthesis is otherwise restricted to myeloid cells in the bone marrow [17, 18]. During granulocyte/monocyte differentiation in the bone marrow, only promyelocytes and promyelomonocytes actively transcribe the MPO gene [17]. The primary 80 kDa MPO translation product undergoes cleavage of the signal peptide and N-linked glycosylation [17], resulting in a 90 kDa apoproMPO which is heme-free and thus enzymatically inactive [17]. During association with endoplasmic reticulum chaperones, calreticulin and calnexin, apoproMPO acquires heme and becomes the enzymatically active precursor proMPO [19], which then enters the Golgi. After exiting the Golgi, a series of proteolytic steps follow during which the propeptide is removed and the protein is cleaved into a heavy (α) subunit (59 kDa) and a light (β) subunit (13.5 kDa) joined together by disulfide bonds [8]. This heavy-light chain complex dimerizes to generate mature, enzymatically active MPO containing a pair of heavy-light protomers and two heme groups [8]. Human and mouse MPO have molecular weights of 146 kDa and 135 kDa, respectively [8, 20].

Mature MPO is stored in azurophilic granules of fully differentiated neutrophils. However, following priming and activation by inflammatory mediators including TLR ligands and cytokines such as GM-CSF and TNF, as well as Ig/Fc receptor-mediated signals [22–24], MPO can be released via multiple mechanisms. Neutrophils can rapidly release MPO by degranulation and by cell death pathways including apoptosis and necrosis [8, 21, 25]. More recently, it has been shown that MPO can be released from neutrophils via the extrusion of NETs [26]. Interestingly, some proMPO is also constitutively secreted by neutrophils via the Golgi [17], but the function and physiological relevance of extracellular proMPO are still to be elucidated.

3. Production of Reactive Intermediates by MPO

In the presence of hydrogen peroxide (H_2O_2) and a low-molecular-weight intermediate (halide: chloride, bromide, or thiocyanate; tyrosine; or nitrite) MPO catalyses the formation of powerful reactive intermediates including hypochlorous (HOCl), hypobromous (HOBr), and hypothiocyanous (HOSCN) acids, tyrosyl radical, and reactive nitrogen intermediates (Figure 1), all of which can have profound effects on cellular function by modifying proteins, lipids, and/or DNA [8]. The H_2O_2 required for MPO function comes mainly from the phagocyte NADPH oxidase during the respiratory burst [8]. Given its abundance in physiological fluids [27], chloride is believed to be the physiological halide and, therefore, a preferred substrate for MPO and subsequent HOCl production in most circumstances.

HOCl is a short-lived, but very potent chlorinating oxidant [28]. It can oxidize/chlorinate a variety of targets including proteins, lipids, and DNA and thus have significant biological effects [28]. Formation of 3-chlorotyrosine (due to HOCl chlorination of tyrosine on proteins) and, more recently described, glutathione sulfonamide (GSA; a product of HOCl-mediated oxidation of glutathione), serves as specific biomarkers of MPO/HOCl production *in vivo* [8, 28–30]. Taurine, a free amino acid present at high concentrations in neutrophils [31], also readily reacts with HOCl to form taurine chloramine, a less reactive, but long-lived oxidant which can contribute to cell damage [8]. More detailed descriptions of the reactions catalysed by MPO and the oxidants it produces are provided elsewhere [8, 32].

4. The MPO/HOCl System in Intracellular and Extracellular Microbial Killing by Neutrophils

Neutrophils are one of the most important front line defenders involved in microbial ingestion and subsequent killing. Several lines of evidence demonstrate that the MPO/HOCl system plays an important role in optimal intracellular killing of bacteria (e.g., *Pseudomonas aeruginosa*) and fungi (e.g., *Candida albicans*) by neutrophils [8, 33, 34]. It should be noted, though, that the clearance of several pathogens including *Staphylococcus aureus* and *Candida glabrata* is not affected by the absence of MPO [8, 34]. In addition, the majority of MPO-deficient patients do not suffer from chronic infections despite the demonstration of a neutrophil microbicidal defect *in vitro* [8]. This suggests the existence of MPO-independent antimicrobial systems such as reactive nitrogen intermediates and proteases which have been shown to contribute to microbicidal activity of neutrophils in the presence as well as in the absence of MPO [32, 35]. In addition, the reduction of microbial killing due to the absence of MPO in humans may be compensated by an enhancement of protective (i.e., antimicrobial) adaptive immunity, as discussed in more detail below. For in-depth discussion about the well recognised and extensively studied role of MPO in intracellular microbial killing by neutrophils, we suggest references to more comprehensive past reviews [32].

Neutrophils are also well known to release NETs, structures composed of decondensed chromatin, histones, and various antimicrobial molecules including elastase and MPO, into the extracellular space [1], thus aiding in the overall elimination and spread of pathogens. NETs can trap extracellular microbes that they come in contact with and, although limited, evidence also exists to suggest that NETs can kill some, but not all, extracellular microbes [36, 37]. Together with elastase, MPO has been demonstrated to associate with nuclear DNA/histones and play a role in NET formation as well as NET-mediated bacterial killing [38–40]. Studies with normal and MPO-deficient human neutrophils showed that MPO contributes to the formation/release of NETs in response to stimulation with PMA or *Candida albicans* [38]. Similarly, the induction of NETs in neutrophils from healthy donors via TNF, IL-8, or IL-1β, in the absence of any infectious stimuli, required the presence of active MPO [41]. A recent study has added to our understanding of how MPO contributes to NET formation inside human neutrophils by showing that MPO activates elastase allowing it to enter the nucleus where it can then associate with DNA/histones [42].

However, MPO is not required for NET formation with all stimuli. For example, in human neutrophils stimulated with *S. aureus* or *E. coli*, inhibition of MPO had no effect on NETs [43]. Reports in which human neutrophils were stimulated with *Pseudomonas aeruginosa* have yielded conflicting results [43, 44], the explanation for which is still to be provided. Furthermore, studies using cells from MPO-deficient animals or inhibitors of MPO activity showed that MPO is not involved in PMA/bacteria-induced NETosis by murine neutrophils [44]. Mouse neutrophils do contain less MPO than their human counterparts [6], which may provide a partial explanation for the discrepancy between the human and murine studies.

In addition to playing a role in NET formation, MPO has been demonstrated to contribute to NET-mediated killing of extracellular microbes. NET-associated MPO is enzymatically active and can produce HOCl in the presence of its substrate, H_2O_2 [39]. Production of HOCl by MPO bound to NETs resulted in the killing of *S. aureus in vitro* and inhibition of MPO or addition of a strong HOCl scavenger methionine reversed this effect [39]. This suggests that HOCl generated by NET-associated MPO may also play an important role in extracellular bacterial killing *in vivo* at sites of inflammation.

5. MPO-Derived Oxidants Cause Tissue Injury in Inflammatory/Autoimmune Diseases

Through the release of various mediators including reactive oxygen species (ROS), proinflammatory cytokines, and proteases, neutrophils play an important role as effector cells in many inflammatory and autoimmune diseases including cardiovascular disease and atherosclerosis, rheumatoid arthritis (RA), and inflammatory diseases of the lung and kidney [1]. Through the formation of reactive oxidating/chlorinating agents, MPO is one of the key neutrophil-derived mediators contributing to organ inflammation and fibrosis in many immune-mediated diseases. As this classical effector function of MPO has been comprehensively described in many other reviews [8, 45], it is not discussed here in detail. Active MPO and/or its products such as HOCl-modified proteins, 3-chlorotyrosine and GSA, are upregulated at sites of inflammation in cardiovascular disease and atherosclerotic lesions, RA joints, and lungs of patients with cystic fibrosis and inflammatory and fibrotic kidney disease [12, 29, 46–49]. This indicates MPO-mediated damage by reactive oxidants, mainly HOCl. Reports showing that there is significant attenuation or exacerbation of disease due to the absence of endogenous or administration of exogenous MPO, respectively, in models of these conditions [50–58], further support the hypothesis that MPO is an important local mediator of inflammation and subsequent organ damage.

MPO-containing NETs have also been implicated in the pathogenesis of several inflammatory diseases including systemic lupus erythematosus (SLE), atherosclerosis, and RA. For example, glomerular NET deposition positively correlates with anti-dsDNA autoantibody levels and the severity of lupus nephritis [59]. Recently, NET-induced macrophage activation and cytokine production have been reported to contribute to the development of atherosclerotic lesions [60]. In addition, lipid oxidation/chlorination by the MPO/HOCl system is suggested to contribute to the pathogenesis of atherosclerosis and SLE [61, 62]. Enhanced formation of NETs, providing a source of citrullinated autoantigens, is also observed in joints of patients with RA [63]. MPO is present on NETs in target organs in SLE, atherosclerosis, and renal vasculitis [14, 59, 60] and it is therefore plausible, although not yet experimentally confirmed, that NET-bound MPO contributes to organ inflammation and injury in those conditions given that NET-associated MPO is enzymatically active and can produce tissue damaging HOCl in the presence of H_2O_2 [39].

6. MPO as an Autoantigen in AAV

In addition to neutrophil-derived inflammatory mediators contributing to tissue damage in inflammatory conditions as effector molecules, neutrophil proteins such as proteinase-3 and MPO play a key role in the development of autoimmune AAV, acting as targets (i.e., autoantigens) against which the pathogenic immune response has been generated. MPO is a common autoantigen in AAV, a disease characterised by inflammation of small blood vessels including glomerular capillaries in the kidney and commonly associated with the presence of pathogenic neutrophil-activating MPO-ANCA [64]. Renal biopsies from vasculitis patients show a prominence of glomerular delayed-type hypersensitivity effectors (T cells, macrophages, and fibrin) and neutrophils, suggesting that cellular immunity, together with MPO-ANCA, plays a significant part in the disease process [65].

Evidence from animal studies, which is supported by human observations and *in vitro* experiments [65–72], suggests that the pathogenesis of MPO-AAV involves 4 major steps, as outlined below. First, MPO-specific autoimmunity develops in secondary lymphoid organs, resulting in the emergence of autoreactive effector CD4 T cells and MPO-ANCA-producing B cells. Although it is not known how autoimmunity to MPO is generated in humans, evidence from animal studies shows that activation of myeloid DCs by NETotic, but not apoptotic or necrotic, neutrophils can result in the generation of MPO-specific autoimmunity and development of renal vasculitis [73]. Of note, the induction of autoimmunity by NET-activated DCs in the animal studies was not restricted to MPO but also resulted in the generation of anti-dsDNA antibodies [73] which are associated with SLE. This is not surprising since NET release by neutrophils would expose a variety of intracellular autoantigens for presentation to DCs. Recently, the immunodominant MPO T cell epitope ($MPO_{409-428}$) was defined in mice [72], and, interestingly, it showed significant overlap with the dominant B cell epitope in AAV patients [74], indicating its relevance to human disease. Importantly, $MPO_{409-428}$ was shown to be nephritogenic since immunisation of mice with $MPO_{409-428}$ resulted in the generation of pathogenic MPO-specific CD4 T cells and ANCA [72].

Second, neutrophil priming by cytokines (e.g., TNF), which may occur after infection-related stimuli, leads to MPO exposure on the cell surface, allowing ANCA to bind and fully activate the neutrophils. Third, ANCA-activated neutrophils lodge in glomeruli [75], causing injury [76] and depositing the autoantigen, MPO [69]. Finally, MPO-specific effector CD4 T cells migrate to inflamed glomeruli where they recognise MPO and direct accumulation of macrophages and fibrin, causing, together with ANCA-induced neutrophil responses, severe and proliferative renal vasculitis (glomerulonephritis; GN) [69, 72]. The antigen presenting cells exposing MPO peptides/MHC-II for recognition by effector CD4 T cells in glomeruli are yet to be identified; however several potential candidates exist including intrinsic glomerular cells such as endothelial cells and podocytes, as well as kidney-infiltrating MPO-positive macrophages and neutrophils. All these cell types can upregulate surface MHC-II and costimulatory molecules in response to proinflammatory stimuli and have been shown to contain MPO in biopsies from patients with AAV [14, 77–80].

In addition to acting as an autoantigen in AAV, MPO may contribute to disease pathogenesis through its enzymatic activity and production of oxidative/chlorinating radicals, although this remains to be confirmed. Extracellular, including NET-associated, MPO is pronounced in glomeruli of AAV patients [14, 26]. Future studies are yet to demonstrate the presence of specific biomarkers of MPO activity such as 3-chlorotyrosine, HOCl-modified proteins, or GSA, to suggest MPO-mediated damage in AAV. Moreover, recent advancements in the development of specific MPO inhibitors for *in vivo* use [81–83] should make it more feasible to investigate whether MPO contributes to renal injury in models of AAV via its enzymatic activity.

7. Nonenzymatic Functions of MPO in Inflammation

MPO actions are mediated predominantly via its enzymatic activity and generation of reactive intermediates. However, evidence exists demonstrating that it can also regulate the function of immune and nonimmune cells via its nonenzymatic effects. For example, by binding to CD11b/CD18 (Mac-1), MPO can induce neutrophil activation in an autocrine fashion including MAPK and NFκB activation, ROS production, surface integrin upregulation, and degranulation [84], as well as decreased apoptosis leading to enhanced inflammation in the lung [85]. In addition, human leukocytes can adhere to MPO via binding to CD11b/CD18 [86] which may also contribute to the proinflammatory effects of MPO by further augmenting leukocyte accumulation at sites of inflammation. Inactive MPO has also been shown to increase macrophage activation such as cytokine production and induction of respiratory burst *in vitro* [87]. These observations are likely to be relevant *in vivo* as well since injection of inactivated MPO into the joints of rats exacerbated symptoms of arthritis [52]. Here, the proinflammatory effects of MPO were reversed by injection of mannan, thus most likely blocking the interaction between extracellular MPO and mannose receptor on macrophages [52]. Furthermore, enzymatically inactive MPO can activate endothelial cells to produce cytokines such as IL-6 and IL-8 [88]. The exact mechanisms by which this occurs are unknown, but MPO-mediated endothelial cell activation is likely to add to the proinflammatory effects of MPO, since the leukocyte-endothelial cell interaction is one of the critical processes in inflammatory responses within tissues.

8. MPO Suppresses the Generation of Adaptive Immunity

In addition to playing an important role at sites of inflammation, neutrophils have been shown to contribute to the development of adaptive immunity. A number of studies have shown that neutrophils can attract and activate immature DCs at sites of inflammation, as well as promote DC trafficking to draining lymph nodes, thus augmenting adaptive immune responses [89–92]. Neutrophils can also rapidly migrate to lymph nodes after antigen injection, mainly via the lymphatics, in a CD11b-, CXCR4-, and, in some cases, CCR7-dependent manner, where they either enhance or suppress the subsequent induction of T cell responses [3, 92–94]. Neutrophil-mediated inhibition of adaptive immunity in mice is supported by studies in humans showing that a subset of human neutrophils can attenuate T cell responses [95]. However, the mechanisms and mediators by which neutrophils inhibit the generation of adaptive immunity in lymph nodes are not well known. Recent studies demonstrating that

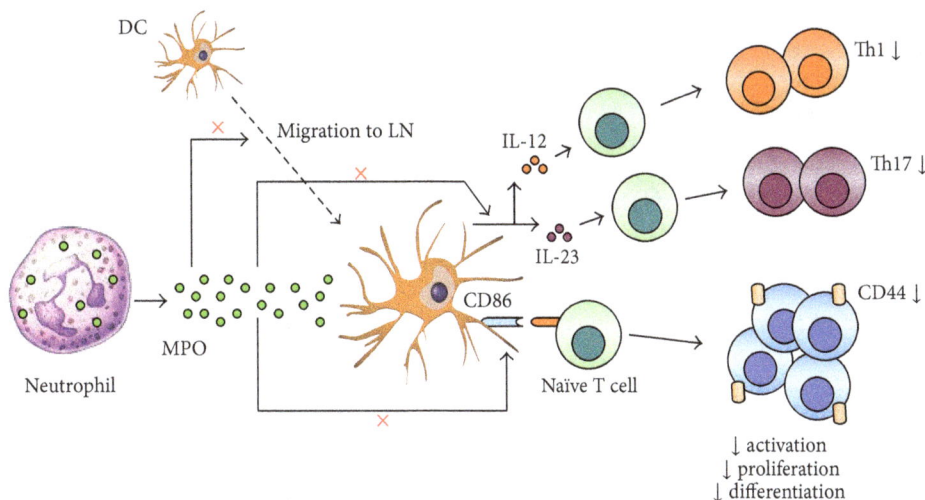

FIGURE 2: *Neutrophil MPO suppresses DC function and adaptive immunity.* Odobasic et al. [21] showed that rapidly infiltrating neutrophils release MPO in draining lymph nodes (LN) after antigen/adjuvant injection. The deposited MPO suppresses various aspects of DC function including costimulatory molecule (e.g., CD86) expression and cytokine (IL-12, IL-23) production and migration, resulting in decreased generation of CD4 T cell responses including T cell activation (CD44 expression), proliferation, and differentiation into Th1 (IFNγ-producing) and Th17 (IL-17A-releasing) effectors.

MPO plays a key role in neutrophil-mediated suppression of adaptive immunity have provided important insights into these important, but underexplored issues [21, 56, 57, 96].

Our group has shown that neutrophils rapidly and transiently infiltrate draining lymph nodes after antigen injection [21], as observed in other models [97]. Four hours after OVA/LPS injection, neutrophils degranulated and deposited MPO in lymph nodes, where it interacted with DCs [21], suggesting that extracellular MPO may affect DC function and subsequent induction of adaptive immunity. Further experiments using MPO-deficient mice or a specific MPO inhibitor, 4-aminobenzoic acid hydrazide (ABAH), showed that MPO, via its enzymatic activity, suppresses various aspects of DC function *in vivo* (Figure 2) including their activation (costimulatory molecule and MHC-II expression, cytokine production), antigen uptake/processing and migration to lymph nodes (by decreasing CCR7 expression), without affecting their apoptosis [21]. MPO-mediated suppression of DC function correlated with decreased generation of adaptive CD4 T cell (particularly Th1) immunity [21]. The suppressive effects of MPO on DCs were confirmed *in vitro* by culturing bone marrow-derived DCs with LPS and either supernatant from wild type (WT) or MPO−/− neutrophils degranulated in the presence or absence of ABAH, or purified enzymatically active native mouse MPO with or without ABAH. Importantly, *in vitro* studies using monocyte-derived DCs and supernatant from degranulated human neutrophils (±ABAH) or purified human MPO showed that MPO has similar inhibitory effects on DCs in humans [21]. Further mechanistic experiments indicated that HOCl and, to a lesser degree, HOBr are the main products involved in MPO-mediated suppression of DC activation *in vitro* [21], consistent with previous studies showing that taurine chloramine (a product formed by the reaction of HOCl and the amino

acid taurine) can decrease DC maturation [98]. HOSCN also had inhibitory effects on DCs, but to a much lesser extent than HOCl and HOBr [21], consistent with HOSCN being a much less reactive oxidant [99]. In contrast, MPO-mediated consumption of nitric oxide, which itself can reduce DC maturation [100], reversed the effects of HOCl on DC activation *in vitro*. Interestingly, Mac-1, an inhibitory receptor on DCs [101], was shown to be involved in the enzymatic MPO-mediated suppression of DC IL-12 production [21]. Although the exact pathways involved in this process are still to be identified, these observations may be explained, in part, by previous reports showing that oxidants (thus potentially MPO-derived products) can induce activating conformational changes in Mac-1 [102], which would be expected to inhibit DC function.

The inhibition of DC function and subsequent generation of adaptive immunity by MPO are relevant to immune-driven diseases since it can result in attenuation of certain T cell-mediated inflammatory conditions. For example, in a model of lupus nephritis, dependent on both autoreactive T cells and humoral immunity [103, 104], we showed that MPO-deficient mice develop more severe renal injury in association with enhanced accumulation of cellular effectors, CD4 T cells, macrophages, and neutrophils [96]. This in turn correlated with enhanced activation of DCs and increased T cell autoimmunity in lymph nodes and spleen. Of note, augmented renal injury was observed in MPO−/− mice despite reduced deposition of humoral mediators of injury (antibody and complement) in glomeruli and decreased presence of markers of oxidative damage, 8-hydroxydeoxyguanosine and GSA [96]. Therefore, in experimental lupus nephritis, MPO-mediated suppression of pathogenic T cell autoimmunity overrides the local damaging effects of MPO in the kidney. These results are concordant with observations in humans showing an increased incidence of lupus nephritis in patients with a polymorphism causing reduced MPO expression [105]. Similarly, in antigen-induced arthritis (AIA), which is very T cell-driven [106], MPO−/− mice developed more severe joint inflammation and damage in association with augmented CD4 T cell responses in the spleen [21]. Furthermore, Brennan et al. demonstrated that MPO−/− mice develop more severe disease in experimental autoimmune encephalomyelitis (EAE), a model of MS, correlating with higher antigen-specific lymphocyte proliferation in draining lymph nodes [13]. Collectively, these studies are supported by a report showing increased incidence of chronic inflammatory conditions in MPO-deficient patients [107], indicating their relevance to humans.

In another murine model of GN induced by a planted foreign antigen (sheep globulin) against the glomerular basement membrane (GBM), our group reported that MPO−/− mice are protected from renal injury in the initial (heterologous) phase of the disease [56] which is mediated by neutrophils but is independent of T cells [108], showing that neutrophil-derived MPO contributes to kidney damage locally. However, during the later (autologous) T cell/macrophage-mediated phase of the disease [109, 110], renal injury was similar between WT and MPO−/− mice, despite enhanced adaptive immunity in the spleen and increased glomerular accumulation of T cells and macrophages in MPO-deficient animals [56]. Together, these experiments suggested that the inhibitory effects of MPO on adaptive immunity in secondary lymphoid organs can also be counterbalanced by the local pathogenic effects of MPO in the target organ.

In other inflammatory conditions though, the injurious local effects of MPO can dominate over its inhibitory effects on immune responses in lymph nodes and spleen, leading to exacerbation of disease, as shown in some models of RA. For example, in collagen-induced arthritis (CIA), mediated by autoreactive T cells and antibody, but also neutrophils [111–113], we demonstrated that disease is attenuated due to MPO deficiency despite enhanced T cell autoimmunity in secondary lymphoid tissues, without an effect on autoantibody levels [57]. This suggested that MPO has dominant proinflammatory local effects in the joints which was confirmed in an acute neutrophil-mediated, T cell-independent KB × N model [114] by showing that joint inflammation and damage were significantly reduced in MPO−/− mice without an effect on circulating cytokines [57].

Overall, these studies indicate that the net impact of MPO on disease development depends on the balance between its local injurious effects in the target organ and inhibitory effects on adaptive immunity in secondary lymphoid tissue and that this balance varies in different autoimmune diseases. Although it is not clearly understood which factors tip this balance in either direction, the above studies do suggest that under conditions where neutrophils play a very important role as effectors of injury in the inflamed organs (e.g., CIA, KB × N arthritis, heterologous anti-GBM GN), the local pathogenic effects of MPO predominate. In contrast, in situations where T cell immunity is the main driver of disease with lesser involvement of neutrophils as effectors (e.g., AIA, lupus nephritis, autologous anti-GBM GN, and

EAE), the immunosuppressive effects of MPO in secondary lymphoid organs predominate, tipping the balance towards MPO-mediated attenuation of disease.

9. MPO Deficiency in Humans

Hereditary MPO deficiency in humans is not rare, with reported prevalence in the United States and Europe ranging from 1 : 1000 to 1 : 4000 [7, 115–118]. Patients lacking MPO are more susceptible to fungal infections, particularly those caused by Candida albicans [118–120]. This is in line with murine studies [33] and the MPO/HOCl system being critical for the direct killing of the fungus and C. albicans-induced NET formation [38, 53, 118]. Although reports exist demonstrating that MPO-deficient patients can have a higher incidence of severe infections [107, 121], the majority of patients lacking MPO have been shown not to be particularly susceptible to chronic infections [8]. Similar to humans, MPO knockout mice exhibit higher susceptibility to some, but not all infections including those caused by Candida glabrata, S. aureus, and S. pneumoniae [8, 34]. This may be due to several factors: (i) MPO-deficiency increases the expression and activity of inducible NO synthase resulting in augmented levels of NO and reactive nitrogen intermediates which have been shown to play a role in the killing of microbes by neutrophils in the presence and in the absence of MPO [32, 35], (ii) the lack of the MPO/HOCl system results in increased activity of antimicrobial neutrophil granule proteases such as elastase and cathepsin-G [122–124], (iii) neutrophils from MPO-deficient patients have increased phagocytosis and degranulation [125, 126], and (iv) the absence of MPO augments the generation of adaptive immunity, as shown by us and others [13, 21, 56, 96]. Therefore, decreased microbial killing due to the absence of MPO/HOCl may be compensated for by other systems involved in pathogen clearance, including increased expression reactive nitrogen intermediates, enhanced activity and release of proteases from neutrophil granules, augmented phagocytic activity of neutrophils, and increased adaptive immunity against the invading microbes.

Although the clinical consequences of MPO deficiency in humans have not been thoroughly investigated, some studies have found that patients with total or subtotal lack of MPO have an increased incidence of chronic inflammatory conditions [107, 121] which are known to be mediated by the adaptive immune system. Similarly, patients with a genetic polymorphism resulting in decreased expression of MPO have a higher risk of developing autoimmune lupus nephritis [105], and MS and diabetes patients have been reported to have lower MPO activity in their blood leukocytes [127, 128]. These observations may be, in part, explained by studies showing increased development of adaptive immune responses and T cell-driven inflammatory conditions in MPO-deficient animals [13, 21, 56, 96], as discussed above.

10. Conclusion

Neutrophils use MPO to mediate many of their multifaceted functions that they have in the immune system (summarised

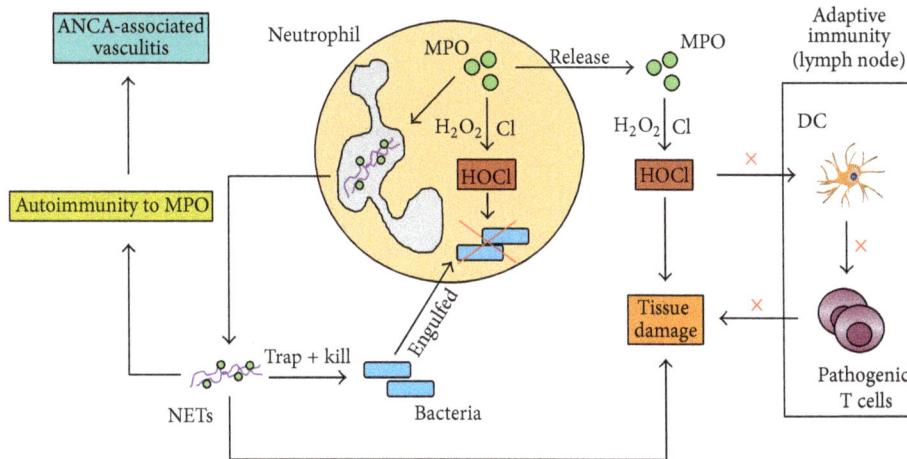

FIGURE 3: *Summary of MPO involvement in neutrophil functions in innate and adaptive immunity.* MPO is involved in microbe clearance by neutrophils both intracellularly (via the production of HOCl) and extracellularly (via the release of NETs). On the other hand, the release of MPO-containing NETs can result in the generation of autoimmunity against MPO and subsequent development of ANCA-associated vasculitis. HOCl that is produced outside of activated neutrophils following MPO release can cause significant tissue damage. In contrast, MPO that is released by neutrophils in lymph nodes can inhibit DC activation and thus generation of adaptive T cell responses, thus attenuating organ injury. HOCl, hypochlorous acid; H_2O_2, hydrogen peroxide; Cl, chloride; NETs, neutrophil extracellular traps; DC, dendritic cell; ANCA, anti-neutrophil cytoplasmic antibody.

in Figure 3). Through the production of HOCl in the presence of H_2O_2 and chloride, MPO plays an important role in the killing of microbes which have been engulfed by neutrophils. MPO can also associate with nuclear DNA/histones and contribute to the formation/release of NETs which trap and sometimes kill (via MPO-produced HOCl) extracellular bacteria. On the other hand, stimulation of DCs by NET-bound MPO can result in the generation of MPO-specific autoimmunity and subsequent development of AAV. MPO release and subsequent formation of HOCl in the extracellular environment following neutrophil activation have been shown to contribute to tissue inflammation and damage. Importantly, MPO deposited by neutrophils in lymph nodes can inhibit DC activation and subsequent generation of adaptive T cell immunity thus leading to attenuation of immune-mediated tissue injury. Future studies will not only further our understanding about these already described functions of MPO but are also likely to uncover novel roles of this neutrophil enzyme in the regulation of cellular events that take place during the course of innate and adaptive immune responses.

Conflict of Interests

The authors declare that there is no conflict of interests regarding the publication of this paper.

References

[1] T. N. Mayadas, X. Cullere, and C. A. Lowell, "The multifaceted functions of neutrophils," *Annual Review of Pathology: Mechanisms of Disease*, vol. 9, pp. 181–218, 2014.

[2] A. Schreiber and R. Kettritz, "The neutrophil in antineutrophil cytoplasmic autoantibody-associated vasculitis," *Journal of Leukocyte Biology*, vol. 94, no. 4, pp. 623–631, 2013.

[3] C.-W. Yang, B. S. I. Strong, M. J. Miller, and E. R. Unanue, "Neutrophils influence the level of antigen presentation during the immune response to protein antigens in adjuvants," *Journal of Immunology*, vol. 185, no. 5, pp. 2927–2934, 2010.

[4] K. Agner, "Verdoperoxidase. A ferment isolated from leukocytes," *Acta Chemica Scandinavica*, vol. 2, supplement 8, pp. 1–62, 1941.

[5] J. Schultz and K. Kaminker, "Myeloperoxidase of the leucocyte of normal human blood. I. Content and localization," *Archives of Biochemistry and Biophysics*, vol. 96, no. 3, pp. 465–467, 1962.

[6] P. G. Rausch and T. G. Moore, "Granule enzymes of polymorphonuclear neutrophils: a phylogenetic comparison," *Blood*, vol. 46, no. 6, pp. 913–919, 1975.

[7] A. Bos, R. Wever, and D. Roos, "Characterization and quantification of the peroxidase in human monocytes," *Biochimica et Biophysica Acta*, vol. 525, no. 1, pp. 37–44, 1978.

[8] B. S. van der Veen, M. P. de Winther, and P. Heeringa, "Myeloperoxidase: molecular mechanisms of action and their relevance to human health and disease," *Antioxidants & Redox Signaling*, vol. 11, no. 11, pp. 2899–2937, 2009.

[9] K. E. Brown, E. M. Brunt, and J. W. Heinecke, "Immunohistochemical detection of myeloperoxidase and its oxidation products in Kupffer cells of human liver," *American Journal of Pathology*, vol. 159, no. 6, pp. 2081–2088, 2001.

[10] M. R. Rodrigues, D. Rodriguez, M. Russo, and A. Campa, "Macrophage activation includes high intracellular myeloperoxidase activity," *Biochemical and Biophysical Research Communications*, vol. 292, no. 4, pp. 869–873, 2002.

[11] R. M. Nagra, B. Becher, W. W. Tourtellotte et al., "Immunohistochemical and genetic evidence of myeloperoxidase involvement in multiple sclerosis," *Journal of Neuroimmunology*, vol. 78, no. 1-2, pp. 97–107, 1997.

[12] E. Malle, G. Waeg, R. Schreiber, E. F. Gröne, W. Sattler, and H.-J. Gröne, "Immunohistochemical evidence for the myeloperoxidase/H$_2$O$_2$/halide system in human atherosclerotic lesions: colocalization of myeloperoxidase and hypochlorite-modified proteins," *European Journal of Biochemistry*, vol. 267, no. 14, pp. 4495–4503, 2000.

[13] M.-L. Brennan, A. Gaur, A. Pahuja, A. J. Lusis, and W. F. Reynolds, "Mice lacking myeloperoxidase are more susceptible to experimental autoimmune encephalomyelitis," *Journal of Neuroimmunology*, vol. 112, no. 1-2, pp. 97–105, 2001.

[14] K. M. O'Sullivan, C. Y. Lo, S. A. Summers et al., "Renal participation of myeloperoxidase in antineutrophil cytoplasmic antibody (ANCA)-associated glomerulonephritis," *Kidney International*, vol. 88, no. 5, pp. 1030–1046, 2015.

[15] V. L. Shepherd and J. R. Hoidal, "Clearance of neutrophil-derived myeloperoxidase by the macrophage mannose receptor," *American Journal of Respiratory Cell and Molecular Biology*, vol. 2, no. 4, pp. 335–340, 1990.

[16] S. Sugiyama, Y. Okada, G. K. Sukhova, R. Virmani, J. W. Heinecke, and P. Libby, "Macrophage myeloperoxidase regulation by granulocyte macrophage colony-stimulating factor in human atherosclerosis and implications in acute coronary syndromes," *The American Journal of Pathology*, vol. 158, no. 3, pp. 879–891, 2001.

[17] M. Hansson, I. Olsson, and W. M. Nauseef, "Biosynthesis, processing, and sorting of human myeloperoxidase," *Archives of Biochemistry and Biophysics*, vol. 445, no. 2, pp. 214–224, 2006.

[18] A. Tobler, C. W. Miller, K. R. Johnson, M. E. Selsted, G. Rovera, and H. P. Koeffler, "Regulation of gene expression of myeloperoxidase during myeloid differentiation," *Journal of Cellular Physiology*, vol. 136, no. 2, pp. 215–225, 1988.

[19] W. M. Nauseef, S. J. McCormick, and M. Goedken, "Coordinated participation of calreticulin and calnexin in the biosynthesis of myeloperoxidase," *The Journal of Biological Chemistry*, vol. 273, no. 12, pp. 7107–7111, 1998.

[20] M. Shafran and S. Lyslova, "Purification and properties of myeloperoxidase from mice leukocytes," *Voprosy Meditsinskoĭ Khimii*, vol. 21, pp. 629–633, 1975.

[21] D. Odobasic, A. R. Kitching, Y. Yang et al., "Neutrophil myeloperoxidase regulates T-cell-driven tissue inflammation in mice by inhibiting dendritic cell function," *Blood*, vol. 121, no. 20, pp. 4195–4204, 2013.

[22] Y. Dang, G. M. Lowe, S. W. Edwards, and D. W. Galvani, "The effects of GM-CSF on myeloperoxidase release in normal and myelodysplastic neutrophils," *Leukemia Research*, vol. 17, no. 12, pp. 1037–1044, 1993.

[23] J. U. Holle, M. Windmöller, C. Lange, W. L. Gross, K. Herlyn, and E. Csernok, "Toll-like receptor TLR2 and TLR9 ligation triggers neutrophil activation in granulomatosis with polyangiitis," *Rheumatology*, vol. 52, no. 7, pp. 1183–1189, 2013.

[24] W. W. Chatham, A. Turkiewicz, and W. D. Blackburn Jr., "Determinants of neutrophil HOCl generation: ligand-dependent responses and the role of surface adhesion," *Journal of Leukocyte Biology*, vol. 56, no. 5, pp. 654–660, 1994.

[25] B. J. Bentwood and P. M. Henson, "The sequential release of granule constituents from human neutrophils," *Journal of Immunology*, vol. 124, no. 2, pp. 855–862, 1980.

[26] K. Kessenbrock, M. Krumbholz, U. Schönermarck et al., "Netting neutrophils in autoimmune small-vessel vasculitis," *Nature Medicine*, vol. 15, no. 6, pp. 623–625, 2009.

[27] H. Fliss, "Oxidation of proteins in rat heart and lungs by polymorphonuclear leukocyte oxidants," *Molecular and Cellular Biochemistry*, vol. 84, no. 2, pp. 177–188, 1988.

[28] C. C. Winterbourn, "Biological reactivity and biomarkers of the neutrophil oxidant, hypochlorous acid," *Toxicology*, vol. 181-182, pp. 223–227, 2002.

[29] D. T. Harwood, A. J. Kettle, S. Brennan, and C. C. Winterbourn, "Simultaneous determination of reduced glutathione, glutathione disulphide and glutathione sulphonamide in cells and physiological fluids by isotope dilution liquid chromatography-tandem mass spectrometry," *Journal of Chromatography B: Analytical Technologies in the Biomedical and Life Sciences*, vol. 877, no. 28, pp. 3393–3399, 2009.

[30] D. T. Harwood, A. J. Kettle, and C. C. Winterbourn, "Production of glutathione sulfonamide and dehydroglutathione from GSH by myeloperoxidase-derived oxidants and detection using a novel LC-MS/MS method," *Biochemical Journal*, vol. 399, no. 1, pp. 161–168, 2006.

[31] D. B. Learn, V. A. Fried, and E. L. Thomas, "Taurine and hypotaurine content of human leukocytes," *Journal of Leukocyte Biology*, vol. 48, no. 2, pp. 174–182, 1990.

[32] S. J. Klebanoff, A. J. Kettle, H. Rosen, C. C. Winterbourn, and W. M. Nauseef, "Myeloperoxidase: a front-line defender against phagocytosed microorganisms," *Journal of Leukocyte Biology*, vol. 93, no. 2, pp. 185–198, 2013.

[33] Y. Aratani, H. Koyama, S.-I. Nyui, K. Suzuki, F. Kura, and N. Maeda, "Severe impairment in early host defense against Candida albicans in mice deficient in myeloperoxidase," *Infection and Immunity*, vol. 67, no. 4, pp. 1828–1836, 1999.

[34] Y. Aratani, F. Kura, H. Watanabe et al., "Differential host susceptibility to pulmonary infections with bacteria and fungi in mice deficient in myeloperoxidase," *Journal of Infectious Diseases*, vol. 182, no. 4, pp. 1276–1279, 2000.

[35] V. Brovkovych, X.-P. Gao, E. Ong et al., "Augmented inducible nitric oxide synthase expression and increased NO production reduce sepsis-induced lung injury and mortality in myeloperoxidase-null mice," *American Journal of Physiology—Lung Cellular and Molecular Physiology*, vol. 295, no. 1, pp. L96–L103, 2008.

[36] S. Bruns, O. Kniemeyer, M. Hasenberg et al., "Production of extracellular traps against aspergillus fumigatus in vitro and in infected lung tissue is dependent on invading neutrophils and influenced by hydrophobin roda," *PLoS Pathogens*, vol. 6, no. 4, Article ID e1000873, 2010.

[37] V. Brinkmann, U. Reichard, C. Goosmann et al., "Neutrophil extracellular traps kill bacteria," *Science*, vol. 303, no. 5663, pp. 1532–1535, 2004.

[38] K. D. Metzler, T. A. Fuchs, W. M. Nauseef et al., "Myeloperoxidase is required for neutrophil extracellular trap formation: implications for innate immunity," *Blood*, vol. 117, no. 3, pp. 953–959, 2011.

[39] H. Parker, A. M. Albrett, A. J. Kettle, and C. C. Winterbourn, "Myeloperoxidase associated with neutrophil extracellular traps is active and mediates bacterial killing in the presence of hydrogen peroxide," *Journal of Leukocyte Biology*, vol. 91, no. 3, pp. 369–376, 2012.

[40] V. Papayannopoulos, K. D. Metzler, A. Hakkim, and A. Zychlinsky, "Neutrophil elastase and myeloperoxidase regulate the formation of neutrophil extracellular traps," *Journal of Cell Biology*, vol. 191, no. 3, pp. 677–691, 2010.

[41] R. S. Keshari, A. Jyoti, M. Dubey et al., "Cytokines induced neutrophil extracellular traps formation: implication for the inflammatory disease condition," *PLoS ONE*, vol. 7, no. 10, Article ID e48111, 2012.

[42] K. D. Metzler, C. Goosmann, A. Lubojemska, A. Zychlinsky, and V. Papayannopoulos, "A myeloperoxidase-containing complex regulates neutrophil elastase release and actin dynamics during NETosis," *Cell Reports*, vol. 8, no. 3, pp. 883–896, 2014.

[43] H. Parker, M. Dragunow, M. B. Hampton, A. J. Kettle, and C. C. Winterbourn, "Requirements for NADPH oxidase and myeloperoxidase in neutrophil extracellular trap formation differ depending on the stimulus," *Journal of Leukocyte Biology*, vol. 92, no. 4, pp. 841–849, 2012.

[44] K. Akong-Moore, O. A. Chow, M. von Köckritz-Blickwede, and V. Nizet, "Influences of chloride and hypochlorite on neutrophil extracellular trap formation," *PLoS ONE*, vol. 7, no. 8, Article ID e42984, 2012.

[45] K. Friedrichs, S. Baldus, and A. Klinke, "Fibrosis in atrial fibrillation—role of reactive species and MPO," *Frontiers in Physiology*, vol. 3, article 214, 2012.

[46] P. P. Bradley, R. D. Christensen, and G. Rothstein, "Cellular and extracellular myeloperoxidase in pyogenic inflammation," *Blood*, vol. 60, no. 3, pp. 618–622, 1982.

[47] A. J. Kettle, T. Chan, I. Osberg et al., "Myeloperoxidase and protein oxidation in the airways of young children with cystic fibrosis," *American Journal of Respiratory and Critical Care Medicine*, vol. 170, no. 12, pp. 1317–1323, 2004.

[48] E. Malle, C. Woenckhaus, G. Waeg, H. Esterbauer, E. F. Gröne, and H.-J. Gröne, "Immunological evidence for hypochlorite-modified proteins in human kidney," *The American Journal of Pathology*, vol. 150, no. 2, pp. 603–615, 1997.

[49] L. K. Stamp, I. Khalilova, J. M. Tarr et al., "Myeloperoxidase and oxidative stress in rheumatoid arthritis," *Rheumatology*, vol. 51, no. 10, Article ID kes193, pp. 1796–1803, 2012.

[50] R. J. Johnson, W. G. Couser, E. Y. Chi, S. Adler, and S. J. Klebanoff, "New mechanism for glomerular injury. Myeloperoxidase-hydrogen peroxide-halide system," *The Journal of Clinical Investigation*, vol. 79, no. 5, pp. 1379–1387, 1987.

[51] R. J. Johnson, S. J. Klebanoff, R. F. Ochi et al., "Participation of the myeloperoxidase-H_2O_2-halide system in immune complex nephritis," *Kidney International*, vol. 32, no. 3, pp. 342–349, 1987.

[52] D. L. Lefkowitz, M. P. Gelderman, S. R. Fuhrmann et al., "Neutrophilic myeloperoxidase-macrophage interactions perpetuate chronic inflammation associated with experimental arthritis," *Clinical Immunology*, vol. 91, no. 2, pp. 145–155, 1999.

[53] A. Lehners, S. Lange, G. Niemann et al., "Myeloperoxidase deficiency ameliorates progression of chronic kidney disease in mice," *American Journal of Physiology—Renal Physiology*, vol. 307, no. 4, pp. F407–F417, 2014.

[54] R. A. Matthijsen, D. Huugen, N. T. Hoebers et al., "Myeloperoxidase is critically involved in the induction of organ damage after renal ischemia reperfusion," *The American Journal of Pathology*, vol. 171, no. 6, pp. 1743–1752, 2007.

[55] T. S. McMillen, J. W. Heinecke, and R. C. LeBoeuf, "Expression of human myeloperoxidase by macrophages promotes atherosclerosis in mice," *Circulation*, vol. 111, no. 21, pp. 2798–2804, 2005.

[56] D. Odobasic, A. R. Kitching, T. J. Semple, and S. R. Holdsworth, "Endogenous myeloperoxidase promotes neutrophil-mediated renal injury, but attenuates T cell immunity inducing crescentic glomerulonephritis," *Journal of the American Society of Nephrology*, vol. 18, no. 3, pp. 760–770, 2007.

[57] D. Odobasic, Y. Yang, R. C. M. Muljadi et al., "Endogenous myeloperoxidase is a mediator of joint inflammation and damage in experimental arthritis," *Arthritis and Rheumatology*, vol. 66, no. 4, pp. 907–917, 2014.

[58] V. Rudolph, R. P. Andrié, T. K. Rudolph et al., "Myeloperoxidase acts as a profibrotic mediator of atrial fibrillation," *Nature Medicine*, vol. 16, no. 4, pp. 470–474, 2010.

[59] E. Villanueva, S. Yalavarthi, C. C. Berthier et al., "Netting neutrophils induce endothelial damage, infiltrate tissues, and expose immunostimulatory molecules in systemic lupus erythematosus," *Journal of Immunology*, vol. 187, no. 1, pp. 538–552, 2011.

[60] A. Warnatsch, M. Ioannou, Q. Wang, and V. Papayannopoulos, "Inflammation. Neutrophil extracellular traps license macrophages for cytokine production in atherosclerosis," *Science*, vol. 349, no. 6245, pp. 316–320, 2015.

[61] B. Shao, C. Tang, A. Sinha et al., "Humans with atherosclerosis have impaired ABCA1 cholesterol efflux and enhanced high-density lipoprotein oxidation by myeloperoxidase," *Circulation Research*, vol. 114, no. 11, pp. 1733–1742, 2014.

[62] C. K. Smith, A. Vivekanandan-Giri, C. Tang et al., "Neutrophil extracellular trap-derived enzymes oxidize high-density lipoprotein: an additional proatherogenic mechanism in systemic lupus erythematosus," *Arthritis and Rheumatology*, vol. 66, no. 9, pp. 2532–2544, 2014.

[63] R. Khandpur, C. Carmona-Rivera, A. Vivekanandan-Giri et al., "NETs are a source of citrullinated autoantigens and stimulate inflammatory responses in rheumatoid arthritis," *Science Translational Medicine*, vol. 5, no. 178, Article ID 178ra40, 2013.

[64] S. M. Flint, E. F. McKinney, and K. G. C. Smith, "Emerging concepts in the pathogenesis of antineutrophil cytoplasmic antibody-associated vasculitis," *Current Opinion in Rheumatology*, vol. 27, no. 2, pp. 197–203, 2015.

[65] M. A. Cunningham, X. R. Huang, J. P. Dowling, P. G. Tipping, and S. R. Holdsworth, "Prominence of cell-mediated immunity effectors in 'pauci-immune' glomerulonephritis," *Journal of the American Society of Nephrology*, vol. 10, no. 3, pp. 499–506, 1999.

[66] A. M. Coughlan, S. J. Freeley, and M. G. Robson, "Animal models of anti-neutrophil cytoplasmic antibody-associated vasculitis," *Clinical and Experimental Immunology*, vol. 169, no. 3, pp. 229–237, 2012.

[67] P.-Y. Gan, S. R. Holdsworth, A. R. Kitching, and J. D. Ooi, "Myeloperoxidase (MPO)-specific CD4$^+$ T cells contribute to MPO-anti-neutrophil cytoplasmic antibody (ANCA) associated glomerulonephritis," *Cellular Immunology*, vol. 282, no. 1, pp. 21–27, 2013.

[68] R. Kettritz, "How anti-neutrophil cytoplasmic autoantibodies activate neutrophils," *Clinical and Experimental Immunology*, vol. 169, no. 3, pp. 220–228, 2012.

[69] A.-J. Ruth, A. R. Kitching, R. Y. Q. Kwan et al., "Anti-neutrophil cytoplasmic antibodies and effector CD4$^+$ cells play nonredundant roles in anti-myeloperoxidase crescentic glomerulonephritis," *Journal of the American Society of Nephrology*, vol. 17, no. 7, pp. 1940–1949, 2006.

[70] H. Xiao, P. Heeringa, P. Hu et al., "Antineutrophil cytoplasmic autoantibodies specific for myeloperoxidase cause glomerulonephritis and vasculitis in mice," *Journal of Clinical Investigation*, vol. 110, no. 7, pp. 955–963, 2002.

[71] L. Harper, D. Radford, T. Plant, M. Drayson, D. Adu, and C. O. S. Savage, "IgG from myeloperoxidase-antineutrophil cytoplasmic antibody-positive patients stimulates greater activation of primed neutrophils than IgG from proteinase 3-antineutrophil cytosplasmic antibody-positive patients," *Arthritis & Rheumatism*, vol. 44, no. 4, pp. 921–930, 2001.

[72] J. D. Ooi, J. Chang, M. J. Hickey et al., "The immunodominant myeloperoxidase T-cell epitope induces local cell-mediated injury in antimyeloperoxidase glomerulonephritis," *Proceedings of the National Academy of Sciences of the United States of America*, vol. 109, no. 39, pp. E2615–E2624, 2012.

[73] S. Sangaletti, C. Tripodo, C. Chiodoni et al., "Neutrophil extracellular traps mediate transfer of cytoplasmic neutrophil antigens to myeloid dendritic cells toward ANCA induction and associated autoimmunity," *Blood*, vol. 120, no. 15, pp. 3007–3018, 2012.

[74] A. J. Roth, J. D. Ooi, J. J. Hess et al., "Epitope specificity determines pathogenicity and detectability in anca-associated vasculitis," *Journal of Clinical Investigation*, vol. 123, no. 4, pp. 1773–1783, 2013.

[75] M. P. Kuligowski, R. Y. Q. Kwan, C. Lo et al., "Antimyeloperoxidase antibodies rapidly induce α4-integrin-dependent glomerular neutrophil adhesion," *Blood*, vol. 113, no. 25, pp. 6485–6494, 2009.

[76] H. Xiao, P. Heeringa, P. Hu et al., "Antineutrophil cytoplasmic autoantibodies specific for myeloperoxidase cause glomerulonephritis and vasculitis in mice," *Journal of Clinical Investigation*, vol. 110, no. 7, pp. 955–963, 2002.

[77] A. Goldwich, M. Burkard, M. Ölke et al., "Podocytes are non-hematopoietic professional antigen-presenting cells," *Journal of the American Society of Nephrology*, vol. 24, no. 6, pp. 906–916, 2013.

[78] C. Iking-Konert, S. Vogt, M. Radsak, C. Wagner, G. M. Hänsch, and K. Andrassy, "Polymorphonuclear neutrophils in Wegener's granulomatosis acquire characteristics of antigen presenting cells," *Kidney International*, vol. 60, no. 6, pp. 2247–2262, 2001.

[79] P. A. Knolle, T. Germann, U. Treichel et al., "Endotoxin down-regulates T cell activation by antigen-presenting liver sinusoidal endothelial cells," *Journal of Immunology*, vol. 162, no. 3, pp. 1401–1407, 1999.

[80] D. V. Ostanin, E. Kurmaeva, K. Furr et al., "Acquisition of antigen-presenting functions by neutrophils isolated from mice with chronic colitis," *Journal of Immunology*, vol. 188, no. 3, pp. 1491–1502, 2012.

[81] A.-K. Tide, T. Sjögren, M. Svensson et al., "2-Thioxanthines are mechanism-based inactivators of myeloperoxidase that block oxidative stress during inflammation," *The Journal of Biological Chemistry*, vol. 286, no. 43, pp. 37578–37589, 2011.

[82] W. Zheng, R. Warner, R. Ruggeri et al., "PF-1355, A mechanism-based myeloperoxidase inhibitor, prevents immune complex vasculitis and anti-glomerular basement membrane glomerulonephritis," *Journal of Pharmacology and Experimental Therapeutics*, vol. 353, no. 2, pp. 288–298, 2015.

[83] C. Liu, R. Desikan, Z. Ying et al., "Effects of a novel pharmacologic inhibitor of myeloperoxidase in a mouse atherosclerosis model," *PLoS ONE*, vol. 7, no. 12, Article ID e50767, 2012.

[84] D. Lau, H. Mollnau, J. P. Eiserich et al., "Myeloperoxidase mediates neutrophil activation by association with CD11b/CD18 integrins," *Proceedings of the National Academy of Sciences of the United States of America*, vol. 102, no. 2, pp. 431–436, 2005.

[85] D. El Kebir, L. József, W. Pan, and J. G. Filep, "Myeloperoxidase delays neutrophil apoptosis through CD11b/CD18 integrins and prolongs inflammation," *Circulation Research*, vol. 103, no. 4, pp. 352–359, 2008.

[86] M. W. Johansson, M. Patarroyo, F. Oberg, A. Siegbahn, and K. Nilsson, "Myeloperoxidase mediates cell adhesion via the alpha M beta 2 integrin (Mac-1, CD11b/CD18)," *Journal of Cell Science*, vol. 110, part 9, pp. 1133–1139, 1997.

[87] K. Grattendick, R. Stuart, E. Roberts et al., "Alveolar macrophage activation by myeloperoxidase: a model for exacerbation of lung inflammation," *American Journal of Respiratory Cell and Molecular Biology*, vol. 26, no. 6, pp. 716–722, 2002.

[88] D. L. Lefkowitz, E. Roberts, K. Grattendick et al., "The endothelium and cytokine secretion: the role of peroxidases as immunoregulators," *Cellular Immunology*, vol. 202, no. 1, pp. 23–30, 2000.

[89] S. Bennouna, S. K. Bliss, T. J. Curiel, and E. Y. Denkers, "Cross-talk in the innate immune system: neutrophils instruct recruitment and activation of dendritic cells during microbial infection," *The Journal of Immunology*, vol. 171, no. 11, pp. 6052–6058, 2003.

[90] S. Bennouna and E. Y. Denkers, "Microbial antigen triggers rapid mobilization of TNF-alpha to the surface of mouse neutrophils transforming them into inducers of high-level dendritic cell TNF-alpha production," *The Journal of Immunology*, vol. 174, no. 8, pp. 4845–4851, 2005.

[91] F. C. Weber, T. Németh, J. Z. Csepregi et al., "Neutrophils are required for both the sensitization and elicitation phase of contact hypersensitivity," *Journal of Experimental Medicine*, vol. 212, no. 1, pp. 15–22, 2015.

[92] H. R. Hampton, J. Bailey, M. Tomura, R. Brink, and T. Chtanova, "Microbe-dependent lymphatic migration of neutrophils modulates lymphocyte proliferation in lymph nodes," *Nature Communications*, vol. 6, article 7139, 2015.

[93] C. Beauvillain, P. Cunin, A. Doni et al., "CCR7 is involved in the migration of neutrophils to lymph nodes," *Blood*, vol. 117, no. 4, pp. 1196–1204, 2011.

[94] C. V. Gorlino, R. P. Ranocchia, M. F. Harman et al., "Neutrophils exhibit differential requirements for homing molecules in their lymphatic and blood trafficking into draining lymph nodes," *The Journal of Immunology*, vol. 193, no. 4, pp. 1966–1974, 2014.

[95] J. Pillay, V. M. Kamp, E. Van Hoffen et al., "A subset of neutrophils in human systemic inflammation inhibits T cell responses through Mac-1," *Journal of Clinical Investigation*, vol. 122, no. 1, pp. 327–336, 2012.

[96] D. Odobasic, R. C. Muljadi, K. M. O'Sullivan et al., "Suppression of autoimmunity and renal disease in pristane-induced lupus by myeloperoxidase," *Arthritis & Rheumatology*, vol. 67, no. 7, pp. 1868–1880, 2015.

[97] V. Abadie, E. Badell, P. Douillard et al., "Neutrophils rapidly migrate via lymphatics after *Mycobacterium bovis* BCG intradermal vaccination and shuttle live bacilli to the draining lymph nodes," *Blood*, vol. 106, no. 5, pp. 1843–1850, 2005.

[98] J. Marcinkiewicz, B. Nowak, A. Grabowska, M. Bobek, L. Petrovska, and B. Chain, "Regulation of murine dendritic cell functions in vitro by taurine chloramine, a major product of the neutrophil myeloperoxidase-halide system," *Immunology*, vol. 98, no. 3, pp. 371–378, 1999.

[99] C. L. Hawkins, "The role of hypothiocyanous acid (HOSCN) in biological systems," *Free Radical Research*, vol. 43, no. 12, pp. 1147–1158, 2009.

[100] H. Xiong, C. Zhu, F. Li et al., "Inhibition of interleukin-12 p40 transcription and NF-κB activation by nitric oxide in murine macrophages and dendritic cells," *Journal of Biological Chemistry*, vol. 279, no. 11, pp. 10776–10783, 2004.

[101] E. M. Behrens, U. Sriram, D. K. Shivers et al., "Complement receptor 3 ligation of dendritic cells suppresses their stimulatory capacity," *The Journal of Immunology*, vol. 178, no. 10, pp. 6268–6279, 2007.

[102] E. Blouin, L. Halbwachs-Mecarelli, and P. Rieu, "Redox regulation of β2-integrin CD11b/CD18 activation," *European Journal of Immunology*, vol. 29, no. 11, pp. 3419–3431, 1999.

[103] T. K. Nowling and G. S. Gilkeson, "Mechanisms of tissue injury in lupus nephritis," *Arthritis Research and Therapy*, vol. 13, no. 6, article 250, 2011.

[104] W. H. Reeves, P. Y. Lee, J. S. Weinstein, M. Satoh, and L. Lu, "Induction of autoimmunity by pristane and other naturally occurring hydrocarbons," *Trends in Immunology*, vol. 30, no. 9, pp. 455–464, 2009.

[105] H. Bouali, P. Nietert, T. M. Nowling et al., "Association of the G-463A myeloperoxidase gene polymorphism with renal disease in African Americans with systemic lupus erythematosus," *Journal of Rheumatology*, vol. 34, no. 10, pp. 2028–2034, 2007.

[106] D. Pohlers, K. Nissler, O. Frey et al., "Anti-CD4 monoclonal antibody treatment in acute and early chronic antigen-induced arthritis: influence on T helper cell activation," *Clinical and Experimental Immunology*, vol. 135, no. 3, pp. 409–415, 2004.

[107] D. Kutter, P. Devaquet, G. Vanderstocken, J. M. Paulus, V. Marchal, and A. Gothot, "Consequences of total and subtotal myeloperoxidase deficiency: risk or benefit ?" *Acta Haematologica*, vol. 104, no. 1, pp. 10–15, 2000.

[108] M. P. Kuligowski, A. R. Kitching, and M. J. Hickey, "Leukocyte recruitment to the inflamed glomerulus: a critical role for platelet-derived P-selectin in the absence of rolling," *Journal of Immunology*, vol. 176, no. 11, pp. 6991–6999, 2006.

[109] X. R. Huang, S. R. Holdsworth, and P. G. Tipping, "Evidence for delayed-type hypersensitivity mechanisms in glomerular crescent formation," *Kidney International*, vol. 46, no. 1, pp. 69–78, 1994.

[110] P. G. Tipping, X. R. Huang, M. Qi, G. Y. Van, and W. W. Tang, "Crescentic glomerulonephritis in CD4- and CD8-deficient mice: requirement for CD4 but not CD8 cells," *The American Journal of Pathology*, vol. 152, no. 6, pp. 1541–1548, 1998.

[111] J. L. Eyles, M. J. Hickey, M. U. Norman et al., "A key role for G-CSF-induced neutrophil production and trafficking during inflammatory arthritis," *Blood*, vol. 112, no. 13, pp. 5193–5201, 2008.

[112] C. Mauri, C.-Q. Q. Chu, D. Woodrow, L. Mori, and M. Londei, "Treatment of a newly established transgenic model of chronic arthritis with nondepleting anti-CD4 monoclonal antibody," *The Journal of Immunology*, vol. 159, no. 10, pp. 5032–5041, 1997.

[113] L. Svensson, J. Jirholt, R. Holmdahl, and L. Jansson, "B cell-deficient mice do not develop type II collagen-induced arthritis (CIA)," *Clinical and Experimental Immunology*, vol. 111, no. 3, pp. 521–526, 1998.

[114] B. T. Wipke and P. M. Allen, "Essential role of neutrophils in the initiation and progression of a murine model of rheumatoid arthritis," *The Journal of Immunology*, vol. 167, no. 3, pp. 1601–1608, 2001.

[115] R. Cramer, M. R. Soranzo, and P. Dri, "Incidence of myeloperoxidase deficiency in an area of northern Italy: histochemical, biochemical and functional studies," *British Journal of Haematology*, vol. 51, no. 1, pp. 81–87, 1982.

[116] M. Kitahara, H. J. Eyre, Y. Simonian, C. L. Atkin, and S. J. Hasstedt, "Hereditary myeloperoxidase deficiency," *Blood*, vol. 57, no. 5, pp. 888–893, 1981.

[117] C. Larrocha, M. Fernandez de Castro, G. Fontan, A. Viloria, J. L. Fernández-Chacón, and C. Jiménez, "Hereditary myeloperoxidase deficiency: study of 12 cases," *Scandinavian Journal of Haematology*, vol. 29, no. 5, pp. 389–397, 1982.

[118] M. F. Parry, R. K. Root, J. A. Metcalf, K. K. Delaney, L. S. Kaplow, and W. J. Richar, "Myeloperoxidase deficiency: prevalence and clinical significance," *Annals of Internal Medicine*, vol. 95, no. 3, pp. 293–301, 1981.

[119] R. I. Lehrer and M. J. Cline, "Leukocyte myeloperoxidase deficiency and disseminated candidiasis: the role of myeloperoxidase in resistance to *Candida* infection," *Journal of Clinical Investigation*, vol. 48, no. 8, pp. 1478–1488, 1969.

[120] C. Nguyen and H. P. Katner, "Myeloperoxidase deficiency manifesting as pustular candidal dermatitis," *Clinical Infectious Diseases*, vol. 24, no. 2, pp. 258–260, 1997.

[121] D. Kutter, "Prevalence of myeloperoxidase deficiency: population studies using Bayer-Technicon automated hematology," *Journal of Molecular Medicine*, vol. 76, no. 10, pp. 669–675, 1998.

[122] T. O. Hirche, J. P. Gaut, J. W. Heinecke, and A. Belaaouaj, "Myeloperoxidase plays critical roles in killing *Klebsiella pneumoniae* and inactivating neutrophil elastase: effects on host defense," *The Journal of Immunology*, vol. 174, no. 3, pp. 1557–1565, 2005.

[123] B. Korkmaz, T. Moreau, and F. Gauthier, "Neutrophil elastase, proteinase 3 and cathepsin G: physicochemical properties, activity and physiopathological functions," *Biochimie*, vol. 90, no. 2, pp. 227–242, 2008.

[124] B. Shao, A. Belaaouaj, C. L. M. J. Verlinde, X. Fu, and J. W. Heinecke, "Methionine sulfoxide and proteolytic cleavage contribute to the inactivation of cathepsin G by hypochlorous acid: an oxidative mechanism for regulation of serine proteinases by myeloperoxidase," *Journal of Biological Chemistry*, vol. 280, no. 32, pp. 29311–29321, 2005.

[125] P. Dri, R. Cramer, R. Menegazzi, and P. Patriarca, "Increased degranulation of human myeloperoxidase-deficient polymorphonuclear leucocytes," *British Journal of Haematology*, vol. 59, no. 1, pp. 115–125, 1985.

[126] O. Stendahl, B. I. Coble, C. Dahlgren, J. Hed, and L. Molin, "Myeloperoxidase modulates the phagocytic activity of polymorphonuclear neutrophil leukocytes. Studies with cells from a myeloperoxidase-deficient patient," *The Journal of Clinical Investigation*, vol. 73, no. 2, pp. 366–373, 1984.

[127] G. Ramsaransing, A. Teelken, V. M. Prokopenko, A. V. Arutjunyan, and J. De Keyser, "Low leucocyte myeloperoxidase activity in patients with multiple sclerosis," *Journal of Neurology Neurosurgery and Psychiatry*, vol. 74, no. 7, pp. 953–955, 2003.

[128] K. Uchimura, A. Nagasaka, R. Hayashi et al., "Changes in superoxide dismutase activities and concentrations and myeloperoxidase activities in leukocytes from patients with diabetes mellitus," *Journal of Diabetes and its Complications*, vol. 13, no. 5-6, pp. 264–270, 1999.

8

Preparation and Biological Activity of the Monoclonal Antibody against the Second Extracellular Loop of the Angiotensin II Type 1 Receptor

Mingming Wei,[1,2] Chengrui Zhao,[3] Suli Zhang,[1,2] Li Wang,[4] Huirong Liu,[1,2] and Xinliang Ma[1,2,5]

[1]*Department of Physiology and Pathophysiology, School of Basic Medical Sciences, Capital Medical University, Beijing 100069, China*
[2]*Beijing Key Laboratory of Metabolic Disorders Related Cardiovascular Diseases, Capital Medical University, Beijing 100069, China*
[3]*Department of Physiology, Basic Medical Department, Fenyang College of Shanxi Medical University, Fenyang, Shanxi 032200, China*
[4]*Department of Pathology, Shanxi Medical University, Taiyuan, Shanxi 030001, China*
[5]*Department of Emergency Medicine, Thomas Jefferson University, 1025 Walnut Street, College Building, Suite 808, Philadelphia, PA 19107, USA*

Correspondence should be addressed to Huirong Liu; liuhr2000@126.com and Xinliang Ma; maxinliang@ccmu.edu.cn

Academic Editor: Xiao-Feng Yang

The current study was to prepare a mouse-derived antibody against the angiotensin II type 1 receptor (AT1-mAb) based on monoclonal antibody technology, to provide a foundation for research on AT1-AA-positive diseases. Balb/C mice were actively immunized with the second extracellular loop of the angiotensin II type 1 receptor (AT$_1$R-ECII). Then, mouse spleen lymphocytes were fused with myeloma cells and monoclonal hybridomas that secreted AT1-mAb were generated and cultured, after which those in logarithmic-phase were injected into the abdominal cavity of mice to retrieve the ascites. Highly purified AT1-mAb was isolated from mouse ascites after injection with 1×10^7 hybridomas. A greater amount of AT1-mAb was purified from mouse ascites compared to the cell supernatant of hybridomas. AT1-mAb purified from mouse ascites constricted the thoracic aorta of mice and increased the beat frequency of neonatal rat myocardial cells via the AT$_1$R, identical to the effects of AT1-AA extracted from patients' sera. Murine blood pressure increased after intravenous injection of AT1-mAb via the tail vein. High purity and good biological activity of AT1-mAb can be obtained from mouse ascites after intraperitoneal injection of monoclonal hybridomas that secrete AT1-mAb. These data provide a simple tool for studying AT1-AA-positive diseases.

1. Introduction

Angiotensin II (Ang II) receptors are a class of G-protein-coupled receptors that exist in four subtypes: AT$_1$R–AT$_4$R. The angiotensin II type 1 receptor (AT$_1$R) is mainly expressed in vascular smooth muscle cells (VSMCs), endothelial cells, and myocardial fibroblasts [1] and as such plays a prominent role in regulating the cardiovascular system. Ang II can activate the AT$_1$R, thereby increasing vascular tension, causing vasoconstriction, and increasing the force of cardiac muscular contractions. However, excessive activation of AT$_1$R can cause cardiovascular pathologies such as hypertension

[2], vascular injury [3], arrhythmia [4], and myocardial hypertrophy [5].

Preeclampsia is a serious type of pregnancy-induced hypertension that clinically manifests itself in the form of high blood pressure and proteinuria after 20 weeks of pregnancy. Numerous studies have reported that excessive AT$_1$R activation is an important mechanism underlying the occurrence and development of preeclampsia. Angiotensin II 1 type autoantibodies (AT1-AA) are agonists of AT$_1$R that can cause excessive activation [6] by interacting with the second extracellular loop of the AT$_1$R (AT$_1$R-ECII) [7], thereby causing high blood pressure and proteinuria, which are the typical signs and symptoms of preeclampsia in pregnant rats. These findings suggest that AT1-AA may play an important role in the pathology of preeclampsia [8]. Therefore, evaluating the functions of AT1-AA and its underlying mechanisms and targets has become a major research focus. However, obtaining enough highly purified AT1-AA to establish animal models has been a considerable problem, as to date only limited amounts of antisera from clinical patients with preeclampsia have been isolated. To study the pathophysiological roles of AT1-AA, it is important to establish a more simple and productive method for the preparation of these autoantibodies.

In the present study, we prepared a mouse-derived antibody against the AT_1R-ECII (AT1-mAb) using monoclonal antibody technology. Then, we identified the biological activities of AT1-mAb and compared them to AT1-AA purified from preeclamptic patients. This research is aim to find a simple and effective way to gain AT1-mAb to study AT1-AA positive disease, so as to provide basis for clinical treatment.

2. Materials and Methods

2.1. Experimental Animals and Materials. Our experiments were approved by the Institutional Animal Care and Use Committee of Capital Medical University (Beijing, China) and conformed to the Guiding Principles in the Use and Care of Animals published by the National Institutes of Health (NIH Publication number 85-23, revised 1996). Animals were provided by Vital River, License: SCXK (Beijing), 2012-0001. Before the experiments, the mice were fed *ad libitum* and maintained in 12-hour light/dark cycles. Healthy, 12-week-old Balb/C mice ($n = 60$; 45 females, 15 males; body weight, 18–20 g) were used for preparation of ascites (vehicle group: $n = 10$, hybridomas (10^7) group: $n = 10$, females), isolated vascular ring experiment ($n = 20$; 15 females, 5 males), and experiments *in vivo* ($n = 20$; 10 females, 10 males), and 0–3-day-old newborn Wistar rats ($n = 30$; weight, 4–6 g) were used for neonatal rat cardiomyocytes beat frequency experiment. We observed these rats at least twice daily. They were given pentobarbital sodium (150 mg/kg) [9] by intraperitoneal injection (IP) to reduce anxiety for surgical anesthesia. Once the experiment was completed, all Balb/C mice were euthanized by decapitation at the guillotine (a physical method was suggested by AVMA Guidelines on Euthanasia).

2.2. Purification of AT1-AA from Patients' Sera. Six preeclampsia women were recruited from the Taiyuan Central Hospital (Taiyuan, Shanxi province, China) (Table 1). This investigation was conducted according to the principles expressed in the Declaration of Helsinki. This research protocol was approved by the Ethics Committee for the Protection of Human Subjects of Taiyuan Central Hospital. All patients had given written consent. Before serum was collected, 10 mL fasting blood samples were collected from these six subjects through cubital veins and stand at room temperature for 1 hour and then centrifuged at 3000 rpm for 15 min. The sera were isolated and stored at 20°C for purification of AT1-AA [10] over Protein G affinity column (Sweden).

TABLE 1: Clinical data of patients with preeclampsia subjects.

Patients	Preeclampsia ($n = 6$)
Maternal age (years)	30 (27–34)
Gestational age at sampling (weeks)	37.5 (35–40)
Ethnic background	Han
SBP (mmHg)	152 ± 11
DBP (mmHg)	105 ± 6
Proteinuria (mg/day)	478 ± 33.5

SBP, systolic blood pressure; DBP, diastolic blood pressure.

2.3. Hybridoma Preparation. Peptides against the human AT_1R-ECII antigen epitope (murine and human AT_1R-ECII share 92% homology, Supplementary Figure 1 (see Supplementary Material available online at http://dx.doi.org/10.1155/2016/1858252)) were synthesized (I-H-R-N-V-F-F-I-E-N-T-N-I-T-V-C-A-F-H-Y-E-S-Q-N-S-T; GenBank AAB34644.1) at 98% purity. The peptides coupled to keyhole limpet hemocyanin (KLH) protein were used as immunogens, and those coupled to bovine serum albumin (BSA) were used as the control. This peptide was used as an antigen to immunize the mice to prepare sera containing high titers of polyclonal antibodies, and then the cells were fused to generate the hybridoma cell lines (Beijing B&M Biotech Co., Ltd.). In total, 40 strains of monoclonal hybridoma cell lines were generated, and the 5 strains that secreted the highest titers of AT1-mAb in the cell culture supernatant were identified by Biotin-Avidin Enzyme-Linked Immunosorbent Assay (BA-ELISA). Specific hybridomas were frozen in liquid nitrogen until use.

2.4. Hybridoma Culture. (1) For thawing, the hybridomas were quickly placed in a CryoTube at 37°C in a constant-temperature water bath, transferred to 10 mL Roswell Park Memorial Institute (RPMI) 1640 medium (HyClone, China), and centrifuged at 3000 rpm for 10 min at 4°C after mixing, after which the supernatant was removed. (2) For culturing, the cells were grown in RPMI supplemented with 10% fetal bovine serum (Gibco, USA). After 24 h, the supernatant was removed and fresh culture medium was added to the cells. (3) For subculturing, cells in logarithmic growth phase were cultured for about 3 days until 80–90% confluency, after which the supernatant was collected and frozen at −20°C until purification. The remaining cells were also collected and used for ascites preparation. (4) For cryopreservation and storage of cells, half-adherent cells were centrifuged at 1000 rpm for 5 min. Then, the supernatant was removed and the cells were cryopreserved in fetal bovine serum : RPMI : dimethyl sulfoxide (DMSO) at a ratio of 5 : 4 : 1.

2.5. Extraction of AT1-mAb from Hybridoma Culture Supernatant and Mouse Ascites. (1) Extraction of AT1-mAb from hybridoma culture supernatant: the proteins in the hybridoma culture supernatant were concentrated at a ratio of 5 : 1 and filtered using a 0.45 μm filter, and the IgG of the hybridoma culture supernatant was purified over a protein G affinity column. (2) Extraction of AT1-mAb from mouse ascites: incomplete Freund's adjuvant (0.02 mL/g, Sigma, St. Louis, MO, USA) was injected into the abdominal cavity of all Balb/C mice. Three days later, 1×10^5–1×10^9 hybridomas suspended in 0.4 mL phosphate-buffered saline (PBS) were introduced into mouse abdominal cavity by IP injection with a 1 mL syringe. Ascites formation was observed by weighed and abdominal shape at every week, ascites fluid was collected in the second week, and the supernatant was collected after centrifugation at 1000 rpm for 5 min and diluted in PBS and affinity purified with immobilized Protein G. And all mice were euthanized by decapitation at the 4th week, when they cannot generate much more ascites.

2.6. Specificity Identification of the AT1-mAb. (1) The purified antibodies were resolved on a 15% sodium dodecyl sulfate-polyacrylamide gel electrophoresis (SDS-PAGE) gel, and the gel was stained with Coomassie Brilliant Blue. (2) The specificity of the antibodies purified from the hybridoma culture supernatant and mouse ascites was determined by BA-ELISA [11], with the wavelength of detection set at 405 nm to provide the optical density (OD) (Spectra Max Plus; Molecular Devices, Sunnyvale, CA): P/N = (positive OD − blank OD)/(negative OD − blank OD); P/N > 2.1 was identified as the positive sample; P/N < 1.5 was identified as the negative sample. The procedure is as follows: 1 μg/mL AT_1R-ECII peptide dissolved in Na_2CO_3 solution (0.1 mol/L, pH 11.0) was coated in 96-well microtiter plates and incubated overnight at 4°C. The wells were saturated with 1% PMT buffer (1% (w/v) bovine serum albumin, 0.1% (v/v) Tween 20 in phosphate-buffered saline (PBS-T), pH 7.4) at 37°C for 1 h. After washing the plates with PBS-T for 3 times, 5 μL samples diluted in 45 μL PMT were added to the plates and incubated at 37°C for 1.5 h. After 3 times' washing, biotinylated rabbit anti-mouse IgG antibodies and biotinylated goat anti-human IgG antibodies (1 : 4500 dilutions in PMT; Zhong Shan Jin Qiao, Beijing, China) were added to the wells and incubated at 37°C for 1 h. After 3 times' washing, the streptavidin-peroxidase conjugate (1 : 3000, Vector, CA) was added to the wells and incubated at 37°C for 1 h. Finally, 2,2-azino-di(3-ethylbenzothiazoline) sulfonic acid- (ABTS-) H_2O_2 (Roche, Basel, Switzerland) substrate buffer was applied and reacted in the dark at 37°C for 0.5 h.

2.7. The Biological Activity and Functional Identification of AT1-mAb. (1) For the cultivation of primary neonatal rat myocardial cells, we rapidly removed hearts from 0–3-day-old newborn Wistar rats into PBS, cut them into pieces, and washed away the blood cells for 2-3 times with PBS. 35 mg trypsin and 25 mg collagenase type II were dissolved in 30 mL PBS. These digestive enzymes were filtered by 0.22 μm filters and then stand at 37°C. The heart tissue was added into 5 mL beaker and digested in 3 mL enzyme solution for 3–5 min with sustained shaking at 37°C. The supernatant was aspirated into low-glucose Dulbecco's Modified Eagle's medium (DMEM) with 10% fetal bovine serum to terminate digestion. Finally, the cells were centrifuged through a 200-mesh filter and centrifuged at 1000 rpm for 5 min and placed in 10 cm dish. After 2 hours, the supernatant was aspirated and packed in 6-well plates, the adherent cells were fibroblast cells. After culturing for 5 days, the beat of the myocardial cells was observed under a microscope. The

AT_1R blocker valsartan (Sigma, Y0001132) and AT_2R blocker PD123319 (Sigma, P186) were added to the myocardial cell culture medium. After 10 minutes, purified AT1-mAb was added to the culture medium, and the beat frequency of the myocardial cells was recorded. (2) For isolated vascular ring technology [12], the sodium pentobarbital was used for surgical anesthesia before isolating aortic rings from the mice. The mice were euthanized by decapitation after thoracic aortas were isolated immediately, and a 2 mm vascular ring was removed and affixed to an internal System-610M Multi Myograph bath sensor (Danish Myo Technology A/S Inc., Denmark). The bath contained 5 mL hydroxyethyl piper-azine ethanesulfonic acid 4-(2-hydroxyethyl)piperazine-1-ethanesulfonic acid (HEPES; 144 mM NaCl, 5.8 mM KCl, 1.2 mM $MgCl_2N_6H_2O$, 2.5 mM $CaCl_2$, 11.1 mM glucose, and 5 mM HEPES) solution (pH, 7.38–7.40) into which a 95% O_2/5% CO_2 gas mixture was continually bubbled. We allowed a 1 h equilibration period before the start of the experiment, and the HEPES solution was replaced every 15 min. Using the vascular ring transducer system, vascular ring tension changes were collected and recorded with LabChart 7 software. The initial passive vascular tension was determined by vascular standardization. HEPES buffer containing 60 mM potassium (144 mM NaCl, 60 mM KCl, 1.2 mM $MgCl_2N_6H_2O$, 2.5 mM $CaCl_2$, 11.1 mM glucose, and 5 mM HEPES; pH, 7.38–7.40) was used for a precontracted vasoactive test. The contractile responses of the vascular rings (tension) to different drugs were defined as a percentage of average contractile intensity to KCl (KCl% = detected drugs/ΔKCl × 100%). (3) The tail-cuff method was used to measure blood pressure in mice, and the position of the mouse was fixed by using a mouse holder maintained on a 37°C hot plate, while a small mouse tail blood flow sensor was placed at the mouse tail root; we then waited until the heart rate stabilized at approximately 375 beats/min. After the blood began to flow smoothly and steadily, we measured systolic blood pressure five times per animal using software of noninvasive automated sphygmomanometer (Japan) and recorded the mean overall blood pressure.

2.8. Statistical Analysis. Using SPSS 16.0 (Chicago, IL, USA) for statistical analysis, between-group comparisons were performed with t-tests, and comparisons among groups were performed with one-way ANOVA, followed by Tukey's post hoc test ($^*P$ < 0.05, $^{**}P$ < 0.01). All of the bar graphs are shown as the mean ± standard error of the mean (SEM).

3. Results

3.1. Concentration of AT1-mAb Is Higher in Mouse Ascites Than in Hybridoma Supernatant. Hybridoma supernatant was collected after 3 days of culture. The results of the bicin-choninic acid (BCA) assay revealed that the concentration of the monoclonal antibodies purified from the supernatant was 3.75×10^{-6} mol/L. Different amounts of hybridomas were injected into the abdominal cavity of mice (1×10^5, 1×10^6, 1×10^7, 1×10^8, and 1×10^9), and different concentrations (2.5×10^{-6}, 9.3×10^{-6}, 3×10^{-5}, 1.32×10^{-5}, and 1.49×10^{-5} mol/L) of monoclonal antibodies were obtained. The

(a)

(b)

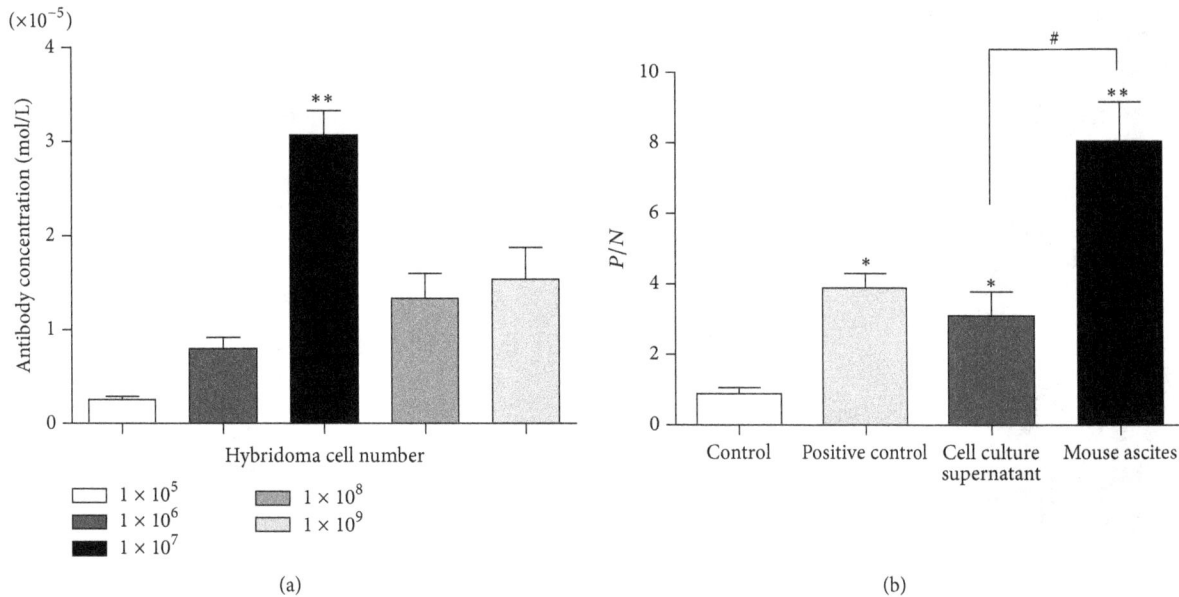

FIGURE 1: Concentration of AT1-mAb purified from mouse ascites was higher than that from hybridoma supernatant. (a) Concentration of monoclonal antibody that was purified from mouse ascites ($^{**}P < 0.01$ versus 1×10^{-5}, 1×10^{-6}, 1×10^{-8}, and 1×10^{-9}, $n = 8$). (b) Content of AT1-mAb that was purified from the cellular supernatant of hybridomas compared with that from mouse ascites, and positive control was the AT1-AA purified from preeclampsia sera. $^{#}P < 0.05$ versus cellular supernatant; $^{*}P < 0.05$ versus control; $^{**}P < 0.01$ versus control. Data represent the mean $\pm$ SEM; $n = 8$.

highest concentration of monoclonal antibodies purified from mouse ascites was from the group that was injected with 1×10^{7} hybridomas ($P < 0.01$ versus 1×10^{-5}, 1×10^{-6}, 1×10^{-8}, and 1×10^{-9}; $n = 8$) (Figure 1(a)). The BA-ELISA results showed that the monoclonal antibodies purified from hybridoma supernatants and mouse ascites were AT1-mAb, AT1-AA purified from preeclampsia sera was used as positive control, and the sera from AT1-AA-negative Balb/C mice were used as control (P/N values: positive control, 3.96 ± 1.9 versus 0.88 ± 0.43 for controls; $P < 0.05$; hybridoma cell culture supernatant, 3.11 ± 1.81 versus 0.88 ± 0.43 for controls; $P < 0.05$; mouse ascites, 8.07 ± 3.32 versus 0.88 ± 0.43 for controls; $P < 0.01$; $n = 8$); the content of AT1-mAb purified from mouse ascites was higher than that purified from the hybridoma supernatant (P/N: 8.07 ± 3.12 versus 3.11 ± 1.81 for the supernatant; $P < 0.05$; $n = 8$) (Figure 1(b)) and we extracted the whole protein from the neonatal rat cardiomyocytes, which express the AT_1R; the Western blot showed that both AT1-AA and AT1-mAb can recognize AT_1R at the same location specifically (Supplementary Figure 2).

3.2. AT1-mAb Purified from Mouse Ascites Belongs to the IgG Immunoglobulin Class. SDS-PAGE was used to analyze the purity of hybridoma supernatant and mouse ascites. The results showed that the antibody extracted from hybridoma supernatant showed that there were several other bands in addition to the heavy and light chain (Figure 2(b)); compared to IgG control (Figure 2(a)), the heavy and light chain of purified AT1-mAb were 55 kDa and 25 kDa (Figure 2(c)),

which revealed that the antibody extracted from mouse ascites belongs to the IgG immunoglobulin class.

3.3. AT1-mAb Purified from Mouse Ascites Increases the Beat Frequency of Newborn Rat Cardiomyocytes. As shown in Figure 3 (the picture of the newborn rat cardiomyocytes, Figure 3(a)), when 10^{-8} mol/L AT1-mAb (purified from mouse ascites) was added to the culture medium, the beat frequency of the newborn rat cardiomyocytes increased, similar to the effect caused by AT1-AA (10^{-8} mol/L) extracted from patients' sera (AT1-mAb, 77.67 ± 19.67 versus 57.08 ± 5.29 before treatment; AT1-AA, 84.33 ± 8.33 versus 60.67 ± 3.79 before treatment; $P < 0.05$; $n = 6$); Ang II (10^{-7} mol/L), the endogenous AT_1R agonist, also increased the beat frequency of the rat cardiomyocytes (99.71 ± 22.14 versus 58.36 ± 5.75 before treatment; $P < 0.05$; $n = 6$); AT_1R blocker valsartan (10^{-7} mol/L) could block the beating frequency increase caused by AT1-mAb, although the AT_2R blocker PD123319 (10^{-7} mol/L) did not have an inhibitory effect (94.08 ± 2.89 versus 72.03 ± 5.77 before treatment; $P < 0.05$; $n = 6$) (Figure 3(b)). These data reveal that AT1-mAb can increase the beat frequency of newborn rat cardiomyocytes by activating the AT_1R, but not AT_2R.

3.4. AT1-mAb Purified from Mouse Ascites Induces Contraction of the Thoracic Aorta. The results in Figure 4 show that both 10^{-7} mol/L Ang II and 10^{-8} mol/L AT1-mAb purified from mouse ascites could induce vasoconstriction. Compared to negative IgG group (Figure 4(a)), the effect

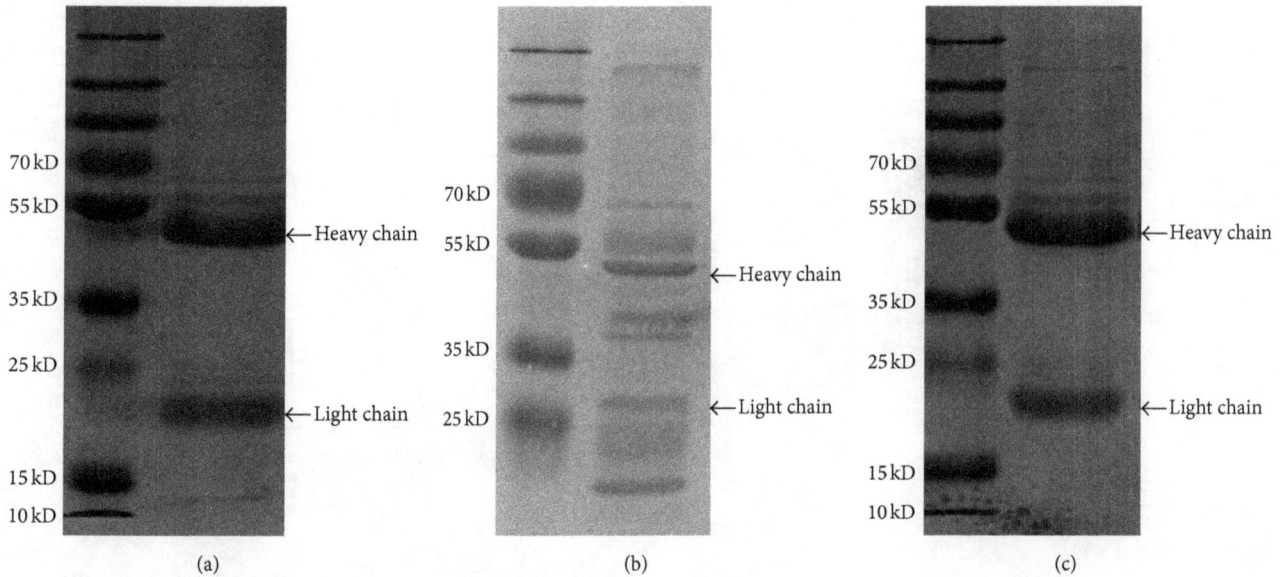

FIGURE 2: Purity of AT1-mAb from hybridoma supernatant and mouse ascites. (a) IgG control; (b) the antibody extracted from hybridoma supernatant; (c) the antibody extracted from mouse ascites.

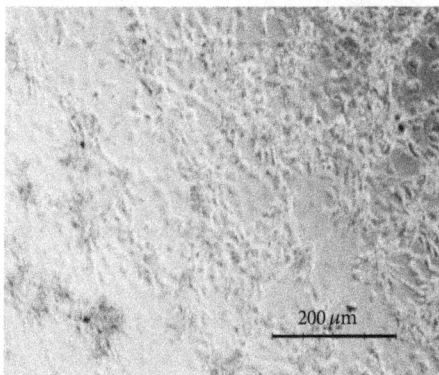

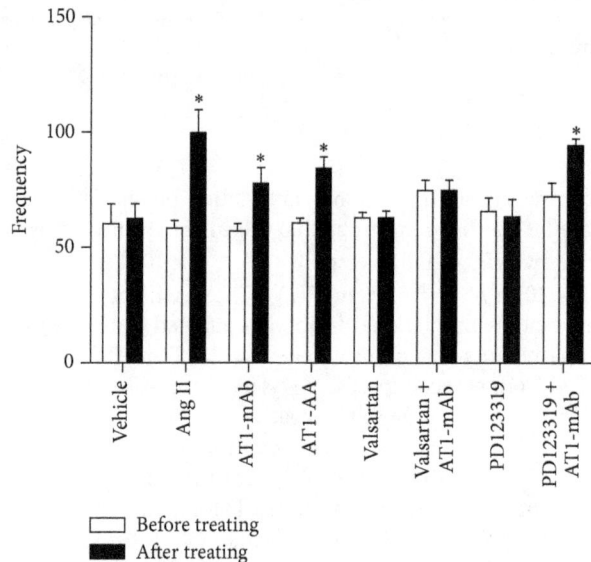

FIGURE 3: Biological activity of AT1-mAb was identified by changes in beat frequency of neonatal rat myocardial cells. (a) Cultured neonatal rat myocardial cells. Scale bar = 200 μm. (b) Different processing factors had different effects on beating frequency of cultured neonatal rat myocardial cells *in vitro*. $^*P < 0.05$ versus before treating. Data represent the mean ± SEM; $n = 6$.

of AT1-mAb on vascular function was the same as that caused by AT1-AA (10^{-8} mol/L) extracted from patients' sera (tension values: Ang II, Figure 4(b), 52.71% ± 20.86% versus 3.72% ± 2.26% for negative IgG; AT1-mAb, Figure 4(c), 37.51% ± 16.42% versus 3.72% ± 2.26% for negative IgG; AT1-AA, Figure 4(f), 40.50% ± 19.20% versus 3.72% ± 2.26% for negative IgG; $P < 0.05$; $n = 6$. When valsartan (10^{-7} mol/L) was added first, the vasoconstriction caused by AT1-mAb was blocked (Figure 4(d), $P > 0.05$; $n = 6$). However, when PD123319 (10^{-7} mol/L) was added first, the vasoconstriction caused by AT1-mAb could not be blocked (Figure 4(e), 28.93% ± 10.04% versus 3.72% ± 2.26% for negative IgG; $P < 0.05$; $n = 6$). Statistical graph of isolated vascular ring is Figure 4(g). These results demonstrate that AT1-mAb exerts its biological functions by activating the AT_1R, but not the AT_2R.

3.5. AT1-mAb Directly Increases the Blood Pressure of Pregnant Mice. Twelve-week-old healthy adult females and males were caged together, and ultrasonography showed successful

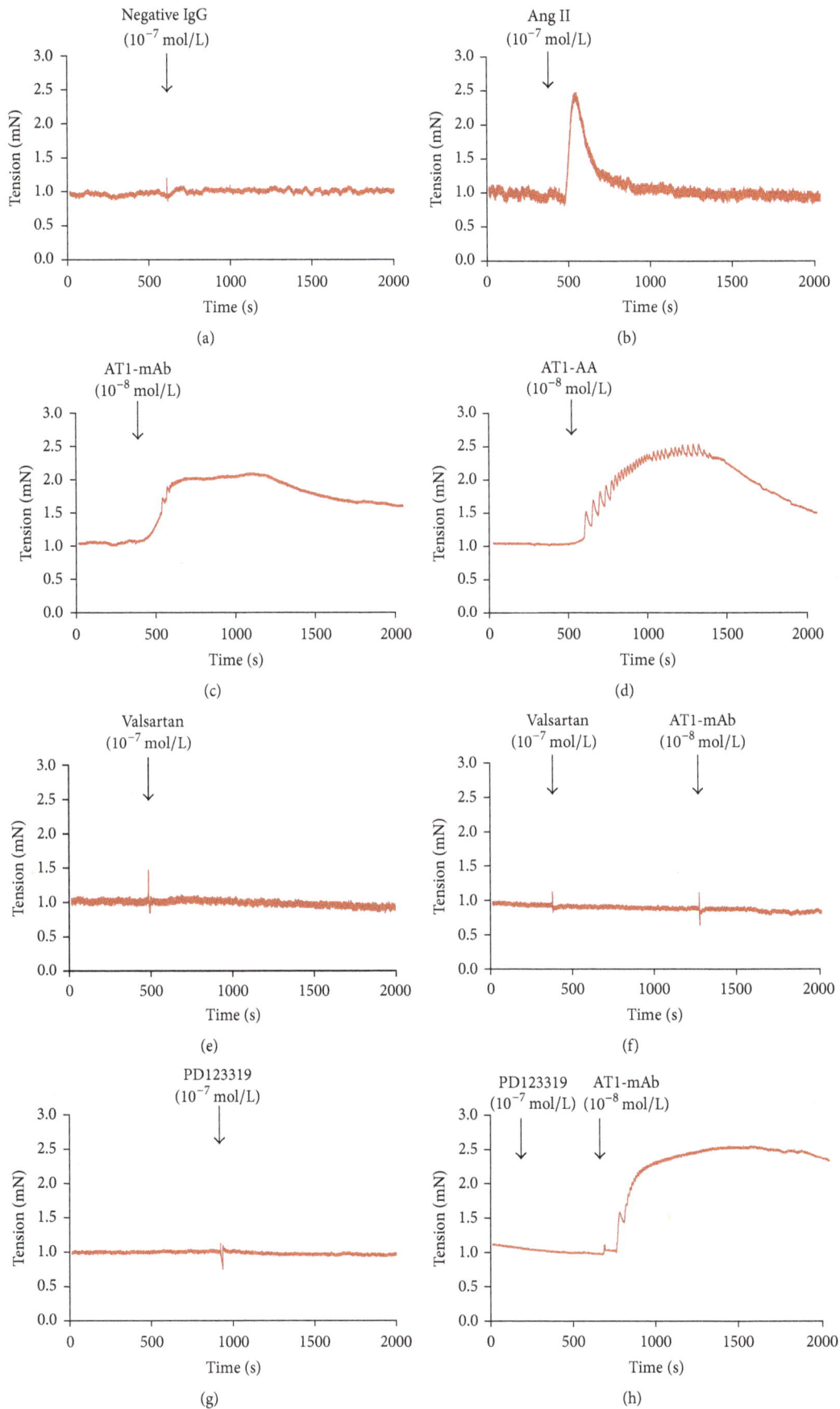

FIGURE 4: Continued.

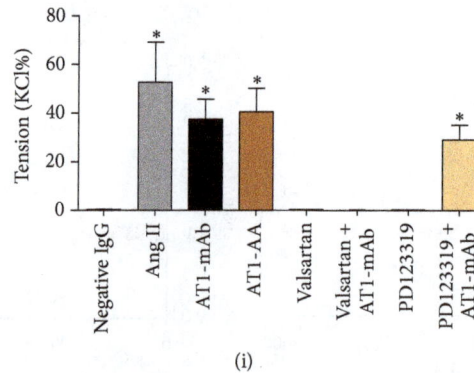

(i)

FIGURE 4: Biological activity of AT1-mAb was identified by isolated thoracic aorta ring technology. (a) Negative IgG isolated from healthy mouse serum; (b) Agonist of AT_1R, Ang II; (c) AT1-mAb; (d) for AT1-AA exert the same effect on the contractile force of mouse thoracic aorta; (e) blocking agent for AT_1R, valsartan; (f) valsartan + AT1-mAb; (g) blocking agent for AT_2R, PD123319; (h) PD123319 + AT1-mAb; and (i) statistical graph of isolated vascular ring. $^*P < 0.05$ versus negative IgG. Data represent the mean ± SEM; $n = 6$.

pregnancy. On the 13th day of gestation, AT1-mAb ($20\ \mu g/g$) [13] was injected into the pregnant mice through the tail vein, and an equal dose of normal saline was injected into the mice in the control group (control group, Figure 5(a); AT1-mAb group, Figure 5(b)). The content of the AT1-mAb in pregnant mice sera was tested on days 14, 16, and 18 of gestation. The levels of AT1-mAb began to rise from the 14th day of gestation and were maintained to the 18th day (OD on day 14 of gestation: 0.27 ± 0.05 versus 0.12 ± 0.02 for saline; day 16 of gestation, 0.26 ± 0.05 versus 0.14 ± 0.016 for saline; day 18 of gestation, 0.25 ± 0.03 versus 0.13 ± 0.02 for saline; $P < 0.05$; $n = 6$; Figure 5(c)). On alternate days, blood pressures were measured using mouse tail sensors. The systolic blood pressures of AT1-mAb-positive pregnant mice were significantly higher than those of mice in the control group on days 14, 16, and 18 of gestation (118.46 ± 5.82 versus 92.94 ± 7.64 mmHg for saline on day 14 of gestation: 129.78 ± 8.92 versus 98.08 ± 10.81 for saline on day 16 of gestation; and 137.69 ± 4.73 versus 97.10 ± 9.17 for saline on day 18 of gestation; $P < 0.05$; $n = 6$; Figure 5(d)).

4. Discussion

A large number of studies have identified AT1-AA as a harmful factor that exists in several diseases associated with cardiovascular disturbances, especially in patients with preeclampsia [14]. It plays an agonistic role by specifically interacting with AT_1R-ECII. However, other unknown pathological mechanisms of AT1-AA action need to be further explored. Obtaining AT1-AA is the primary goal in establishing AT1-AA-positive animal model and studying the pathological significance of and mechanisms underlying this antibody in diseases such as preeclampsia [15]. Currently, isolating antibody from the sera of preeclamptic patients is a basic approach to obtaining AT1-AA; however, it is crucial to acquire other sources of AT1-AA because of the limited availability of clinical patients' sera, collection difficulties, and large losses when purification is not timely [16]. Active immunization is an alternate method for obtaining AT1-AA, which involve mixing synthetic AT_1R-ECII with incomplete

Freund's adjuvant to retrieve the antigen and injecting it into the animals by subcutaneous injection with a booster injection administered at 2-week intervals. Typically, it is possible to procure high titer until the 8th week [17]. Therefore, active immunization requires a relatively long time and a large dose of antigen peptides. In addition, the retrieved antibodies are usually polyclonal in nature. Therefore, it is important to obtain AT1-mAb with high potency and specificity to allow the study of the pathologic roles of AT1-AA [18]. Monoclonal antibody technology was used in the present experiment. The synthetic peptide AT_1R-ECII was used to actively immunize Balb/C mice through subcutaneous injection, and then single B lymphocytes capable of secreting AT1-mAb were hybridized with unlimited proliferating myeloma cells to obtain hybrid cells that could be immortalized and secrete AT1-mAb. The hybridomas were selected using ELISA, and AT1-mAb was extracted from mouse ascites after hybridomas were inoculated into Balb/C mice for 2 weeks. Our results showed that AT1-mAb can be extracted from hybridoma supernatants and mouse ascites, the content of AT1-mAb purified from mouse ascites was higher than that purified from the hybridoma supernatant, and the AT1-mAb purified from mouse ascites belongs to the IgG immunoglobulin class. Additionally, compared to extracting AT1-mAb from hybridoma supernatants, extracting AT1-mAb from mouse ascites is of higher potency and less cost. Therefore, we chose the mouse ascites method for preparing purified AT1-mAb.

Numerous studies have shown that there are a variety of G-protein-coupled receptors, including AT_1R, on the surface of mouse vascular endothelial cells [19] and smooth muscle cells [20], as well as on neonatal rat cardiomyocytes [21]. Ang II, an endogenous agonist of the AT_1R, binds to AT_1R and causes a positive inotropic effect, such as the increased beat frequency of cardiomyocytes and induction of vasoconstriction [22]. Therefore, after the specificity of the AT1-mAb purified from mouse ascites was confirmed, neonatal rat cardiomyocyte experiments and isolated vascular ring technology were used to evaluate the biological activity of AT1-mAb. When AT1-mAb was added to the culture medium of neonatal rat cardiomyocytes, the beat frequencies

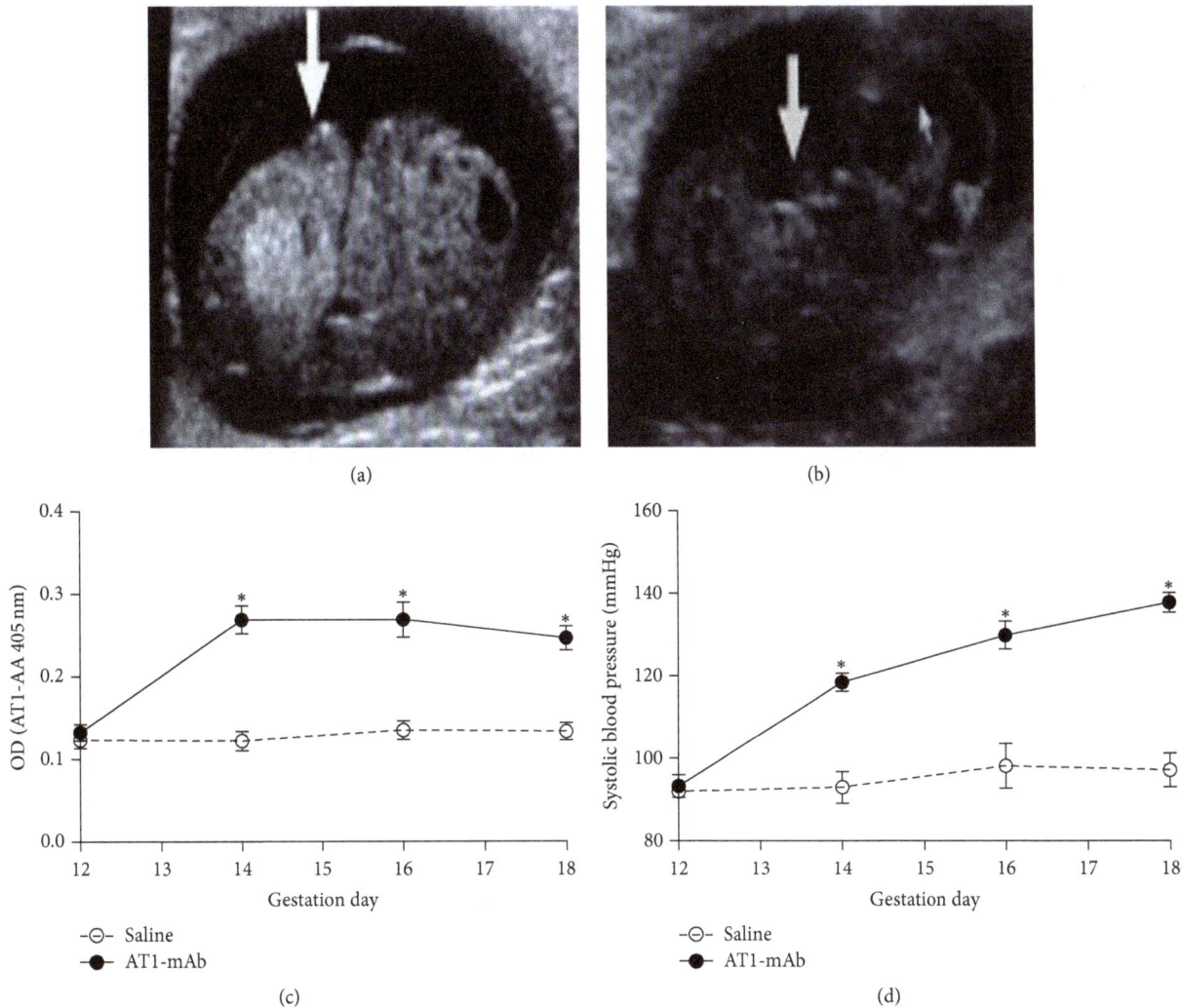

FIGURE 5: Elevated blood pressure of pregnant mice caused by AT1-mAb. (a) Control group; (b) AT1-mAb group; (c) content of AT1-mAb in sera of mice; (d) systolic blood pressure levels in the pregnant mouse model. $^*P < 0.05$ versus saline. Data represent the mean $\pm$ SEM; $n = 6$.

of cardiomyocytes were significantly increased, similar to the effect of AT1-AA isolated from patients' sera. When the AT_1R blocker valsartan was added to the medium first, the cell surface receptors were blocked by blocking the effect of AT1-mAb on beat frequency in rat neonatal cardiomyocytes; the AT_2R blocker PD123319 did not have a blocking effect. Furthermore, similar to AT1-AA purified from patients' sera, AT1-mAb purified from mouse ascites caused observable vasoconstriction in mouse thoracic aorta. If the AT_1R blocker valsartan was added prior to giving AT1-mAb treatment in the isolated vascular ring, vasoconstriction was completely blocked, whereas the AT_2R blocker PD123319 did not block the effect. All of the above observations demonstrate that AT1-mAb purified from mouse ascites does not bind to AT_2R but rather specifically activates AT_1R, thereby exerting its agonist-like biological effects. In addition, compared to the instantaneous vasoconstrictor effect caused by Ang II, AT1-mAb and AT1-AA caused continued contraction in mouse thoracic aorta, which suggests that activation of AT_1R without desensitization may be an important mechanism whereby

AT1-AA produces pathological and damaging effects. Additional studies are required to further explore this putative mechanism.

Finally, to confirm that AT1-mAb plays a biological role in vivo, we injected AT1-mAb into Balb/C mice via the tail vein on the 13th day of gestation. Researchers demonstrated that the half-life of clinically sourced AT1-AA is about 10 days, so that the AT1-AA can be retained in the body for a long period, and thus mouse blood pressure may also be maintained at a high level after AT1-AA injection [23]. In addition, when pregnant mice were given an injection of AT1-mAb purified from ascites, blood pressure on day 14 of gestation was increased and continued until the end of the experiment. This suggests that AT1-mAb extracted from ascites simulated patient-derived antibodies both in vitro and in vivo.

In summary, we prepared AT1-mAb with high specificity, high concentration, and biological activity by inoculating hybridomas that secrete AT1-mAb into the mouse abdominal cavity (Figure 6). Preparation of AT1-mAb is required to

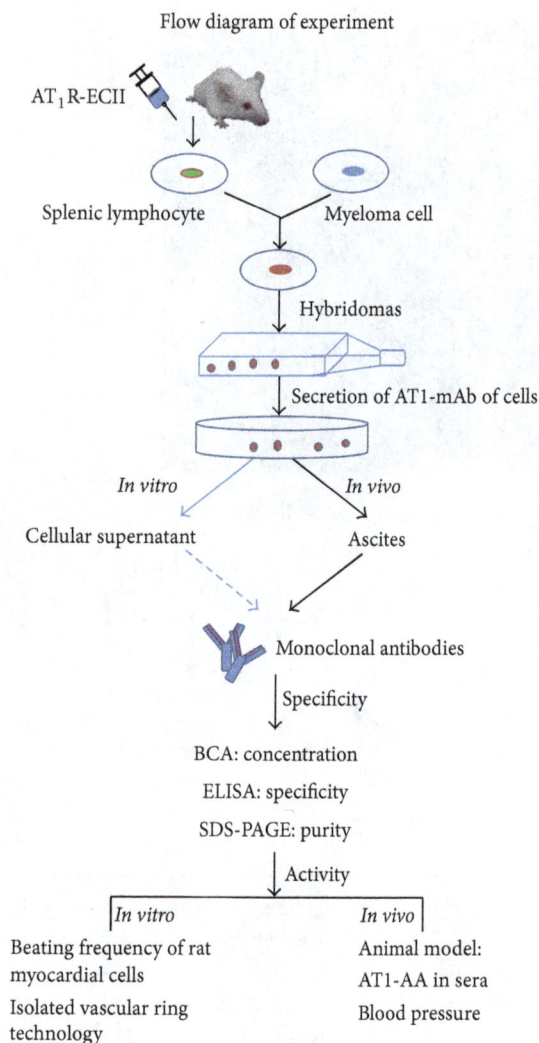

FIGURE 6: Flowchart of experimental procedures.

establish AT1-AA-positive animal models and will be a useful tool for the research of clinical diseases that manifest a high titer of AT1-AA, such as preeclampsia.

Conflict of Interests

The authors declare that there is no conflict of interests regarding the publication of this paper.

Authors' Contribution

Huirong Liu, Xinliang Ma, and Suli Zhang designed the research; Mingming Wei, Chengrui Zhao, and Li Wang performed the research and analyzed the data; and Mingming Wei and Suli Zhang wrote the paper.

Acknowledgments

This research was supported by three funders: (1) The Beijing Natural Science Foundation of China (Grant no. 7152017; http://www.nsfc.gov.cn/); (2) National Natural Science Foundation of China (no. 81300694; http://isisn.nsfc.gov.cn/) (these funders played a role in study design, data collection and analysis, decision to publish, or preparation of the paper); (3) 973 Project Prophase Research Initiative (2014CB560704 to HL; http://www.bjedu.gov.cn/). This funder had no role in study design, data collection and analysis, decision to publish, or preparation of the paper. The authors thank Jianyu Shang for technical help, and they thank Jinghui Lei and Wenlong Xia for help in writing.

References

[1] M. de Gasparo, K. J. Catt, T. Inagami, J. W. Wright, and T. Unger, "International union of pharmacology. XXIII. The angiotensin II receptors," *Pharmacological Reviews*, vol. 52, no. 3, pp. 415–472, 2000.

[2] D. X. Liu, Y. Q. Zhang, B. Hu, J. Zhang, and Q. Zhao, "Association of AT1R polymorphism with hypertension risk: an update meta-analysis based on 28,952 subjects," *Journal of the Renin-Angiotensin-Aldosterone System*, vol. 16, no. 4, pp. 898–909, 2015.

[3] A. C. Montezano, A. N. D. Cat, F. J. Rios, and R. M. Touyz, "Angiotensin II and vascular injury," *Current Hypertension Reports*, vol. 16, article 431, 2014.

[4] R. R. Blanco, H. Austin, R. N. Vest III et al., "Angiotensin receptor type 1 single nucleotide polymorphism 1166A/C is associated with malignant arrhythmias and altered circulating miR-155 levels in patients with chronic heart failure," *Journal of Cardiac Failure*, vol. 18, no. 9, pp. 717–723, 2012.

[5] S. Yasuno, K. Kuwahara, H. Kinoshita et al., "Angiotensin II type 1a receptor signalling directly contributes to the increased arrhythmogenicity in cardiac hypertrophy," *British Journal of Pharmacology*, vol. 170, no. 7, pp. 1384–1395, 2013.

[6] H. Welter, A. Huber, S. Lauf et al., "Angiotensin II regulates testicular peritubular cell function via AT1 receptor: a specific situation in male infertility," *Molecular and Cellular Endocrinology*, vol. 393, no. 1-2, pp. 171–178, 2014.

[7] K. Wenzel, A. Rajakumar, H. Haase et al., "Angiotensin II type 1 receptor antibodies and increased angiotensin II sensitivity in pregnant rats," *Hypertension*, vol. 58, no. 1, pp. 77–84, 2011.

[8] I. Bogdan, L. Schärer, R. Rüdlinger, and J. Hafner, "Epidermodysplasia verruciformis in two brothers developing aggressive squamous cell carcinoma," *Dermatologic Surgery*, vol. 33, no. 12, pp. 1525–1528, 2007.

[9] Y. Y. Ji, Z. D. Wang, S. F. Wang et al., "Ischemic preconditioning ameliorates intestinal injury induced by ischemia-reperfusion in rats," *World Journal of Gastroenterology*, vol. 21, no. 26, pp. 8081–8088, 2015.

[10] S. L. Zhang, R. H. Zheng, L. H. Yang et al., "Angiotensin type 1 receptor autoantibody from preeclamptic patients induces human fetoplacental vasoconstriction," *Journal of Cellular Physiology*, vol. 228, no. 1, pp. 142–148, 2013.

[11] S. L. Zhang, X. Zhang, L. H. Yang et al., "Increased susceptibility to metabolic syndrome in adult offspring of angiotensin type 1 receptor autoantibody-positive rats," *Antioxidants & Redox Signaling*, vol. 17, no. 5, pp. 733–743, 2012.

[12] L. Ma, K. Wang, J. Shang et al., "Anti-peroxynitrite treatment ameliorated vasorelaxation of resistance arteries in aging rats: involvement with NO-sGC-cGKs pathway," *PLoS ONE*, vol. 9, no. 8, Article ID e104788, 2014.

[13] C. C. Zhou, Y. J. Zhang, R. A. Irani et al., "Angiotensin receptor agonistic autoantibodies induce pre-eclampsia in pregnant mice," *Nature Medicine*, vol. 14, no. 8, pp. 855–862, 2008.

[14] H.-P. Wang, W.-H. Zhang, X.-F. Wang et al., "Exposure to AT1 receptor autoantibodies during pregnancy increases susceptibility of the maternal heart to postpartum ischemia-reperfusion injury in rats," *International Journal of Molecular Sciences*, vol. 15, no. 7, pp. 11495–11509, 2014.

[15] X. Yang, F. Wang, W. B. Lau et al., "Autoantibodies isolated from preeclamptic patients induce endothelial dysfunction via interaction with the angiotensin II AT1 receptor," *Cardiovascular Toxicology*, vol. 14, no. 1, pp. 21–29, 2014.

[16] W. J. Li, Y. Q. Chen, S. H. Li et al., "Agonistic antibody to angiotensin ii type 1 receptor accelerates atherosclerosis in apoe$^{-/-}$ mice," *American Journal of Translational Research*, vol. 6, no. 6, pp. 678–690, 2014.

[17] L. Song, S.-L. Zhang, K.-H. Bai et al., "Serum agonistic autoantibodies against type-1 angiotensin II receptor titer in patients with epithelial ovarian cancer: a potential role in tumor cell migration and angiogenesis," *Journal of Ovarian Research*, vol. 6, article 22, 2013.

[18] J. Yang, L. Li, J. Y. Shang et al., "Angiotensin II type 1 receptor autoantibody as a novel regulator of aldosterone independent of preeclampsia," *Journal of Hypertension*, vol. 33, no. 5, pp. 1046–1056, 2015.

[19] J. L. Gorman, S. T. K. Liu, D. Slopack et al., "Angiotensin II evokes angiogenic signals within skeletal muscle through coordinated effects on skeletal myocytes and endothelial cells," *PLoS ONE*, vol. 9, no. 1, Article ID e85537, 2014.

[20] E. Goupil, D. Fillion, S. Clément et al., "Angiotensin II type I and prostaglandin F2α receptors cooperatively modulate signaling in vascular smooth muscle cells," *The Journal of Biological Chemistry*, vol. 290, no. 5, pp. 3137–3148, 2015.

[21] L. Lin, C. Y. Tang, J. F. Xu et al., "Mechanical stress triggers cardiomyocyte autophagy through angiotensin II type 1 receptor-mediated p38MAP kinase independently of angiotensin II," *PLoS ONE*, vol. 9, no. 2, Article ID e89629, 2014.

[22] G. P. Diniz, M. S. Carneiro-Ramos, and M. L. M. Barreto-Chaves, "Angiotensin type 1 receptor mediates thyroid hormone-induced cardiomyocyte hypertrophy through the Akt/GSK-3β/mTOR signaling pathway," *Basic Research in Cardiology*, vol. 104, no. 6, pp. 653–667, 2009.

[23] Y. Xia and R. E. Kellems, "Angiotensin receptor agonistic autoantibodies and hypertension: preeclampsia and beyond," *Circulation Research*, vol. 113, no. 1, pp. 78–87, 2013.

9

Monocyte Activation in Immunopathology: Cellular Test for Development of Diagnostics and Therapy

Ekaterina A. Ivanova[1] and Alexander N. Orekhov[2,3,4]

[1]Department of Development and Regeneration, KU Leuven, 3000 Leuven, Belgium
[2]Institute of General Pathology and Pathophysiology, Moscow 125315, Russia
[3]Institute for Atherosclerosis Research, Skolkovo Innovation Center, Moscow 121609, Russia
[4]Department of Biophysics, Biological Faculty, Moscow State University, Moscow 119991, Russia

Correspondence should be addressed to Ekaterina A. Ivanova; kate.ivanov@gmail.com

Academic Editor: Oscar Bottasso

Several highly prevalent human diseases are associated with immunopathology. Alterations in the immune system are found in such life-threatening disorders as cancer and atherosclerosis. Monocyte activation followed by macrophage polarization is an important step in normal immune response to pathogens and other relevant stimuli. Depending on the nature of the activation signal, macrophages can acquire pro- or anti-inflammatory phenotypes that are characterized by the expression of distinct patterns of secreted cytokines and surface antigens. This process is disturbed in immunopathologies resulting in abnormal monocyte activation and/or bias of macrophage polarization towards one or the other phenotype. Such alterations could be used as important diagnostic markers and also as possible targets for the development of immunomodulating therapy. Recently developed cellular tests are designed to analyze the phenotype and activity of living cells circulating in patient's bloodstream. Monocyte/macrophage activation test is a successful example of cellular test relevant for atherosclerosis and oncopathology. This test demonstrated changes in macrophage activation in subclinical atherosclerosis and breast cancer and could also be used for screening a panel of natural agents with immunomodulatory activity. Further development of cellular tests will allow broadening the scope of their clinical implication. Such tests may become useful tools for drug research and therapy optimization.

1. Introduction

Immunopathology is associated with the most common life-threatening disorders, including atherosclerosis and related cardiovascular diseases, cancer, and chronic inflammation. A number of diseases, such as lupus erythematosus, rheumatoid arthritis, or HIV infections, are characterized by pronounced immunopathologies; others, such as atherosclerosis and cancer, by less obvious latent pathological changes in the immune system. Such changes may represent early events in the disease initiation and development and might therefore be especially interesting for timely diagnostics and for development of preventive treatment.

The role of the immune system dysfunction in cancer is currently well recognized [1]. Altered macrophage plasticity and polarization can contribute both to the malignancy development and to the tumor vascularization [2]. In that regard, comprehensive analysis of the macrophage population diversity would be necessary for developing adequate therapeutic approaches and monitoring the therapy efficiency.

Recent studies have revealed many aspects of the complex and important role of macrophages in the pathogenesis of atherosclerosis [3]. Formation of the atherosclerotic plaque begins with monocyte activation and transformation into macrophages that reside in the subendothelial area of the blood vessel wall and accumulate lipids in their cytoplasm becoming foam cells. This lipid trapping is performed by means of uncontrolled phagocytosis. At the same time, certain types of macrophages are implicated in tissue repair, and these cells have been found in regressing plaques in mouse models [4, 5]. Therefore, different types of macrophages are responsible for the plaque initiation, growth, and, eventually, regression [6–8]. Correspondingly, anti-inflammatory agents are considered as an important component of antiatherosclerotic therapy [9]. Here again, the analysis of macrophage phenotypic diversity could improve the understanding of the pathological process and assessment of the therapy efficiency.

According to current epidemiological data, atherosclerosis-related diseases and cancer are the two greatest contributors to the overall mortality in the developed countries [10, 11]. Given that these diseases are tightly associated with immunopathology, development of comprehensive diagnostic methods and therapeutic approaches to modulate the immune system appears to be of the greatest importance. However, the existing diagnostic methods are imperfect and their improvement remains challenging. Likewise, no drugs are available to date that allow targeted immune correction in atherosclerosis. It is clear that changes in cytokine expression and phenotypic features of macrophages may reflect the disease progression state. These features may therefore be used for monitoring the pathological process and treatment efficiency.

2. Cellular Tests for Diagnostics and Drug Research

In many pathological conditions, the analysis of different types of cells circulating in the bloodstream can provide valuable information about the disease progression. During the recent years, a number of cell types have been isolated and studied for possible application in diagnostics and drug development.

Circulating tumor cells (CTCs) can be extracted from patient's blood and used to analyze the expression of relevant genes and surface markers. For instance, successful isolation and molecular characterization have been described for metastatic breast cancer [12], metastatic colorectal cancer [13], and lung cancer [14]. This strategy is especially useful in cases of advanced metastatic cancer, where the patients could benefit from a personalized treatment. The analysis of CTCs has a great diagnostic potential but can also help in revealing the possible drug resistance of the tumor and designing the optimal therapy [15]. Many current studies are focused on the improvement of CTC-based analyses and their clinical implementation.

Peripheral blood mononuclear cells (PBMCs) are relatively easily obtainable cells that can be used for monitoring a wide spectrum of conditions and pathologies. The analysis of mRNA profiles of isolated PBMCs could be used for evaluation of metabolic changes [16]. PBMCs can also be kept in short-term culture and used for studying cytokine production induced by stimulation. For instance, changes in proinflammatory cytokine production by isolated PBMCs have been described in such conditions as allergies, alterations of immune response, and immunization [17–19]. Studies on PBMCs have demonstrated that vascular endothelial growth factor (VEGF) production was decreased in women with preeclampsia [20]. Isolated PBMCs can serve as a relevant system for testing various drugs, especially related to inflammation [21]. Recently, the potential of macrophage-based test

system for diagnostics and treatment of atherosclerosis has been explored [22].

Atherosclerosis is associated with life-threatening cardiovascular diseases [7]. Atherosclerosis progression is usually slow, and the disease often remains asymptomatic until the ischemia of organs and tissues becomes evident. This may happen due to the obstruction of a blood vessel with growing atherosclerotic plaque or the embolism caused by a thrombus formed on a destabilized plaque. Therefore, the first manifestations of the disease are often lethal [23, 24]. Diagnostic of preclinical (asymptomatic) atherosclerosis is therefore especially important. However, it is hindered by the absence of clinical symptoms and complaints and by the fact that the spectrum of risk factors is very wide, including genetic predisposition, lifestyle and diet patterns, chronic inflammation, and metabolic factors. Immunopathology is likely to be one of the mechanisms underlying atherosclerosis development starting from the early stages, and its assessment can therefore have an important diagnostic value.

3. Monocyte/Macrophage Diversity and Functions

Monocytes and macrophages are the key players in the innate immune system. These cells can eliminate pathogens by phagocytosis, release of reactive oxygen species, production of proinflammatory cytokines, and modulation of the T-cell immune response [25]. Macrophages are present in all organs and tissues and represent the first line of immune defence, responsible for removal of foreign agents and pathogens. They participate in all stages of the inflammatory process. The pool of macrophages remains constant in every tissue, and the cells are renewed from the population of circulating monocytes [26], although the results of recent studies suggest that these cells are also capable of self-renewal [27]. It has been known for a long time that changes in the phagocytic activity of macrophages might be dependent on changes in the peripheral blood monocyte population, and alterations of the monocyte pool lead to various pathological conditions [28]. Proliferation of promonocytes, which can be stimulated by systemic inflammatory stimuli, leads to the increase of the number of circulating monocytes [29, 30]. Monocytes and macrophages, together with their precursors and dendritic cells, form the mononuclear phagocyte system (MPS) [31], although the identity of the dendritic cells remains disputed [32, 33]. The development, maintenance, differentiation, and function of MPS are regulated mostly by colony-stimulating factor 1 (CSF-1) in homeostatic conditions [34] and by granulocyte-macrophage colony-stimulating factor (GM-CSF) during inflammation [35]. Inflammatory signals and various pathological conditions, including atherosclerosis development, stimulate the inactive circulating monocytes to become activated macrophages that can be distinguished by their phenotypic properties. Macrophages can acquire different functional phenotypes influenced by the surrounding microenvironment in a process known as macrophage polarization.

Studies of macrophage population revealed significant heterogeneity and plasticity of this cell type. Reaching consensus on macrophage classification was challenging due to the high variety of activation types, dependence of the results on the particular experimental setup, and differences of macrophage activation profiles between humans and animal models. Recently, a group of leading immunologists have summarized the current knowledge on the issue and drawn recommendations for conducting and reporting the experiments involving macrophage polarization [36]. Initially, two main classes of macrophages, M1 and M2, have been defined which could be obtained by activation of macrophages by proinflammatory interferon γ (IFN-γ) and lipopolysaccharide (LPS) or by interleukin-4 (IL-4), respectively [37–39]. A simplified scheme of macrophage polarization is presented in Figure 1.

M1 macrophages are characterized by the production of proinflammatory cytokines tumor necrosis factor-α (TNFα), IL-1β, IL-6, IL-12, and proteolytic enzymes, as well as by the expression of Fc-γ receptors on the cell surface [40, 41]. Polarization towards the proinflammatory phenotype can be induced *in vitro* by toll-like receptor (TLR) ligands, including TNFα, lipopolysaccharide (LPS), and interferon γ (IFN-γ) that might also play a role in the pathogenesis of atherosclerosis [42]. It has been demonstrated that M1 macrophages are present in the atherosclerotic plaques where they maintain the local inflammatory process and promote the extracellular matrix degradation contributing to the formation of unstable plaques that can induce thrombus formation and are therefore especially dangerous [43–45].

The subpopulation of M2 macrophages was further divided into several subtypes depending on the activation stimuli (Figure 1): M2a (activated by IL-4), M2b (activated by immune complexes), and M2c (activated by IL-10) [46]. Each of these subtypes is characterized by a distinct pattern of cytokine and surface marker expression which can also vary between the species. It has been proposed therefore to refer to different subtypes of macrophages indicating the activation type (e.g., M(IL-4) instead of M2a) [36]. M2a macrophages have strong anti-inflammatory properties and can be regarded as tissue-repairing cells [47]. They have poor phagocytic capacity and participate in the formation of extracellular matrix by stimulating production of collagen. They express IL-1 receptor antagonist (IL-1ra) and secrete CCL18, transforming growth factor β (TGF-β), and remodelling enzymes. M2b and M2c macrophages express different chemokine receptors, produce IL-10, and can modulate inflammation but do not synthesize the extracellular matrix and can therefore be regarded as regulatory macrophages [48]. Anti-inflammatory macrophages were also shown to express mannose receptor (CD206), stabilin-1, and decoy receptor IL-1RII on the surface [49–51]. M2 phenotype can also be induced by T regulatory cells [52]. However, the heterogeneity of this population requires further studies and standardization of the nomenclature. For the sake of simplicity, later in this work, we will refer to the IL-4-activated M2a macrophages as "M2 phenotype."

The production and release of the proinflammatory cytokines, such as IL-1β and IL-18, are dependent on the

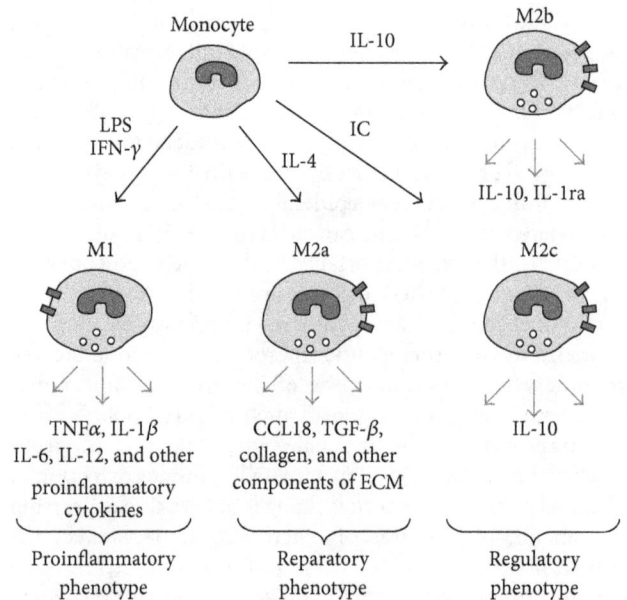

FIGURE 1: Simplified scheme of macrophage polarization. Activation of monocytes is followed by the polarization of macrophages to acquire proinflammatory phenotype (M1) or anti-inflammatory phenotypes (M2a–M2c) depending on the activation stimuli. Each phenotype is characterized by the secretion of a distinct pattern of pro- or anti-inflammatory cytokines and other molecules. For instance, M1 macrophages release TNFα, IL-1β, IL-6, IL-12, and other proinflammatory cytokines, whereas M2a macrophages produce CCL18, TGF-β, collagen, and other extracellular matrix components. LPS: bacterial lipopolysaccharides; IC: immune complexes; IFN-γ: interferon gamma; IL: interleukin; TNFα: tumor necrosis factor-alpha; TGF-β: transforming growth factor beta; CCL18: CC chemokine ligand 18.

macrophage inflammasome status [53, 54]. Inflammasome is a caspase-activating complex formed by several proteins, including caspase-1, which is responsible for cytokine maturation. Active caspase-1 can also be released from the activated cells and may contribute to the damage of neighbouring cells [55]. The inflammasome activation has been reported in various pathological conditions and infections. In can be induced by danger- and pathogen-associated molecular patterns (DAMPs and PAMPs) [56–59]. Importantly, inflammasome is activated in atherosclerosis in response to cholesterol accumulation in the blood vessel wall and formation of cholesterol crystals in foam cells [60]. On the other hand, atherogenesis can be associated with ongoing infections with various pathogens, such as *Chlamydia pneumonia* and *Helicobacter pylori*, which can induce the inflammasome activation [61–63]. There might exist other factors that contribute to the inflammasome activation and atherosclerosis progression, including the formation of uric acid crystals [64] and impaired autophagy [65]. Therefore, the inflammasome activation and release of proinflammatory cytokines and caspase-1 are relevant for atherosclerosis progression and can be regarded as important markers of the pathological process.

4. Cellular Tests Based on Monocyte/Macrophage Phenotypic Changes in Atherosclerosis

Development of a reliable monocyte/macrophage-based functional test remains challenging due to several technical problems. Isolation of monocytes from blood can lead to their activation. A number of different isolation methods have been proposed during the recent years. The traditional method implies cell adhesion, which leads to monocytes activation and is therefore widely criticized. Another method is fluorescence-activated cell sorting (FACS), which is fast and accurate but requires labelling of cells with specific antibodies, which can also lead to activation. A pure fraction of monocytes/macrophages can be isolated using magnetic separation. In this method, unspecific activation can also occur due to possible phagocytosis of paramagnetic particles. So far, the only method that can extract nonactivated monocytes is elutriation [66, 67]. It requires, however, special equipment and is impossible to introduce into routine clinical practice. Because of these technical problems, recent studies focused on the identification of molecular markers that could substitute for functional tests in diagnostics of immunopathologies.

Studies of monocyte function include the assessment of their motility, adhesion, phagocytic activity, and low-density protein (LDL) uptake [68, 69]. Macrophages can take part in pathological processes via stimulation with circulating soluble activation factors, adhesion to the endothelium, and migration into the tissue where they meet local activation factors. The monocytes' response to these stimuli depends on their priming in circulation and therefore can have a diagnostic potential. The analysis of macrophage pro- and anti-inflammatory phenotypic classes can provide important information on the disease progression, as has been demonstrated for atherosclerosis [22].

A monocyte/macrophage-based assay has recently been designed to evaluate changes in monocyte response to pro- and anti-inflammatory stimuli and to reveal possible bias of the macrophage polarization towards M1 or M2 phenotype. In this method, a pure population of blood monocytes was isolated using magnetic separation [49, 70] (Figure 2). The analysis of macrophage activity was performed by stimulating the cells with LPS, proinflammatory stimulus IFN-γ, and anti-inflammatory stimulus IL-4 [71]. Pro- and anti-inflammatory cytokine production measurement was used as readout. Proinflammatory activity of macrophages was assessed by the levels of secreted TNFα and IL-1β and anti-inflammatory activity by the levels of CCL18 production and IL-1ra expression. Inflammasome activation can also be assessed in this experimental system by measuring the IL-1β expression at mRNA level and comparing the results with the amount of mature IL-1β detected by ELISA. Another evidence of inflammasome activation that can be used as readout is the release of active caspase-1 [55]. Expression and release of the inflammasome-dependent cytokines TNFα and IL-8 should also be measured to provide the control of inflammasome activity. Further characterization of macrophages can be performed by analyzing such markers as

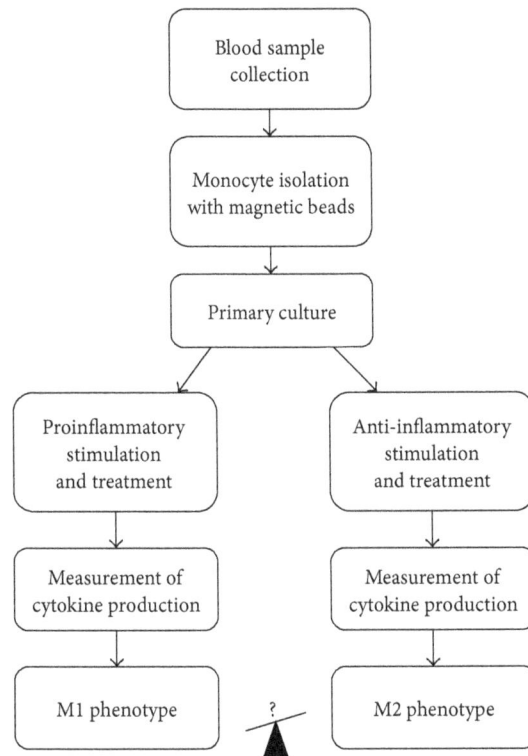

FIGURE 2: General design of the monocyte/macrophage activation assay.

MMR, CD163, TGF-RII, CSFR1, TNFRI, CD16, CD32, CD64, and stabilin-1, as well as the expression of TLR1, TLR2, and TLR4 at mRNA level and on the cell surface. Changes in the expression of these markers correlate with stimulation type and intensity. The described experimental system can provide important information on monocyte activation state and possible skew of the monocyte predisposition towards pro- or anti-inflammatory response. Apart from altered polarization towards one or the other phenotype, pathological conditions can be associated with other phenotypical alterations of monocytes/macrophage, including phagocytosis, migration, and proliferation. Alterations of macrophage phenotype and plasticity associated with atherosclerosis have recently been discussed in a comprehensive review [46].

The described method has been used to analyze activation of monocytes isolated from blood of healthy subjects ($n = 19$), atherosclerosis patients ($n = 22$), and breast cancer patients ($n = 18$). The obtained results demonstrated that production of proinflammatory TNFα was significantly lower in atherosclerosis patients and significantly higher in cancer patients in comparison to healthy subjects. On the other hand, production of anti-inflammatory CCL18 was decreased both in atherosclerosis and in cancer patients [22].

To evaluate the diagnostic potential of macrophages' activation test in asymptomatic atherosclerosis, a study was performed on individuals with predisposition to atherosclerosis ($n = 21$, mean age 63 ± 9 years) and subclinical atherosclerosis ($n = 21$, mean age 62 ± 7 years) in comparison

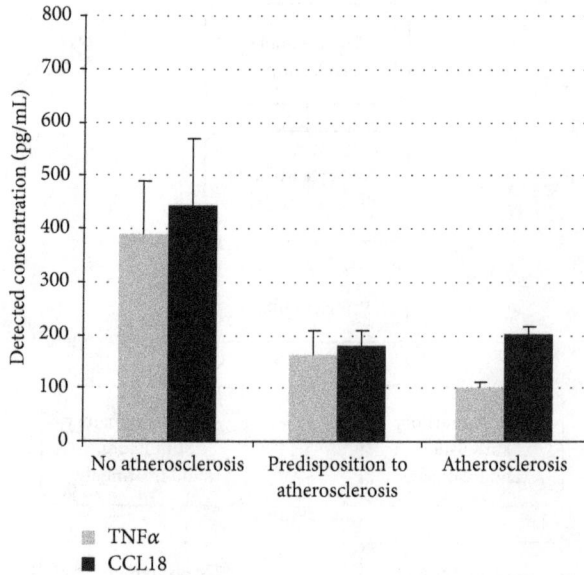

FIGURE 3: Study of monocyte/macrophage activation in subclinical and clinical atherosclerosis. Monocytes were isolated from the blood of subjects from 3 study groups ($n = 20$ in each group). Cells were stimulated with IFN-γ (100 ng/mL) or IL-4 (10 ng/mL). Secretion of TNFα and CCL18 was measured by ELISA.

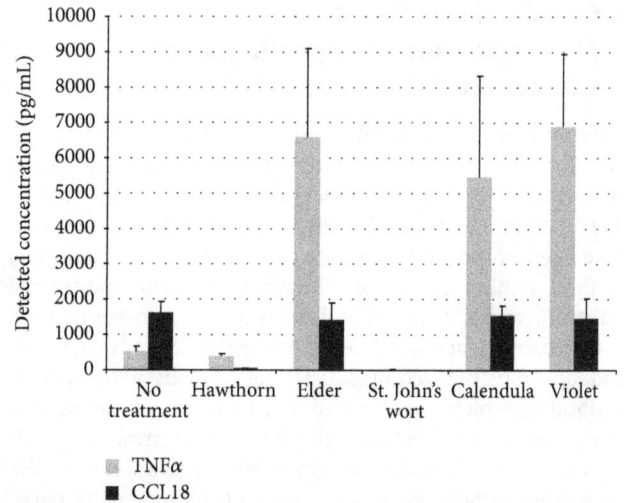

FIGURE 4: Modulation of macrophage polarization by natural agents. Macrophages were isolated from healthy subjects and brought into primary culture. Macrophages were incubated with extracts of various medicinal plants and stimulated with IFN-γ (100 ng/mL) or IL-4 (10 ng/mL). Secretion of TNFα and CCL18 was measured by ELISA.

to healthy subjects ($n = 21$, mean age 60 ± 9 years). Predisposition to atherosclerosis and subclinical atherosclerosis were detected by measuring the age-adjusted carotid intima media thickness (cIMT). The analysis of TNFα and CCL18 production by stimulated macrophages revealed dramatic individual differences between the analyzed subjects that may reflect the individuals' predisposition to immunopathology. Macrophages from subjects with subclinical atherosclerosis were characterized by especially low degree of activation in response to stimuli [22] (Figure 3). Therefore, the ability of macrophages to polarize towards pro- and anti-inflammatory phenotypes was decreased at early stages of atherosclerosis development, although the causative significance of this observation remains unclear.

5. Application of Cellular Tests for Drug Development

Changes of the immune system occur early in many pathological processes, opening the intriguing possibility that patients may benefit from a preventive treatment targeting the underlying immunopathology. Imbalanced macrophage polarization is observed in such conditions as atherosclerosis and cancer. Enhanced monocyte activation may lead to macrophage polarization towards pro- or anti-inflammatory phenotype leading to chronic inflammation and atherosclerosis or to oncopathologies, respectively [22]. Therefore, macrophage depolarization might be exploited for the development of preventive treatment [72]. For instance, it has been demonstrated that depolarization of macrophages from the M2 phenotype was associated with tumor regression [73].

To explore the potential of the macrophage activation test for drug development, the macrophage depolarization effects of herbal extracts were studied on cells obtained from healthy subjects. Plant extracts with immune-modulating properties are widely used in traditional medicine, but their therapeutic potential for modern clinical practice remains to be investigated. The extracts of the following plants with known anti-inflammatory activity were included into the study: flowers of hawthorn (*Crataegus* sp.), elderberry (*Sambucus nigra*), and calendula (*Calendula officinalis*) and herbs of St. John's wort (*Hypericum perforatum*) and violet (*Viola* sp.). Cultured macrophages were exposed to pro- and anti-inflammatory stimuli (IFN-γ and IL-4, resp.), and TNFα and CCL18 production was measured after 6 days. TNFα secretion by IFN-γ-stimulated macrophages treated with elderberry, calendula, and violet extracts was 10–13-fold higher than that of untreated stimulated macrophages. On the other hand, hawthorn and St. John's wort extracts significantly inhibited TNFα secretion. Extracts of hawthorn and St. John's wort also suppressed the secretion of CCL18 by IL-4-stimulated macrophages (Figure 4). Therefore, St. John's wort and hawthorn extracts appear to be natural agents with immune-modulatory properties that could be used for macrophage depolarization. Importantly, natural agents are characterized by relatively good tolerance and minimal side effects and are therefore especially suitable for long-term therapy, which is necessary for successful immune correction.

One of the therapeutic strategies for treatment of atherosclerosis is the inhibition of intracellular cholesterol accumulation. It is well established that hypercholesterolemia is a potent risk factor for atherosclerosis development [74–76]. However, the accumulating evidence demonstrates that atherogenic potential depends not so much on the total level of cholesterol as on the nature of cholesterol-containing

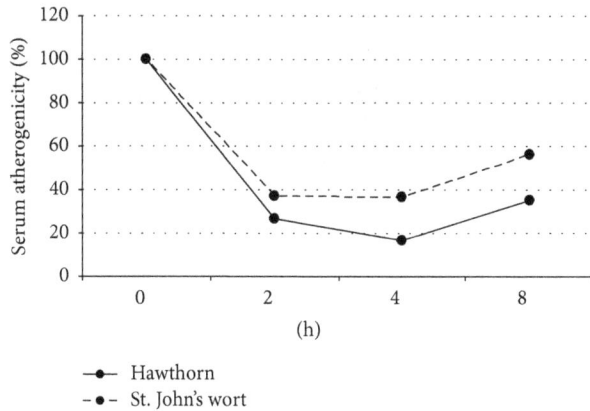

FIGURE 5: Study of serum atherogenicity in cellular assay. Four patients with atherosclerosis were given water extracts of 8 g of hawthorn berries or 3 g St. John's wort herb. Blood samples were collected before treatment and after 2, 4, and 8 hours and blood serum was added to cultured primary subendothelial intimal cells. Serum atherogenicity was measured as the increase of cholesterol content in cultured cells after 24 h.

lipoprotein particles that serve as a source of cholesterol storage in the arterial wall. Low-density lipoprotein (LDL) and especially its modifications, such as small dense, oxidized, desialylated, or electronegative LDL, play the key role in atherogenesis, and their levels positively correlate with the disease progression [77–79]. Moreover, modified LDL particles can provoke formation of autoantibodies that initiate the inflammatory response and form highly atherogenic immune complexes with LDL particles [80]. In that regard, LDL composition of blood plasma may be a decisive factor that triggers atherogenesis. The ability of blood serum to induce cholesterol accumulation is referred to as serum atherogenicity. It has been previously demonstrated that serum obtained from atherosclerosis patients caused cholesterol accumulation in cultured cells and therefore was highly atherogenic [81].

Primary culture of human aorta cells can be a useful system for testing various antiatherosclerotic substances. Using this system, atherogenic properties of patient's blood serum can be analyzed before and after drug administration to assess its therapeutic potential [82–84]. Antiatherogenic activity of hawthorn and St. John's wort extracts was tested using the described *ex vivo model*. Serum from study participants was added to cultured subendothelial intimal cells derived from uninvolved human aorta at concentration of 10%, and cholesterol accumulation was measured after 24 h using a previously established method [82]. It was demonstrated that blood serum atherogenicity decreased in study subjects treated with a single dose of hawthorn extract. The observed decrease was 73% and 83% after 2 and 4 hours, respectively, in comparison to the baseline (Figure 5). These results indicate that hawthorn extract may be regarded as a potent antiatherosclerotic agent. On the other hand, St. John's wort extract had no statistically significant effect on cellular cholesterol accumulation.

Taken together, the obtained results demonstrate that the combination of hawthorn and St. John's wort extracts appears promising for the development of antiatherosclerosis therapy. St. John's wort extract was a potent macrophage depolarizing agent, and hawthorn was demonstrated to reduce the serum atherogenicity. Further studies employing macrophage-based cellular test systems will allow identification of novel agents with therapeutic potential.

6. Conclusion

Monocyte/macrophage-based test system is a versatile tool to detect immunopathology, including increased monocyte activation and altered polarization of macrophages towards pro- or anti-inflammatory phenotypes. Alterations in monocyte activation and imbalance in macrophage polarization can be associated with a variety of pathological conditions, including different types of cancer and atherosclerosis. Therefore, the development of immunomodulating therapy might contribute significantly to the improvement of the existing treatment strategies. However, the complexity of the immunopathology requires flexible and reliable methods for diagnostics and monitoring of treatment efficiency. The monocyte/macrophage activation test is one of such methods. It was proven to be suitable for the analysis of immunopathology in subclinical atherosclerosis and breast cancer. This method can also be applied for studying numerous other pathologies, where monocyte/macrophage activation is implicated, including other types of cancer, chronic inflammation, and autoimmune disorders. Given the broad spectrum of cytokines that may be analyzed, the described method can be improved to perform a more detailed study of macrophage activation. The application of monocyte/macrophage activation test for drug research was illustrated by screening a series of medicinal plant extracts for antiatherosclerotic activity. Study of macrophage polarization revealed a potent immunomodulatory activity of hawthorn and St. John's wort extracts that might be beneficial for treatment and prevention of atherosclerosis. Together, these results demonstrate the possibilities of macrophage-based cellular tests for diagnostics and drug research in conditions associated with immunopathology.

Conflict of Interests

The authors declare that there is no conflict of interests regarding the publication of this paper.

Acknowledgment

This work was supported by the Russian Scientific Foundation (Grant no. 14-15-00112).

References

[1] F. Balkwill and A. Mantovani, "Inflammation and cancer: back to Virchow?" *The Lancet*, vol. 357, no. 9255, pp. 539–545, 2001.

[2] S. K. Biswas and A. Mantovani, "Macrophage plasticity and interaction with lymphocyte subsets: cancer as a paradigm," *Nature Immunology*, vol. 11, no. 10, pp. 889–896, 2010.

[3] M. Peled and E. A. Fisher, "Dynamic aspects of macrophage polarization during atherosclerosis progression and regression," *Frontiers in Immunology*, vol. 5, no. 579, 2014.

[4] J. E. Feig, S. Parathath, J. X. Rong et al., "Reversal of hyperlipidemia with a genetic switch favorably affects the content and inflammatory state of macrophages in atherosclerotic plaques," *Circulation*, vol. 123, no. 9, pp. 989–998, 2011.

[5] J. E. Feig, J. X. Rong, R. Shamir et al., "HDL promotes rapid atherosclerosis regression in mice and alters inflammatory properties of plaque monocyte-derived cells," *Proceedings of the National Academy of Sciences of the United States of America*, vol. 108, no. 17, pp. 7166–7171, 2011.

[6] R. Ross, "Atherosclerosis—an inflammatory disease," *The New England Journal of Medicine*, vol. 340, no. 2, pp. 115–126, 1999.

[7] C. Weber and H. Noels, "Atherosclerosis: current pathogenesis and therapeutic options," *Nature Medicine*, vol. 17, no. 11, pp. 1410–1422, 2011.

[8] G. K. Hansson and A. Hermansson, "The immune system in atherosclerosis," *Nature Immunology*, vol. 12, no. 3, pp. 204–212, 2011.

[9] R. Klingenberg and G. K. Hansson, "Treating inflammation in atherosclerotic cardiovascular disease: emerging therapies," *European Heart Journal*, vol. 30, no. 23, pp. 2838–2844, 2009.

[10] R. Beaglehole and R. Bonita, "Global public health: a scorecard," *The Lancet*, vol. 372, no. 9654, pp. 1988–1996, 2008.

[11] J. F. Fries, "Strategies for reduction of morbidity," *The American Journal of Clinical Nutrition*, vol. 55, supplement 6, pp. 1257S–1262S, 1992.

[12] B. Mostert, A. M. Sieuwerts, J. Kraan et al., "Gene expression profiles in circulating tumor cells to predict prognosis in metastatic breast cancer patients," *Annals of Oncology*, vol. 26, no. 3, pp. 510–516, 2015.

[13] B. Mostert, A. M. Sieuwerts, J. Bolt-de Vries et al., "mRNA expression profiles in circulating tumor cells of metastatic colorectal cancer patients," *Molecular Oncology*, vol. 9, no. 4, pp. 920–932, 2015.

[14] V. Hofman, M. Ilie, E. Long et al., "Detection of circulating tumor cells from lung cancer patients in the era of targeted therapy: promises, drawbacks and pitfalls," *Current Molecular Medicine*, vol. 14, no. 4, pp. 440–456, 2014.

[15] B. Polzer, G. Medoro, S. Pasch et al., "Molecular profiling of single circulating tumor cells with diagnostic intention," *EMBO Molecular Medicine*, vol. 6, no. 11, pp. 1371–1386, 2005.

[16] B. Reynés, R. Díaz-Rúa, M. Cifre, P. Oliver, and A. Palou, "Peripheral blood mononuclear cells as a potential source of biomarkers to test the efficacy of weight-loss strategies," *Obesity*, vol. 23, no. 1, pp. 28–31, 2015.

[17] K. L. Bentley-Hewitt, R. K.-Y. Chen, R. E. Lill et al., "Consumption of selenium-enriched broccoli increases cytokine production in human peripheral blood mononuclear cells stimulated ex vivo, a preliminary human intervention study," *Molecular Nutrition & Food Research*, vol. 58, no. 12, pp. 2350–2357, 2014.

[18] V. Bordignon, F. Palamara, G. Altomonte et al., "A laboratory test based on determination of cytokine profiles: a promising assay to identify exposition to contact allergens and predict the clinical outcome in occupational allergic contact dermatitis," *BMC Immunology*, vol. 16, article 4, 2015.

[19] M. M. Venkataswamy, S. N. Madhusudana, S. S. Sanyal et al., "Cellular immune response following pre-exposure and post-exposure rabies vaccination by intradermal and intramuscular routes," *Clinical and Experimental Vaccine Research*, vol. 4, no. 1, pp. 68–74, 2015.

[20] M. G. Cardenas-Mondragon, G. Vallejo-Flores, J. Delgado-Dominguez et al., "Preeclampsia is associated with lower production of vascular endothelial growth factor by peripheral blood mononuclear cells," *Archives of Medical Research*, vol. 45, no. 7, pp. 561–569, 2014.

[21] M. Jenny, M. Klieber, D. Zaknun et al., "In vitro testing for anti-inflammatory properties of compounds employing peripheral blood mononuclear cells freshly isolated from healthy donors," *Inflammation Research*, vol. 60, no. 2, pp. 127–135, 2011.

[22] A. N. Orekhov, I. A. Sobenin, M. A. Gavrilin et al., "Macrophages in immunopathology of atherosclerosis: a target for diagnostics and therapy," *Current Pharmaceutical Design*, vol. 21, no. 9, pp. 1172–1179, 2015.

[23] W. E. Hellings, W. Peeters, F. L. Moll, and G. Pasterkamp, "From vulnerable plaque to vulnerable patient: the search for biomarkers of plaque destabilization," *Trends in Cardiovascular Medicine*, vol. 17, no. 5, pp. 162–171, 2007.

[24] J. A. Schaar, J. E. Muller, E. Falk et al., "Terminology for high-risk and vulnerable coronary artery plaques. Report of a meeting on the vulnerable plaque, June 17 and 18, 2003, Santorini, Greece," *European Heart Journal*, vol. 25, no. 12, pp. 1077–1082, 2004.

[25] N. V. Serbina, T. Jia, T. M. Hohl, and E. G. Pamer, "Monocyte-mediated defense against microbial pathogens," *Annual Review of Immunology*, vol. 26, pp. 421–452, 2008.

[26] R. van Furth and Z. A. Cohn, "The origin and kinetics of mononuclear phagocytes," *The Journal of Experimental Medicine*, vol. 128, no. 3, pp. 415–435, 1968.

[27] M. H. Sieweke and J. E. Allen, "Beyond stem cells: self-renewal of differentiated macrophages," *Science*, vol. 342, no. 6161, Article ID 1242974, 2013.

[28] N. P. Hurst and G. Nuki, "Evidence for defect of complement-mediated phagocytosis by monocytes from patients with rheumatoid arthritis and cutaneous vasculitis," *British Medical Journal*, vol. 282, no. 6282, pp. 2081–2083, 1981.

[29] G. Meuret and G. Hoffmann, "Monocyte kinetic studies in normal and disease states," *British Journal of Haematology*, vol. 24, no. 3, pp. 275–285, 1973.

[30] G. Meuret, J. Bammert, and G. Hoffmann, "Kinetics of human monocytopoiesis," *Blood*, vol. 44, no. 6, pp. 801–816, 1974.

[31] P. R. Taylor and S. Gordon, "Monocyte heterogeneity and innate immunity," *Immunity*, vol. 19, no. 1, pp. 2–4, 2003.

[32] F. Geissmann, S. Gordon, D. A. Hume, A. M. Mowat, and G. J. Randolph, "Unravelling mononuclear phagocyte heterogeneity," *Nature Reviews Immunology*, vol. 10, no. 6, pp. 453–460, 2010.

[33] S. J. Jenkins and D. A. Hume, "Homeostasis in the mononuclear phagocyte system," *Trends in Immunology*, vol. 35, no. 8, pp. 358–367, 2014.

[34] A. Bartocci, D. S. Mastrogiannis, G. Migliorati, R. J. Stockert, A. W. Wolkoff, and E. R. Stanley, "Macrophages specifically regulate the concentration of their own growth factor in the circulation," *Proceedings of the National Academy of Sciences of the United States of America*, vol. 84, no. 17, pp. 6179–6183, 1987.

[35] J. C. Gasson, "Molecular physiology of granulocyte-macrophage colony-stimulating factor," *Blood*, vol. 77, no. 6, pp. 1131–1145, 1991.

[36] P. J. Murray, J. E. Allen, S. K. Biswas et al., "Macrophage activation and polarization: nomenclature and experimental guidelines," *Immunity*, vol. 41, no. 1, pp. 14–20, 2014.

[37] S. Gordon and F. O. Martinez, "Alternative activation of macrophages: mechanism and functions," *Immunity*, vol. 32, no. 5, pp. 593–604, 2010.

[38] C. D. Mills, K. Kincaid, J. M. Alt, M. J. Heilman, and A. M. Hill, "M-1/M-2 macrophages and the Th1/Th2 paradigm," *The Journal of Immunology*, vol. 164, no. 12, pp. 6166–6173, 2000.

[39] S. Gordon and P. R. Taylor, "Monocyte and macrophage heterogeneity," *Nature Reviews Immunology*, vol. 5, no. 12, pp. 953–964, 2005.

[40] A. Gratchev, K. Schledzewski, P. Guillot, and S. Goerdt, "Alternatively activated antigen-presenting cells: molecular repertoire, immune regulation, and healing," *Skin Pharmacology and Applied Skin Physiology*, vol. 14, no. 5, pp. 272–279, 2001.

[41] S. Gordon, "The macrophage," *BioEssays*, vol. 17, no. 11, pp. 977–986, 1995.

[42] F. De Paoli, B. Staels, and G. Chinetti-Gbaguidi, "Macrophage phenotypes and their modulation in atherosclerosis," *Circulation Journal*, vol. 78, no. 8, pp. 1775–1781, 2014.

[43] R. N. Hanna, I. Shaked, H. G. Hubbeling et al., "NR4A1 (Nur77) deletion polarizes macrophages toward an inflammatory phenotype and increases atherosclerosis," *Circulation Research*, vol. 110, no. 3, pp. 416–427, 2012.

[44] M. J. Davies, "Stability and instability: two faces of coronary atherosclerosis. The Paul Dudley White lecture 1995," *Circulation*, vol. 94, no. 8, pp. 2013–2020, 1996.

[45] H. C. Stary, A. B. Chandler, R. E. Dinsmore et al., "A definition of advanced types of atherosclerotic lesions and a histological classification of atherosclerosis. A report from the committee on vascular lesions of the council on arteriosclerosis, American Heart Association," *Circulation*, vol. 92, no. 5, pp. 1355–1374, 1995.

[46] J. Rojas, J. Salazar, M. S. Martínez et al., "Macrophage heterogeneity and plasticity: impact of macrophage biomarkers on atherosclerosis," *Scientifica*, vol. 2015, Article ID 851252, 17 pages, 2015.

[47] T. J. Koh and L. A. DiPietro, "Inflammation and wound healing: the role of the macrophage," *Expert Reviews in Molecular Medicine*, vol. 13, article e23, 2011.

[48] B. D. Fleming and D. M. Mosser, "Regulatory macrophages: setting the threshold for therapy," *European Journal of Immunology*, vol. 41, no. 9, pp. 2498–2502, 2011.

[49] A. Gratchev, J. Kzhyshkowska, K. Duperrier, J. Utikal, F. W. Velten, and S. Goerdt, "The receptor for interleukin-17E is induced by Th2 cytokines in antigen-presenting cells," *Scandinavian Journal of Immunology*, vol. 60, no. 3, pp. 233–237, 2004.

[50] V. Kodelja, C. Müller, O. Politz, N. Hakij, C. E. Orfanos, and S. Goerdt, "Alternative macrophage activation-associated CC-chemokine-1, a novel structural homologue of macrophage inflammatory protein-1α with a Th2- associated expression pattern," *The Journal of Immunology*, vol. 160, no. 3, pp. 1411–1418, 1998.

[51] O. Politz, A. Gratchev, P. A. G. McCourt et al., "Stabilin-1 and -2 constitute a novel family of fasciclin-like hyaluronan receptor homologues," *The Biochemical Journal*, vol. 362, no. 1, pp. 155–164, 2002.

[52] M. M. Tiemessen, A. L. Jagger, H. G. Evans, M. J. C. van Herwijnen, S. John, and L. S. Taams, "CD4$^+$CD25$^+$Foxp3$^+$ regulatory T cells induce alternative activation of human

monocytes/macrophages," *Proceedings of the National Academy of Sciences of the United States of America*, vol. 104, no. 49, pp. 19446–19451, 2007.

[53] F. Martinon, K. Burns, and J. Tschopp, "The inflammasome: a molecular platform triggering activation of inflammatory caspases and processing of proIL-β," *Molecular Cell*, vol. 10, no. 2, pp. 417–426, 2002.

[54] K. J. Moore and I. Tabas, "Macrophages in the pathogenesis of atherosclerosis," *Cell*, vol. 145, no. 3, pp. 341–355, 2011.

[55] A. Sarkar, S. Mitra, S. Mehta, R. Raices, and M. D. Wewers, "Monocyte derived microvesicles deliver a cell death message via encapsulated caspase-1," *PLoS ONE*, vol. 4, no. 9, Article ID e7140, 2009.

[56] M. A. Gavrilin, S. Mitra, S. Seshadri et al., "Pyrin critical to macrophage IL-1β response to *Francisella* challenge," *The Journal of Immunology*, vol. 182, no. 12, pp. 7982–7989, 2009.

[57] M. A. Gavrilin, D. H. A. Abdelaziz, M. Mostafa et al., "Activation of the pyrin inflammasome by intracellular *Burkholderia cenocepacia*," *Journal of Immunology*, vol. 188, no. 7, pp. 3469–3477, 2012.

[58] F. Martinon, A. Mayor, and J. Tschopp, "The inflammasomes: guardians of the body," *Annual Review of Immunology*, vol. 27, pp. 229–265, 2009.

[59] C. A. Janeway Jr. and R. Medzhitov, "Innate immune recognition," *Annual Review of Immunology*, vol. 20, pp. 197–216, 2002.

[60] P. Duewell, H. Kono, K. J. Rayner et al., "NLRP3 inflammasomes are required for atherogenesis and activated by cholesterol crystals," *Nature*, vol. 464, no. 7293, pp. 1357–1361, 2010.

[61] V. V. Valtonen, "Infection as a risk factor for infarction and atherosclerosis," *Annals of Medicine*, vol. 23, no. 5, pp. 539–543, 1991.

[62] A. Luque, M. M. Turu, N. Rovira, J. O. Juan-Babot, M. Slevin, and J. Krupinski, "Early atherosclerotic plaques show evidence of infection by *Chlamydia pneumoniae*," *Frontiers in Bioscience*, vol. 4, no. 7, pp. 2423–2432, 2012.

[63] M. Charakida and D. Tousoulis, "Infections and atheromatous plaque: current therapeutic implications," *Current Pharmaceutical Design*, vol. 19, no. 9, pp. 1638–1650, 2013.

[64] E. Krishnan, "Inflammation, oxidative stress and lipids: the risk triad for atherosclerosis in gout," *Rheumatology*, vol. 49, no. 7, Article ID keq037, pp. 1229–1238, 2010.

[65] B. Razani, C. Feng, T. Coleman et al., "Autophagy links inflammasomes to atherosclerotic progression," *Cell Metabolism*, vol. 15, no. 4, pp. 534–544, 2012.

[66] E. F. Strasser and R. Eckstein, "Optimization of leukocyte collection and monocyte isolation for dendritic cell culture," *Transfusion Medicine Reviews*, vol. 24, no. 2, pp. 130–139, 2010.

[67] S. B. Clarkson and P. A. Ory, "CD16. Developmentally regulated IgG Fc receptors on cultured human monocytes," *The Journal of Experimental Medicine*, vol. 167, no. 2, pp. 408–420, 1988.

[68] S. Krause, A. Pohl, C. Pohl et al., "Ex vivo investigation of blood monocyte and platelet behaviour in pigs maintained on an atherogenic diet," *Experimental and Toxicologic Pathology*, vol. 44, no. 3, pp. 144–146, 1992.

[69] F. P. Bell and R. G. Gerrity, "Evidence for an altered lipid metabolic state in circulating blood monocytes under conditions of hyperlipemia in swine and its implications in arterial lipid metabolism," *Arteriosclerosis and Thrombosis*, vol. 12, no. 2, pp. 155–162, 1992.

[70] A. Gratchev, P. Guillot, N. Hakiy et al., "Alternatively activated macrophages differentially express fibronectin and its splice

variants and the extracellular matrix protein βIG-H3," *Scandinavian Journal of Immunology*, vol. 53, no. 4, pp. 386–392, 2001.

[71] A. Gratchev, J. Kzhyshkowska, K. Köthe et al., "Mφ1 and Mφ2 can be re-polarized by Th2 or Th1 cytokines, respectively, and respond to exogenous danger signals," *Immunobiology*, vol. 211, no. 6–8, pp. 473–486, 2006.

[72] D. M. Mosser and J. P. Edwards, "Exploring the full spectrum of macrophage activation," *Nature Reviews Immunology*, vol. 8, no. 12, pp. 958–969, 2008.

[73] S. M. Pyonteck, L. Akkari, A. J. Schuhmacher et al., "CSF-1R inhibition alters macrophage polarization and blocks glioma progression," *Nature Medicine*, vol. 19, no. 10, pp. 1264–1272, 2013.

[74] E. R. Andreeva, I. M. Pugach, and A. N. Orekhov, "Subendothelial smooth muscle cells of human aorta express macrophage antigen in situ and in vitro," *Atherosclerosis*, vol. 135, no. 1, pp. 19–27, 1997.

[75] E. R. Andreeva, I. M. Pugach, and A. N. Orekhov, "Collagen-synthesizing cells in initial and advanced atherosclerotic lesions of human aorta," *Atherosclerosis*, vol. 130, no. 1-2, pp. 133–142, 1997.

[76] E. J. Mills, B. Rachlis, P. Wu, P. J. Devereaux, P. Arora, and D. Perri, "Primary prevention of cardiovascular mortality and events with statin treatments: a network meta-analysis involving more than 65,000 patients," *Journal of the American College of Cardiology*, vol. 52, no. 22, pp. 1769–1781, 2008.

[77] S. Hirayama and T. Miida, "Small dense LDL: an emerging risk factor for cardiovascular disease," *Clinica Chimica Acta*, vol. 414, pp. 215–224, 2012.

[78] D. Steinberg, S. Parthasarathy, T. E. Carew, J. C. Khoo, and J. L. Witztum, "Beyond cholesterol. Modifications of low-density lipoprotein that increase its atherogenicity," *The New England Journal of Medicine*, vol. 320, no. 14, pp. 915–924, 1989.

[79] A. N. Orekhov, V. V. Tertov, and D. N. Mukhin, "Desialylated low density lipoprotein—naturally occurring modified lipoprotein with atherogenic potency," *Atherosclerosis*, vol. 86, no. 2-3, pp. 153–161, 1991.

[80] A. N. Orekhov, V. V. Tertov, A. E. Kabakov, I. Y. Adamova, S. N. Pokrovsky, and V. N. Smirnov, "Autoantibodies against modified low density lipoprotein. Nonlipid factor of blood plasma that stimulates foam cell formation," *Arteriosclerosis and Thrombosis*, vol. 11, no. 2, pp. 316–326, 1991.

[81] E. I. Chazov, A. N. Orekhov, N. V. Perova et al., "Atherogenicity of blood serum from patients with coronary heart disease," *The Lancet*, vol. 328, no. 8507, pp. 595–598, 1986.

[82] A. N. Orekhov, V. V. Tertov, K. A. Khashimov, S. S. Kudryashov, and V. N. Smirnov, "Evidence of antiatherosclerotic action of verapamil from direct effects on arterial cells," *The American Journal of Cardiology*, vol. 59, no. 5, pp. 495–496, 1987.

[83] S. E. Akopov, A. N. Orekhov, V. V. Tertov, K. A. Khashimov, E. S. Gabrielyan, and V. N. Smirnov, "Stable analogues of prostacyclin and thromboxane A$_2$ display contradictory influences on atherosclerotic properties of cells cultured from human aorta The effect of calcium antagonists," *Atherosclerosis*, vol. 72, no. 2-3, pp. 245–248, 1988.

[84] A. N. Orekhov, V. V. Tertov, S. A. Kudryashov, K. A. Khashimov, and V. N. Smirnov, "Primary culture of human aortic intima cells as a model for testing antiatherosclerotic drugs. Effects of cyclic AMP, prostaglandins, calcium antagonists, antioxidants, and lipid-lowering agents," *Atherosclerosis*, vol. 60, no. 2, pp. 101–110, 1986.

10

Gq-Coupled Receptors in Autoimmunity

Lu Zhang[1] and Guixiu Shi[2]

[1]Department of Nephrology, The First Affiliated Hospital of Xiamen University, Xiamen 361003, China
[2]Department of Rheumatology and Clinical Immunology, The First Affiliated Hospital of Xiamen University, Xiamen 361003, China

Correspondence should be addressed to Guixiu Shi; gshi@xmu.edu.cn

Academic Editor: Xiao-Feng Yang

Heterotrimeric G proteins can be divided into Gi, Gs, Gq/11, and G12/13 subfamilies according to their α subunits. The main function of G proteins is transducing signals from G protein coupled receptors (GPCRs), a family of seven transmembrane receptors. In recent years, studies have demonstrated that GPCRs interact with Gq, a member of the Gq/11 subfamily of G proteins. This interaction facilitates the vital role of this family of proteins in immune regulation and autoimmunity, particularly for Gαq, which is considered the functional α subunit of Gq protein. Therefore, understanding the mechanisms through which Gq-coupled receptors control autoreactive lymphocytes is critical and may provide insights into the treatment of autoimmune disorders. In this review, we summarize recent advances in studies of the role of Gq-coupled receptors in autoimmunity, with a focus on their pathologic role and downstream signaling.

1. Introduction

Many receptors for hormones, neurotransmitters, neuropeptides, chemokines, and autocrine and paracrine signaling molecules interact with heterotrimeric G proteins to exert their actions on target cells [1]; these receptors are considered G protein coupled receptors (GPCRs) [2]. It is estimated that more than 800 GPCRs are encoded in the mammalian genome [3], supporting that GPCRs are common membrane receptors in cells.

Heterotrimeric G proteins consist of an α-subunit, which binds to and hydrolyzes guanosine-5′-triphosphate (GTP), and β- and γ-subunits, which form an indissociable complex [4]. GPCRs transmit extracellular signals into the cell by binding to and activating different intracellular signaling proteins, termed G proteins (G$\alpha\beta\gamma$, families Gi, Gs, Gq/11, G12/13) or arrestins [5]. The Gq proteins, like all heterotrimeric G proteins, are composed of three subunits: Gαq, Gβ, and Gγ [6]. Gαq-GTP and the G$\beta\gamma$ dimer then transmit receptor-generated signals to downstream effector molecules and protein binding partners until the intrinsic GTPase activity of Gα hydrolyzes GTP to GDP and the inactive subunits reassociate [6]; this is called the "active and inactive" cycle. Each of the four major subfamilies of G proteins is associated with different signaling pathways: Gq/11 activates the phospholipase C (PLC) family; Gs stimulates the adenylyl cyclase (AC) pathway; Gi/o inhibits AC; and G12/13 activates small GTPases [4].

The Gq/11 subfamily, including Gq, G11, G14, and G15/16, shares structural similarity, and activation of the α subunit within each protein complex can activate PLC-β [4–7]. Furthermore, all of these four subunits regulate both overlapping and distinct signaling pathways, thereby stimulating inositol lipid (i.e., calcium/protein kinase C (PKC)) signaling through PLC-β isoforms [1, 4–9]. Genetic studies using whole animal models have demonstrated the importance of Gq in cardiac, lung, brain, and platelet functions, helping to define the physiological and pathological processes mediated by the Gq [5, 10].

Recent studies have described all four subtypes of Gq/11 coupled GPCRs, including the muscarinic 1, 3, and 5 (M1, M3, and M5) receptors; bombesin receptor, vasopressin receptor, endothelin receptor, thyrotropin-releasing hormone receptor (TRHR), gonadotropin-releasing hormone receptor (GnRHR), membrane estrogen receptor (mER), chemokine receptors, adrenergic receptors (α1AR), and angiotensin II type 1 receptor (AT(1)R) [11–13]. In the field of immunology, chemokine and hormone receptors have been shown to function as Gq protein-coupled GPCRs. These GqPCRs are expressed on lymphocytes and are regulated by their ligands in the immune system [14–18]. Abnormal regulation of these receptors may be associated with the pathogenesis of autoimmunity and a variety of autoimmune diseases induced by autoreactive lymphocytes, leading to morbidity and mortality in individuals with autoimmune disorders [19–24].

2. The Diversity of Gq-Coupled Receptors in Autoimmunity

Gq is the most commonly studied subclass of the Gq/11 subfamily in the field of immunology [18] and is mainly coupled to sex hormone receptors and some chemokine receptors, which are differentially expressed in certain types of lymphocytes [6, 18] (Table 1).

2.1. The GnRHRs and mERs. Gonadotropin-releasing hormone (GnRH) is the primary hormone associated with reproduction; GnRH is known to exert its actions largely through two related Gq/11 protein receptors [25]. The interaction between GnRH and its cognate type I receptor (GnRHR) in the pituitary results in the activation of Gq, PLC-β, phospholipase A2 (PLA2), and phospholipase D (PLD) [2]. Sequential activation of phospholipases generates the second messengers inositol 1, 4,5-tris-phosphate (IP3), diacylglycerol (DAG), and arachidonic acid (AA), which are required for Ca^{2+} mobilization. Further activation of various protein kinase C isoforms (PKCs) induces sequential activation of mitogen-activated protein kinases (MAPKs) [26] and promotes nuclear transcription. GnRHR mRNA and protein have been found in the pituitary, lymphocytes, mononuclear cells, and various types of cancer cells [23]. Many autoimmune diseases, particularly systemic lupus erythematosus (SLE), exhibit gender-specific differences, and GnRHRs have been shown to function as immunostimulatory hormone receptors, playing pivotal roles in the observed gender-specific differences in immunity and/or autoimmunity [27].

Acute treatment with GnRH increases the expression of *GnRHR* mRNA in murine thymocytes [28]. Studies in mice and rats have shown that GnRH stimulates the expression of hormone-GqPCR and the interleukin- (IL-) 2 receptor, the proliferation of B and T lymphocytes, and the elevation of serum IgG levels [27]. Jacobson [23] measured *GnRHR* mRNA and GnRH binding in lupus-prone mice after in vivo exposure to GnRH or vehicle. Their results showed that even vehicle-treated females expressed more GnRHR in immune cells than did vehicle-treated males; gender differences were confirmed, with females expressing Gq-coupled hormone receptor mRNA and protein more than males [26]. In mice given GnRH, GnRH (through GqPCR) exacerbated lupus in vivo in females only [27]. Additional studies have shown that GnRH (through GqPCR) stimulates T/B lymphocyte proliferation in vitro in females only [29]. These differences in expression and activation of GnRHR through GqPCR on lymphocytes contribute to the observed gender differences in immunity and/or autoimmunity.

In addition to the pivotal function of intracellular estrogen receptors in autoimmunity, researchers have also shown that mERs can stimulate Gq-coupled GPCRs through PKC and calcium pathways [30]. Rider and Abdou [31] suggested that estrogen acting through Gq-mERs enhances T-cell activation in women with lupus, resulting in amplified T/B-cell interactions, B-cell activation, and autoantibody production.

Thus, the gender differences in GnRH and estrogen production and function can be directly associated with Gq protein receptor expression, which plays a critical role in maintaining the balance of T/B lymphocytes and affects the morbidity of autoimmune diseases that predominantly affect women.

2.2. The Chemokine Receptors. Chemokine receptors are expressed on T cells, B cells, monocytes, macrophages, and dendritic cells [32]. Chemokine receptors and their ligand axis play pivotal roles in leukocyte migration, differentiation, adhesion, and activation [32, 33]. Many chemokine receptors have been implicated in the pathogenesis of autoimmune connective tissue diseases such as SLE, rheumatoid arthritis (RA), and systemic sclerosis (SS) [19–21, 32, 34–37]. However, previous studies have demonstrated the indispensable role of chemokine receptors in autoimmune diseases, highlighting the role of Gi protein-coupled chemokine receptors (rather than Gq-coupled receptors) in directing the migration of immune cells, which mostly signal through the canonical AC pathway [19, 36].

In a cell-based study, Arai and Charo [32] showed that monocyte chemotactic protein- (MCP-) 1-related chemokine receptors (mainly CC family receptors) interact with multiple subtypes of G proteins in a cell type-specific manner and that the third intracellular loop of CC type receptors mediates Gq coupling.

Moreover, many studies have shown that chemokine receptors can interact with multiple G-protein subtypes; the coupling is cell type-specific [32]. Shi and colleagues [38] showed that chemokine receptors can be divided into CD38-dependent and -independent subclasses, depending on whether CD38 is needed for the chemotaxis of the ligand. CD38-dependent chemokine receptors couple to Gq, indicating that there is indeed a novel Gq protein-coupled alternative signaling pathway separate from the canonical Gi-coupled classic pathway.

Autoimmunity-associated chemokine receptors mainly include the CC family (CCR5 and CCR7) and the CXC family (CXCR3, CXCR4, CXCR5, and CXCR7) [19, 20, 34, 36–41]. To date, most chemokine receptors, such as CXCR4 and CXCR5 on T cells and B cells, have been shown to be induced by Gi in the classic pathway, while CCR7 and CXCR4 have been shown to be dependent on Gq pathways only on dendritic cells (DCs) [38]. Hence, the dependence of autoimmune diseases on the specific Gq coupled chemokine receptor alone is still unclear. Since this chemokine receptor is engaged and activated in lymphocytes by GPCRs, it is possible that these Gq-coupled receptors may interact functionally with Gi to regulate chemotaxis in lymphocytes during the effector stage [42].

TABLE 1: Gq-coupled GPCRs in autoimmunity.

Type	AID	Cell type	Disease model	Function in general	References
GnRHR	SLE	Lymphocytes Mononuclear cells Cancer cells	Lupus-prone mice	Through high level of GnRH stimulates the expression of hormone-GqPCR and the interleukin- (IL-) 2 receptor, the proliferation of B and T lymphocytes, and the elevation of serum IgG levels	[23, 26–29]
mER	SLE	T/B lymphocytes	Lupus patients	Amplify T/B-cell interactions, B-cell activation, and autoantibody production	[30, 31]
Chemokine receptor	SLE RA SS	T lymphocytes DCs Monocytes Neutrophils (CD38-dependent)	Gnαq−/− mice	(1) Compete with T-cell receptor stop signals and determine the duration of T-cell-APC interactions, form more stable conjugates, and enhance proliferation and cytokine production (2) DCs and monocytes' migration to inflammatory sites and lymph nodes	[15, 19–21, 32, 38, 42, 48]
AT(1)R	Autoimmune-regulated cardiomyopathy and HTN	T lymphocytes	Gq TG mice	Unbalance between T-cell-induced inflammation and T-cell suppressor responses for the regulation of pathological process	[43, 44]
α1-AR	HTN	Lymphocytes	HTN patients	High levels of autoantibodies against the second extracellular loop of α1-adrenoceptor (α1-AR) in patients with hypertension	[11, 45, 46]

AID: autoimmune disease; HTN: hypertension; APC: antigen-presenting cell.

2.3. Others. AT(1)R, one of the best-studied GPCRs, signals through Gq to transduce signals on lymphocytes in autoimmune-regulated cardiomyopathy and hypertension [43]. Experimental findings support the concept that the balance between T cell-induced inflammation and T cell suppressor responses is critical for the regulation of blood pressure levels; autoantibodies to these receptors can exacerbate the pathological process [44]. High levels of autoantibodies against the second extracellular loop of α1-adrenoceptor (α1-AR) are also found in patients with hypertension, suggesting an important role of α1-AR and AT(1)R autoimmunity in the pathogenesis and management of hypertension, particularly in patients having high levels of receptor-associated autoantibodies [11, 45, 46]. However, the precise mechanism is still unknown.

3. How Do Gq-Coupled Receptors Play a Role in Autoimmunity?

Autoimmunity comprises a variety of autoreactive lymphocytes characterized by the loss of tolerance to a variety of autoantigens and imbalanced humoral and cellular immunity in biological systems [19, 23, 47]. Gq-coupled GPCRs on different lymphocytes can transduce a series of extracellular

signals into the nucleus to regulate immune function. Immune responses are coordinated by the extracellular ligand to GPCR on lymphocytes, and activated intracellular Gq protein then activates enzymes, second messengers, protein kinases, and nuclear translocation, consequently inducing the migration, activation, and apoptosis of lymphocytes [48]. This well-orchestrated function of hematopoietic cells is complex; however, it is clear that Gq-coupled receptors and the signaling molecules that reside downstream of these receptors are critical to these functions.

3.1. Induction of T-Cell Proliferation by GqPCR

3.1.1. GnRHR. Women are more likely to actively express GnRH and GnRHR than men, as described above, particularly during the reproductive period, at which time immune responses are different [26, 30]. Furthermore, in the spleen and thymus, the expression of G proteins on mononuclear cells differs in a gender-dependent manner [23]. GnRHR exhibits direct immunostimulatory properties, and lymphocytes produce GnRH and express GnRHR [23, 26, 49]. The G protein Gαq/11 regulates the transduction of signals from multiple hormones from specific cell surface receptors to a variety of intracellular effectors, including the AC pathway, PLC-β, and the ion channel pathway [49]. Jacobson et al. [26] demonstrated that antisense nucleotides to Gαq/11 inhibit hormone and GnRHR signaling, suppressing the proliferation of T cells from female mice after in vitro culture. Additional studies have shown that antisense oligonucleotides to Gq-coupled GPCRs can also be effective in vivo for ameliorating murine lupus; specifically, antisense oligonucleotides directed against Gαq in female lupus-prone mice effectively reduce serum IgG levels, anti-DNA antibody levels, hematuria, and proteinuria, even in terms of the histopathology of renal biopsies [27]. Thus, these studies demonstrate the utility of GnRH inhibitors to modulate GqPCR activation in mice and suggest a novel potential target for the treatment of lupus.

3.1.2. Chemokine Receptors.

Molon et al. [48] have shown that signals mediated by chemokine receptors may compete with T-cell receptor stop signals and determine the duration of T-cell antigen-presenting cell interactions. During T-cell stimulation by antigen-presenting cells, T-cell chemokine receptors coupled to Gq and/or G11 protein are recruited to the immunological synapse. When chemokine receptors are sequestered at the immunological synapse, T cells become insensitive to chemotactic gradients, form more stable conjugates, and enhance proliferation and cytokine production. Thus, chemokine receptor trapping at the immunological synapse enhances T-cell activation by improving T-cell antigen-presenting cell attractions and impeding the "distraction" of successfully engaged T cells by other chemokine sources. Ngai et al. [15] suggested that optimal activation of the T-cell receptor requires signaling through chemokine receptor-Gq and that removal of Gαq locks cells into a migratory phenotype, making the cell less responsive to T-cell receptor signaling. Previous studies have shown that activation of Gαq inhibits migration through an Lck-SHP-1 pathway, priming cells for activation through the T-cell receptor-CD3 complex [42]. Thus, these novel GqPCR signaling pathways are involved in mediating the threshold of chemotaxis and T-cell receptor activation, playing an irreplaceable role in immunity and autoimmunity.

3.2. Induction of DC and Monocyte Migration by GqPCRs.

A Gi-coupled classic pathway activates T lymphocytes and alternative Gq-dependent chemokine receptors, promoting the migration of DCs and monocytes. Furthermore, Gq, similar to CD38, regulates extracellular calcium entry in chemokine-stimulated cells. Gq-deficient (Gnaq–/–) DCs and monocytes are unable to migrate to inflammatory sites and lymph nodes in vivo, demonstrating that this alternative Gq-coupled chemokine receptor signaling pathway is critical for the initiation of immune responses [32, 38].

4. The Diversity of Gq-Coupled GPCRs Mediates Activation of Signal-Regulated Pathways

Binding partners to GqPCR distinct from PLC-β include novel activators (Ric-8A and tubulin), candidate effectors (RhoGEFs, PI3K, GPCR kinases (GRKs), Btk, and complex regulator of G-protein signaling (RGS) proteins), regulators (RGS proteins and GRKs), and scaffold/adaptor proteins (EBP50/NHERF1, CDP/CD81, caveolin-1, and TPR1) [1, 4, 6, 50]. Downstream of these signaling proteins, signals through GPCR to Gq family members exhibit unexpected differences in signaling pathways and the regulation of gene expression profiles [8, 50].

4.1. Gq-Related PLC-β and PKC/Calcium Pathways.

PLC-β is the most well-known downstream effector molecule of GqPCR (Figure 1). The canonical pathway for the Gq/11 family is the activation of PLC-β enzymes, which catalyze the hydrolysis of the minor membrane phospholipid phosphatidylinositol bisphosphate (PIP2) to release IP3 and DAG [4–7, 13, 14]. These second messengers serve to propagate and amplify the GqPCR-mediated signal with calcium mobilization following release from IP3-regulated intracellular stores and DAG-mediated stimulation of PKC activity [4, 5]. Inositol lipids, DAG, PKC, and calcium each participate in multiple signaling networks, linking Gq family members through a host of different cellular events [1]. This pathway has been widely studied as a marker of GqPCR signaling [8]. As the aforementioned chemokine receptors, there are classic (Gi) and alternative (Gq) coupled GPCR pathways depending on the specific type of the chemokines and chemokine-stimulated cells [38]. The Gi is through AC pathway mentioned in the introduction part. The Gq activates the PLC family that can regulate the extracellular calcium entry in chemokine-stimulated cell and also subsequently influence the downstream effectors such as PI3K/Akt for survival of the cell.

4.2. The PI3K-Akt-Mammalian Target of Rapamycin (mTOR) Pathway.

Multiple reports have documented the negative influence of Gq-coupled receptors on the growth factor-directed activation of PI3K and Akt isoforms [1, 4–7, 13]. One report showed that Gαq directly inhibits the PI3K p110a catalytic subunit in vitro [51]. In addition, a previous study also showed that Gαq represses Akt activation in fibroblast cell lines [52–54] and cardiomyocytes [55, 56]; however, overexpression of Gαq in cardiomyocytes leads to cardiac hypertrophy and cardiomyocyte apoptosis [10, 57].

PI3K can be activated by the $\beta\gamma$ dimers released from Gi-coupled receptors [5]. In contrast, Gq normally inhibits PI3K activation and prevents activation of Akt [6, 7, 10, 14, 38]. Furthermore, Gαq inhibits the activation of the PI3K-Akt pathway, as has been demonstrated in Gnαq–/– mice. Indeed, by measurement of the phosphorylation of Akt at Ser473 (phospho-Akt), a phosphorylation site under the control of PI3K demonstrated that the level of phospho-Akt was higher in Gnαq–/– mice than in WT B cells [58]. Furthermore, deletion of phosphatase and tensin homolog (PTEN), an inhibitor of PI3K, also promotes mature B-cell survival [59] and can rescue autoreactive B cells from anergy [60]. Interestingly, the autoreactive prone marine zone-like B (MZB) cell compartment is also expanded in mice expressing activated p110 or lacking PTEN [61]. In the absence of Gαq, B cells constitutively express higher levels of activated Akt

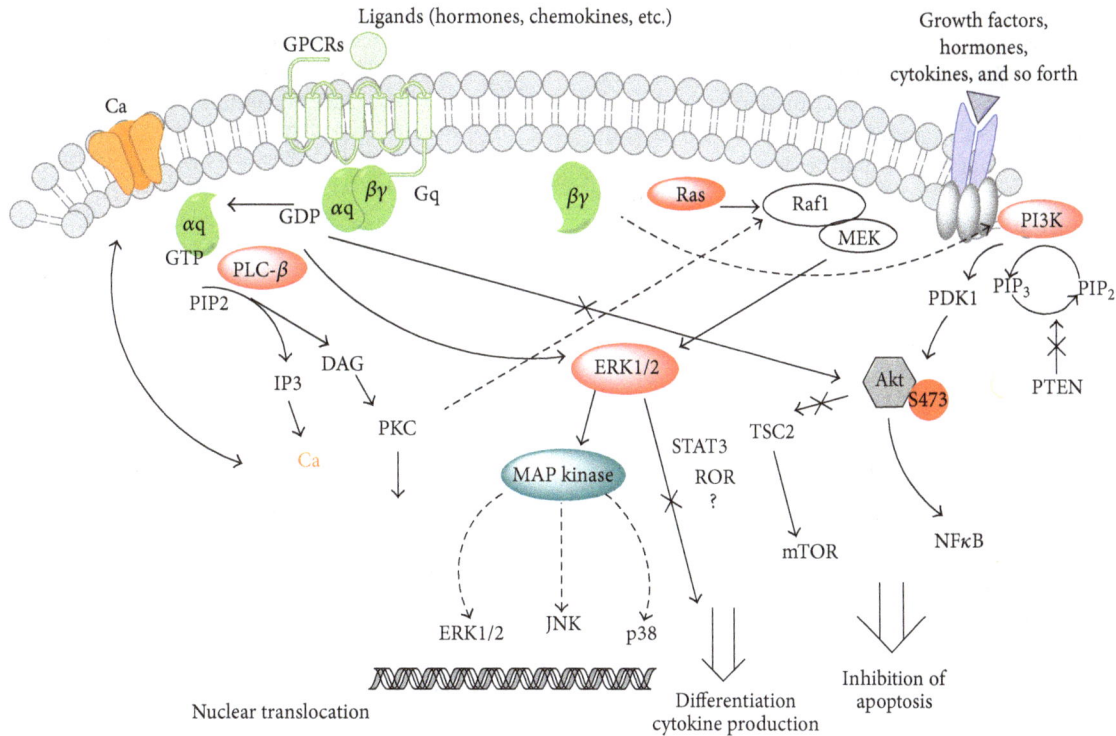

FIGURE 1: Signaling pathways demonstrating the link between Gq-coupled receptors and induction of autoimmunity. The figure shows the major signaling pathways that are believed to regulate the extracellular signals transduce into lymphocytes, which include the classic PLC-β/PKC pathway (left) and inhibition of the PI3K-Akt pathway to maintain normal immune tolerance (right) while Gq can also facilitate the activation of the ERK-MAPK pathway, regulating the differentiation of lymphocytes and controlling the expression of cytokines (middle).

and preferentially survive BCR-induced cell death signals and BAFF (B-cell-activating factor of the TNF family, also known as BLyS, for B lymphocyte stimulator) withdrawal in vitro and in vivo [10, 58, 62]. The B cells isolated from multiple models of autoimmunity have been reported to express elevated levels of phospho-Akt [62], and perturbations in the PI3K/Akt axis can lead to the development of autoimmunity [51, 62].

4.3. The MAPK/ERK Pathway. In addition to PLC-β and PI3K, many studies have demonstrated that Gq-coupled receptors can also regulate other intracellular signaling molecules, such as members of the MAPK family [6, 7, 50, 57]. The MAPK signaling cascade is one of the most ancient and evolutionarily conserved signaling pathways and responds to a broad range of extracellular and intracellular changes [63–67]. Among the MAPKs, p38 MAPK regulates the expression of tumor necrosis factor- (TNF-) α, interferon- (IFN-) γ, and other cytokines via transcriptional and posttranscriptional mechanisms. Therefore, inhibiting p38 MAPK may abrogate TNF-α, providing potential anti-inflammatory effects [65, 68, 69]. Predominant Th1 and Th17 cytokine production are characteristic of many organ-specific autoimmune diseases, and the dysregulation of p38 MAPK activity specifically in autoreactive lymphocytes appears to enhance IL-17 and IFN-γ expression [66, 70–72]. Additionally, the ERK pathway can be activated by the small G protein Ras via the Raf group of MAP kinase kinase kinases (MKKKs) [66]. Solid evidence has supported that

endothelin-dependent ERK/MAPK activation depends on the GqPCR/PLC-β/Ca^{2+}/Src signaling cascade [64]. Taken together, these studies have shown that GqPCR and Gαq are involved in the activation of ERK.

Thus, complex GPCR signaling should be studied as a concerted network at the systems level [73]. The detailed "cross-talk" mechanism between these GqPCR pathways still needs to be explored in the future.

5. Perspectives

In this review, we have outlined current evidence supporting the biological, pathological, and cell signaling functions of Gq-coupled GPCRs in autoimmunity. This discussion reinforced the idea of cell signaling diversity and challenged the established paradigm that Gq-coupled GPCR signals in immunology are functionally redundant. Moreover, studies of traditional pathways alone do not account for many Gq-mediated responses; Gαq-linked signaling suggests that GqPCRs have complex roles in signal transduction that are not yet fully understood.

Our previous studies have shown that Gq is associated with immune diseases and has pivotal roles in autoimmunity [17, 18, 24, 33, 38, 72, 74]. Gq is downregulated in RA's patients and relates to the disease's activity [74]; it can control the RA's progress via Th17 differentiation [72]. While Gq-containing G proteins can regulate B-cell selection and survival and are required to prevent B-cell-dependent autoimmunity [38], the deficiency of Gq can enhance the T-cell's survival [17] and influence the migration of DCs and neutrophils. Based on our unpublished data it is also related to autoinflammatory diseases. Therefore, we are interested in clarifying the role of Gq-coupled GPCRs in immune tolerance and autoimmunity, with the aim of improving therapeutic approached. Nonetheless, there are still some limitations to the available data describing the role of Gq-coupled GPCRs in autoreactive lymphocytes. Further studies using in vitro-derived lymphocytes may not accurately reflect the situations occurring in vivo. Moreover, the aforementioned studies involved different races and small patient populations, which may also have influenced the final results.

To date, many studies have focused on Gq-coupled membrane receptors and, to a lesser extent, G11. However, relatively little is known about G14 and G15/16. Future studies of autoimmunity may improve our understanding of the unique cell signaling roles and properties of other Gq/11 family proteins, including G14 and G15/16. Taken together, our discussion herein summarizes our current understanding of the complexity of Gq-coupled membrane receptor signaling and highlights many exciting new areas for future investigations in autoimmunity.

Conflict of Interests

The authors declare no conflict of interests.

Acknowledgment

The authors would like to acknowledge financial support from the Natural Science Foundation of China (Grant no. 81471534) to Dr. Guixiu Shi.

References

[1] K. B. Hubbard and J. R. Hepler, "Cell signalling diversity of the Gqα family of heterotrimeric G proteins," *Cellular Signalling*, vol. 18, no. 2, pp. 135–150, 2006.

[2] Z. Naor, "Signaling by G-protein-coupled receptor (GPCR): studies on the GnRH receptor," *Frontiers in Neuroendocrinology*, vol. 30, no. 1, pp. 10–29, 2009.

[3] K. Sisley, R. Doherty, and N. A. Cross, "What hope for the future? GNAQ and uveal melanoma," *The British Journal of Ophthalmology*, vol. 95, no. 5, pp. 620–623, 2011.

[4] S. R. Neves, P. T. Ram, and R. Iyengar, "G protein pathways," *Science*, vol. 296, no. 5573, pp. 1636–1639, 2002.

[5] N. Wettschureck, A. Moers, and S. Offermanns, "Mouse models to study G-protein-mediated signaling," *Pharmacology & Therapeutics*, vol. 101, no. 1, pp. 75–89, 2004.

[6] N. Mizuno and H. Itoh, "Functions and regulatory mechanisms of Gq-signaling pathways," *Neuro-Signals*, vol. 17, no. 1, pp. 42–54, 2009.

[7] G. Sánchez-Fernández, S. Cabezudo, C. García-Hoz et al., "Gαq signalling: the new and the old," *Cellular Signalling*, vol. 26, no. 5, pp. 833–848, 2014.

[8] T. Kawakami and W. Xiao, "Phospholipase C-β in immune cells," *Advances in Biological Regulation*, vol. 53, no. 3, pp. 249–257, 2013.

[9] A. M. Lyon, V. G. Taylor, and J. J. G. Tesmer, "Strike a pose: Gαq complexes at the membrane," *Trends in Pharmacological Sciences*, vol. 35, no. 1, pp. 23–30, 2014.

[10] S. Mishra, H. Ling, M. Grimm, T. Zhang, D. M. Bers, and J. H. Brown, "Cardiac hypertrophy and heart failure development through Gq and CaM kinase II signaling," *Journal of Cardiovascular Pharmacology*, vol. 56, no. 6, pp. 598–603, 2010.

[11] A. Fišerová, M. Starec, M. Kuldová et al., "Effects of D2-dopamine and α-adrenoceptor antagonists in stress induced changes on immune responsiveness of mice," *Journal of Neuroimmunology*, vol. 130, no. 1-2, pp. 55–65, 2002.

[12] S.-M. Lee, Y. Yang, and R. B. Mailman, "Dopamine D1 receptor signaling: Does GαQ-phospholipase C actually play a role?" *The Journal of Pharmacology and Experimental Therapeutics*, vol. 351, no. 1, pp. 9–17, 2014.

[13] B. A. Wilson and M. Ho, "*Pasteurella multocida* toxin as a tool for studying Gq signal transduction," *Reviews of Physiology, Biochemistry and Pharmacology*, vol. 152, pp. 93–109, 2004.

[14] R. S. Misra, G. Shi, M. E. Moreno-Garcia et al., "Gαq-containing G proteins regulate B cell selection and survival and are required to prevent B cell–dependent autoimmunity," *Journal of Experimental Medicine*, vol. 207, no. 8, pp. 1775–1789, 2010.

[15] J. Ngai, T. Methi, K. W. Andressen et al., "The heterotrimeric G-protein α-subunit Gαq regulates TCR-mediated immune responses through an Lck-dependent pathway," *European Journal of Immunology*, vol. 38, no. 11, pp. 3208–3218, 2008.

[16] L. Svensson, P. Stanley, F. Willenbrock, and N. Hogg, "The Galphaq/11 proteins contribute to T lymphocyte migration by promoting turnover of integrin LFA-1 through recycling," *PLoS ONE*, vol. 7, no. 6, Article ID e38517, 2012.

[17] D. Wang, Y. Zhang, Y. He, Y. Li, F. E. Lund, and G. Shi, "The deficiency of Gαq leads to enhanced T-cell survival," *Immunology and Cell Biology*, vol. 92, no. 9, pp. 781–790, 2014.

[18] Y. Wang, Y. Li, and G. Shi, "The regulating function of heterotrimeric G proteins in the immune system," *Archivum Immunologiae et Therapiae Experimentalis*, vol. 61, no. 4, pp. 309–319, 2013.

[19] A. Antonelli, S. M. Ferrari, D. Giuggioli, E. Ferrannini, C. Ferri, and P. Fallahi, "Chemokine (C-X-C motif) ligand (CXCL)10 in autoimmune diseases," *Autoimmunity Reviews*, vol. 13, no. 3, pp. 272–280, 2014.

[20] C. Carvalho, S. L. Calvisi, B. Leal et al., "CCR5-Delta32: implications in SLE development," *International Journal of Immunogenetics*, vol. 41, no. 3, pp. 236–241, 2014.

[21] J. Y. Choi, J. H. Ho, S. G. Pasoto et al., "Circulating follicular helper-like T cells in systemic lupus erythematosus: association with disease activity," *Arthritis & Rheumatology*, vol. 67, no. 4, pp. 988–999, 2015.

[22] G. S. Firestein, "Evolving concepts of rheumatoid arthritis," *Nature*, vol. 423, no. 6937, pp. 356–361, 2003.

[23] J. D. Jacobson, "Gonadotropin-releasing hormone and G proteins: potential roles in autoimmunity," *Annals of the New York Academy of Sciences*, vol. 917, pp. 809–818, 2000.

[24] Y. Li, Y. Wang, Y. He et al., "Gαq gene promoter polymorphisms and rheumatoid arthritis in the Han Chinese population are not associated," *Genetics and Molecular Research*, vol. 12, no. 2, pp. 1841–1848, 2013.

[25] D. Stanislaus, J. H. Pinter, J. A. Janovick, and P. M. Conn, "Mechanisms mediating multiple physiological responses to gonadotropin-releasing hormone," *Molecular and Cellular Endocrinology*, vol. 144, no. 1-2, pp. 1–10, 1998.

[26] J. D. Jacobson, M. A. Ansari, M. Kinealy, and V. Muthukrishnan, "Gender-specific exacerbation of murine lupus by gonadotropin-releasing hormone: potential role of Gα(q/11)," *Endocrinology*, vol. 140, no. 8, pp. 3429–3437, 1999.

[27] M. A. Ansari, M. Dhar, V. Muthukrishnan, T. L. Morton, N. Bakht, and J. D. Jacobson, "Administration of antisense oligonucleotides to Gα$_{Q/11}$ reduces the severity of murine lupus," *Biochimie*, vol. 85, no. 6, pp. 627–632, 2003.

[28] J. D. Jacobson, L. J. Crofford, L. Sun, and R. L. Wilder, "Cyclical expression of GnRH and GnRH receptor mRNA in lymphoid organs," *Neuroendocrinology*, vol. 67, no. 2, pp. 117–125, 1998.

[29] T. L. Morton, M. A. Ansari, and J. D. Jacobson, "Gender differences and hormonal modulation of G proteins Gα$_{q/11}$ expression in lymphoid organs," *Neuroendocrinology*, vol. 78, no. 3, pp. 147–153, 2003.

[30] P. E. Micevych, J. Kuo, and A. Christensen, "Physiology of membrane oestrogen receptor signalling in reproduction," *Journal of Neuroendocrinology*, vol. 21, no. 4, pp. 249–256, 2009.

[31] V. Rider and N. I. Abdou, "Gender differences in autoimmunity: molecular basis for estrogen effects in systemic lupus erythematosus," *International Immunopharmacology*, vol. 1, no. 6, pp. 1009–1024, 2001.

[32] H. Arai and I. F. Charo, "Differential regulation of G-protein-mediated signaling by chemokine receptors," *The Journal of Biological Chemistry*, vol. 271, no. 36, pp. 21814–21819, 1996.

[33] Y. Liu and G. Shi, "Role of G protein-coupled receptors in control of dendritic cell migration," *BioMed Research International*, vol. 2014, Article ID 738253, 11 pages, 2014.

[34] C. A. Flanagan, "Receptor conformation and constitutive activity in CCR5 chemokine receptor function and HIV infection," *Advances in Pharmacology*, vol. 70, pp. 215–263, 2014.

[35] M. Henneken, T. Dörner, G.-R. Burmester, and C. Berek, "Differential expression of chemokine receptors on peripheral blood B cells from patients with rheumatoid arthritis and systemic lupus erythematosus," *Arthritis Research & Therapy*, vol. 7, no. 5, pp. R1001–R1013, 2005.

[36] O. Launay, S. Paul, A. Servettaz et al., "Control of humoral immunity and auto-immunity by the CXCR4/CXCL12 axis in lupus patients following influenza vaccine," *Vaccine*, vol. 31, no. 35, pp. 3492–3501, 2013.

[37] C. K. Wong, P. T. Y. Wong, L. S. Tam, E. K. Li, D. P. Chen, and C. W. K. Lam, "Elevated production of B Cell Chemokine CXCL13 is correlated with systemic lupus erythematosus disease activity," *Journal of Clinical Immunology*, vol. 30, no. 1, pp. 45–52, 2010.

[38] G. Shi, S. Partida-Sánchez, R. S. Misra et al., "Identification of an alternative Gαq-dependent chemokine receptor signal transduction pathway in dendritic cells and granulocytes," *The Journal of Experimental Medicine*, vol. 204, no. 11, pp. 2705–2718, 2007.

[39] L. Bidyalaxmi Devi, A. Bhatnagar, A. Wanchu, and A. Sharma, "A study on the association of autoantibodies, chemokine, and its receptor with disease activity in systemic lupus erythematosus in North Indian population," *Rheumatology International*, vol. 33, no. 11, pp. 2819–2826, 2013.

[40] C. R. Mackay, "Moving targets: cell migration inhibitors as new anti-inflammatory therapies," *Nature Immunology*, vol. 9, no. 9, pp. 988–998, 2008.

[41] G. Trujillo, A. J. Hartigan, and C. M. Hogaboam, "T regulatory cells and attenuated bleomycin-induced fibrosis in lungs of CCR7$^{-/-}$ mice," *Fibrogenesis & Tissue Repair*, vol. 3, article 18, 2010.

[42] J. Ngai, M. Inngjerdingen, T. Berge, and K. Tasken, "Interplay between the heterotrimeric G-protein subunits Galphaq and Galphai2 sets the threshold for chemotaxis and TCR activation," *BMC Immunology*, vol. 10, article 27, 2009.

[43] M. Platten, S. Youssef, E. M. Hur et al., "Blocking angiotensin-converting enzyme induces potent regulatory T cells and modulates TH1- and TH17-mediated autoimmunity," *Proceedings of the National Academy of Sciences of the United States of America*, vol. 106, no. 35, pp. 14948–14953, 2009.

[44] B. Rodríguez-Iturbe, H. Pons, Y. Quiroz, and R. J. Johnson, "The immunological basis of hypertension," *American Journal of Hypertension*, vol. 27, no. 11, pp. 1327–1337, 2014.

[45] S. Nag and S. S. Mokha, "Activation of a Gq-coupled membrane estrogen receptor rapidly attenuates α2-adrenoceptor-induced antinociception via an ERK I/II-dependent, nongenomic mechanism in the female rat," *Neuroscience*, vol. 267, pp. 122–134, 2014.

[46] L. Yan, X. Tan, W. Chen, H. Zhu, J. Cao, and H. Liu, "Enhanced vasoconstriction to α1 adrenoceptor autoantibody in spontaneously hypertensive rats," *Science China Life Sciences*, vol. 57, no. 7, pp. 681–689, 2014.

[47] Y. H. Lee, J.-H. Kim, and G. G. Song, "Chemokine receptor 5 Delta32 polymorphism and systemic lupus erythematosus, vasculitis, and primary Sjogren's syndrome. Meta-analysis of possible associations," *Zeitschrift für Rheumatologie*, vol. 73, no. 9, pp. 848–855, 2014.

[48] B. Molon, G. Gri, M. Bettella et al., "T cell costimulation by chemokine receptors," *Nature Immunology*, vol. 6, no. 5, pp. 465–471, 2005.

[49] J. P. Hapgood, H. Sadie, W. van Biljon, and K. Ronacher, "Regulation of expression of mammalian gonadotrophin-releasing hormone receptor genes," *Journal of Neuroendocrinology*, vol. 17, no. 10, pp. 619–638, 2005.

[50] J. H. Kehrl and S. Sinnarajah, "RGS2: a multifunctional regulator of G-protein signaling," *The International Journal of Biochemistry & Cell Biology*, vol. 34, no. 5, pp. 432–438, 2002.

[51] A. Patke, I. Mecklenbräuker, H. Erdjument-Bromage, P. Tempst, and A. Tarakhovsky, "BAFF controls B cell metabolic fitness through a PKCβ- and Akt-dependent mechanism," *The Journal of Experimental Medicine*, vol. 203, no. 11, pp. 2551–2562, 2006.

[52] R. K. Bommakanti, S. Vinayak, and W. F. Simonds, "Dual regulation of Akt/protein kinase B by heterotrimeric G protein subunits," *The Journal of Biological Chemistry*, vol. 275, no. 49, pp. 38870–38876, 2000.

[53] L. M. Ballou, Y.-P. Jiang, G. Du, M. A. Frohman, and R. Z. Lin, "Ca^{2+}- and phospholipase D-dependent and -independent pathways activate mTOR signaling," *FEBS Letters*, vol. 550, no. 1–3, pp. 51–56, 2003.

[54] L. M. Ballou, H.-Y. Lin, G. Fan, Y.-P. Jiang, and R. Z. Lin, "Activated Gαq inhibits p110α phosphatidylinositol 3-kinase and Akt," *The Journal of Biological Chemistry*, vol. 278, no. 26, pp. 23472–23479, 2003.

[55] A. L. Howes, J. F. Arthur, T. Zhang et al., "Akt-mediated cardiomyocyte survival pathways are compromised by Gαq-induced phosphoinositide 4,5-bisphosphate depletion," *The Journal of Biological Chemistry*, vol. 278, no. 41, pp. 40343–40351, 2003.

[56] M. R. Morissette, A. L. Howes, T. Zhang, and J. H. Brown, "Upregulation of GLUT1 expression is necessary for hypertrophy and survival of neonatal rat cardiomyocytes," *Journal of Molecular and Cellular Cardiology*, vol. 35, no. 10, pp. 1217–1227, 2003.

[57] J. S. Gutkind and S. Offermanns, "A new G_q-initiated MAPK signaling pathway in the heart," *Developmental Cell*, vol. 16, pp. 163–164, 2009.

[58] S. L. Pogue, T. Kurosaki, J. Bolen, and R. Herbst, "B cell antigen receptor-induced activation of Akt promotes B cell survival and is dependent on Syk kinase," *Journal of Immunology*, vol. 165, no. 3, pp. 1300–1306, 2000.

[59] R. Kumar, S. Srinivasan, S. Koduru et al., "Psoralidin, an herbal molecule, inhibits phosphatidylinositol 3-kinase-mediated Akt signaling in androgen-independent prostate cancer cells," *Cancer Prevention Research*, vol. 2, no. 3, pp. 234–243, 2009.

[60] C. D. Browne, C. J. Del Nagro, M. H. Cato, H. S. Dengler, and R. C. Rickert, "Suppression of phosphatidylinositol 3,4,5-trisphosphate production is a key determinant of B cell anergy," *Immunity*, vol. 31, no. 5, pp. 749–760, 2009.

[61] A. N. Anzelon, H. Wu, and R. C. Rickert, "Pten inactivation alters peripheral B lymphocyte fate and reconstitutes CD19 function," *Nature Immunology*, vol. 4, no. 3, pp. 287–294, 2003.

[62] T. Wu and C. Mohan, "The AKT axis as a therapeutic target in autoimmune diseases," *Endocrine, Metabolic & Immune Disorders Drug Targets*, vol. 9, no. 2, pp. 145–150, 2009.

[63] J.-Y. Choe, S.-J. Lee, S.-H. Park, and S.-K. Kim, "Tacrolimus (FK506) inhibits interleukin-1β-induced angiopoietin-1, Tie-2 receptor, and vascular endothelial growth factor through down-regulation of JNK and p38 pathway in human rheumatoid fibroblast-like synoviocytes," *Joint Bone Spine*, vol. 79, no. 2, pp. 137–143, 2012.

[64] H. Cramer, K. Schmenger, K. Heinrich et al., "Coupling of endothelin receptors to the ERK/MAP kinase pathway. Roles of palmitoylation and $G\alpha_q$," *The FEBS Journal*, vol. 268, no. 20, pp. 5449–5459, 2001.

[65] G. Cui, X. Qin, Y. Zhang, Z. Gong, B. Ge, and Y. Q. Zang, "Berberine differentially modulates the activities of ERK, p38 MAPK, and JNK to suppress Th17 and Th1 T cell differentiation in type 1 diabetic mice," *The Journal of Biological Chemistry*, vol. 284, no. 41, pp. 28420–28429, 2009.

[66] C. Dong, R. J. Davis, and R. A. Flavell, "MAP kinases in the immune response," *Annual Review of Immunology*, vol. 20, pp. 55–72, 2002.

[67] D. M. Fuller, M. Zhu, S. Koonpaew, M. I. Nelson, and W. Zhang, "The importance of the erk pathway in the development of linker for activation of T cells-mediated autoimmunity," *Journal of Immunology*, vol. 189, no. 8, pp. 4005–4013, 2012.

[68] A. Mavropoulos, T. Orfanidou, C. Liaskos et al., "p38 Mitogen-activated protein kinase (p38 MAPK)-mediated autoimmunity: lessons to learn from ANCA vasculitis and pemphigus vulgaris," *Autoimmunity Reviews*, vol. 12, no. 5, pp. 580–590, 2013.

[69] A. Mavropoulos, T. Orfanidou, C. Liaskos et al., "P38 MAPK signaling in pemphigus: implications for skin autoimmunity," *Autoimmune Diseases*, vol. 2013, Article ID 728529, 11 pages, 2013.

[70] R. Noubade, D. N. Krementsov, R. Del Rio et al., "Activation of p38 MAPK in CD4 T cells controls IL-17 production and autoimmune encephalomyelitis," *Blood*, vol. 118, no. 12, pp. 3290–3300, 2011.

[71] R. Wei, L. Dong, Q. Xiao, D. Sun, X. Li, and H. Nian, "Engagement of Toll-like receptor 2 enhances interleukin (IL)-17$^+$ autoreactive T cell responses via p38 mitogen-activated protein kinase signalling in dendritic cells," *Clinical and Experimental Immunology*, vol. 178, no. 2, pp. 353–363, 2014.

[72] Y. Liu, D. Wang, F. Li, and G. Shi, "Gαq controls rheumatoid arthritis via regulation of Th17 differentiation," *Immunology and Cell Biology*, vol. 93, no. 7, pp. 616–624, 2015.

[73] M. E. Csete and J. C. Doyle, "Reverse engineering of biological complexity," *Science*, vol. 295, no. 5560, pp. 1664–1669, 2002.

[74] Y. Wang, Y. Li, Y. He et al., "Expression of G protein αq subunit is decreased in lymphocytes from patients with rheumatoid arthritis and is correlated with disease activity," *Scandinavian Journal of Immunology*, vol. 75, no. 2, pp. 203–209, 2012.

11

Electroporated Antigen-Encoding mRNA Is Not a Danger Signal to Human Mature Monocyte-Derived Dendritic Cells

Stefanie Hoyer,[1] **Kerstin F. Gerer,**[1,2] **Isabell A. Pfeiffer,**[1] **Sabrina Prommersberger,**[1,2] **Sandra Höfflin,**[1,2] **Tanushree Jaitly,**[1] **Luca Beltrame,**[3] **Duccio Cavalieri,**[4] **Gerold Schuler,**[1] **Julio Vera,**[1] **Niels Schaft,**[1] **and Jan Dörrie**[1]

[1]*Department of Dermatology, Universitätsklinikum Erlangen, Erlangen, Germany*
[2]*Department of Genetics, Friedrich-Alexander-Universität Erlangen-Nürnberg, Erlangen, Germany*
[3]*Department of Oncology, Istituto di Ricerche Farmacologiche Mario Negri, Milan, Italy*
[4]*Department of Neurosciences, Psychology, Drug Research and Child Health, University of Florence, Florence, Italy*

Correspondence should be addressed to Jan Dörrie; jan.doerrie@uk-erlangen.de

Academic Editor: Smita Nair

For therapeutic cancer vaccination, the adoptive transfer of mRNA-electroporated dendritic cells (DCs) is frequently performed, usually with monocyte-derived, cytokine-matured DCs (moDCs). However, DCs are rich in danger-sensing receptors which could recognize the exogenously delivered mRNA and induce DC activation, hence influencing the DCs' immunogenicity. Therefore, we examined whether electroporation of mRNA with a proper cap and a poly-A tail of at least 64 adenosines had any influence on cocktail-matured moDCs. We used 16 different RNAs, encoding tumor antigens (MelanA, NRAS, BRAF, GNAQ, GNA11, and WT1), and variants thereof. None of those RNAs induced changes in the expression of CD25, CD40, CD83, CD86, and CD70 or the secretion of the cytokines IL-8, IL-6, and TNFα of more than 1.5-fold compared to the control condition, while an mRNA encoding an NF-κB-activation protein as positive control induced massive secretion of the cytokines. To determine whether mRNA electroporation had any effect on the whole transcriptome of the DCs, we performed microarray analyses of DCs of 6 different donors. None of 60,000 probes was significantly different between mock-electroporated DCs and MelanA-transfected DCs. Hence, we conclude that no transcriptional programs were induced within cocktail-matured DCs by electroporation of single tumor-antigen-encoding mRNAs.

1. Introduction

During the last decade, immunotherapy has evolved as a new pillar of cancer treatment [1]. Therapeutic vaccination with dendritic cells (DCs) is a safe and well-established strategy [2–4]. A deeper understanding of DC maturation and activation together with efficient, GMP-compliant and reproducible antigen- (Ag-) loading strategies is the key to success. One technology that has proven suitable in this context is mRNA transfection [3, 5, 6], which can be utilized, on the one hand, to load mature DCs with tumor antigen [7–9], and on the other hand, to deliver maturation and activation signals to the DCs. The latter is usually achieved by using mRNA that encodes DC-activating proteins, like constitutively active inhibitor of kappa B kinase (IKK) [10] or CD40L, alone [11], or combined with a constitutively active TLR [12].

However, since DCs comprise a whole battery of nucleic acid receptors on their surface, in their endosomes, and in their cytoplasm [13, 14], the transfected mRNA itself, independently from the encoded protein, may deliver a maturation signal. Single-stranded (ss)RNA was reported to activate TLR7 and TLR8 on DCs [15–17] and TLR3 can be activated by short double-strand stretches in exogenous mRNA [18, 19]. RIG-I-like receptors (RLR) recognize various viral RNA species in the cytoplasm [20] and may be capable of sensing transfected RNA as well. Bacterial RNA is a potent DC maturation stimulus, but the specific receptors are yet unknown [21].

TABLE 1: mRNAs used for transfection.

Antigen	Description	Abbreviation
MelanA	MelanA (MART1) full length wild type	MelanA
NRAS	NRAS-fragment 40 AA around mutation site 61 with DC-LAMP signal and flag-tag	NRAS-DCL
NRAS Q61K	NRAS-fragment 40 AA around mutation Q61K with DC-LAMP signal and flag-tag	NRAS-DCL K
NRAS Q61R	NRAS-fragment 40 AA around mutation Q61R with DC-LAMP signal and flag-tag	NRAS-DCL R
BRAF	BRAF-fragment 67 AA around mutation site 600 with flag-tag	BRAF
BRAF V600E	BRAF-fragment 67 AA around mutation V600E with flag-tag	BRAF E
BRAF	BRAF-fragment 67 AA around mutation site 600 with DC-LAMP signal and flag-tag	BRAF-DCL
BRAF V600E	BRAF-fragment 67 AA around mutation V600E with DC-LAMP signal and flag-tag	BRAF-DCL E
GNAQ	GNAQ-fragment 47 AA around mutation site 209 with DC-LAMP signal and flag-tag	GQ-DCL
GNAQ Q209P	GNAQ-fragment 47 AA around mutation Q209P with DC-LAMP signal and flag-tag	GQ-DCL P
GNAQ Q209L	GNAQ-fragment 47 AA around mutation Q209L with DC-LAMP signal and flag-tag	GQ-DCL L
GNA11	GNA11-fragment 47 AA around mutation site 209 with DC-LAMP signal and flag-tag	G11-DCL
GNA11 Q209P	GNA11-fragment 47 AA around mutation Q209P with DC-LAMP signal and flag-tag	G11-DCL P
GNA11 Q209L	GNA11-fragment 47 AA around mutation Q209L with DC-LAMP signal and flag-tag	G11-DCL L
WT-1	Wilms tumor 1 full length wild type	WT1
GNAQ	Wilms tumor 1 full length with DC-LAMP signal and flag-tag	WT1-DCL
$IKK\beta$[1]	Constitutively active stabilized $IKK\beta$ to activate NF-κB	$IKK\beta$

[1]Not a tumor antigen, but a DC-activating protein.

In the design of clinical vaccination protocols, it is, however, pivotal to know which maturation program is induced in the DCs and whether and how any additional maturation stimulus might distort the intended mature phenotype of the vaccine DCs. When DCs (usually monocyte-derived ones) are generated, matured, and Ag-loaded for clinical application, one requires a well-defined product, and any remaining insecurity about any factors that influence the phenotype of the DCs should be resolved.

Hence, we took the effort to carefully compare monocyte-derived cytokine-matured DCs that were electroporated without RNA with DCs that were electroporated with various *in vitro*-transcribed mRNAs. We analyzed the DCs' phenotype and cytokine secretion and, for mRNA, encoding the tumor antigen MelanA, a transcriptome analysis was performed, to detect if any of these features would be changed by the introduced mRNA.

2. Materials and Methods

2.1. Cells and Reagents. Monocyte-derived dendritic cells (DCs) were generated from blood, obtained from healthy donors following informed consent and approval by the institutional review board as described before [9]. PBMCs were purified by density centrifugation, and monocytes were separated from the nonadherent fraction (NAF) by plastic adherence and differentiated to DCs over 6 days in DC medium (RPMI 1640 (Lonza, Verviers, Belgium) containing 1% heat-inactivated autologous plasma, 2 mM L-glutamine (Lonza), and 20 mg/L gentamicin (PAA, Pasching, Austria)) with GM-CSF (800 IU/mL; CellGenix, Freiburg, Germany, PeproTech, Hamburg, Germany, and Miltenyi Biotec, Bergisch Gladbach, Germany) and IL-4 (250 IU/mL; CellGenix, PeproTech, and Miltenyi Biotec) in the absence of fetal calf serum, as described before [9]. DCs were matured (mDCs) on day 6 for 24 h with 200 IU/mL IL-1β (CellGenix), 1000 U/mL IL-6 (CellGenix), 10 ng/mL TNFα (Beromun, Boehringer Ingelheim Pharma, Germany), and 1 μg/mL PGE$_2$ (Pfizer, Zurich, Switzerland). mDCs were used for electroporation with mRNA after maturation.

2.2. In Vitro RNA Transcription and Electroporation of DCs. *In vitro* transcription of mRNA from pGEM4Z64A vectors was performed as described previously [9] with Life Technologies mMESSAGE mMACHINE T7 ULTRA kits according to the manufacturer's instructions. DCs were electroporated with different mRNAs (Table 1) as described in [10, 22]. As a control, mDCs were electroporated without mRNA.

2.3. Cell Surface Marker Analysis. mDCs were electroporated as described above, incubated in DC medium at 37°C in a humidified incubator, and harvested 24 h after electroporation. The expression of distinct markers was analyzed by flow cytometry. For the determination of surface marker expression, the following antibodies and their respective isotype controls were used: IgG1-PE, anti-CD25-PE, anti-CD40-PE, anti-CD70-PE, anti-CD80-PE, anti-CD83-PE, anti-CD86-PE (all from BD), and IgG3-PE (eBioscience). Seventy-five to one hundred thousand cells were incubated with antibody for 30 minutes at 4°C in FACS solution, consisting of PBS supplemented with 1% FCS (PAA, GE healthcare) and 0.02% sodium azide (Merck). The cells were then washed once with FACS solution and immunofluorescence was measured using a FACScan cytofluorometer equipped with CellQuest software (BD Biosciences). mDCs were gated on in the forward and side scatter channels and the mean fluorescence intensities (MFIs) were measured. Specific MFI was calculated by subtraction of the MFI of the isotype control.

2.4. Cytokine Secretion Analysis. mDCs were electroporated as described above and were incubated in DC medium at 37°C in a humidified incubator, and supernatants were taken 24 h after electroporation. Cytokine concentrations were analyzed with an Inflammation Cytometric Bead Array (BD, Heidelberg, Germany) following the manufacturer's instructions.

2.5. Statistical Analysis. We performed a 1-way ANOVA with multiple comparison test (according to Dunnet/Tukey) with a confidence level of 0.05 using GraphPad Prism V6.02 to determine statistically significant differences for the surface staining data (Figure 2) with the unadjusted mean fluorescence intensities, the percentage values of positive cells, and the cytokine concentrations (Figures 3 and 4). For the data in Figures 2 and 3, the multicomparison was performed according to Dunnet against the mock condition. For the data in Figure 4, all conditions were compared to each other according to Tukey.

2.6. Cryoconservation of Cell Pellets. mDCs were electroporated as described above, were incubated in DC medium at 37°C in a humidified incubator, and were harvested 4 h after electroporation. One to two hundred thousand cells were centrifuged for 10 min at 10.000 rpm at 4°C and the supernatant was removed. The cell pellet was frozen and stored in liquid nitrogen until microarray analysis.

2.7. Microarray Analysis. Cryoconserved electroporated mDCs were sent to Miltenyi Biotec for microarray analysis. Cells were lysed, mRNA was isolated and reverse-transcribed to cDNA, the cDNA was amplified, and Cy3 was labeled and then hybridized to Agilent Whole Human Genome Oligo Microarrays (8 × 60 K). Fluorescence signals of the hybridized Agilent Microarrays were detected using Agilent's Microarray Scanner System (Agilent Technologies). The Agilent Feature Extraction Software (FES) was used to read out and process the microarray image files. The resulting text files produced by FES were then processed for quality control, removing control probes and probes flagged as unreliable by the scanning software. The raw data underwent background correction to eliminate background noise and local fluctuations. To this end, the normal-exponential convolution method was used (Normexp). Next, the data were normalized to correct chip-related variations in the signal intensity (e.g., labeling and hybridization inefficiencies). To this end, the quantile method with offset = 16 was applied to the data.

Unadjusted p values were calculated with Student's t-test and the Benjamini Hochberg method for False Discovery Rate was used to adjust the p value and find differentially expressed genes. Data processing and analysis were performed in the software R computing environment (version 3.0.2) using the Bioconductor (version 3.1) package "limma"

(linear models for microarray and RNA-seq data) described in [23].

3. Results

3.1. mRNA Electroporation into Human Cocktail-Matured, Monocyte-Derived DCs Results in a High Transfection Efficiency. To formally show that mRNA electroporation results in protein expression in the cocktail-matured, monocyte-derived DCs, we generated these DCs and electroporated them either without RNA (mock) or with RNA encoding the tumor antigen MelanA (Figure 1). These DCs were produced by a highly standardized and validated process, which is approved for DC generation for clinical applications [24]. Hence, the product is very well known considering the phenotype of the DCs. Therefore, we did not include a typical DC-specific marker in these experiments but rather focused on maturation and activation markers on these DCs. The DCs displayed a mature phenotype, which was not altered by transfection with MelanA-encoding mRNA (Figures 1(a) and 1(b)). Four and twenty-four hours after electroporation, the intracellular MelanA expression was determined by flow cytometry. As shown in Figure 1(c), MelanA expression was detected at both time-points. The transfection efficiency at 4 h was >95% (Figure 1(c); left panel). Due to the transiency of mRNA transfection, the MelanA expression had decreased at the 24 h time-point (Figure 1(c); right panel). These data show that the electroporated mRNA enters the cytoplasm of the vast majority of the mature DCs very efficiently.

3.2. mRNA Electroporation into Human Cocktail-Matured, Monocyte-Derived DCs Has No Influence on the Phenotype of These Cells. As it was suggested that introduction of mRNA could trigger intracellular TLRs or other receptors [15–21], we examined whether mRNA electroporation has an influence on the phenotype of cocktail-matured, monocyte-derived DCs. We electroporated these DCs either without RNA (Figure 2; mock) or with a panel of 16 different RNAs encoding tumor antigens, or parts thereof (MelanA, NRAS, BRAF, GNAQ, GNA11, and WT1), either mutated or not, and either linked to the lysosomal targeting signal DC-LAMP or not (Table 1). Twenty-four hours after electroporation, the surface expression of CD25, CD40, CD86, CD70, and CD83 was determined by flow cytometry. When looking at mean fluorescence intensities (MFIs), electroporations with the 16 different RNAs encoding different tumor antigens resulted in differences in cell surface marker expression of less than 1.5-fold compared to mock-electroporated DCs (Figure 2(a)). No large differences in expression of these markers were observed when looking at percent positive cells (Figure 2(b)). According to a 1-way ANOVA with multiple comparison test, no statistically significant differences were present within the surface staining data ($p > 0.05$). We did not measure expression of MHC-class II, as we had observed before that there are no big changes on human monocyte-derived DCs, even after activation of NF-κB (data not shown).

From these data, we can conclude that the introduction of mRNA into human cocktail-matured, monocyte-derived

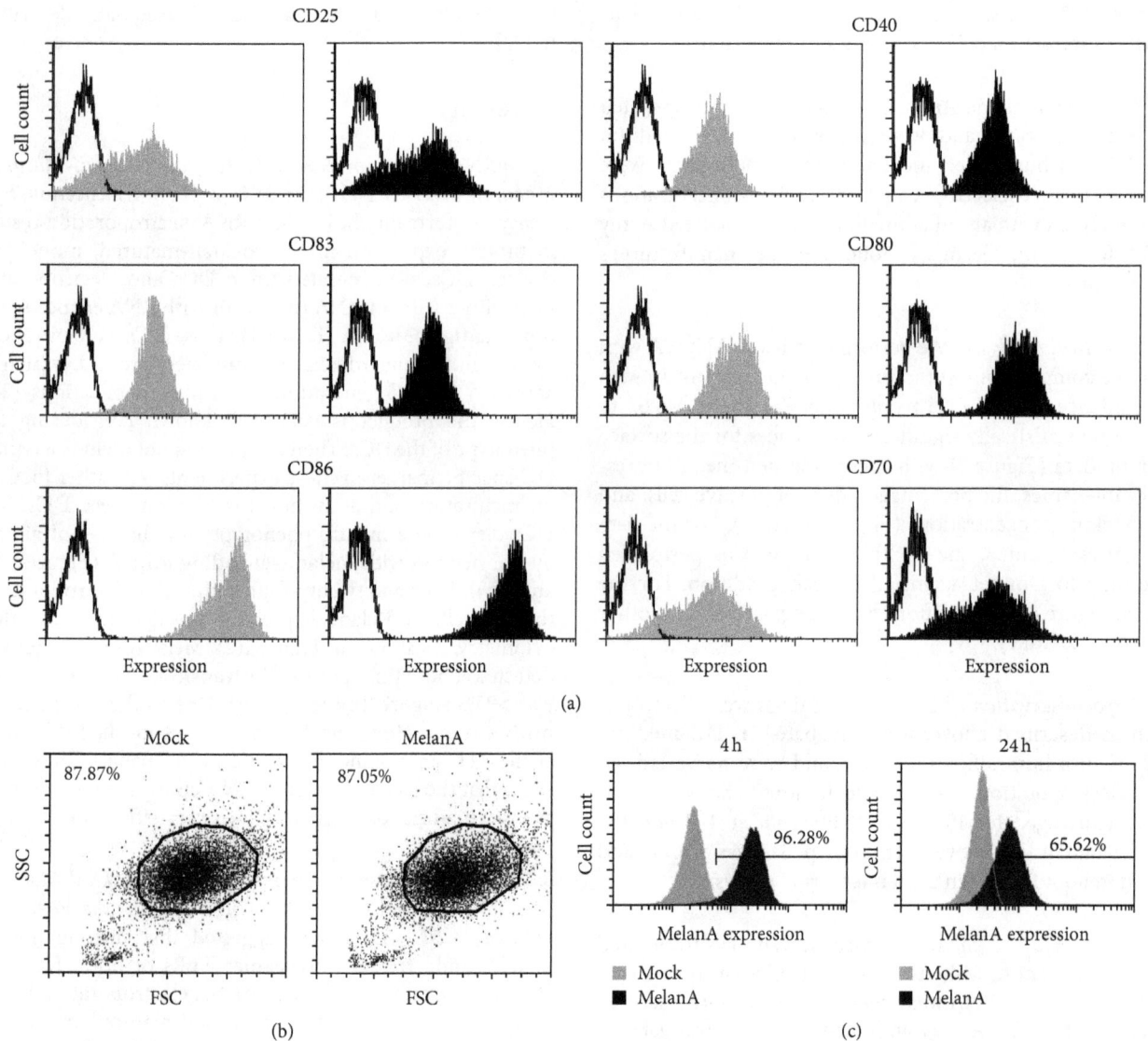

(a)

(b)

(c)

FIGURE 1: MelanA is expressed in cocktail-matured, monocyte-derived DCs after mRNA electroporation. DCs were either electroporated without mRNA (mock; gray histogram) or with mRNA encoding the tumor antigen MelanA (MelanA; black histogram). (a) Surface marker expression of CD25, CD40, CD83, CD86, CD70, and CD80 on mock-electroporated and MelanA-RNA-electroporated DCs 24 h after electroporation is shown (black lines; respective isotype controls). One representative of ≥4 experiments is shown. (b) Gating of mock-electroporated (Mock) or MelanA-RNA-electroporated (MelanA) DCs was performed according to forward and side scatter. (c) Four and twenty-four hours after electroporation, the intracellular MelanA expression was determined by flow cytometry. The percentage of positive cells is indicated. One representative of >10 experiments is shown.

DCs by electroporation did not result in a relevant change of the phenotype of these cells.

3.3. mRNA Electroporation into Human Cocktail-Matured, Monocyte-Derived DCs Has No Influence on the Cytokine Secretion by These Cells. Next, we investigated whether mRNA electroporation has an influence on the cytokine secretion of cocktail-matured, monocyte-derived DCs. We electroporated DCs either without RNA (Figure 3; Mock) or with the 16 different RNAs encoding tumor antigens

and harvested the supernatants of the cells 24 h after electroporation to determine the cytokine secretion in a cytometric bead array. Within 24 h after electroporation, the DCs hardly any IL-1β, IL-10, and IL-12p70 (data not shown) but produced measurable quantities of IL-8, IL-6, and TNFα (Figure 3). However, mock-electroporated DCs also secreted these cytokines, and the electroporations with the 16 different RNAs, encoding different tumor antigens, resulted in a difference in cytokine secretion of maximum 1.5-fold compared to mock-electroporated DCs (Figure 3). According to a 1-way ANOVA with multiple comparison test,

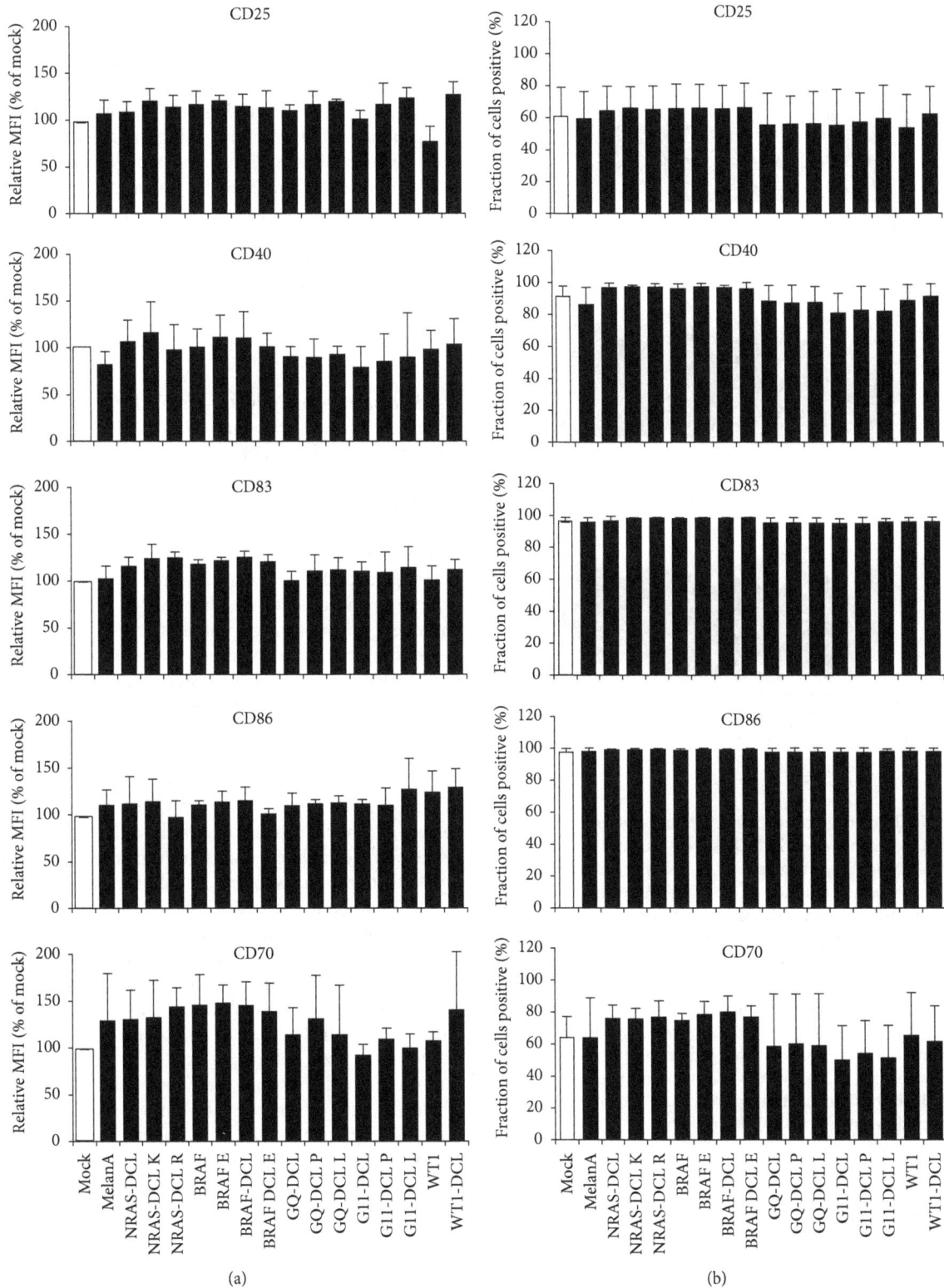

FIGURE 2: No difference in phenotype between mock- and mRNA-electroporated DCs. DCs were either electroporated without RNA (Mock) or a panel of 16 RNAs encoding different tumor antigens, either mutated or not and either linked to the lysosomal targeting signal DC-LAMP or not (see Table 1). Twenty-four hours after electroporation, the surface expression of CD25, CD40, CD86, CD70, and CD83 was determined by flow cytometry. Surface marker expression of mock-electroporated DCs was put at 100% and marker expression after electroporation of the mRNAs was put in relation to that (a), or percent positive cells are shown (b). Shown are averages of at least 3 independent experiments. Error bars indicate the standard deviation (SD). According to a 1-way ANOVA with multiple comparison test, no statistically significant differences were present within the surface staining data ($p > 0.05$).

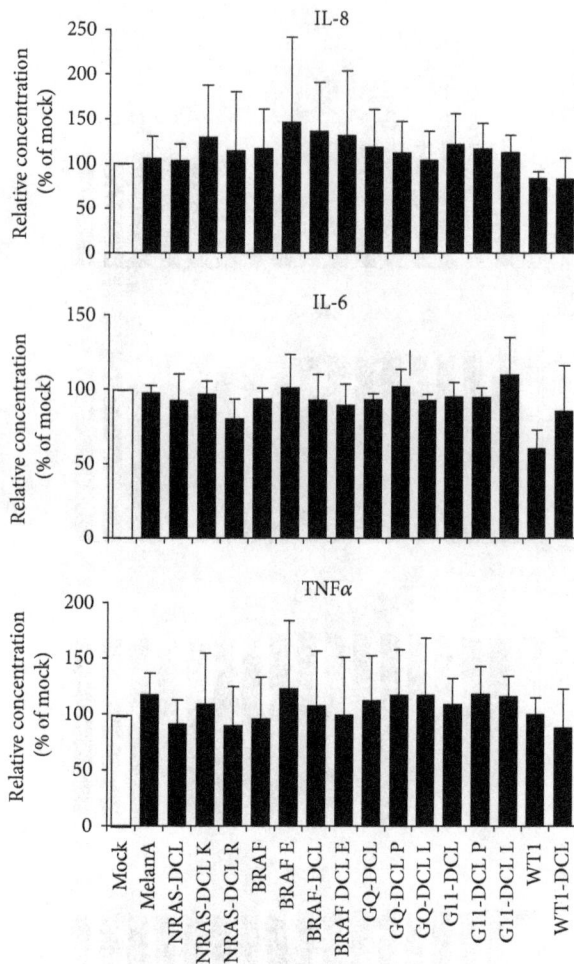

FIGURE 3: No difference in cytokine secretion between mock- and MelanA-RNA-electroporated DC. DCs were electroporated either without RNA (Mock) or with a panel of 16 RNAs encoding different tumor antigens, either mutated or not, and either linked to the lysosomal targeting signal DC-LAMP or not (see Table 1). Twenty-four hours after electroporation, supernatants of the cells were taken and the cytokine secretion by the cells was determined in a cytometric bead array. Cytokine secretion of mock-electroporated DCs was defined as 100% and concentrations after electroporation of the mRNAs were put in relation to that. Shown are averages of at least 3 independent experiments. Error bars indicate the standard deviation (SD). According to a 1-way ANOVA with multiple comparison test, no statistically significant differences were present within the cytokine secretion data ($p > 0.05$).

no statistically significant differences were present within the cytokine secretion data ($p > 0.05$).

These data show that the electroporated mRNAs also had no relevant influence on cytokine secretion by human cocktail-matured, monocyte-derived DCs.

Due to the fact that the secretion of IL-8, IL-6, and TNFα was clear but at low quantities, we wanted to formally prove that our DCs were able to produce these cytokines at higher quantities, when properly activated under similar conditions. Therefore, we electroporated the mature DCs either without RNA or with RNAs encoding MelanA combined or not

with RNA encoding a constitutively active form of IKKβ, which is, on the protein level, able to activate the NF-κB pathway in the DCs [10]. Indeed, we saw that transfection with constitutively active IKKβ resulted in high IL-8, IL-6, and TNFα secretion (Figure 4), proving that our DCs can produce these cytokines at high quantities. In addition, there was no difference between the cytokine secretion by mock-transfected and MelanA-transfected DCs (Figure 4), again showing that mRNA transfection *per se* did not induce cytokine production in DCs. The 1-way ANOVA with multiple comparison test showed that the IKKβ-transfected DCs were highly significantly different from the mock and MelanA conditions but that the mock and MelanA conditions were not.

3.4. Microarray Analysis Reveals No Differentially Expressed Genes between Mock- and MelanA-Transfected DCs. Although we found no obvious differences in the expression of a handful of surface markers and the secretion of half a dozen of cytokines upon mRNA electroporation, we still could not exclude that the exogenous mRNA would induce signaling within the DCs, which, by chance, would regulate other target genes and modulate the expression of other factors. To explore in more detail whether mRNA electroporation has any effect on the transcriptome of the DCs, we performed GeneChip microarray analyses with matured DCs (mDCs) of 6 independent donors, which had either been mock-electroporated or electroporated with MelanA RNA. DCs were harvested and frozen 4 h after electroporation, and samples were hybridized to Agilent Whole Human Genome Oligo Microarrays (8 × 60 K). Fluorescence signals of the hybridized Agilent Microarrays were determined, preprocessed, and normalized. Afterwards, differentially expressed genes were calculated and significance was examined by Student's t-test and subsequent adjustment using the Benjamini Hochberg method for False Discovery Rate. These calculations were performed using the limma (linear models for microarray and RNA-seq data) software package for the Bioconductor R computing environment [23] (see Section 2). The expression levels of all the microarray probes are compared directly in Figure 5 to depict the degree of difference between the two sample groups. The scatter plot shows that the individual values are close to the identity function (Figure 5), except for a small number of outliers, of which none was significant (Figure 5). Indeed, none of the probes showed a significant difference between mock-electroporated DCs and MelanA-electroporated DCs, and the adjusted p values were all above 0.99995, indicating that no differentially expressed genes (DEGs) were present. This suggests that the difference at the transcriptional level between mock-electroporated DCs and MelanA-electroporated DCs is negligible.

4. Discussion

In this study, we have shown that electroporation of antigen-encoding RNA into matured monocyte-derived dendritic cells (moDCs) had no influence on the phenotype of these

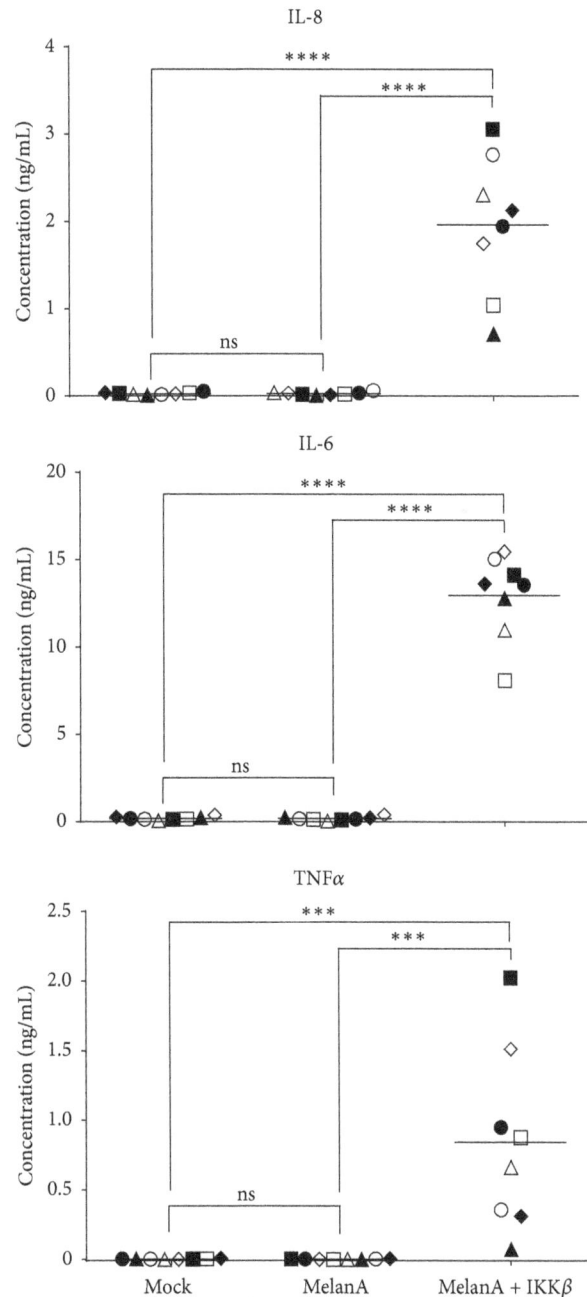

FIGURE 4: Massive cytokine secretion after electroporation with mRNA encoding a DC-activating protein. DCs were electroporated either without RNA (Mock) or with RNA encoding the tumor antigen MelanA (MelanA) or MelanA and constitutively active stabilized mutated IKKβ. Twenty-four hours after electroporation, supernatants of the cells were taken and the cytokine secretion by the cells was determined in a cytometric bead array. The cytokine concentrations in the supernatants are depicted. Each symbol represents an individual donor, tested in an independent experiment ($n = 8$). The horizontal bars show the average values. p values were calculated by the 1-way ANOVA with multiple comparison test (according to Tukey) with a confidence level of 0.05; ns: $p > 0.05$, $***p \leq 0.001$, and $****p \leq 0.0001$.

DCs and on the cytokine secretion by these DCs and even that there was no influence of the RNA on the transcriptome of the DCs. This is pivotal information for the use of mRNA-electroporated moDCs in a clinical setting, since it is necessary to generate vaccines of consistent quality by a stable production process, no matter what antigen-encoding RNA is used for electroporation, and it shows that

our matured moDCs are of a robust phenotype. Since we [9] and others [8, 11, 25] observed that DCs, which were antigen-electroporated after cytokine-maturation, seemed to perform better, we limited our analysis to DCs matured and electroporated in that order. Hence, we cannot say anything about the influence of mRNA electroporation into DCs prior to maturation and can only speculate that immature

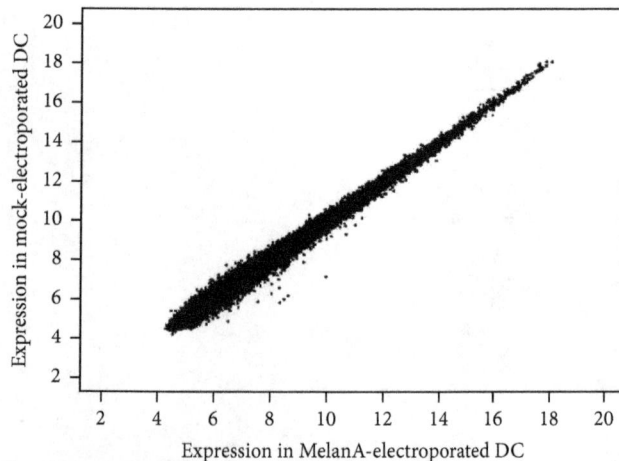

FIGURE 5: No difference in microarray analysis between mock- and MelanA-RNA-electroporated DCs. Scatter plot of the probe set expression levels for MelanA-RNA-electroporated DCs versus Mock-electroporated DCs samples. Data from 6 samples per experimental condition were processed for background correction and normalization. In the figure, the average probe intensity for each experimental condition is visualized.

DCs might be more susceptible for mRNA-mediated signals. However, this should be investigated in separate studies and is beyond the scope of this paper.

Other researchers have indeed observed mRNA-induced maturation of DCs, however under different experimental conditions [19, 26]. Ceppi and coworkers, who worked with porcine monocyte-derived DCs, observed that DC activation can occur after exogenous delivery of mRNA. Lipofection of mRNA induced maturation of immature porcine DCs, that is, MHC class II and CD80/CD86 upregulation [19]. An important element therein is the lipofection-induced production of type I IFN by the DCs, which also showed evidence of maturation. The DC activation was caused by the double-stranded secondary structures formed by the transfected mRNA, and the effect depended on the quantity of lipofected mRNA [19]. It is well established that viral or synthetic double-stranded RNA (dsRNA) acts as a danger signal to DCs, inducing them to produce IFNα/β and to mature [27]. Furthermore, it was reported that mRNA lipofection has the capacity to activate DCs (human moDCs) [26]. These authors noted the upregulation of activation markers, like CD25, CD80, CD83, CD86, MHC class I, and MHC class II, and cytokine production, like IL-12, IFNα, and TNFα [26].

Although our different antigen-encoding mRNAs can fold and form dsRNA stretches according to the Mfold Web Server (http://unafold.rna.albany.edu/?q=mfold/RNA-Folding-Form) [28] and thus in theory can also stimulate dsRNA-sensing receptors, we did not observe any DC activation. This can be explained by two main differences of our experiments compared to the experimental setup used by Ceppi et al. and Ni et al.

We used moDCs, which had been matured with a cocktail containing IL-1β, TNFα, IL-6, and PGE$_2$ before the mRNA was introduced, while in the other publications the mRNA

was introduced into immature DCs. It might be that the weak stimulus of the introduced mRNA is just not able to change the robust mature phenotype of the cytokine-matured DCs. However, sensing of RNA by receptors should still induce a difference in the transcriptome.

Therefore, it is more plausible that our antigen-encoding RNAs are simply not sensed by the corresponding receptors, because they do not reach the compartments containing these receptors. Indeed it was shown that the RNA must reach the active TLRs in the endolysosomal compartment to be recognized by TLR7, TLR8, and TLR9 and that self-nucleic acids do not enter the TLR-sensing compartment under normal physiological conditions (reviewed in [13]). Only after entering the endolysosomal compartment, the TLRs are activated upon cleavage by resident pH-dependent proteases. This mechanism prevents that self-nucleic acids at different locations in the cell are recognized by the TLRs. Once activated, the TLRs themselves cannot distinguish between foreign and self-nucleic acids; however, the latter do not encounter the active receptors [29]. Normal "naked" mRNA is rapidly degraded by endolysosomal RNas before the receptor is activated. However, if the RNA is protected by lipids, which is the case with lipofection in the publications of Ceppi et al. and Ni et al., or stabilized by protamine [30], or protected by virus particles (reviewed in [13]), it is stable enough to enter the endolysosomal compartment where it is recognized by the activated TLRs resulting in an activation of the DCs.

5. Conclusion

Taken together, our data show that electroporation of mature monocyte-derived DCs with antigen-encoding RNA does not deliver a danger signal to the DCs and does not result in a change of the DCs. This is important knowledge for the scientific community using these DCs in vaccination trials, where a stable and robust cell type is needed.

Disclosure

Stefanie Hoyer, Kerstin F. Gerer, Isabell A. Pfeiffer, Sabrina Prommersberger, Sandra Höfflin, and Tanushree Jaitly share first authorship. Niels Schaft and Jan Dörrie share senior authorship.

Conflict of Interests

The authors declare that there is no conflict of interests regarding the publication of this paper.

Acknowledgments

The authors thank Stefanie Baumann and Verena Wellner for excellent technical assistance and the medical staff for acquisition of donor material. This work was partially financed by the *Deutsche Forschungsgemeinschaft* (DFG; SFB 643 Project C1) and the *Bundesministerium für Bildung und*

Forschung (BMBF; project DCmutaVacc, *Förderkennzeichen* 01GU1107A).

References

[1] C. L. Sawyers, C. Abate-Shen, K. C. Anderson et al., "AACR cancer progress report 2013," *Clinical Cancer Research*, vol. 19, no. 20, supplement, pp. S4–S98, 2013.

[2] K. Palucka and J. Banchereau, "Dendritic-cell-based therapeutic cancer vaccines," *Immunity*, vol. 39, no. 1, pp. 38–48, 2013.

[3] G. Schuler, "Dendritic cells in cancer immunotherapy," *European Journal of Immunology*, vol. 40, no. 8, pp. 2123–2130, 2010.

[4] R. M. Steinman, "Dendritic cells: understanding immunogenicity," *European Journal of Immunology*, vol. 37, supplement 1, pp. S53–S60, 2007.

[5] S. Kreiter, M. Diken, A. Selmi, Ö. Türeci, and U. Sahin, "Tumor vaccination using messenger RNA: prospects of a future therapy," *Current Opinion in Immunology*, vol. 23, no. 3, pp. 399–406, 2011.

[6] D. Benteyn, C. Heirman, A. Bonehill, K. Thielemans, and K. Breckpot, "mRNA-based dendritic cell vaccines," *Expert Review of Vaccines*, vol. 14, no. 2, pp. 161–176, 2015.

[7] X. Liao, Y. Li, C. Bonini et al., "Transfection of RNA encoding tumor antigens following maturation of dendritic cells leads to prolonged presentation of antigen and the generation of high-affinity tumor-reactive cytotoxic T lymphocytes," *Molecular Therapy*, vol. 9, no. 5, pp. 757–764, 2004.

[8] A. Michiels, S. Tuyaerts, A. Bonehill et al., "Electroporation of immature and mature dendritic cells: Implications for dendritic cell-based vaccines," *Gene Therapy*, vol. 12, no. 9, pp. 772–782, 2005.

[9] N. Schaft, J. Dörrie, P. Thumann et al., "Generation of an optimized polyvalent monocyte-derived dendritic cell vaccine by transfecting defined RNAs after rather than before maturation," *Journal of Immunology*, vol. 174, no. 5, pp. 3087–3097, 2005.

[10] I. A. Pfeiffer, S. Hoyer, K. F. Gerer et al., "Triggering of NF-κB in cytokine-matured human DCs generates superior DCs for T-cell priming in cancer immunotherapy," *European Journal of Immunology*, vol. 44, no. 11, pp. 3413–3428, 2014.

[11] D. M. Calderhead, M. A. Debenedette, H. Ketteringham et al., "Cytokine maturation followed by CD40L mRNA electroporation results in a clinically relevant dendritic cell product capable of inducing a potent proinflammatory CTL response," *Journal of Immunotherapy*, vol. 31, no. 8, pp. 731–741, 2008.

[12] S. Van Lint, S. Wilgenhof, C. Heirman et al., "Optimized dendritic cell-based immunotherapy for melanoma: the TriMix-formula," *Cancer Immunology, Immunotherapy*, vol. 63, no. 9, pp. 959–967, 2014.

[13] E. Brencicova and S. S. Diebold, "Nucleic acids and endosomal pattern recognition: how to tell friend from foe?" *Frontiers in Cellular and Infection Microbiology*, vol. 4, article 37, 2013.

[14] A. Szabo and E. Rajnavolgyi, "Collaboration of Toll-like and RIG-I-like receptors in human dendritic cells: tRIGgering antiviral innate immune responses," *American Journal of Clinical and Experimental Immunology*, vol. 2, no. 3, pp. 195–207, 2013.

[15] S. S. Diebold, T. Kaisho, H. Hemmi, S. Akira, and C. R. e Sousa, "Innate antiviral responses by means of TLR7-mediated recognition of single-stranded RNA," *Science*, vol. 303, no. 5663, pp. 1529–1531, 2004.

[16] J. M. Lund, L. Alexopoulou, A. Sato et al., "Recognition of single-stranded RNA viruses by Toll-like receptor 7," *Proceedings of the National Academy of Sciences of the United States of America*, vol. 101, no. 15, pp. 5598–5603, 2004.

[17] F. Heil, H. Hemmi, H. Hochrein et al., "Species-specific recognition of single-stranded RNA via toll-like receptor 7 and 8," *Science*, vol. 303, no. 5663, pp. 1526–1529, 2004.

[18] K. Karikó, H. Ni, J. Capodici, M. Lamphier, and D. Weissman, "mRNA is an endogenous ligand for Toll-like receptor 3," *The Journal of Biological Chemistry*, vol. 279, no. 13, pp. 12542–12550, 2004.

[19] M. Ceppi, N. Ruggli, V. Tache, H. Gerber, K. C. McCullough, and A. Summerfield, "Double-stranded secondary structures on mRNA induce type I interferon (IFN α/β) production and maturation of mRNA-transfected monocyte-derived dendritic cells," *Journal of Gene Medicine*, vol. 7, no. 4, pp. 452–465, 2005.

[20] H. Kumar, T. Kawai, and S. Akira, "Pathogen recognition by the innate immune system," *International Reviews of Immunology*, vol. 30, no. 1, pp. 16–34, 2011.

[21] F. Eberle, M. Sirin, M. Binder, and A. H. Dalpke, "Bacterial RNA is recognized by different sets of immunoreceptors," *European Journal of Immunology*, vol. 39, no. 9, pp. 2537–2547, 2009.

[22] J. Dörrie, N. Schaft, I. Müller et al., "Introduction of functional chimeric E/L-selectin by RNA electroporation to target dendritic cells from blood to lymph nodes," *Cancer Immunology, Immunotherapy*, vol. 57, no. 4, pp. 467–477, 2008.

[23] M. E. Ritchie, B. Phipson, D. Wu et al., "limma powers differential expression analyses for RNA-sequencing and microarray studies," *Nucleic Acids Research*, vol. 43, no. 7, p. e47, 2015.

[24] M. Erdmann, J. Dörrie, N. Schaft et al., "Effective clinical-scale production of dendritic cell vaccines by monocyte elutriation directly in medium, subsequent culture in bags and final antigen loading using peptides or RNA transfection," *Journal of Immunotherapy*, vol. 30, no. 6, pp. 663–674, 2007.

[25] A. Bonehill, C. Heirman, S. Tuyaerts et al., "Messenger RNA-electroporated dendritic cells presenting MAGE-A3 simultaneously in HLA class I and class II molecules," *Journal of Immunology*, vol. 172, no. 11, pp. 6649–6657, 2004.

[26] H. Ni, J. Capodici, G. Cannon et al., "Extracellular mRNA induces dendritic cell activation by stimulating tumor necrosis factor-alpha secretion and signaling through a nucleotide receptor," *The Journal of Biological Chemistry*, vol. 277, no. 15, pp. 12689–12696, 2002.

[27] M. Cella, M. Salio, Y. Sakakibara, H. Langen, I. Julkunen, and A. Lanzavecchia, "Maturation, activation, and protection of dendritic cells induced by double-stranded RNA," *Journal of Experimental Medicine*, vol. 189, no. 5, pp. 821–829, 1999.

[28] M. Zuker, "Mfold web server for nucleic acid folding and hybridization prediction," *Nucleic Acids Research*, vol. 31, no. 13, pp. 3406–3415, 2003.

[29] M. C. Tal and A. Iwasaki, "Autophagy and innate recognition systems," *Current Topics in Microbiology and Immunology*, vol. 335, no. 1, pp. 107–121, 2009.

[30] A. E. Sköld, J. J. van Beek, S. P. Sittig et al., "Protamine-stabilized RNA as an ex vivo stimulant of primary human dendritic cell subsets," *Cancer Immunology, Immunotherapy*, vol. 64, no. 11, pp. 1461–1473, 2015.

12

Luciferase mRNA Transfection of Antigen Presenting Cells Permits Sensitive Nonradioactive Measurement of Cellular and Humoral Cytotoxicity

Tana A. Omokoko,[1,2] Uli Luxemburger,[1,3] Shaheer Bardissi,[2] Petra Simon,[1,2] Magdalena Utsch,[4] Andrea Breitkreuz,[1,2] Özlem Türeci,[1,4] and Ugur Sahin[1,3]

[1]*Division of Translational and Experimental Oncology, Department of Medicine III, Johannes Gutenberg University, Freiligrathstrasse 12, 55131 Mainz, Germany*
[2]*BioNTech Cell & Gene Therapies GmbH, An der Goldgrube 12, 55131 Mainz, Germany*
[3]*BioNTech AG, An der Goldgrube 12, 55131 Mainz, Germany*
[4]*Ganymed Pharmaceuticals AG, An der Goldgrube 12, 55131 Mainz, Germany*

Correspondence should be addressed to Tana A. Omokoko; tana.omokoko@biontechcells.de

Academic Editor: Andrew Geall

Immunotherapy is rapidly evolving as an effective treatment option for many cancers. With the emerging fields of cancer vaccines and adoptive cell transfer therapies, there is an increasing demand for high-throughput *in vitro* cytotoxicity assays that efficiently analyze immune effector functions. The gold standard ^{51}Cr-release assay is very accurate but has the major disadvantage of being radioactive. We reveal the development of a versatile and nonradioactive firefly luciferase *in vitro* transcribed (IVT) RNA-based assay. Demonstrating high efficiency, consistency, and excellent target cell viability, our optimized luciferase IVT RNA is used to transfect dividing and nondividing primary antigen presenting cells. Together with the long-lasting expression and minimal background, the direct measurement of intracellular luciferase activity of living cells allows for the monitoring of killing kinetics and displays paramount sensitivity. The ability to cotransfect the IVT RNA of the luciferase reporter and the antigen of interest into the antigen presenting cells and its simple read-out procedure render the assay high-throughput in nature. Results generated were comparable to the ^{51}Cr release and further confirmed the assay's ability to measure antibody-dependent cell-mediated cytotoxicity and complement-dependent cytotoxicity. The assay's combined simplicity, practicality, and efficiency tailor it for the analysis of antigen-specific cellular and humoral effector functions during the development of novel immunotherapies.

1. Introduction

Cancer immunotherapy is emerging as an important contributor to the armamentarium of future oncology treatments [1–4]. This was heralded by the advent of checkpoint inhibitors, which have made a paradigm shifting difference in the outcome of cancer treatment, resulting in sustained effects and long term survival [5, 6]. Checkpoint inhibitors only unleash the effector functions of preformed T cell specificities. This has motivated the reassessment of vaccination approaches as a complementary concept [7]. As a parallel development,

due to maturation of technology and promising clinical data, the interest in redirecting adoptively transferred T cells by recombinant T cell receptors (TCRs) and chimeric antigen receptors (CARs) has moved into the spotlight [8, 9], as has the pursuit of cancer-cell surface directed antibodies recruiting and activating immune effectors such as FcR positive immune cells (ADCC) or the complement cascade (CDC).

One of the many technical challenges in immunotherapy development is the assessment of cytotoxicity induced by immune effectors, whether engineered or therapeutically elicited, in biological assays. Such assays are required for different stages of immunotherapeutic product development, including but not limited to high-throughput discovery/selection of clinical lead candidates, mechanism-of-action or pharmacodynamics, biomarker studies accompanying clinical trial protocols, and potency assays for release of immunotherapeutic compounds.

Biological cytotoxicity assays for immunotherapeutic concepts may be more challenging as compared to those for chemical compounds due to various reasons. These include the use of difficult-to-label target cells, or, regarding reporter gene transfection-based assays, the use of difficult-to-transfect targets such as primary human professional antigen presenting cells (APCs). These have to be modified to efficiently express not only the reporter gene but also the antigen of interest when measuring the cytotoxicity of cytotoxic T lymphocytes (CTLs).

Many cytotoxicity assays assess the integrity of target cell membranes after coincubation with killing reagents, for example, CTLs or monoclonal antibodies (mAbs). The Chromium-51- (^{51}Cr-) release assay, first described in 1968 [10], is still the gold-standard but has the drawback of being radioactive and consequently hazardous. Newer nonradioactive assays using vital dyes [11], fluorescent dyes [12, 13], and combinations thereof [14] as well as bioluminescence-based assays [15, 16] have various disadvantages ranging from suboptimal labelling of targets to spontaneous release by leaky cells and inacceptable labor intensiveness [14, 17, 18].

A commonly used nonradioactive reporter gene is the luciferase enzyme [19–21]. When expressed in living cells, luciferase produces bioluminescence through a photogenic reaction in which it catalyzes the oxygenation of luciferin taken up from a substrate buffer that is added to the wells in the presence of intracellular oxygen and ATP.

Existing plasmid-based approaches using luciferase for the assessment of cytotoxicity such as the one described by Brown et al. [22] have the drawbacks of insufficient transfection efficiencies and significant decreases in vitality when using nondividing primary cells [23].

Therefore, the objective of the project presented here was to develop an efficient nonradioactive firefly luciferase-based cytotoxicity assay system compatible with dividing and primary nondividing APCs and suitable for high-throughput screening of cytotoxicity of immunotherapeutic formats. More specifically, the assay should robustly allow the assessment of antigen-specific CTL responses, antibody-dependent cell-mediated cytotoxicity (ADCC), and complement-dependent cytotoxicity (CDC).

To this end, instead of using a plasmid-based reporter gene delivery, a gene-encoding RNA was used. RNA is a versatile format to not only deliver the nonradioactive firefly luciferase reporter into the target cells, but also allow the antigen to be recognized by the respective immune effectors. Gene-encoding RNA for engineering of cells has the advantages of being easy to produce in large amounts by *in vitro* transcription (IVT) and easy to deliver by electroporation without compromising cell viability and, since it does not need to enter the nucleus, it is also an efficient system to transfect both dividing and nondividing cells. Furthermore,

this approach circumvents transcriptional regulation issues faced when using DNA plasmids [23–26].

As previously reported, we have developed a plasmid construct (pST1-*Insert*-2BglobinUTR-A120-Sap1), which upon *in vitro* transcription gives rise to a 3′ modified RNA with optimized stability and translational efficiency [27]. This is achieved by fusing the cDNA of the gene of interest to the plasmid's cassette featuring two sequential human beta-globin 3′ untranslated regions (UTRs) and a 120-nucleotide long poly(A) tail with an unmasked 3′ end.

Taking advantage of our plasmid construct, this paper presents a sensitive, rapid, and simple-to-perform luciferase IVT RNA-based bioassay applicable for high-throughput screening of cytotoxicity mediated by antigen-specific CTLs or ADCC- or CDC-inducing mAbs.

2. Materials and Methods

2.1. Cells and Cell Lines. The human erythromyeloblastoid leukaemia cell line K562 stably transfected with human HLA-A*0201 (referred to as K562-A2) was cultured under standard conditions [28]. Endogenously human Claudin 18.2 (hCLDN18.2) expressing human gastric cancer cell lines NUGC-4 and KATO-III were maintained in RPMI 1640 (Life Technologies) supplemented with 10% foetal calf serum (Biofluid Inc., Gaithersburg, MD, USA) at 37°C, 5% CO_2, and RPMI 1640 supplemented with 20% foetal calf serum at 37°C, 7.5% CO_2, respectively. The CHO-K1 cell line stably expressing hCLDN18.2 was cultured in DMEM-F12 (Life Technologies), supplemented with 10% foetal calf serum, 1% Penicillin-Streptomycin (Life Technologies), and 1.5 mg/mL Geneticin (GE Healthcare Life Sciences) at 37°C, 7.5% CO_2. Peripheral blood mononuclear cells (PBMCs) were isolated by Ficoll-Hypaque (Amersham Biosciences, Uppsala, Sweden) density gradient centrifugation from buffy coats obtained from healthy blood bank donors. Monocytes were enriched from PBMCs with anti-CD14 microbeads (Miltenyi Biotec, Bergisch-Gladbach, Germany). Immature (iDCs) and mature dendritic cells (mDCs) were generated as previously described [27]. The monospecific CTL cell line IVSB specific for the HLA-A*0201-restricted tyrosinase-derived epitope $tyr_{368-376}$ [29, 30] was cultured as previously described [31].

2.2. In Vitro Expansion of Human T Cells. CD8$^+$ T cells were purified from PBMC of human cytomegalovirus (CMV)$^+$ donors by positive magnetic cell sorting (Miltenyi Biotec) and expanded by coculturing 2×10^6 effectors with 3×10^5 autologous DCs either electroporated with IVT RNA or pulsed with overlapping peptide pool for 1 week in complete medium supplemented with 5% AB serum, 10 U/mL IL-2, and 5 ng/mL IL-7.

For nonspecific expansion, 2×10^6 per well naïve CD8$^+$ T cells purified from CMV$^-$ donors were stimulated in OKT3 mAb coated 24-well plates (Janssen-Cilag GmbH, Neuss). Coating was performed using 300 μL/well PBS-diluted mAb (10 μg/mL) for 2 h at 37°C. After 24 h of culture, 50 U/mL IL-2 was added to the stimulated CTLs. On day 3, the cells were resuspended in fresh medium supplemented with 50 U/mL

IL-2 and cultured for another 4 days in 24-well plates without OKT3.

2.3. Peptides and Peptide Pulsing of Stimulator Cells.

Pools of N- and C-terminally free 15-mer peptides (all peptides purchased from JPT Peptide Technologies GmbH) with 11 amino acid overlaps corresponding to sequences of CMV-pp65 and HIV-gag (referred to as antigen pool), the latter used as negative control, were dissolved in DMSO to a final concentration of 0.5 mg/mL. The HLA-A*0201 restricted peptides derived from the CMV-pp65 (pp65$_{495-503}$, NLVP-MVATV), tyrosinase (tyr$_{368-376}$, YMDGTMSQV), and SSX2 (SSX2$_{41-49}$, KASEKIFYV) antigens were reconstituted in PBS 10% DMSO. For pulsing, stimulator cells were incubated for 1 h at 37°C in culture medium using concentrations of 1–3 μg/mL, where not otherwise indicated.

2.4. Vectors for In Vitro Transcription.

A plasmid for *in vitro* transcription of the synthetic firefly luciferase reporter gene (*luc2*) was constructed based on the previously described pST1-insert-2hBgUTR-A(120) vector, which allows the generation of RNA with optimized stability and translational efficacy [27]. The *luc2* gene was subcloned from the pGL4.14[luc2/Hygro] vector (Promega Corporation, Madison, WI, USA) and an internal EciI restriction site deleted by site-directed mutagenesis (Agilent) using the oligo luc2mut sense (5′-CTA CCA GGC ATC CGA CAG GGC TAC GGC CTG ACA GAA AC-3′) and the reverse complement (Eurofins Genomics).

The pST1-2hBgUTR-A(120)-IVT vectors containing enhanced green fluorescent protein (eGFP) and the full-length TCR alpha and beta chains of the pp65$_{495-503}$-specific and HLA-A*0201-restricted TCR-8-CMV#14 have been previously described [27, 31]. The pp65 antigen-encoding vector pST1-sec-pp65-MITD-2hBgUTR-A(120) features a signal sequence for routing to the endoplasmic reticulum and the MHC class I transmembrane and cytoplasmic domains to improve MHC class I and II presentation [32].

2.5. Generation of IVT RNA and Transfer into Cells.

IVT RNA was generated as previously described [27] and added to cells suspended in X-VIVO 15 medium (Lonza) in a precooled 4 mm gap sterile electroporation cuvette (Bio-Rad). Electroporation was performed with a Gene-Pulser-II apparatus (Bio-Rad; human iDC: 276 V/150 μF; human mDC: 290 V/150 μF; CD8$^+$ T cells: 450 V/250 μF; K562-A2, CHO and NUGC-4: 200 V/300 μF; KATO III: 250 V/475 μF).

2.6. Flow Cytometric Analysis.

Flow cytometric analysis was performed on a FACS-Calibur analytical flow cytometer using CellQuest-Pro software (BD Biosciences). DC maturation markers were detected by staining with PE-labelled anti-CD83 and APC-labelled anti-HLA-DR antibodies (BD Biosciences).

2.7. Luciferase-Based CTL Cytotoxicity Assay.

APCs were electroporated with 10–50 μg of *luc2* IVT RNA. For coelectroporation experiments, *luc2* IVT RNA and either pp65

or control RNA were electroporated into the target cells simultaneously. After electroporation, cells were resuspended in prewarmed culture medium and incubated overnight at 37°C and 5% CO_2. 20 h later, cells were diluted to a final concentration of 2×10^6 cells/mL in culture medium containing 1–3 μg/mL specific peptide (pool) or control peptide (pool) and were incubated for 1 h at 37°C and 5% CO_2. After pulsing with peptides, cells were washed and resuspended in complete culture medium and 1×10^4 cells per well were plated in triplicate in 50 μL into white 96-well flat-bottom plates (Thermo Scientific). CD8$^+$ effector cells were washed, counted, and cocultured in different E : T ratios in a final volume of 100 μL per well at 37°C and 5% CO_2 for 3 h. Minimal and maximal lysis control wells contained 1×10^4 target cells alone in a total volume of 100 μL and 90 μL, respectively. After the specified time 50 μL of a D-luciferin substrate solution containing 3.6 mg/mL D-luciferin (BD Biosciences Pharmingen), 150 mM HEPES (Life Technologies) and 1.2 mU/μL Adenosine 5′-Triphosphatase (Sigma-Aldrich) were added to each well to a final volume of 150 μL. Maximum lysis control wells were treated with 10 μL 2% Triton X-100/PBS prior to addition of substrate. 96-well plates were incubated for another hour at 37°C and 5% CO_2. After a total coincubation time of 4 h, the intracellular luciferase activity of living cells was measured using a Tecan Infinite M200 reader (Tecan Group AG, Crailsheim, Germany). Percent specific lysis was calculated as follows:

$$\left(1 - \frac{CPS_{experimental} - CPS_{minimal}}{CPS_{maximal} - CPS_{minimal}}\right) \times 100. \quad (1)$$

2.8. ^{51}Cr-Release Assay.

Autologous DCs were loaded with 3 μg/mL pp65 peptide pool or control peptide and labelled with 100 μCi of ^{51}Cr (NEN Life Science) for 90 min at 37°C and 5% CO_2. ^{51}Cr labelled DCs were washed and resuspended in complete culture medium and 1×10^4 targets per 200 μL per well coincubated in triplicate with effector T cells at different E : T ratios for 4 h. A total of 60 μL of the supernatant was harvested, and released ^{51}Cr was measured with a scintillation counter. Spontaneous release was also determined. Percent specific lysis was calculated using the following equation:

$$\frac{experimental\ release - spontaneous\ release}{maximum\ release - spontaneous\ release} \times 100. \quad (2)$$

2.9. Luciferase-Based ADCC Assay.

Target cells were electroporated using 7 μg of *luc2* IVT RNA. After electroporation, cells were resuspended in 2.4 mL prewarmed culture medium. 2×10^4 KATO-III cells or 2.5×10^4 NUGC-4 cells per 50 μL per well were plated independently in triplicate into white 96-well flat-bottom plates (NUNC) and were incubated for 4–6 h at 37°C, 7.5%, and 5% CO_2, respectively. Different IMAB 362 concentrations ranging from 0.06 ng/mL to 200 μg/mL and Ficoll-Paque-purified PBMCs from healthy donors were added to each well (E : T ratio of 40 : 1). KATO-III and NUGC-4 cell-containing plates were incubated for 24 h at 37°C, 7.5%, and 5% CO_2, respectively. After overnight incubation, 10 μL 8% Triton X-100/PBS solution was added to the maximum lysis control wells and 10 μL PBS to the other wells. Finally, 50 μL D-luciferin substrate solution containing 3.2 mg/mL D-luciferin, 160 mM HEPES, and 0.64 mU/μL Adenosine 5'-Triphosphatase was added to each well to a final volume of 160 μL and plates were incubated for 90 min at room temperature (RT) in the dark. Bioluminescence was measured using a luminometer (Infinite M200, TECAN). Percentage of specific lysis was calculated using the formula described above for the luciferase-based CTL cytotoxicity assay.

2.10. Luciferase-Based CDC Assay.

CHO-K1~hCLDN18.2 cells were electroporated using 7 μg of luc2 IVT RNA and resuspended in 2.4 mL prewarmed culture medium. 5×10^4 cells per 50 μL per well were plated in triplicate into white 96-well flat-bottom plates (NUNC) and were incubated for 24 h at 37°C, 7.5% CO_2. 44% human serum from healthy donors was prepared in RPMI medium supplemented with 20 mM HEPES. IMAB 362 antibody was diluted in human serum to final assay concentrations ranging from 31.6 ng/mL to 10 μg/mL. 50 μL of different IMAB 362 antibody concentrations were added to the target cells to achieve an end concentration of 20% (v/v) serum. The 96-well plate was incubated for 80 min at 37°C, 7.5% CO_2. After incubation, 10 μL 8% Triton X-100/PBS solution was added to control for maximum lysis and 10 μL PBS to the remaining wells. D-Luciferin substrate solution was added to each well as described above for the ADCC assay. Plates were incubated for 45 min at RT in the dark and then measured in a luminometer (Infinite M200, TECAN). Specific lysis was calculated as described above for the ADCC assay.

3. Results and Discussion

3.1. Electroporation of Firefly Luciferase IVT RNA into Dividing and Nondividing APCs Is Nontoxic and Leads to Strong and Long-Lasting Gene Expression.

One of the key elements for the performance of a cytotoxicity assay system is the labelling of the target cell population with a reporter system without affecting cell viability. This limitation is pronounced when using nondividing cells, such as primary human APCs, frequently required in the context of immunotherapy drug development. Plasmid-based reporter gene assays are of low efficiency and do not provide a good solution [22]. Instead of using a plasmid-based delivery approach, the use of a luciferase gene-encoding mRNA was investigated here.

The firefly luciferase (luc2) gene was cloned into the pST1-2hBgUTR-A(120)-EciI vector and in vitro transcribed from this construct with a stability optimized 3' end (Figure 1(a)). 5.4 μg of this IVT RNA was electroporated into K562 leukemic cells stably transfected with the human HLA-A*0201 gene (hereinafter referred to as K562-A2) [28]. In addition, difficult-to-transfect nondividing primary human cells, namely, iDCs and mDCs, were also used as targets (Figure 1(b)). Luminescence after D-luciferin substrate addition was instantly detected and strongly increased between 2 and 8 h after electroporation. Signals reached

maximum levels after 10 to 24 h in all cell types. K562-A2 cells showed the highest signal levels. Activity in primary cells was also very robust, and a 2–4-fold higher maximum luciferase activity was detected in mDCs compared to iDCs. High and durable expression levels were achieved with an approximately 80% signal intensity still being detectable 36 h after electroporation into K562-A2 cells and mDCs, and 24 h in the case of iDCs. Luciferase expression kinetics exhibited batch consistency within each cell type and were not affected by the use of higher luc2 IVT RNA amounts (data not shown).

To assess the viability of the target cells, 10 μg RNA encoding luciferase and eGFP were electroporated into human iDCs and mDCs generated from the same donor. Both iDCs and mDCs displayed excellent viability, ranging from 85 to 95% in the 72 h after electroporation with reporter RNA as determined by flow cytometry (Figure 1(c)). 80–90% of all living DCs expressed eGFP stably over 72 h illustrating high transfection efficiency. This gives the IVT RNA approach an advantage over plasmid based assays, which show low efficiencies when used with nondividing primary APCs, probably a consequence of using more stringent electrical settings [23]. Both iDCs and mDCs retained their phenotypes after electroporation as demonstrated by the sustained levels of the maturation markers HLA-DR and CD83 in luc2 transfected cells compared to controls for as long as 72 hours after electroporation. As expected, mDCs showed a higher expression of both markers (Figure 1(c)).

In summary, the data demonstrate high, stable, and long-lasting expression of luc2 reporter IVT RNA in dividing as well as nondividing primary APCs, without compromising the viability or immunological phenotype of the target cells.

3.2. Optimization of the Assay Parameters Enhances and Prolongs Luciferase Signals Whilst Minimizing Background and Reveals a Strict Luminescence to Cell Number Correlation.

As a next step, the implementation of the IVT RNA-based reporter-gene engineering of target cells into a robust cytotoxicity assay with a favorable signal-to-noise ratio and a high sensitivity was investigated.

For K562-A2 cells electroporated with 20 μg of luc2 IVT RNA, a D-luciferin substrate concentration of 1.2 mg/mL achieved the highest signals (Figure 2(a)). These signals were prolonged and stable, allowing continuous detection of living cells after a single administration of substrate for at least 4 h (Figure 2(b)). Bioluminescence dropped to levels close to zero following Triton X-100 detergent-mediated cell lysis, demonstrating responsiveness of the technique to cytotoxic events (Figure 2(b)). The rapid reduction of background signals from dying cells is further accelerated by the addition of ATPase to the substrate buffer, which results in the immediate hydrolysis of ATP released from these cells and ceasing of luciferase activity following cell death (data not shown). The stability of the signal over 4 hours and the direct assessment of cell death allow both endpoint measurements and the determination of killing kinetics, which is superior to many other assays such as the ^{51}Cr and the Europium release assays, that only allow the former [17, 18, 33].

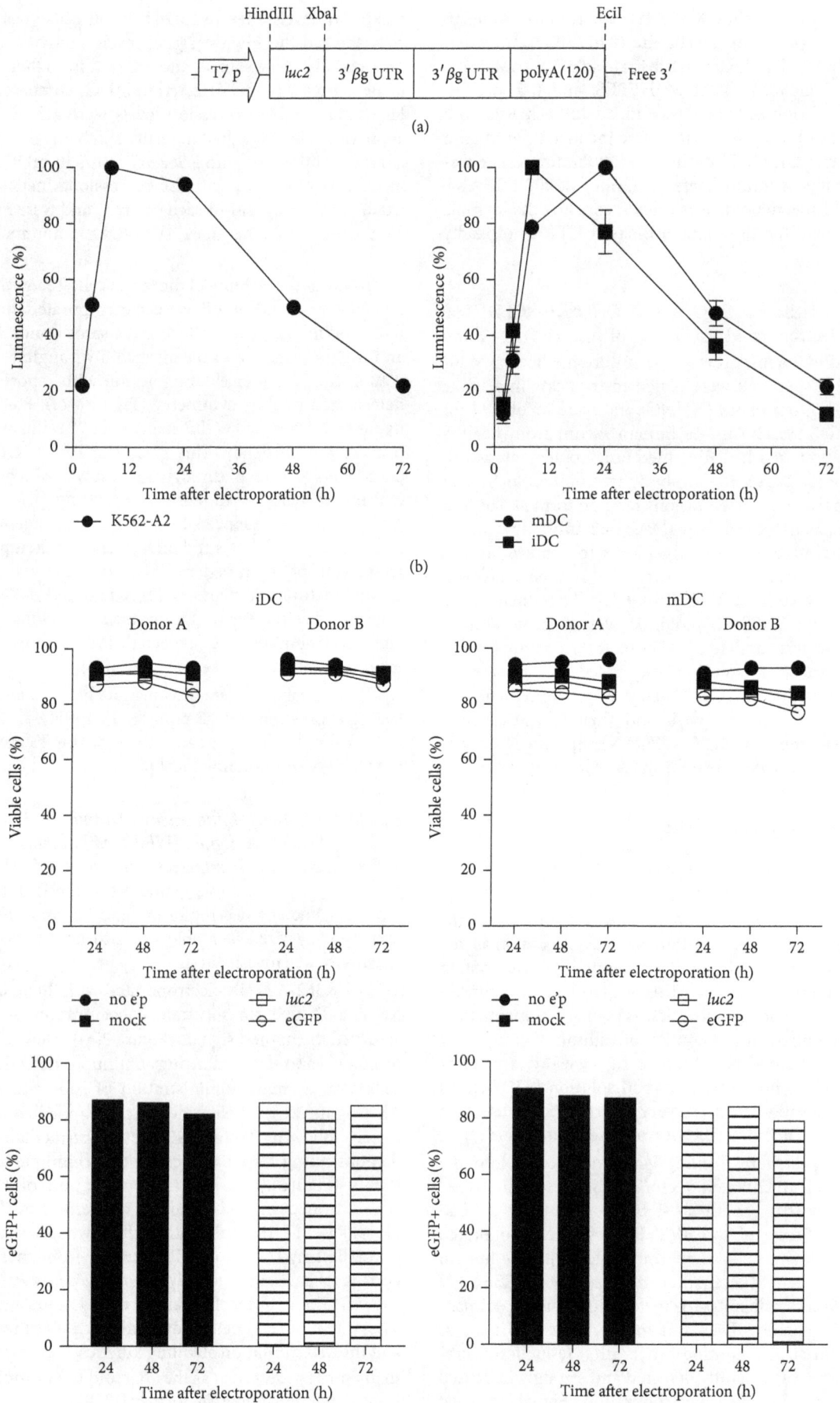

FIGURE 1: Continued.

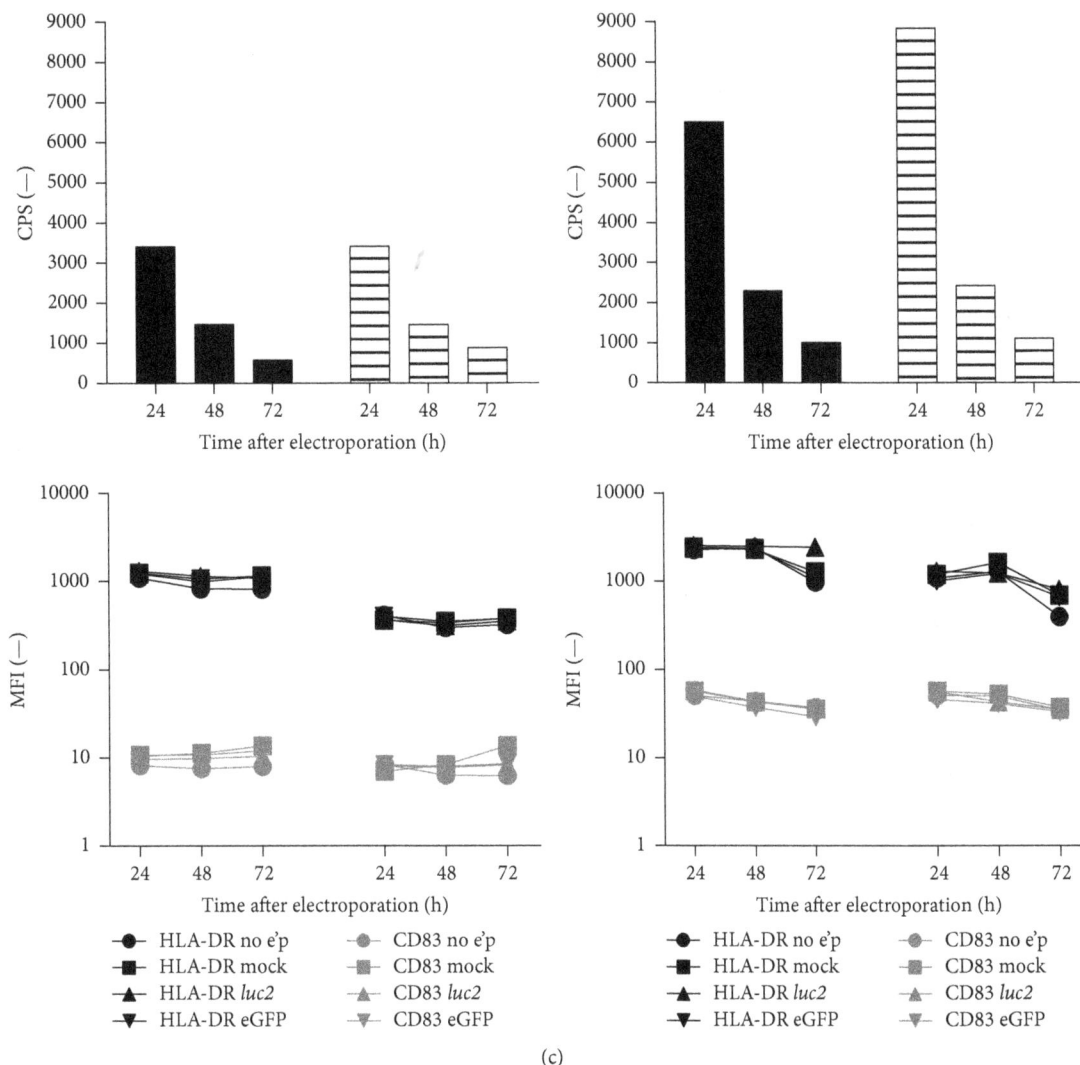

(c)

FIGURE 1: Electroporation of firefly luciferase IVT RNA into DCs and K562-A2 cells is nontoxic and leads to strong and long-lasting gene expression without affecting target cell phenotype. (a) Optimised *luc2* reporter vector: composed of a gene-optimized synthetic firefly luciferase reporter gene cloned in front of two human β-globin 3′ untranslated regions (UTRs) fused head to tail and an unmasked free poly(A) tail of 120 bp. (b) Kinetics of *luc2* expression in K562-A2 cells ($n = 1$), human iDCs ($n = 3$), and mDCs ($n = 3$). Cells transfected with 8 pmol of *luc2*-encoding IVT RNA were harvested at different time points to measure luminescence from 1×10^4 cells (Bright-Glo Luciferase Assay Kit for 96-well plates (Promega)). Results are the mean ± SD luminescence. Percent luminescence is relative to the highest luminescence signal obtained in each experiment. (c) Viability, reporter gene expression of iDCs and mDCs after eGFP and *luc2* electroporation and phenotype after electroporation are depicted in descending order, respectively. iDCs (left panel) and mDCs (right panel) of 2 different donors were transfected with 10 μg eGFP- or *luc2*-encoding IVT RNA. Negative controls: cells electroporated without RNA (mock) and unelectroporated (no e′p) cells. Cells were harvested at different time points. Viability and HLA-DR, CD83, and eGFP expression levels were determined by flow cytometry. Luciferase activity of 1×10^4 viable cells was measured by luminescence in triplicate.

Electroporation of K562-A2 cells with increasing amounts of *luc2* IVT RNA displayed a dose-dependent increase in luminescence (Figure 2(c)).

The strict linear dependence between the detectable bioluminescence and transfected cell numbers further verified the sensitivity of the method (Figure 2(d)).

Next, these conditions were tested on nondividing primary cells, namely, human monocyte-derived iDCs and mDCs. Addition of D-luciferin to human iDCs and mDCs

24 h after their electroporation with *luc2* IVT RNA also demonstrated a linear correlation between cell number and bioluminescence (Figure 2(e)). Luciferase activity from as few as 1,000 cells was more than 24-fold higher than background levels, implying that luminescence from such few cells suffices for accurate reporter gene detection (Figure 2(e)).

The equipment and the read-out conditions of the assay greatly affect the specific signal, background reading, and the cross-talk between wells. In our hands, white polystyrene

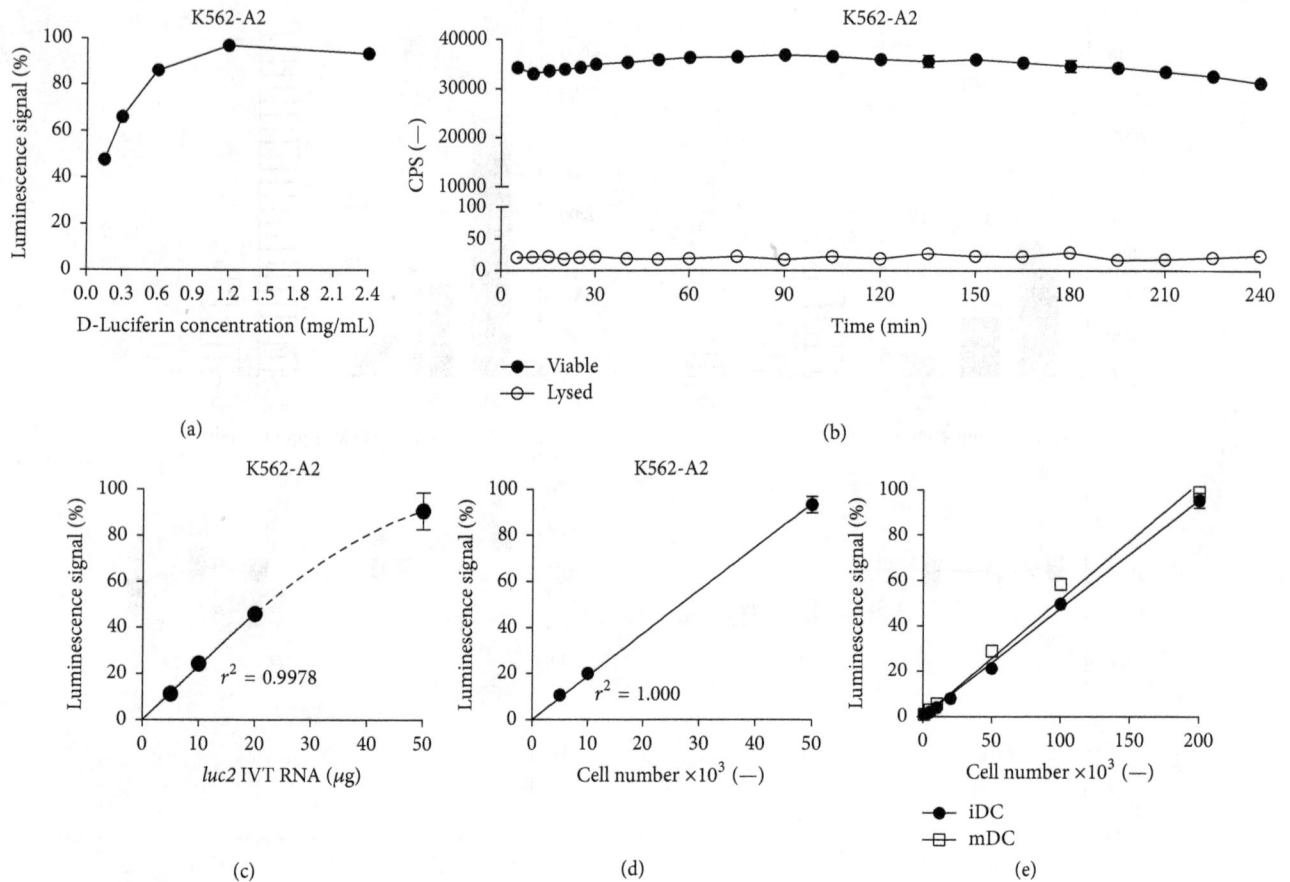

(a)

(b)

(c)

(d)

(e)

FIGURE 2: Optimization of the assay parameters enhances and prolongs luciferase signals whilst minimizing background reading and reveals a strict luminescence to cell number correlation. (a) Optimal D-luciferin substrate concentration. 1×10^6 K562-A2 cells were transfected with 20 μg $luc2$ IVT RNA. After 24 h, luminescence of 5×10^4 cells per well was measured following addition of D-luciferin in different concentrations. (b) Stable bioluminescence upon D-luciferin substrate addition and immediate abolition of signals following total cell lysis. 2.5×10^6 K562-A2 cells were transfected with 50 μg $luc2$ IVT RNA. 24 h after transfection, luminescence of 5×10^4 viable or 0.2% Triton X-100 treated cells was repeatedly measured after a single administration of 1.2 mg/mL D-luciferin substrate. Graph represents mean $\pm$ SD luminescence ($n = 3$). (c) Luminescence is dependent on $luc2$ IVT RNA dose. 1×10^6 K562-A2 cells were transfected with different amounts of $luc2$ IVT RNA. 24 h after transfection, luminescence of 5×10^4 cells per well was measured. (d) Luminescence is linearly dependent on the number of transfected K562-A2 cells. 1×10^6 K562-A2 cells were transfected with 50 μg $luc2$ IVT RNA. 24 h after transfection, 1.2 mg/mL D-luciferin was added and luminescence of different amounts of cells was measured. (e) Luminescence is linearly dependent on the number of transfected primary cells. Human iDCs and mDCs were electroporated with 50 μg $luc2$ IVT RNA. 24 h after transfection, 1.2 mg/mL D-luciferin was added and luminescence of different amount of cells was measured. Cell number and signal intensity correlation ($p < 0.0001$, $r^2 = 0.9984$ (iDC) and 0.9923 (mDC)). Graphs (a), (c), (d), and (e) represent mean $\pm$ SD luminescence ($n = 3$) relative to the highest luminescence signal obtained within each experiment.

flat-bottom plates that reflect light and maximize the output signal and the more cost-efficient Tecan Infinite M200 luminescence plate reader (Tecan, Crailsheim, Germany) resulted in an excellent signal-to-noise ratio, achieving specific signals with multiple logs above background (Table 1; Figure 2(b)). That, along with the advancements in plate readers, such as the automatic regulation of temperature and reagent addition, further promotes the automation of this assay for high-throughput screening. It should be noted that one can easily modify the assay according to one's needs, for example, target cell type and amount of cells usually available, by choosing a suitable plate reader and adjusting the amount of luciferase IVT RNA used for electroporation.

3.3. Luciferase IVT RNA Electroporation Permits Assessment of Antigen-Specific CTL Activity Comparable to the ^{51}Cr Release and Superior in the Ability to Monitor Killing Kinetics.

Having optimized the key performance parameters of the assay system, the CMV-pp65 model antigen was used to measure primary antigen-specific CTL responses, as is frequently required in vaccine approaches. To generate the respective reagents, effector T cells from a CMV$^+$ donor were expanded by coculture with pp65 antigen pool loaded autologous iDCs. Simultaneously, mDCs of the donor were generated and electroporated with $luc2$ IVT RNA. 20 h after transfection, the autologous target cells were loaded with either pp65 antigen pool or control antigen pool before being cocultured with

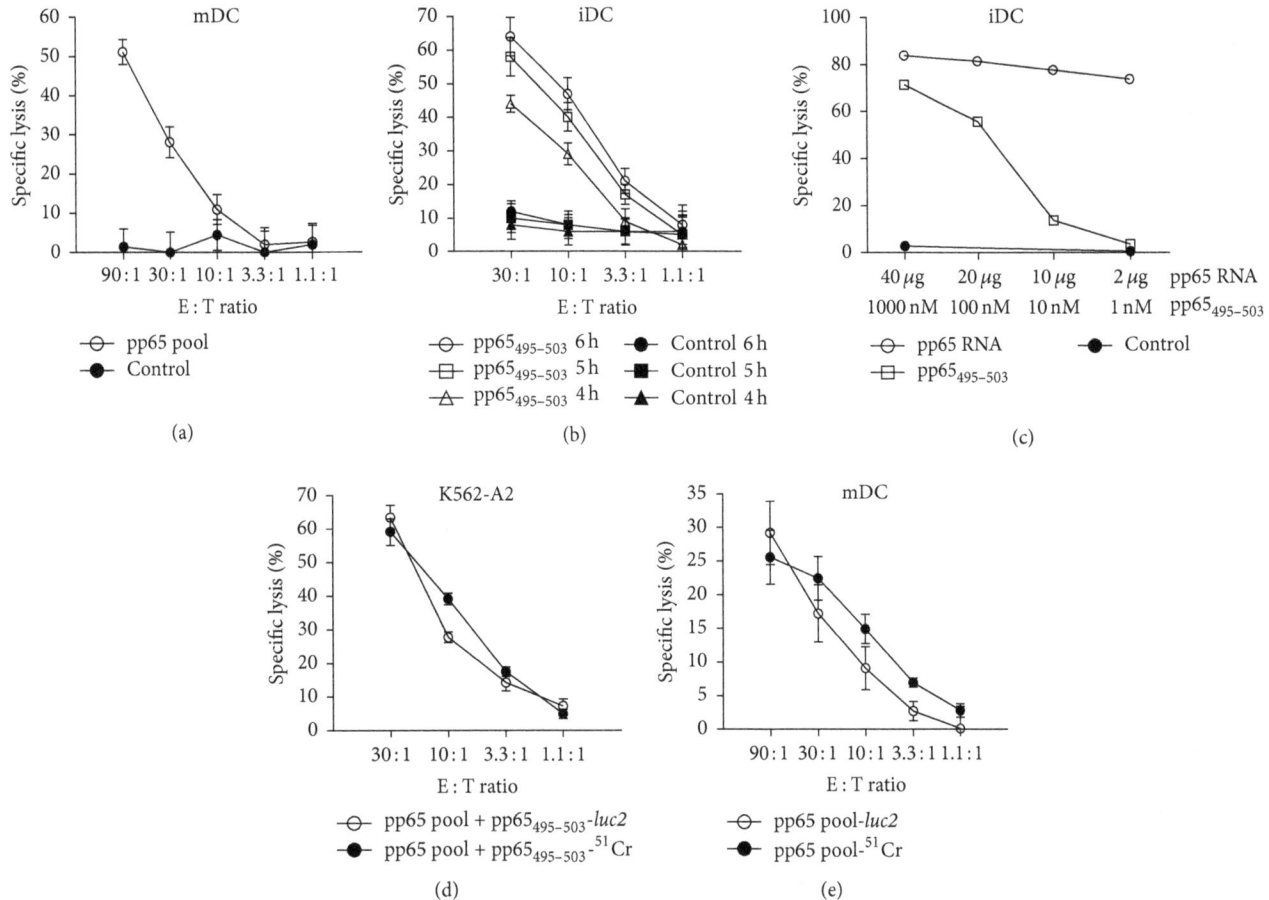

FIGURE 3: Luciferase IVT RNA electroporation permits assessment of antigen-specific CTL activity comparable to the ^{51}Cr release and superior in the ability to monitor killing kinetics. (a) Cytolytic activity of primary CMV-pp65-specific T cells. CMV$^+$ donor-derived CD8$^+$ T cells were expanded for one week and used to assess the killing of autologous mDCs transfected with 50 μg *luc2* RNA and loaded with overlapping peptide pools representing either CMV-pp65 or HIV-gag as control. Specific lysis was determined after 4 h incubation of peptide-loaded target cells with CD8$^+$ effector cells using different E : T ratios. (b) Kinetics of killing mediated by TCR-transfected CD8$^+$ T cells. OKT3-stimulated CD8$^+$ T cells of a CMV$^-$ HLA-A*0201$^+$ donor were transfected with 20 μg TCR-8-CMV#14 alpha and beta chain IVT RNAs. Autologous iDCs transfected with 20 μg *luc2* RNA were loaded with either peptide pp65$_{495-503}$ or tyr$_{368-376}$ as control. iDCs and CD8$^+$ T cells were cocultured at different E : T ratios and specific killing was assessed at different time points. (c) Dose-dependent killing of target cells using different antigen formats. OKT3-stimulated CD8$^+$ T cells from a CMV$^-$ HLA-A*0201$^+$ donor were electroporated with 20 μg TCR-8-CMV-#14 IVT RNA. Autologous iDCs were cotransfected with 20 μg *luc2* IVT RNA and decreasing amounts of a CMV-pp65 antigen-encoding IVT RNA or were *luc2* transfected and subsequently pulsed with titrated amounts of peptide pp65$_{495-503}$. iDC transfected with *luc2* IVT RNA and pulsed with 1000 nM SSX2$_{41-49}$ peptide served as a control. Effector and target cells were incubated at an E : T ratio of 19 : 1. ((d) and (e)) Comparability of the *luc2* IVT RNA assay with the ^{51}Cr assay. Cytotoxicity of CMV-pp65-specific CD8$^+$ T cells of a HLA-A*0201$^+$ CMV$^+$ donor against (d) K562-A2 cells or (e) autologous mDCs was assessed after one week antigen-specific expansion using the *luc2* IVT RNA assay in comparison to the ^{51}Cr assay. 20 h after *luc2* RNA electroporation, target cells were loaded with pp65$_{495-503}$ peptide either alone or together with 100 μCi of ^{51}Cr. 1×10^4 peptide-loaded targets were incubated at different E : T ratios with CD8$^+$ effector cells for 4 h. Cytotoxicity was determined via measurement of luminescence after addition of D-luciferin substrate or via measurement of released ^{51}Cr after harvesting of supernatant. All graphs represent the mean ± SD lysis ($n = 3$).

the CD8$^+$ effectors at different E : T ratios for 4 h. The calculated specific lysis of pp65 pulsed target cells increased with increasing E : T ratios, while target cells pulsed with control peptides were not lysed, illustrating the assays ability to detect and quantify antigen-specific CTL immune responses (Figure 3(a)).

In order to assess the assay's capacity of directly determining the kinetics of CTL-mediated killing, OKT3-stimulated

CD8$^+$ T cells from a CMV$^-$ HLA-A*0201$^+$ donor were electroporated with IVT RNA encoding a previously isolated T cell receptor (TCR-8-CMV-#14) directed against the immunodominant CMV-pp65-derived HLA-A*0201-restricted peptide pp65$_{495-503}$ [31]. Autologous iDCs were transfected with *luc2* IVT RNA and 20 h later loaded with either the specific or a control peptide. Effector and target cells were incubated at different E : T ratios. D-Luciferin was

TABLE 1: White opaque flat-bottom plates together with the Infinite M200 (Tecan) plate reader result in a robust signal-to-noise ratio.

Parameter	Experiment	Outcome
Plate opacity	White opaque versus transparent	Specific luciferase signals obtained from white opaque plates were 2-3-fold higher
Plate design	Flat-bottom versus V-shaped bottom	Only negligible well-to-well cross-talk was observed when flat-bottom plates were used
Plate reader	Wallac VICTOR2 (Perkin Elmer) versus Infinite M200 (Tecan) versus GENios Pro (Tecan)	Signals from the Infinite M200 device were 4-fold and signals from the GENios Pro 20-fold higher than those detected with the Wallac VICTOR2

added once after 3 h. Following that, multiple luminescence readouts were taken at different time points and descriptive killing kinetics could be recorded (Figure 3(b)). For each E : T ratio, the specific lysis increased over time, with the 30 : 1 ratio showing the highest specific lysis at all time points, while control peptide loaded iDCs were not lysed.

Other popular flow cytometry based cytotoxicity assays monitor, for example, caspase activation or granzyme B substrate cleavage in target cells [34]. These alternatives have the ability to quantify target cell death at the single-cell level. However, one needs to carefully determine the best time for such endpoint measurements, as markers of apoptosis such as caspase activity are only transiently present. This may be challenging especially with regard to T cell populations with unknown or low frequency antigen-specific effectors. Due to the long-lasting signals, the luciferase assay, on the other hand, provides the opportunity to take multiple measurements over a longer time period.

A further advantage of using gene-encoding RNA is that, together with the luciferase reporter gene IVT RNA, any other antigen (or vaccine) IVT RNA of interest can be cotransfected. OKT3-stimulated CD8$^+$ T cells from a CMV$^-$ HLA-A*0201$^+$ donor were electroporated with the same TCR-8-CMV-#14 IVT RNA. Autologous iDCs were cotransfected with luc2 IVT RNA and decreasing amounts of a pp65 antigen-encoding IVT RNA or were luc2 transfected and subsequently pulsed with titrated amounts of the pp65$_{495-503}$ peptide. In addition to illustrating the efficient cotransfection of luciferase and varying amounts of antigen IVT RNA, the results show the sensitive recognition of antigen via the TCR with 74% specific lysis being detected using 2 μg of pp65 RNA for transfection (Figure 3(c)). In the context of this cotransfection ability, it should be noted that the use of a full-length antigen-encoding IVT RNA would allow the detection of CTL responses specific for naturally processed epitopes that are presented on the surface of the APCs.

The ^{51}Cr-release assay is widely used and is considered as the gold standard approach to assess T cell and natural killer cell-mediated cytotoxicity [32, 35–37]. The efficiency of the luciferase IVT RNA assay was thus further confirmed by a direct comparison with the ^{51}Cr-release assay using either K562-A2 cells or primary DCs as target cells. For the former, which were stably transfected with HLA-A*0201 (Figure 3(d)), effector T cells of a CMV$^+$ HLA-A*0201$^+$ donor were expanded using peptide loaded autologous iDCs. K562-A2 cells were electroporated with luc2 IVT RNA. 20 h later, half of the cells were loaded with pp65 antigen pool and pp65$_{495-503}$ peptide alone and the other half were simultaneously labelled with ^{51}Cr. For the primary DCs (Figure 3(e)), effector T cells from a CMV$^+$ donor were expanded using peptide loaded autologous iDCs. In parallel, autologous mDCs were electroporated with luc2 IVT RNA. 20 h later, half of the cells were loaded with pp65 antigen pool or control antigen pool alone and the other half were concurrently labelled with ^{51}Cr. In both settings, peptide-loaded targets and CD8$^+$ effector cells were then incubated at different E : T ratios for 4 h before luminescence and released chromium were measured. The IVT RNA-based assay yielded specific lysis levels that were as sensitive as, and almost identical to, the ^{51}Cr assay, with 60% and ~20% specific lysis of the K562-A2 cells (Figure 3(d)) and autologous mDCs (Figure 3(e)), respectively, at an E : T ratio of 30 : 1.

3.4. Luciferase IVT RNA Electroporation Permits a Highly Sensitive Assessment of Antigen-Specific CTL Activity. Having proven the robustness of the system, the capability of the assay to detect low-frequency antigen-specific T cells was examined. The monospecific CTL cell line IVSB recognizing the HLA-A*0201-restricted tyrosinase-derived epitope tyr$_{368-376}$ was used [29, 30]. Decreasing amounts of IVSB T cells were spiked into peripheral blood lymphocytes (PBLs). The specific lysis of autologous iDCs pulsed with the tyr$_{368-376}$ peptide was assessed. Since specific lysis is calculated using internal maximum and minimum references (see Section 2), iDCs plus PBLs without IVSB T cells were used as the minimum lysis reference in this experiment. Luciferase signals were analyzed after 5, 6, and 9 h of coincubation (Figure 4). After 5 h, the cytotoxic activity of 0.37% antigen-specific T cells corresponding to 740 IVSB cells in a total of 200,000 PBLs was easily detected based on the specific lysis of tyr$_{368-376}$ peptide pulsed target cells (Figure 4). When the incubation time was prolonged to 9 h, the detection

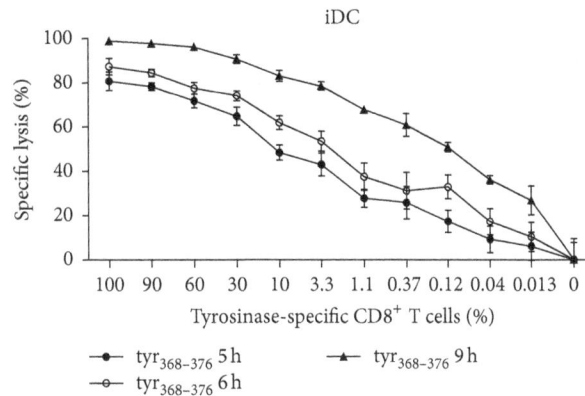

FIGURE 4: Luciferase IVT RNA electroporation permits a highly sensitive assessment of antigen-specific CTL activity. Titrated amounts of IVSB cells were spiked into PBLs and the specific lysis of autologous iDCs pulsed with the $tyr_{368-376}$ peptide was assessed using an E : T ratio of 20 : 1. Luciferase signals were analysed after increasing coincubation times. Results are the mean ± SD (n = 3).

limit was improved to as few as 26 antigen-specific T cells, corresponding to a frequency of 0.013% of PBLs.

The results confirm the suitability of the developed assay to sensitively detect cytotoxicity induced by very rare antigen-specific T cells, as is the case with *ex vivo* tumor-antigen specific effector cells in the blood of cancer patients.

In summary, the data indicates that the luciferase IVT RNA assay performs at least as well as the ^{51}Cr assay and is superior in its sensitivity, nonradioactivity, easy read-out procedure, and the monitoring of killing kinetics.

3.5. The Luciferase IVT RNA-Based Assay Efficiently Assesses mAb-Induced ADCC and CDC of Tumor Cell Lines.

In addition to T cell-mediated cytotoxicity, other effector functions have also been shown to participate in antitumor responses [38]. The assay was therefore adopted to assess ADCC and CDC, which are mediated by the recruitment and activation of either FcR positive effector cells or complement factors by the Fc domains of cell-bound mAbs [39]. To this end, IMAB 362, a therapeutic mAb in advanced clinical development directed against the pan-cancer cell surface antigen Claudin 18.2 (CLDN18.2), which exerts tumor cell death via ADCC and CDC, was used [40–43]. KATO-III and NUGC-4 tumor cells endogenously expressing CLDN18.2 or CHO-K1 cells stably expressing the antigen were electroporated with *luc2* IVT RNA. To measure ADCC, IMAB 362 was added to the KATO-III (Figure 5(a)) and NUGC-4 (Figure 5(b)) target cells 4–6 h after *luc2* electroporation. The cells were then incubated with human PBMCs at a 40 : 1 E : T ratio for 24 h; then D-luciferin substrate was added for luminescence measurement. For the assessment of CDC, 24 h after *luc2* electroporation, the CHO-K1 cells were incubated with IMAB 362, diluted in human serum, for 80 minutes as a source of complement factors. Thereafter, D-luciferin was added for the signal read-out (Figure 5(c)).

Specific lysis via ADCC and CDC was found to be dependent on the IMAB 362 concentration. Dose-response curves

were sigmoid with a good dynamic range. For IMAB 362-induced ADCC-mediated specific lysis of KATO-III cells, as few as 1.19 ng/mL antibody was sufficient to induce 25% killing (Figure 5(a)). For NUGC-4 cells, 24 ng/mL antibody induced 14 to 76% ADCC-mediated lysis among the different donors (Figure 5(b)). The maximum specific cell lysis was approximately 80% in both cell lines and was reached at concentrations of 9.88 μg/mL IMAB 362. Robust CDC was measured at a concentration of 1000 ng/mL and reached a maximum of up to 99% lysis of CHO-K1 cells at an IMAB 362 concentration of 3.16 μg/mL (Figure 5(c)).

The data demonstrates that the luciferase IVT RNA cytotoxicity assay may be used for both ADCC and CDC assessment. This may be very useful for high-throughput testing in the discovery and selection process of therapeutic mAb candidates as well as the assessment of immune cell and humoral responses in clinical vaccine development [44, 45].

4. Conclusions

This paper reports the establishment of a highly suitable nonradioactive IVT RNA firefly luciferase-based cytotoxicity assay. By directly measuring intracellular luciferase activity, the assay efficiently assesses effector cell cytotoxicity mediated by antigen-specific CTLs when using cell lines and primary nondividing APCs as targets. The results generated were comparable to the gold-standard ^{51}Cr-release assay. Taking advantage of an optimized IVT RNA reporter, the approach is extremely sensitive and rapid and has a simple read-out procedure, rendering it applicable for high-throughput screening. In further support of this, the assay allows for the cotransfection of luciferase and the antigen-encoding RNA into the APCs followed by the subsequent monitoring of killing kinetics. The assay was adopted for the evaluation of ADCC and CDC by a cancer cell surface antigen directed mAb. Together, the properties of the developed assay render it an attractive approach for measuring cytotoxicity *in vitro*,

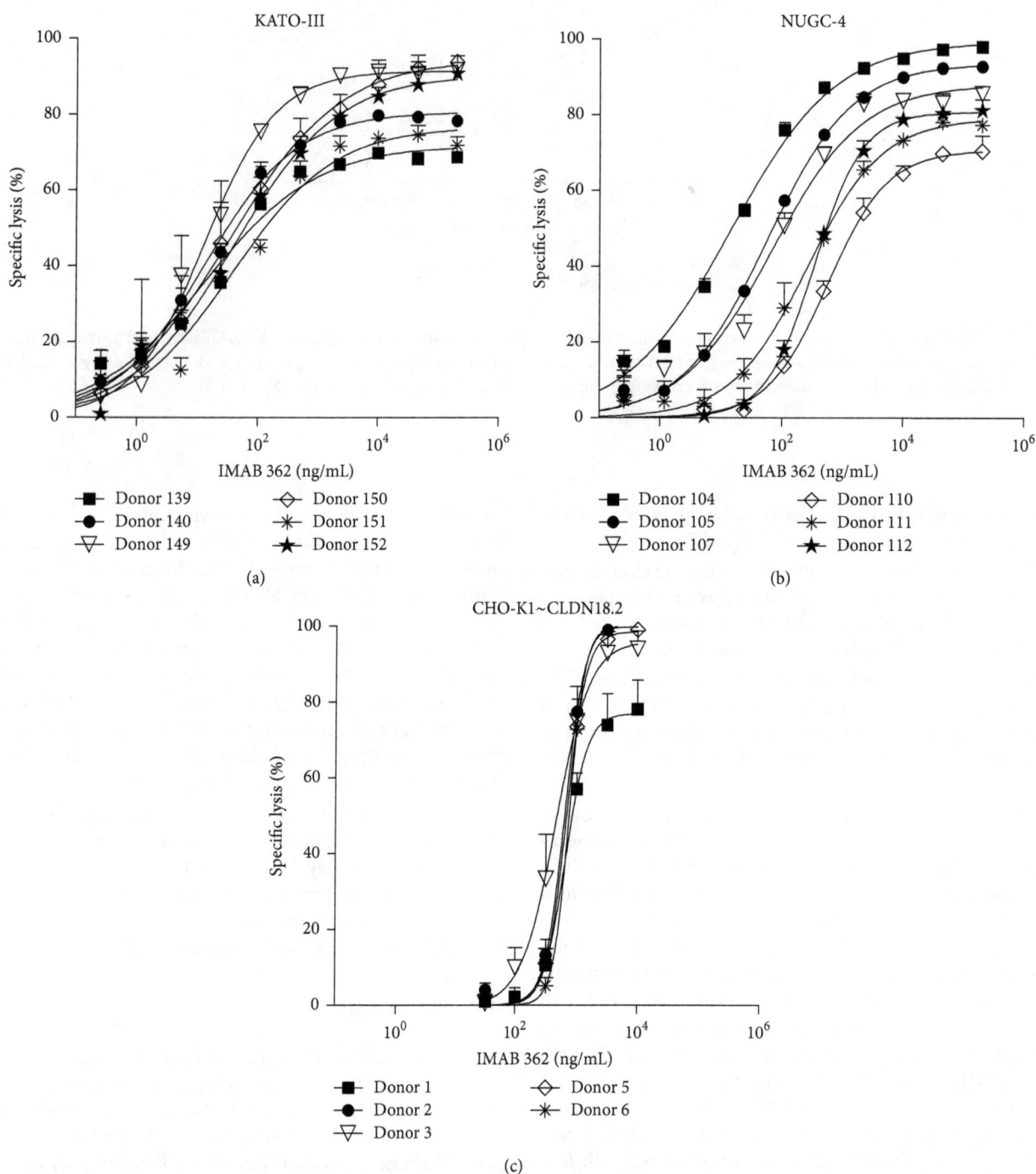

(a)

(b)

(c)

FIGURE 5: The luciferase IVT RNA-based assay efficiently assesses mAb-induced ADCC and CDC of tumour cell lines. ADCC assay using (a) KATO-III and (b) NUGC-4 cells. KATO-III and NUGC-4 cells endogenously expressing hCLDN18.2 were transfected with 7 μg *luc2* IVT RNA and seeded into 96-well plates independently. 4 h later, IMAB 362 at different concentrations and human PBMCs (E : T ratio = 40 : 1) from 6 different donors were added to the target cells and incubated for 24 h. ADCC was determined 40 and 45 min after addition of D-luciferin substrate to the KATO-III and NUGC-4 cells, respectively. (c) CDC assay. CHO-K1 cells stably expressing hCLDN18.2 were transfected with 7 μg *luc2* IVT RNA and seeded into 96-well plates. 24 h later, cells were incubated for 80 min with IMAB 362 diluted in human serum (final concentration of 20%) from 6 different healthy donors. CDC was determined 45 min after addition of D-luciferin substrate. Results are the mean ± SD ($n = 3$).

tailored for the use in the rapidly advancing tumor vaccine development, tumor-specific TCR, and mAb discovery fields.

Conflict of Interests

Ugur Sahin is associated with BioNTech RNA Pharmaceuticals GmbH (Mainz, Germany), a company that develops RNA-based cancer vaccines. Özlem Türeci and Ugur Sahin are inventors on patent applications featuring proprietary IVT RNA templates used in the process.

Authors' Contribution

Tana A. Omokoko and Uli Luxemburger contributed equally to the first authorship. Özlem Türeci and Ugur Sahin contributed equally to the last authorship.

Acknowledgments

The authors thank Dr. Mustafa Diken for technical assistance and Dr. Tim Beissert for critical reading of the paper.

References

[1] J. D. Wolchok and T. A. Chan, "Cancer: antitumour immunity gets a boost," *Nature*, vol. 515, no. 7528, pp. 496–498, 2014.

[2] E. G. Phimister and C. J. Melief, "Mutation-specific T cells for immunotherapy of gliomas," *The New England Journal of Medicine*, vol. 372, no. 20, pp. 1956–1958, 2015.

[3] M. Sznol and D. L. Longo, "Release the hounds! Activating the T-cell response to cancer," *The New England Journal of Medicine*, vol. 372, no. 4, pp. 374–375, 2015.

[4] S. Kreiter, M. Vormehr, N. van de Roemer et al., "Mutant MHC class II epitopes drive therapeutic immune responses to cancer," *Nature*, vol. 520, no. 7549, pp. 692–696, 2015.

[5] A. M. Eggermont, M. Maio, and C. Robert, "Immune checkpoint inhibitors in melanoma provide the cornerstones for curative therapies," *Seminars in Oncology*, vol. 42, no. 3, pp. 429–435, 2015.

[6] P. Sharma and J. P. Allison, "The future of immune checkpoint therapy," *Science*, vol. 348, no. 6230, pp. 56–61, 2015.

[7] D. T. Le, E. Lutz, J. N. Uram et al., "Evaluation of ipilimumab in combination with allogeneic pancreatic tumor cells transfected with a GM-CSF gene in previously treated pancreatic cancer," *Journal of Immunotherapy*, vol. 36, no. 7, pp. 382–389, 2013.

[8] S. A. Rosenberg and N. P. Restifo, "Adoptive cell transfer as personalized immunotherapy for human cancer," *Science*, vol. 348, no. 6230, pp. 62–68, 2015.

[9] T. Omokoko, P. Simon, Ö. Türeci, and U. Sahin, "Retrieval of functional TCRs from single antigen-specific T cells: toward individualized TCR-engineered therapies," *OncoImmunology*, vol. 4, no. 7, Article ID e1005523, 2015.

[10] K. T. Brunner, J. Mauel, J. C. Cerottini, and B. Chapuis, "Quantitative assay of the lytic action of immune lymphoid cells on 51-Cr-labelled allogeneic target cells in vitro; inhibition by isoantibody and by drugs," *Immunology*, vol. 14, no. 2, pp. 181–196, 1968.

[11] D. S. Heo, J.-G. Park, K. Hata, R. Day, R. B. Herberman, and T. L. Whiteside, "Evaluation of tetrazolium-based semiautomatic colorimetric assay for measurement of human antitumor cytotoxicity," *Cancer Research*, vol. 50, no. 12, pp. 3681–3690, 1990.

[12] C. Korzeniewski and D. M. Callewaert, "An enzyme-release assay for natural cytotoxicity," *Journal of Immunological Methods*, vol. 64, no. 3, pp. 313–320, 1983.

[13] K. Blomberg, C. Granberg, I. Hemmilä, and T. Lövgren, "Europium-labelled target cells in an assay of natural killer cell activity. I. A novel non-radioactive method based on time-resolved fluorescence," *Journal of Immunological Methods*, vol. 86, no. 2, pp. 225–229, 1986.

[14] R. Lichtenfels, W. E. Biddison, H. Schulz, A. B. Vogt, and R. Martin, "CARE-LASS (calcein-release-assay), an improved fluorescence-based test system to measure cytotoxic T lymphocyte activity," *Journal of Immunological Methods*, vol. 172, no. 2, pp. 227–239, 1994.

[15] S. P. M. Crouch, R. Kozlowski, K. J. Slater, and J. Fletcher, "The use of ATP bioluminescence as a measure of cell proliferation and cytotoxicity," *Journal of Immunological Methods*, vol. 160, no. 1, pp. 81–88, 1993.

[16] M. A. Karimi, E. Lee, M. H. Bachmann et al., "Measuring cytotoxicity by bioluminescence imaging outperforms the standard chromium-51 release assay," *PLoS ONE*, vol. 9, no. 2, Article ID e89357, 2014.

[17] H. Schäfer, A. Schäfer, A. F. Kiderlen, K. N. Masihi, and R. Burger, "A highly sensitive cytotoxicity assay based on the release of reporter enzymes, from stably transfected cell lines," *Journal of Immunological Methods*, vol. 204, no. 1, pp. 89–98, 1997.

[18] P. Von Zons, P. Crowley-Nowick, D. Friberg, M. Bell, U. Koldovsky, and T. L. Whiteside, "Comparison of europium and chromium release assays: cytotoxicity in healthy individuals and patients with cervical carcinoma," *Clinical and Diagnostic Laboratory Immunology*, vol. 4, no. 2, pp. 202–207, 1997.

[19] A. R. Brasier, J. E. Tate, and J. F. Habener, "Optimized use of the firefly luciferase assay as a reporter gene in mammalian cell lines," *BioTechniques*, vol. 7, no. 10, pp. 1116–1122, 1989.

[20] W. R. Jacobs Jr., R. G. Barletta, R. Udani et al., "Rapid assessment of drug susceptibilities of *Mycobacterium tuberculosis* by means of luciferase reporter phages," *Science*, vol. 260, no. 5109, pp. 819–822, 1993.

[21] C. H. Contag and M. H. Bachmann, "Advances in in vivo bioluminescence imaging of gene expression," *Annual Review of Biomedical Engineering*, vol. 4, pp. 235–260, 2002.

[22] C. E. Brown, C. L. Wright, A. Naranjo et al., "Biophotonic cytotoxicity assay for high-throughput screening of cytolytic killing," *Journal of Immunological Methods*, vol. 297, no. 1-2, pp. 39–52, 2005.

[23] V. F. I. van Tendeloo, P. Ponsaerts, F. Lardon et al., "Highly efficient gene delivery by mRNA electroporation in human hematopoietic cells: superiority to lipofection and passive pulsing of mRNA and to electroporation of plasmid cDNA for tumor antigen loading of dendritic cells," *Blood*, vol. 98, no. 1, pp. 49–56, 2001.

[24] S. Van Meirvenne, L. Straetman, C. Heirman et al., "Efficient genetic modification of murine dendritic cells by electroporation with mRNA," *Cancer Gene Therapy*, vol. 9, no. 9, pp. 787–797, 2002.

[25] D. A. Mitchell and S. K. Nair, "RNA-transfected dendritic cells in cancer immunotherapy," *The Journal of Clinical Investigation*, vol. 106, no. 9, pp. 1065–1069, 2000.

[26] S. Kreiter, M. Diken, A. Selmi, Ö. Türeci, and U. Sahin, "Tumor vaccination using messenger RNA: prospects of a

future therapy," *Current Opinion in Immunology*, vol. 23, no. 3, pp. 399–406, 2011.

[27] S. Holtkamp, S. Kreiter, A. Selmi et al., "Modification of antigen-encoding RNA increases stability, translational efficacy, and T-cell stimulatory capacity of dendritic cells," *Blood*, vol. 108, no. 13, pp. 4009–4017, 2006.

[28] C. M. Britten, R. G. Meyer, T. Kreer, I. Drexler, T. Wölfel, and W. Herr, "The use of HLA-A*0201-transfected K562 as standard antigen-presenting cells for CD8+ T lymphocytes in IFN-γ ELISPOT assays," *Journal of Immunological Methods*, vol. 259, no. 1-2, pp. 95–110, 2002.

[29] T. Wölfel, A. van Pel, V. Brichard et al., "Two tyrosinase non-apeptides recognized on HLA-A2 melanomas by autologous cytolytic T lymphocytes," *European Journal of Immunology*, vol. 24, no. 3, pp. 759–764, 1994.

[30] J. C. A. Skipper, R. C. Hendrickson, P. H. Gulden et al., "An HLA-A2-restricted tyrosinase antigen on melanoma cells results from posttranslational modification and suggests a novel pathway for processing of membrane proteins," *The Journal of Experimental Medicine*, vol. 183, no. 2, pp. 527–534, 1996.

[31] P. Simon, T. A. Omokoko, A. Breitkreuz et al., "Functional TCR retrieval from single antigen-specific human T cells reveals multiple novel epitopes," *Cancer Immunology Research*, vol. 2, no. 12, pp. 1230–1244, 2014.

[32] S. Kreiter, A. Selmi, M. Diken et al., "Increased antigen presentation efficiency by coupling antigens to MHC class I trafficking signals," *Journal of Immunology*, vol. 180, no. 1, pp. 309–318, 2008.

[33] E. Jäger, Y. Nagata, S. Gnjatic et al., "Monitoring CD8 T cell responses to NY-ESO-1: correlation of humoral and cellular immune responses," *Proceedings of the National Academy of Sciences of the United States of America*, vol. 97, no. 9, pp. 4760–4765, 2000.

[34] L. Zaritskaya, M. R. Shurin, T. J. Sayers, and A. M. Malyguine, "New flow cytometric assays for monitoring cell-mediated cytotoxicity," *Expert Review of Vaccines*, vol. 9, no. 6, pp. 601–616, 2010.

[35] B. M. Carreno, V. Magrini, M. Becker-Hapak et al., "A dendritic cell vaccine increases the breadth and diversity of melanoma neoantigen-specific T cells," *Science*, vol. 348, no. 6236, pp. 803–808, 2015.

[36] A. Gros, P. F. Robbins, X. Yao et al., "PD-1 identifies the patient-specific CD8+ tumor-reactive repertoire infiltrating human tumors," *The Journal of Clinical Investigation*, vol. 124, no. 5, pp. 2246–2259, 2014.

[37] A. H. Long, W. M. Haso, J. F. Shern et al., "4-1BB costimulation ameliorates T cell exhaustion induced by tonic signaling of chimeric antigen receptors," *Nature Medicine*, vol. 21, no. 6, pp. 581–590, 2015.

[38] R. Clynes, Y. Takechi, Y. Moroi, A. Houghton, and J. V. Ravetch, "Fc receptors are required in passive and active immunity to melanoma," *Proceedings of the National Academy of Sciences of the United States of America*, vol. 95, no. 2, pp. 652–656, 1998.

[39] J. G. van de Winkel and C. L. Anderson, "Biology of human immunoglobulin G Fc receptors," *Journal of leukocyte biology*, vol. 49, no. 5, pp. 511–524, 1991.

[40] O. Tuereci, S. Woell, S. Jacobs, R. Mitnacht-Kraus, and U. Sahin, "Abstract 2903. IMAB362, a novel first-in-class monoclonal antibody for treatment of pancreatic cancer," *Cancer Research*, vol. 74, no. 19, supplement, p. 2903, 2014.

[41] U. Sahin, S. Al-Batran, W. Hozaeel et al., "IMAB362 plus zoledronic acid (ZA) and interleukin-2 (IL-2) in patients (pts) with advanced gastroesophageal cancer (GEC): clinical activity and safety data from the PILOT phase I trial," *Journal of Clinical Oncology*, vol. 33, supplement, abstract e15079, 2015.

[42] T. Trarbach, M. Schuler, Z. Zvirbule et al., "Efficacy and safety of multiple doses of IMAB362 in patients with advanced gastroesophageal cancer: results of a phase II study," *Annals of Oncology*, vol. 25, supplement 4, p. 218, 2014.

[43] M. Schuler, Z. Zvirbule, F. Lordick et al., "Safety, tolerability, and efficacy of the first-in-class antibody IMAB362 targeting claudin 18.2 in patients with metastatic gastroesophageal adenocarcinomas," *Journal of Clinical Oncology*, vol. 31, p. 4080, 2013.

[44] I. Hoerr, R. Obst, H.-G. Rammensee, and G. Jung, "In vivo application of RNA leads to induction of specific cytotoxic T lymphocytes and antibodies," *European Journal of Immunology*, vol. 30, no. 1, pp. 1–7, 2000.

[45] B. Weide, J.-P. Carralot, A. Reese et al., "Results of the first phase I/II clinical vaccination trial with direct injection of mRNA," *Journal of Immunotherapy*, vol. 31, no. 2, pp. 180–188, 2008.

13

Association of Sicca Syndrome with Proviral Load and Proinflammatory Cytokines in HTLV-1 Infection

Clara Mônica Lima,[1,2,3] **Silvane Santos,**[2,4,5] **Adriana Dourado,**[2]
Natália B. Carvalho,[2] **Valéria Bittencourt,**[2] **Marcus Miranda Lessa,**[1,3]
Isadora Siqueira,[2,6] **and Edgar M. Carvalho**[1,2,4,6]

[1]*Postgraduate Program in Health Sciences, Federal University of Bahia School of Medicine, 40025-010 Salvador, BA, Brazil*
[2]*Immunology Service, Professor Edgard Santos University Hospital, Federal University of Bahia, 40110-060 Salvador, BA, Brazil*
[3]*Department of Otolaryngology, Federal University of Bahia, 40110-060 Salvador, BA, Brazil*
[4]*National Institute of Science and Technology of Tropical Diseases (CNPq/MCT), 40110-060 Salvador, BA, Brazil*
[5]*Department of Biological Sciences, State University of Feira de Santana (UEFS), 44036-900 Feira de Santana, BA, Brazil*
[6]*Gonçalo Moniz Research Center, Oswaldo Cruz Foundation (FIOCRUZ), 40296-710 Salvador, BA, Brazil*

Correspondence should be addressed to Edgar M. Carvalho; imuno@ufba.br

Academic Editor: Enrico Maggi

The *Sjögren* syndrome has been diagnosed in patients with HTLV-1 associated myelopathy and dry mouth and dry eyes are documented in HTLV-1 carriers. However the diagnosis of *Sjögren* syndrome in these subjects has been contested. In this cross-sectional study, we evaluated the role of immunological factors and proviral load, in sicca syndrome associated with HTLV-1 in patients without myelopathy. Subjects were recruited in the HTLV-1 Clinic, from 2009 to 2011. The proviral load and cytokine levels (IFN-γ, TNF-α, IL-5, and IL-10) were obtained from a database containing the values presented by the subjects at admission in the clinic. Of the 272 participants, 59 (21.7%) had sicca syndrome and in all of them anti-*Sjögren* syndrome related antigen A (SSA) and antigen B (SSB) were negatives. The production of TNF-α and IFN-γ was higher in the group with sicca syndrome ($P < 0.05$) than in HTLV-1 infected subjects without sicca syndrome. Our data indicates that patients with sicca syndrome associated with HTLV-1 do not have *Sjögren* syndrome. However the increased production of TNF-α and IFN-γ in this group of patients may contribute to the pathogenesis of sicca syndrome associated with HTLV-1.

1. Introduction

The human T lymphotropic virus type 1 (HTLV-1) infection is distributed worldwide with high prevalence in Central Africa, Central and South America, and South west of Japan [1]. Adult T cell leukemia/lymphoma (ATL), HTLV-1 associated myelopathy or tropical spastic paraparesis (HAM/TSP), and infective dermatitis are etiologically associated with HTLV-1 [2]. The HTLV-1 infects predominantly not only T cells but also B cells and myeloid cell lineage inducing cell activation and proliferation [3]. In such case it is possible that HTLV-1 infecting or activating autoreactive cells might induce the appearance of autoimmune diseases. Actually many reports in the last 20 years showed an association

between rheumatoid arthritis, polymyositis, *Sjögren* syndrome, and systemic lupus erythematosus with HTLV-1 [4–6]. HTLV-1 infection was documented in up to 30% of patients with rheumatoid arthritis in endemic areas for this virus, and *Sjögren* syndrome was reported between 30 and 60% in patients who had HAM/TSP [7–9]. *Sjögren* syndrome is a chronic autoimmune disease of the exocrine glands that affects the salivary and lacrimal glands through a lymphocytic infiltrate, leading to xerostomia (dry mouth) and xeroftalmia (dry eye). However, more recently the association between autoimmune diseases and HTLV-1 has been contested [10, 11]. There is no doubt that a large number of HTLV-1 infected individuals have dry mouth, dry eyes, and arthropathy, but synovitis and polyarthritis are rare

[12, 13]. Lymphocyte infiltration has been documented in salivary glands of HTLV-1 infected subjects indicating its participation in the pathogenesis of salivary glands destruction [14]. But occurrence of autoantibodies characteristic of *Sjögren* syndrome was not observed in patients with the sicca syndrome associated with HTLV-1 infection [10]. Moreover arthritis is not a common finding in patients with sicca syndrome associated with HTLV-1 [15]. Therefore the pathogenesis of sicca syndrome related to HTLV-1 is not clear and the possibility that an autoimmune disease may account for the occurrence of it has been argued.

The role of the inflammatory response and proviral load in the pathogenesis of clinical manifestations related to HTLV-1 has been well documented. Proinflammatory cytokines and chemokines are higher in supernatants of peripheral blood mononuclear cells (PBMCs) culture and in serum of HAM/TSP than HTLV-1 carriers [16, 17] and there is an association of high proviral load with HAM/TSP [18–20]. In patients with HTLV-1 associated periodontal disease, mRNA for tax was present in the periodontal tissue and there was an increased expression of IL-1β and IFN-γ and a decrease in the expression of IL-10 and regulatory T cells in this tissue [21, 22]. Furthermore, both proviral load and production of proinflammatory cytokines are higher in patients with neurogenic bladder associated with HTLV-1 but who do not fulfill the criteria for HAM/TSP, as well as in children with infective dermatitis, than in HTLV-1 carriers, which indicates that these variables are associated with diseases related to HTLV-1 [23, 24]. The aim of this study was to evaluate if there was an association between the levels of cytokines, proviral load, and anti-*Sjögren* syndrome related antigen A (SSA) and anti-*Sjögren* syndrome related antigen B (SSB) antibodies with sicca syndrome associated with HTLV-1.

2. Material and Methods

2.1. Subjects and Diagnosis Criteria. This is a cross-sectional study comparing proviral load and cytokine levels among HTLV-1 infected subjects with or without sicca syndrome. Participants of this study include 272 HTLV-1 infected subjects with age range from 18 to 60 years, of both genders, followed at the HTLV-1 Multidisciplinary Clinic of the Hospital Universitário Professor Edgard Santos in Salvador, Bahia, Brazil. Subjects admitted to the clinic are referred from blood banks or from other clinics due to a positive serology for HTLV-1 and HTLV-2, by enzyme-limited immunosorbent assay (Murex HTLV-I + II Abbot, Dartford, UK). The diagnosis of HTLV-1 is confirmed by Western blot (HTLV Blot 2.4, Genelab, Singapore). The inclusion criteria for participation in the study were the presence of a positive serology for HTLV-1 confirmed by Western blot. Exclusion criteria were presence of human immune deficiency virus (HIV) and diagnosis of HAM/TSP based on the Osame motor disability score (OMDS) ≥ 1. Moreover 27 patients were excluded due to coinfection with hepatitis B or hepatitis C virus. All subjects answered a questionnaire regarding dry mouth and dry eyes and had clinical examination. Dry mouth was determined by oral examination and the salivary flux by the Saxon test [25]. Sicca syndrome was defined by the documentation of dry

mouth and abnormal Saxon test. The majority of the patients also complained of dry eyes.

2.2. Evaluation of Autoantibodies. Serum samples were screened for antinuclear antibodies by immunofluorescence and anti-SSA and anti-SSB by ELISA as previously described [26, 27].

2.3. Immunologic Studies. Cytokines were determined in supernatants of unstimulated PBMCs cultures as previously described [23]. Briefly, PBMCs were obtained from heparinized venous blood by density gradient centrifugation with Ficoll-hypaque (GE Healthcare Bio-Sciences Uppsala Sweden). The mononuclear cells were then washed in saline and after being adjusted to the concentration of 3×10^6 cells/mL were resuspended in RPMI 1640 (Life Technologies Gibco BRL, Gran Island, New York) supplemented with 10% of fetal bovine serum and antibiotics. Unstimulated cells were incubated for 72 hours at 37°C 5% CO_2 and the supernatants were harvested. Determination of IFN-γ, TNF-α, IL-5, and IL-10 was performed by ELISA using reagents from BD Biosciences Pharmingen, San Jose, CA.

2.4. HTLV-1 Proviral Load. DNA was extracted from 10^6 PBMCs using proteinase K and salting-out method. The HTLV-1 proviral load was quantified using a real-time Taq-Man PCR method as previously described using the ABI Prism 7700 Sequence detector system (Applied Biosystems) [28]. Albumin DNA was used as an endogenous reference. The normalized value of the HTLV-1 proviral load was calculated as the ratio of (HTLV-1 DNA average copy number/albumin DNA average copy number) $\times 2 \times 10^6$ and expressed as the number of HTLV-1 copies per 10^6 PBMCs.

2.5. Statistical Analysis. The comparison between the ages in the 2 groups was performed by Student's t-test. The comparison between proportions was performed by Fisher exact test. The data on cytokine levels and proviral load were expressed as median and interquartile (IQ) range and were analyzed by the Kruskal-Wallis test. The correlation between proviral load and cytokine levels was performed by the correlation of Spearmen. The GraphPad Prism 5 (San Diego, CA) was used to perform the statistical evaluation and P values < 0.05 were considered statistically significant.

3. Results

Of the 272 participants of the study, 59 (21.7%) had sicca syndrome. The age, gender, and ethnic group of HTLV-1 infected subjects with sicca syndrome and without sicca syndrome are shown in Table 1. There was no difference regarding age in the two groups ($P = 0.847$) and the female gender predominates in both groups without statistical significance. There were more blacks in the group with sicca syndrome ($P = 0.03$).

The diagnosis of sicca syndrome was based on oral examination and a reduction in the salivary fluid by Saxon test [25]. Regarding other diseases related to HTLV-1, overactive bladder a manifestation considered as an oligosymptomatic

TABLE 1: Demographic characteristics of patients with and without sicca syndrome associated with HTLV-1 infection.

	Without sicca syndrome (n = 213; 88.3%)		With sicca syndrome (n = 59; 21.7%)		P value
Gender					0.100
Male, n (%)	94	44.1%	19	32.2%	
Female, n (%)	119	55.9%	40	67.8%	
Age	Mean	SD	Mean	SD	0.847
	46.90	12.13	46.54	14.22	
Race					0.03
White, n (%)	48	23.2%	13	23.6%	
Mulate, n (%)	94	45.4%	15	27.3%	
Black, n (%)	62	30.0%	27	49.1%	
Other, n (%)	3	1.4%	0	0.0%	

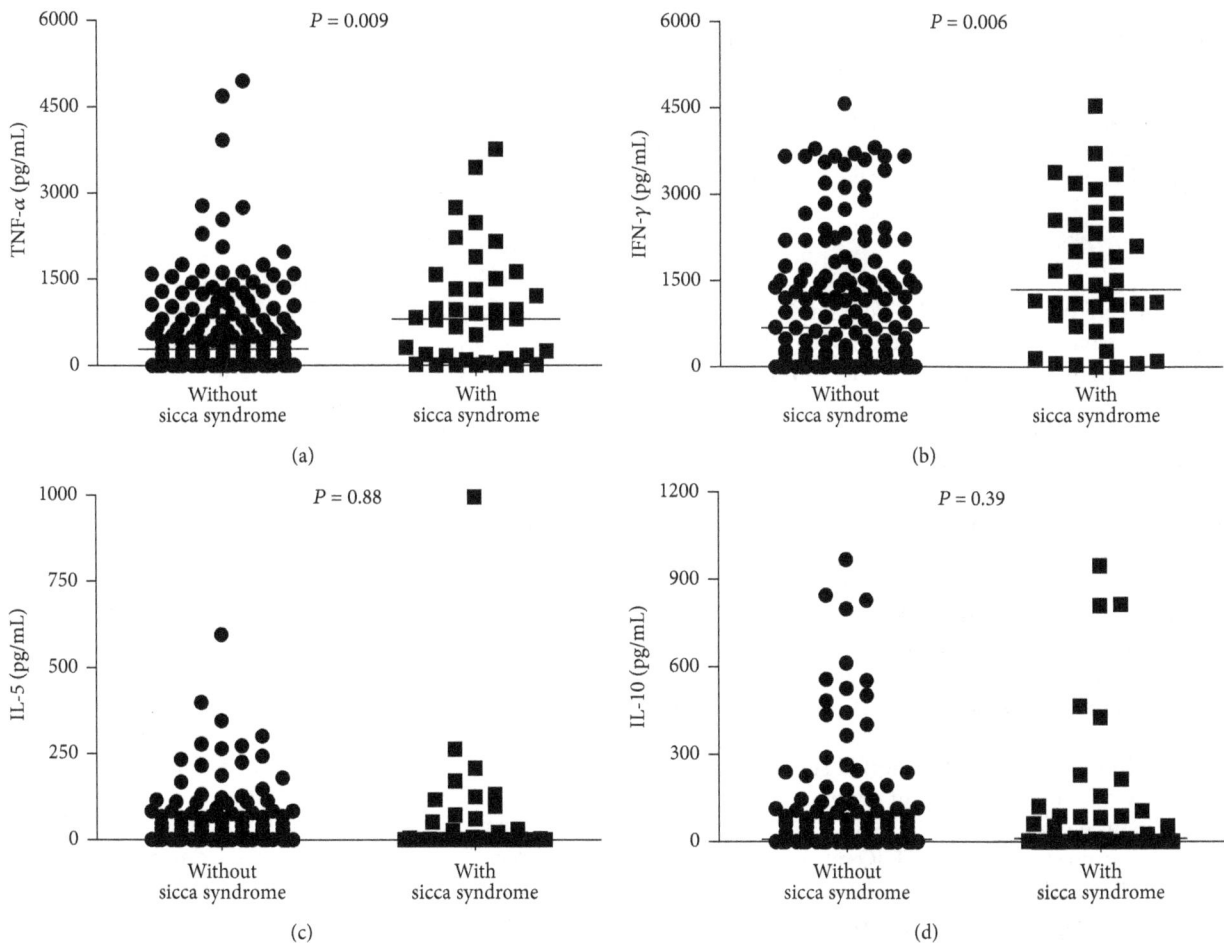

FIGURE 1: Levels of TNF-α (a), IFN-γ (b), IL-5 (c), and IL-10 (d) produced by PBMC from HTLV-1 infected individuals with and without sicca syndrome. Cytokines data represent the values in unstimulated cultures. The levels of cytokines were measured by ELISA.

form of HAM/TSP was documented in 11 (18.6%) of the patients with sicca syndrome and in 26 (12.2%) in the patients without sicca syndrome ($P > 0.5$). There was also no difference regarding polyarthralgia in the 2 groups and synovitis was detected in only 2 patients. One patient had mixed connective tissue disease and sicca syndrome and the other had a seronegative rheumatic arthritis and did not have sicca syndrome.

The spontaneous cytokines (TNF-α, IFN-γ, IL-5, and IL-10) levels in supernatants of PBMCs are shown in Figure 1.

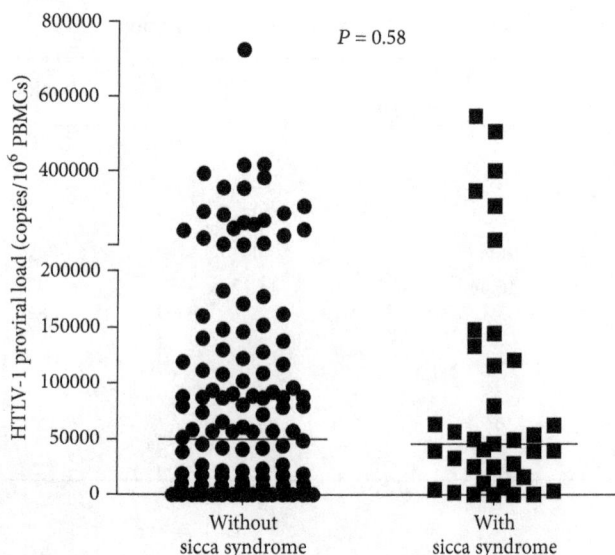

FIGURE 2: HTLV-1 proviral load of HTLV-1 infected individuals with and without sicca syndrome. Proviral load was quantified by real-time TaqMan PCR method and the normalized value of the proviral load was calculated as the ratio of (HTLV-1 DNA average copy number/albumin DNA average copy number) $\times$ 2×10^6 and expressed as the number of HTLV-1 copies per 10^6 PBMCs.

The levels of TNF-α in patients with sicca syndrome (median 803 pg/mL, IQ range 116–1,498) were higher ($P < 0.009$, Figure 1(a)) than that observed in patients without sicca syndrome (median 281 pg/mL, IQ range 0–946). The production of IFN-γ in patients with sicca syndrome (median 1,352 pg/mL, IQ range 717–2,477) was higher ($P = 0.006$, Figure 1(b)) than in the group without sicca syndrome (median 682 pg/mL, IQ range 42–1,604). No difference was observed in the median of the IL-5 levels ($P = 0.88$, Figure 1(c)) in the group with sicca syndrome (1 pg/mL, IQ range 0–61) and that without sicca syndrome (median 0 pg/mL, IQ range 0–62). The production of IL-10 (Figure 1(d)) did not differ between groups ($P = 0.39$). Cytokine levels were undetectable or were very low in supernatants of PBMCs of patients with sicca syndrome.

The proviral load in HTLV-1 infected subjects with and without sicca syndrome is shown in Figure 2. There was no difference between proviral load ($P = 0.58$) in patients with sicca syndrome (median 45,554, IQ range 13,171–126,803 copies/10^6 cells) and in patients without sicca syndrome (median 49,861 copies/10^6 cells, IQ range 2,184–128,187). There was a direct correlation between proviral load and IFN-γ and proviral load and TNF-α when values obtained in the whole sample were analyzed (Figure 3). However no correlation was observed when data from patients with sicca syndrome or without sicca syndrome were analyzed isolately.

Antinuclear antibodies and anti-SSA and anti-SSB antibodies were determined in the two groups. Anti-SSA and anti-SSB antibodies were absent in all subjects. Antinuclear antibodies were detected in 2 subjects, one in the group with and another in the group without sicca syndrome.

4. Discussion

In the present study we show that the proinflammatory cytokines IFN-γ and TNF-α were higher in HTLV-1 infected patients with sicca syndrome than in HTLV-1 infected subjects without sicca syndrome, indicating that the exacerbated proinflammatory response observed in HTLV-1 infection may play a role in the destruction of the salivary and lacrimal glands observed during this viral infection. Moreover our data indicate that autoimmune rheumatic diseases are rarely associated with HTLV-1 and that there is no evidence of Sjögren syndrome in HTLV-1 infected subjects without HAM/TSP.

The prevalence of Sjögren-like syndrome in HTLV-1 infected subjects ranges in accordance with the population studied. Initial studies showed that this association was mainly found in patients with HAM/TSP [7, 8]. However in a cross-sectional study evaluating the frequency of clinical manifestations in HTLV-1 carriers and in seronegative controls, the prevalence of dry mouth was 20.8% in carriers, while it was 11.3% in non-HTLV-1-infected subjects [13]. Poetker et al. also showed a prevalence of 22.5% of dry mouth in HTLV-1 carriers referred from blood banks recently diagnosed with HTLV-1 [12]. Herein, based on the complaint and documentation of dry mouth in the oral examination and a decrease in salivary output determined by Saxon test, the frequency of sicca syndrome in HTLV-1 infected subjects without HAM/TSP was similar to that previously found in a study performed in a HTLV-1 Clinic with small number of participants [29]. HAM/TSP and ATL are the more severe diseases related to HTLV-1, but other recognized manifestations associated with this viral infection include uveitis, chronic periodontitis, urinary manifestations of overactive bladder, sicca syndrome, and HTLV-1 associated arthropathy [2, 13, 30, 31]. It is worthwhile to emphasize that for many years HTLV-1 infection was considered a low morbidity infection as less than 5% of the infected subjects develop HAM/TSP or ATL. In this study we showed that sicca syndrome is frequent even in patients without HAM/TSP.

The documentation of a lymphocytic infiltration and the tax gene expression in the salivary gland of patients with dry mouth infected by the virus are the main evidences that salivary gland destruction in HTLV-1 infection is mediated by T cells [21, 32, 33]. Additionally HTLV-1 was expressed in salivary gland of transgenic mice that express the tax gene and presents a picture similar to Sjögren syndrome [34]. However more recently as autoantibodies related to Sjögren syndrome have not been documented in such patients, the occurrence of Sjögren syndrome associated with HTLV-1 has been argued [10, 35]. Herein patients with dry mouth and dry eyes did not present either anti-SSA or anti-SSB antibodies. This gives support to the concept that, rather than Sjögren syndrome, HTLV-1 infected subjects have a sicca syndrome due to destruction of the salivary glands.

The pathogenesis of the clinical manifestations related to HTLV-1 has been mainly studied in patients with HAM/TSP and is likely multifactorial. The neurologic disease has been associated with high proviral load [18–20] and increased levels of proinflammatory cytokines including IL-1, IL-6,

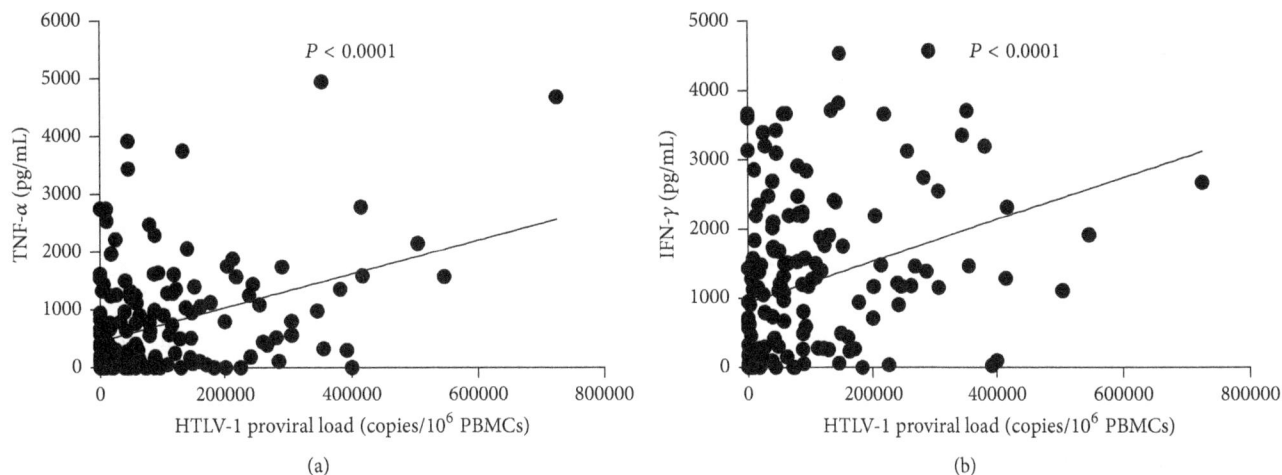

FIGURE 3: Correlation between proviral load and cytokine levels in HTLV-1 infected subjects. There was a direct correlation between proviral load and TNF-α levels (a) and between proviral load and IFN-γ levels (b) when data from all participants of the study were analyzed.

TNF-α, and IFN-γ [36, 37]. In such case there is a passage of T cells from blood to the central nervous system and the tissue damage is mediated by an exaggerated and nonmodulated immunologic response [38, 39]. Giving support to the role of an exaggerated inflammatory response in the pathogenesis of manifestations due to HTLV-1, high levels of proinflammatory cytokines have been documented in other diseases associated with HTLV-1, as in patients with neurogenic bladder who do not fulfill the criteria for HAM/TSP [23], in patients with chronic periodontal disease associated with HTLV-1 [22], and in children with infective dermatitis, a disease associated with development of HAM/TSP [24].

The previous documentation that salivary glands in HTLV-1 infected subjects are infiltrated by lymphocytes and the present study showing an increased production of TNF-α and IFN-γ in patients with HTLV-1 associated with sicca syndrome indicate that viral factors and an increased inflammatory response participate in the pathogenesis of sicca syndrome associated with HTLV-1.

Conflict of Interests

The authors declare that they have no conflict of interests.

Acknowledgments

The authors are grateful to the staff and patients of HTLV-1 Clinic of the Professor Edgard Santos University Hospital. They also thank Cristiano Franco for secretarial assistance.

References

[1] A. Gessain and O. Cassar, "Epidemiological aspects and world distribution of HTLV-1 infection," *Frontiers in Microbiology*, vol. 3, article 388, 2012.

[2] F. A. Proietti, A. B. F. Carneiro-Proietti, B. C. Catalan-Soares, and E. L. Murphy, "Global epidemiology of HTLV-I infection and associated diseases," *Oncogene*, vol. 24, no. 39, pp. 6058–6068, 2005.

[3] M. Yoshida, "Multiple viral strategies of HTLV-1 for dysregulation of cell growth control," *Annual Review of Immunology*, vol. 19, pp. 475–496, 2001.

[4] S. Ijichi, T. Matsuda, I. Maruyama et al., "Arthritis in a human T lymphotropic virus type I (HTLV-I) carrier," *Annals of the Rheumatic Diseases*, vol. 49, no. 9, pp. 718–721, 1990.

[5] O. S. Morgan, C. Mora, P. Rodgers-Johnson, and G. Char, "HTLV-1 and polymyositis in Jamaica," *The Lancet*, vol. 334, no. 8673, pp. 1184–1187, 1989.

[6] S. R. Pinheiro, M. A. Lana-Peixoto, A. B. Proietti, F. Oréfice, M. V. Lima-Martins, and F. A. Proietti, "HTLV-I associated uveitis, myelopathy, rheumatoid arthritis and Sjögren's syndrome," *Arquivos de Neuro-Psiquiatria*, vol. 53, no. 4, pp. 777–781, 1995.

[7] H. Nakamura, K. Eguchi, T. Nakamura et al., "High prevalence of Sjögren's syndrome in patients with HTLV-I associated myelopathy," *Annals of the Rheumatic Diseases*, vol. 56, no. 3, pp. 167–172, 1997.

[8] L. Cartier, J. L. Castilio, J. G. Cea, and R. Villagra, "Chronic dacryosialadenitis in HTLV I associated myelopathy," *Journal of Neurology Neurosurgery and Psychiatry*, vol. 58, no. 2, pp. 244–246, 1995.

[9] S. Motokawa, T. Hasunuma, K. Tajima et al., "High prevalence of arthropathy in HTLV-I carriers on a Japanese island," *Annals of the Rheumatic Diseases*, vol. 55, no. 3, pp. 193–195, 1996.

[10] A. K. Ferraz-Chaoui, A. M. Atta, M. L. S. Atta, B. Galvão-Castro, and M. B. Santiago, "Study of autoantibodies in patients with keratoconjunctivitis sicca infected by the human T cell lymphotropic virus type 1," *Rheumatology International*, vol. 30, no. 6, pp. 775–778, 2010.

[11] R. T. Bailer, A. Lazo, V. Harisdangkul et al., "Lack of evidence for human T cell lymphotrophic virus type I or II infection in patients with systemic lupus erythematosus or rheumatoid arthritis," *The Journal of Rheumatology*, vol. 21, no. 12, pp. 2217–2224, 1994.

[12] S. K. W. Poetker, A. F. Porto, S. P. Giozza et al., "Clinical manifestations in individuals with recent diagnosis of HTLV type I infection," *Journal of Clinical Virology*, vol. 51, no. 1, pp. 54–58, 2011.

[13] M. F. Caskey, D. J. Morgan, A. F. Porto et al., "Clinical manifestations associated with HTLV type I infection: a cross-sectional study," *AIDS Research and Human Retroviruses*, vol. 23, no. 3, pp. 365–371, 2007.

[14] L. Cartier, C. Vergara, and E. Ramírez, "Viral Tax protein expression in salivary glands of patients infected with human t-cell lymphotropic virus type I and Sicca Syndrome," *Revista Medica de Chile*, vol. 133, no. 10, pp. 1183–1190, 2005.

[15] M. M. N. de Carvalho, S. P. Giozza, A. L. M. A. dos Santos, E. M. de Carvalho, and M. I. Araújo, "Frequency of rheumatic diseases in individuals infected with HTLV-1," *Revista Brasileira de Reumatologia*, vol. 46, no. 5, pp. 315–322, 2006.

[16] E. M. Carvalho, O. Bacellar, A. F. Porto, S. Braga, B. Galvão-Castro, and F. Neva, "Cytokine profile and immunomodulation in asymptomatic human T-lymphotropic virus type 1-infected blood donors," *Journal of Acquired Immune Deficiency Syndromes*, vol. 27, no. 1, pp. 1–6, 2001.

[17] J. B. Guerreiro, S. B. Santos, D. J. Morgan et al., "Levels of serum chemokines discriminate clinical myelopathy associated with human T lymphotropic virus type 1 (HTLV-1)/tropical spastic paraparesis (HAM/TSP) disease from HTLV-1 carrier state," *Clinical and Experimental Immunology*, vol. 145, no. 2, pp. 296–301, 2006.

[18] M. Nagai, K. Usuku, W. Matsumoto et al., "Analysis of HTLV-I proviral load in 202 HAM/TSP patients and 243 asymptomatic HTLV-I carriers: high proviral load strongly predisposes to HAM/TSP," *Journal of NeuroVirology*, vol. 4, no. 6, pp. 586–593, 1998.

[19] M. F. R. Grassi, V. N. Olavarria, R. D. A. Kruschewsky et al., "Human T cell lymphotropic virus type 1 (HTLV-1) proviral load of HTLV-associated myelopathy/tropical spastic paraparesis (HAM/TSP) patients according to new diagnostic criteria of HAM/TSP," *Journal of Medical Virology*, vol. 83, no. 7, pp. 1269–1274, 2011.

[20] S. Olindo, A. Lézin, P. Cabre et al., "HTLV-1 proviral load in peripheral blood mononuclear cells quantified in 100 HAM/TSP patients: a marker of disease progression," *Journal of the Neurological Sciences*, vol. 237, no. 1-2, pp. 53–59, 2005.

[21] X. Mariette, F. Agbalika, D. Zucker-Franklin et al., "Detection of the tax gene of HTLV-I in labial salivary glands from patients with Sjögren's syndrome and other diseases of the oral cavity," *Clinical and Experimental Rheumatology*, vol. 18, no. 3, pp. 341–347, 2000.

[22] G. P. Garlet, S. P. Giozza, E. M. Silveira et al., "Association of human T lymphotropic virus 1 amplification of periodontitis severity with altered cytokine expression in response to a standard periodontopathogen infection," *Clinical Infectious Diseases*, vol. 50, no. 3, pp. e11–e18, 2010.

[23] S. B. Santos, P. Oliveira, T. Luna et al., "Immunological and viral features in patients with overactive bladder associated with human T-cell lymphotropic virus type 1 infection," *Journal of Medical Virology*, vol. 84, no. 11, pp. 1809–1817, 2012.

[24] M. C. F. Nascimento, J. Primo, A. Bittencourt et al., "Infective dermatitis has similar immunological features to human T lymphotropic virus-type 1-associated myelopathy/tropical spastic paraparesis," *Clinical and Experimental Immunology*, vol. 156, no. 3, pp. 455–462, 2009.

[25] P. F. Kohler and M. E. Winter, "A quantitative test for xerostomia. The Saxon test, an oral equivalent of the Schirmer test," *Arthritis and Rheumatism*, vol. 28, no. 10, pp. 1128–1132, 1985.

[26] P. J. Maddison, R. P. Skinner, P. Vlachoyiannopoulos, D. M. Brennand, and D. Hough, "Antibodies to nRNP, Sm, Ro(SSA) and La(SSB) detected by ELISA: their specificity and interrelations in connective tissue disease sera," *Clinical and Experimental Immunology*, vol. 62, no. 2, pp. 337–345, 1985.

[27] S. Blomberg, L. Ronnblom, A. C. Wallgren, B. Nilsson, and A. Karlsson-Parra, "Anti-SSA/Ro antibody determination by enzyme-linked immunosorbent assay as a supplement to standard immunofluorescence in antinuclear antibody screening," *Scandinavian Journal of Immunology*, vol. 51, no. 6, pp. 612–617, 2000.

[28] A. Dehée, R. Césaire, N. Désiré et al., "Quantitation of HTLV-I proviral load by a TaqMan real-time PCR assay," *Journal of Virological Methods*, vol. 102, no. 1-2, pp. 37–51, 2002.

[29] J.-C. Vernant, G. Buisson, J. Magdeleine et al., "T-lymphocyte alveolitis, tropical spastic paresis, and Sjögren syndrome," *The Lancet*, vol. 331, no. 8578, p. 177, 1988.

[30] S. P. Giozza, S. B. Santos, M. Martinelli, M. A. Porto, A. L. Muniz, and E. M. Carvalho, "Salivary and lacrymal gland disorders and HTLV-1 infection," *Revue de Stomatologie et de Chirurgie Maxillo-Faciale*, vol. 109, no. 3, pp. 153–157, 2008.

[31] E. L. Murphy, B. Wang, R. A. Sacher et al., "Respiratory and urinary tract infections, arthritis, and asthma associated with HTLV-I and HTLV-II infection," *Emerging Infectious Diseases*, vol. 10, no. 1, pp. 109–116, 2004.

[32] X. Mariette, F. Agbalika, M.-T. Daniel et al., "Detection of human T lymphotropic virus type I tax gene in salivary gland epithelium from two patients with Sjögren's syndrome," *Arthritis and Rheumatism*, vol. 36, no. 10, pp. 1423–1428, 1993.

[33] T. Sumida, F. Yonaha, T. Maeda et al., "Expression of sequences homologous to HTLV-I tax gene in the labial salivary glands of Japanese patients with Sjögren's syndrome," *Arthritis and Rheumatism*, vol. 37, no. 4, pp. 545–550, 1994.

[34] J. E. Green, S. H. Hinrichs, J. Vogel, and G. Jay, "Exocrinopathy resembling Sjogren's syndrome in HTLV-1 tax transgenic mice," *Nature*, vol. 341, no. 6237, pp. 72–74, 1989.

[35] M. M. Carvalho, A. E. Novaes, E. M. Carvalho, and M. I. Araújo, "Doenças reumáticas auto-imunes em indivíduos infectados pelo HTLV-1," *Revista Brasileira de Reumatologia*, vol. 46, no. 5, pp. 334–339, 2006.

[36] Y. Nishiura, T. Nakamura, K. Ichinose et al., "Increased production of inflammatory cytokines in cultured CD4$^+$ cells from patients with HTLV-I-associated myelopathy," *The Tohoku Journal of Experimental Medicine*, vol. 179, no. 4, pp. 227–233, 1996.

[37] S. B. Santos, A. F. Porto, A. L. Muniz et al., "Exacerbated inflammatory cellular immune response characteristics of HAM/TSP is observed in a large proportion of HTLV-I asymptomatic carriers," *BMC Infectious Diseases*, vol. 4, article 7, 2004.

[38] Y. Kuroda, M. Matsui, H. Takashima, and K. Kurohara, "Granulocyte-macrophage colony-stimulating factor and interleukin-1 increase in cerebrospinal fluid, but not in serum, of HTLV-I-associated myelopathy," *Journal of Neuroimmunology*, vol. 45, no. 1-2, pp. 133–136, 1993.

[39] N. Nishimoto, K. Yoshizaki, N. Eiraku et al., "Elevated levels of interleukin-6 in serum and cerebrospinal fluid of HTLV-I-associated myelopathy/tropical spastic paraparesis," *Journal of the Neurological Sciences*, vol. 97, no. 2-3, pp. 183–193, 1990.

14

Annexin A1 and the Resolution of Inflammation: Modulation of Neutrophil Recruitment, Apoptosis, and Clearance

Michelle Amantéa Sugimoto,[1,2,3] **Juliana Priscila Vago,**[2,3,4]
Mauro Martins Teixeira,[3] **and Lirlândia Pires Sousa**[1,2,3,4]

[1] *Programa de Pós-Graduação em Ciências Farmacêuticas, Faculdade de Farmácia, Universidade Federal de Minas Gerais, 31270-901 Belo Horizonte, MG, Brazil*

[2] *Departamento de Análises Clínicas e Toxicológicas, Faculdade de Farmácia, Universidade Federal de Minas Gerais, 31270-901 Belo Horizonte, MG, Brazil*

[3] *Laboratório de Imunofarmacologia, Departamento de Bioquímica e Imunologia, Instituto de Ciências Biológicas, Universidade Federal de Minas Gerais, 31270-901 Belo Horizonte, MG, Brazil*

[4] *Programa de Pós-Graduação em Biologia Celular, Departamento de Morfologia, Instituto de Ciências Biológicas, Universidade Federal de Minas Gerais, 31270-901 Belo Horizonte, MG, Brazil*

Correspondence should be addressed to Lirlândia Pires Sousa; lipsousa72@gmail.com

Academic Editor: Nicolas Demaurex

Neutrophils (also named polymorphonuclear leukocytes or PMN) are essential components of the immune system, rapidly recruited to sites of inflammation, providing the first line of defense against invading pathogens. Since neutrophils can also cause tissue damage, their fine-tuned regulation at the inflammatory site is required for proper resolution of inflammation. Annexin A1 (AnxA1), also known as lipocortin-1, is an endogenous glucocorticoid-regulated protein, which is able to counterregulate the inflammatory events restoring homeostasis. AnxA1 and its mimetic peptides inhibit neutrophil tissue accumulation by reducing leukocyte infiltration and activating neutrophil apoptosis. AnxA1 also promotes monocyte recruitment and clearance of apoptotic leukocytes by macrophages. More recently, some evidence has suggested the ability of AnxA1 to induce macrophage reprogramming toward a resolving phenotype, resulting in reduced production of proinflammatory cytokines and increased release of immunosuppressive and proresolving molecules. The combination of these mechanisms results in an effective resolution of inflammation, pointing to AnxA1 as a promising tool for the development of new therapeutic strategies to treat inflammatory diseases.

1. Introduction

Inflammation is a crucial physiological response for the maintenance of tissue homeostasis, protecting the host against invading microorganisms, foreign substances, or host self-disturbers, such as the molecules derived from damaged cells [1]. After the host has been incited, important microcirculatory events occur in response to local release of proinflammatory mediators, such as histamine, prostaglandins, leukotrienes, cytokines, and chemokines, leading to higher vascular permeability and increased leukocyte recruitment [1]. Leukocytes, such as neutrophils and macrophages, play a key role in inflammatory response, by releasing further inflammatory mediators and acting as effector cells and phagocytes to remove the inflammatory agent/stimuli [2].

Despite the important roles of neutrophils for effective host defense, these cells can also cause tissue damage requiring appropriate regulation [3, 4]. Continuous inflammatory stimuli can lead to aggressive and/or prolonged inflammatory responses, which may be detrimental to the host, leading to chronic inflammation [5]. The efficient removal of the inciting agent by phagocytes is the first signal for triggering proper resolution, through inhibition of proinflammatory mediators production and activation of their catabolism, resulting in the ceasing of further leukocyte recruitment [6]. After that, proresolving pathways are activated in order to restore tissue structure, function, and homeostasis [7, 8]. In this context, anti-inflammatory and proresolving molecules such as specialized lipid mediators (lipoxin A4, resolvins, maresins, and protectins), peptides/proteins (melanocortins, galectins, and annexin A1), and several other substances of different natures are released at the site of inflammation [7, 9, 10]. These endogenous mediators are known for their ability to decrease endothelial activation, reduce leukocyte infiltration, and activate neutrophil apoptosis, which ensures their secure removal by scavenger macrophages through a process called efferocytosis (phagocytosis of apoptotic cells) [4].

Annexin A1 (AnxA1) is an important glucocorticoid- (GC-) regulated protein, which contributes to the resolution of inflammation through various ways (Figure 1). AnxA1 limits neutrophil recruitment and production of proinflammatory mediators. Moreover, AnxA1 acts by inducing neutrophil apoptosis, modulating monocyte recruitment, and enhancing the clearance of apoptotic cells by macrophages. Emerging evidence suggests that AnxA1 also induces macrophage reprogramming toward a resolving phenotype, another key event to restore tissue homeostasis. In this review, we summarize several physiological and potential therapeutic actions of AnxA1 on inflammation resolution. In particular, this review highlights recent advances on the actions of this endogenous mediator and its potential clinical utility.

2. Annexin A1: General Aspects

Endogenous mediators of inflammation, such as AnxA1, are potential therapeutic tools to control inflammatory diseases. Although whether clinical use of proresolving strategies will be useful for treating inflammatory maladies or will show significant undesirable effects remains to be elucidated, it is believed these will be effective and have fewer side effects due to their ability to mimic or induce natural pathways of the resolution phase of inflammation [8, 12].

Annexin superfamily is composed of 13 members, grouped in view of their unique Ca^{2+}-binding-site architecture, which enables them to peripherally attach to negatively charged membrane surfaces [13–15]. AnxA1, also known as annexin I or lipocortin I, was originally identified as a GC-induced protein active on phospholipase- (PL-) A2 inhibition and prevention of eicosanoid synthesis [16–18]. It was subsequently recognized as an endogenous modulator of the inflammatory response, through several studies, mainly those led by Dr. Flower and Dr. Perretti [19, 20]. This 37 kDa protein consists in a homologous core region of 310 amino acid residues, representing almost 90% of the structure, attached to a unique N-terminal region [15]. In addition to mediating membrane binding, Ca^{2+} ions can also induce a conformational change that leads to the exposure of the bioactive N-terminal domain [15, 21, 22]. In fact, studies on the anti-inflammatory activity of AnxA1 revealed not only that the different functions of the protein lie within the unique N-terminus, but also that synthetic peptides from the N-terminal domain may mimic the pharmacological property of the whole protein, specifically binding to formyl peptide receptors (FPRs) [12].

In inflammatory conditions intact AnxA1 (37 kDa) can be cleaved by proteinase-3 and neutrophil elastase generating the 33 kDa cleaved isoform, which is believed to be inactive, and peptides derived from the AnxA1 N-terminus [23–25]. The main cleavage sites on AnxA1 are located at A^{11}, V^{22}, and V^{36}, as identified by cleavage assays coupled to mass spectrometric analyses [25]. Investigation of the $AnxA1_{2-50}$ peptide revealed a novel cleavage site at position 25, probably unmasked due to the simpler conformation of the peptide, compared with the full-length AnxA1 [26]. In fact, the substitution of the mentioned cleavage sites allowed the generation of metabolically stable forms of AnxA1 and its peptide, respectively, named SuperAnxA1 (SAnxA1) [27] and cleavage-resistant $AnxA1_{2-50}$ (CR-$AnxA1_{2-50}$) [26]. The proinflammatory nature of AnxA1 cleavage products is supported by reports of increased levels of the 33 kDa fragment in human and animal inflammatory samples, including bronchoalveolar lavage fluids [28–30] and exudates [11, 25, 31, 32]. For instance, using a model of acute pleurisy, our research group has shown increased levels of the 33 kDa breakdown product of AnxA1 during the time points of high neutrophil infiltration into the pleural cavity followed by regain of the intact form during the resolving phase of the pleurisy [11]. However, what the biological functions of this and other AnxA1-generated peptides are is still unclear, and this matter deserves further investigation.

Evidence for physiological function of AnxA1 in modulating inflammation emerged from studies involving AnxA1-null mice and AnxA1 neutralization strategies. AnxA1-null mice are viable and have a normal phenotype until they are challenged with inflammatory stimuli when they show stronger and more prolonged inflammatory reaction when compared to the wild-type (WT) [33–40]. Resistance to glucocorticoid treatment and aberrant inflammation in AnxA1-deficient mice provided initial evidence for the physiological relevance of the protein [33]. In the absence of AnxA1, the inflammatory response is exacerbated as demonstrated by increased neutrophil extravasation following zymosan-induced peritonitis [35] and endotoxin-induced uveitis [37]. In addition, animals lacking this protein exhibited exacerbated arthritis severity [34] and allergic response in ovalbumin-induced conjunctivitis [39]. AnxA1 KO mice also showed increased atherosclerotic lesion size with an overall increase in lesional macrophages and neutrophils [40]. Moreover, our research group has shown the prevention of spontaneous and dexamethasone-driven resolution of inflammation by using an AnxA1 neutralizing strategy [11]. Aside from the physiological role of the endogenous protein, pharmacological treatment with both human recombinant AnxA1 and its N-terminal peptides exerts anti-inflammatory and proresolving effects in a variety of experimental models, highlighting their therapeutic potential for inflammation resolution [11, 26, 27, 41] and wound repair [42].

AnxA1 exerts many of its anti-inflammatory and proresolving actions through the formyl peptide receptor type

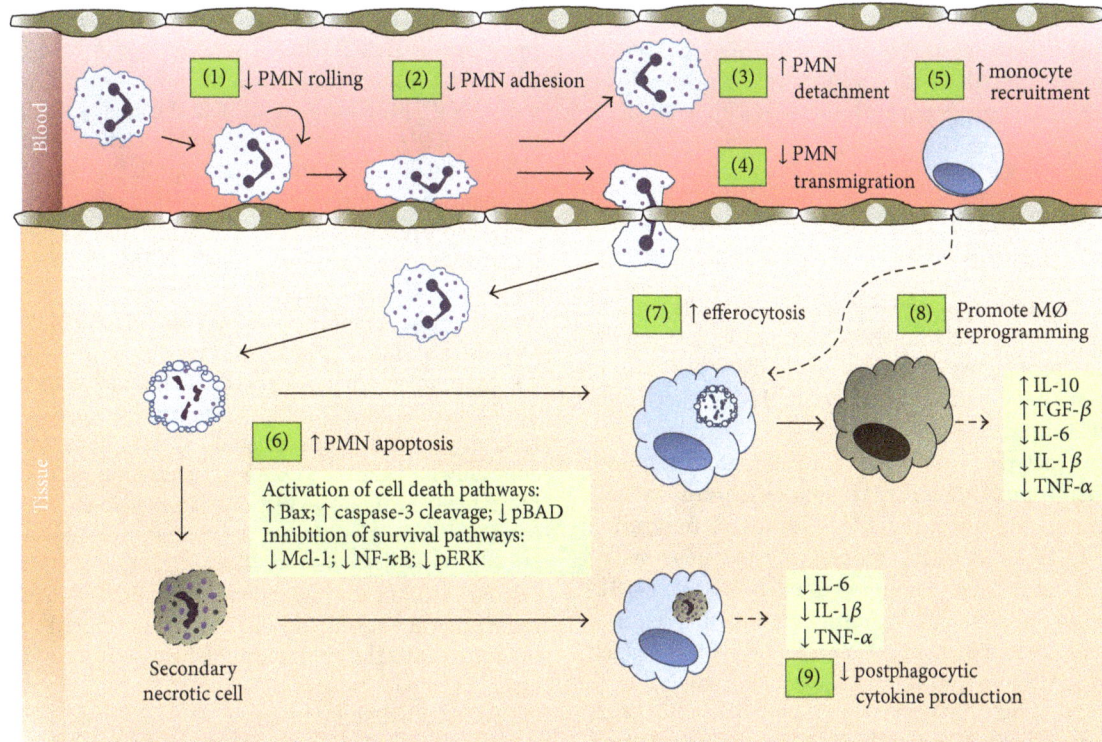

FIGURE 1: Cellular events associated with the anti-inflammatory and proresolving effects of annexin A1 (AnxA1) and its mimetic N-terminal peptides. AnxA1 modulates a wide range of cellular and molecular steps of the inflammatory response and is deeply involved in the endogenous mechanisms that are activated to bring about proper resolution. Pharmacological administration of AnxA1 results in decreased neutrophil rolling (1) and adhesion (2) to endothelium, increased detachment of adherent cells (3), and inhibition of neutrophil transmigration (4). In addition, AnxA1 is able to induce apoptosis, overriding the prosurvival signals that cause prolonged lifespan of neutrophils at the inflammatory site (6). Endogenous and exogenous AnxA1 also promote monocyte recruitment (5) and clearance of apoptotic neutrophils by macrophages (7). Phagocytosis of apoptotic neutrophils by macrophages is coupled with release of anti-inflammatory signals, including transforming growth factor-β, and lower levels of proinflammatory cytokines (8). Besides, AnxA1 is related to macrophage reprogramming toward a proresolving phenotype (8). Initial *in vitro* studies using AnxA1 knock-down leucocytes demonstrate that AnxA1 prevents proinflammatory cytokine production after phagocytosis of secondary necrotic cells. This effect provides an important fail-safe mechanism countering inflammatory responses when the timely clearance of apoptotic cells has failed (9).

2/lipoxin A4 receptor (FPR2/ALX). This receptor, along with FPR1 and FPR3, composes a family of seven-transmembrane domain G protein-coupled receptors which share significant sequence homology [43]. FPR2/ALX receptor is shared by a variety of other peptide/protein and lipid ligands, mediating diverse biological functions of relevance for host defence and inflammation. Interestingly, FPR2/ALX agonists are associated with both proinflammatory (e.g., serum amyloid A and cathelicidin) and proresolving (e.g., AnxA1 and LXA$_4$) signalling pathways [43, 44]. However, how FPR2/ALX can promote both inflammatory response and limit its duration and intensity still remains to be fully elucidated. It is noteworthy that distinct FPR2/ALX domains are required for signalling by different agonists [45]. Using FPR2/ALX transfected cells and chimeric FPR1 and FPR2 clones, Bena and col. (2012) identified that while AnxA1-mediated signalling involves the N-terminal region and extracellular loop II of FPR2/ALX, SAA interacts with the extracellular loops I and II of the same receptor [45]. Otherwise, LXA$_4$ has been shown to activate FPR2/ALX by interacting with extracellular loop III and the associated transmembrane domain [46].

The versatility of FPR2/ALX receptors also seems to rely on the activation of receptor dimmers in a biased fashion. AnxA1 was found to activate FPR2/ALX homodimerization but not the proinflammatory SAA [47]. In contrast to the full-length AnxA1, the short AnxA1 derived peptide Ac2–26 is able to activate all members of the human FPR family [48] and induce FPR2/ALX-FPR1 heterodimerization [47]. These observations suggest that short AnxA1 mimetic peptides might fulfill other functions at variance to those reported for the parental protein [49]. However, a good degree of selectivity was retained by longer AnxA1 derived anti-inflammatory sequences such as AnxA1$_{2-50}$ [26].

Interestingly, the promiscuity of FPR2/ALX seems to be linked to a network of resolution mediators as discussed by Brancaleone and col. (2011) [50]. In fact, the authors provide strong evidence that the engagement of FPR2/ALX by selective agonists (such as LXA$_4$ and antiflammin 2) would induce AnxA1 phosphorylation and mobilization in human PMN [50]. In a similar vein, the proresolving mediator Resolvin E1 (RvE1) stimulates endogenous LXA$_4$ production [51, 52]. Moreover, it has been shown that proresolving mediators such as resolvins and LXA_4 induce further anti-inflammatory molecules *in vivo*, such as interleukin- (IL-) 10 [41]. Taken together, these data suggest that a proresolving cascade may be operating during resolution with FPR2/ALX playing a central role in this process.

3. Anti-Inflammatory and Proresolving Actions of AnxA1

3.1. AnxA1 Regulates Neutrophil Recruitment to the Inflammatory Site. During inflammation neutrophils are rapidly recruited to the infected or injured tissue. However, due to the potential tissue-damaging effects of PMN, their fine-tuned regulation at the inflammatory site is required [53]. Indeed, exacerbated or overshooting inflammatory response with high neutrophil influx may account for chronic inflammatory diseases [5]. Thus, restricting leukocyte infiltration to the tissue is an essential process for spontaneous or pharmacological-induced resolution of inflammation [4, 8].

Neutrophil trafficking to the site of inflammation requires adhesion and transmigration through blood vessels, which is orchestrated by molecules on leukocytes (e.g., $\beta1$, $\beta2$ integrins, and L-selectin) and on endothelial cells (e.g., vascular cell adhesion molecule-1, intercellular adhesion molecule-1, and E-selectin). The leukocyte adhesion cascade is a tightly regulated process, subjected to both positive and negative regulators [71]. For example, anti-inflammatory and proresolving mediators, such as AnxA1, are well documented to counterregulate excessive neutrophil accumulation (an anti-inflammatory action). Human PMN interaction with endothelial cells during the early stage of inflammation promotes modulation of AnxA1 in several ways, such as induction of gene expression [35] and mobilization and cell surface externalization of intracellular AnxA1 [72, 73]. In turn, the externalized protein acts as a brake for PMN adhesion to the microvascular wall, preventing overexuberant cell transmigration to the inflammatory site [4, 27, 72, 74]. Dalli and col. (2008) [75] reinforced the anti-inflammatory properties of PMN-derived microparticles containing functionally active AnxA1. Released upon adhesion to endothelial cells, these microparticles inhibit neutrophil/endothelium interaction under flow, *in vitro*, and PMN recruitment to an air pouch inflamed with IL-1β, *in vivo* [75]. Moreover, microparticles derived from WT but not from AnxA1-deficient neutrophils were able to inhibit IL-1β-induced leukocyte trafficking [75].

Several studies using exogenously administered AnxA1 have provided further evidence for the modulating role of AnxA1 on neutrophil trafficking. *In vivo* observations produced through intravital microscopy techniques indicated that AnxA1 and Ac2–26 administration to mice during zymosan-induced peritonitis produced detachment of adherent neutrophils from the vascular wall with consequent inhibition of neutrophil extravasation across mouse mesenteric postcapillary venules (Table 1) [56]. Supporting these first findings, *in vitro* studies showed that recombinant AnxA1 and its mimetic peptides display inhibitory effects on neutrophil rolling [26, 27, 54, 55] adhesion to endothelial monolayer [26, 27, 40, 48, 54, 55] and transmigration [48].

Shedding of L-selectin appears to be one of the molecular mechanisms that mediate the effects of AnxA1 and its N-terminal peptides on neutrophil recruitment. Walther and col. (2000) [48] have described the ability of the AnxA1 peptide Ac9–25 to cause transient calcium fluxes and L-selectin shedding in human neutrophils. After that, the same mechanism was linked to the inhibitory effects of Ac2–26 on PMN capture and rolling in a flow chamber assay [54]. Similarly, promotion of L-selectin shedding was demonstrated for human recombinant AnxA1 [57, 58], an effect mediated by cell surface metalloprotease ("sheddase") [58]. Recently, Drechsler and col. (2015) [40] brought further insights into the mechanisms behind the antimigratory effects of Ac2–26. According to the authors, the peptide dose dependently reduces the affinity of activated neutrophils for vascular cell adhesion molecule-1 (VCAM-1) and intercellular adhesion molecule-1 (ICAM-1), a response abrogated in cells harvested from FPR2 knockout mice. They demonstrated that Ac2–26 inhibits the adhesiveness of $\beta1$ and $\beta2$ integrins by downmodulating their affinity and valency, but without changing their cell surface expression. It was also demonstrated that Ac2–26 interferes with the chemokine-driven activation of Rap1, an essential step in integrin activation [76, 77].

Pederzoli-Ribeil and col. (2010) [27] combined *in vitro* and *in vivo* experimental strategies to show that AnxA1 and its mutant cleavage-resistant form, SAnxA1, are able to augment rolling velocity and reduce adhesion of PMN to endothelial cells through FPR2 receptors. Furthermore, Dalli and col. (2013) [26] demonstrated the anti-inflammatory actions of the longer acetylated AnxA1 peptide AnxA1$_{2-50}$ and its cleavage-resistant form, CR-AnxA1$_{2-50}$. Both displayed antimigratory effects *in vivo*, reducing leukocyte adhesion to inflamed cremaster venule, neutrophil migration into dermal air pouches in response to IL-1β, and neutrophil migration into peritoneum in response to zymosan.

In vivo anti-inflammatory and antimigratory properties of the short AnxA1 peptide Ac2–26 have also been extensively demonstrated, as exemplified by its ability to inhibit carrageenan-induced PMN adhesion to the vasculature and extravasation into the peritoneal fluid [74]. The peptide was also able to prevent neutrophil recruitment in myotoxin-induced peritonitis [78] and during lung inflammation induced by intestinal ischemia/reperfusion [79]. Moreover, Ac2–26 showed potential benefits in an ocular model by inhibiting neutrophil influx, protein leak, chemical mediator release, and COX-2 expression during endotoxin-induced uveitis [37]. The Ac2–26 peptide also demonstrated antimigratory effects in a model of ovalbumin-induced allergic conjunctivitis, significantly reducing the clinical signs of conjunctivitis through the inhibition of leukocyte influx and cytokines and chemokines release, effects correlated with inhibition of the ERK pathway [39]. Interestingly, increased levels of ERK phosphorylation were associated with exacerbated allergic response observed in AnxA1-deficient mice in comparison to WT animals [39]. Reinforcing the involvement of AnxA1 pathway in neutrophil recruitment, AnxA1-null mice demonstrated a higher extent of neutrophil extravasation in animal models of peritonitis [35, 74], allergic conjunctivitis [39], and uveitis [37].

TABLE 1: *In vitro* and *in vivo* evidence for anti-inflammatory and proresolving properties of annexin A1 and its fragments.

Agent	Experimental model	Outcome/effect on resolution	References
	Inhibition of neutrophil recruitment		
AnxA1	Neutrophil/endothelial interaction (*in vitro*)	↓ PMN capture, rolling, and adhesion ↓ PMN transmigration	[27, 48, 54, 55]
	Neutrophil/endothelial interaction (*in vivo*)	↓ PMN rolling, adhesion, and emigration ↑ Detachment of adherent PMN	[27, 56]
	Human PMN	↑ L-selectin shedding	[57, 58]
	IL-1β inflamed air pouch	↓ PMN migration	[26, 59]
	Carrageenan-induced paw edema	↓ edema ↓ leukocyte infiltration	[27]
SAnxA1	Neutrophil/endothelial interaction (*in vitro*)	↓ PMN capture, rolling, and adhesion	[27]
	Neutrophil/endothelial interaction (*in vivo*)	↓ PMN rolling and adhesion	[27]
	fMLP induced skin edema	↓ MPO activity	[27]
	Carrageenan-induced paw edema	↓ edema ↓ leukocyte infiltration	[27]
AnxA1$_{2-50}$	Neutrophil/endothelial interaction (*in vitro*)	↓ PMN rolling and adhesion	[26]
	Neutrophil/endothelial interaction (*in vivo*)	↓ PMN adhesion	[26]
	IL-1β inflamed air pouch	↓ PMN recruitment	[26]
Ac2–26	Neutrophil/endothelial interaction (*in vitro*)	↓ PMN capture, rolling, and adhesion ↑ L-selectin shedding	[40, 54]
	Human PMN activated with CCL5	↓ β integrin activation	[40]
	Neutrophil/endothelial interaction (*in vivo*)	↓ PMN adhesion and emigration ↑ detachment of adherent PMN	[56]
Ac1–26	Neutrophil/endothelial interaction (*in vitro*)	↓ PMN transmigration	[48]
Ac9–25	Neutrophil/endothelial interaction (*in vitro*)	↓ PMN adhesion and transmigration ↑ L-selectin shedding	[48]
AF-2	Neutrophil/endothelial interaction (*in vitro*)	↓ PMN adhesion ↓ β2 integrin expression	[60, 61]
	Induction of neutrophil apoptosis		
AnxA1	Human PMN	↑ apoptosis (↓ pBAD)	[57]
AnxA1$_{2-50}$	Human neutrophils stimulated with SAA	↑ apoptosis	[26]
Ac2–26	Human neutrophils stimulated with SAA	↑ apoptosis (↑ caspase-3 cleavage; JNK dependent)	[47]
	Acute pleurisy	↑ apoptosis (↑ Bax; ↑ caspase-3 cleavage; ↓ Mcl-1; ↓ NF-κB; ↓ pERK)	[11]
	Skin allograft model	↑ skin allograft survival ↑ apoptosis ↓ neutrophil transmigration	[62]
	Enhancement of monocyte recruitment and efferocytosis		
Ac2–7	Transmigration assay (*in vitro*)	Stimulating human monocyte chemotaxis	[63]
AnxA1	Chemotaxis assays	Human monocyte chemoattractant	[64]
	Administration to mouse peritoneum	↑ monocyte recruitment	[64]
	Phagocytosis of apoptotic leukocytes	↑ efferocytosis ↑ binding of apoptotic cells to MØ	[65, 66]
Ac2–26	Phagocytosis of apoptotic neutrophils	↑ phagocytosis Inducing actin reorganization ↑ TGF-β release ↓ IL-8 release	[67]
AnxA1$_{2-50}$	Zymosan-induced peritonitis	↑ efferocytosis	[26]

TABLE 1: Continued.

Agent	Experimental model	Outcome/effect on resolution	References
	Macrophage reprogramming		
AnxA1	Human MØ cell line	Induced M2-like polarization	[44]
	Human monocytes	↑ IL-10	[47]
	LPS stimulated THP-1 MØ	↓ IL-6, TNF, and IL-1β	[66]
	MØ from NASH livers	↓ M1 polarization (↓ iNOS, IL-12p40) ↑ IL-10	[68]
	Intraperitoneal injection	↑ IL-10	[47]
	Phagocytosis of apoptotic neurons by microglial cells	↓ phagocytosis of healthy cells ↓ NO production	[69]
Ac2–26	Endotoxin-challenged monocytes	↓ IL-6 signalling ↓ TNF-α release	[70]

AnxA1: annexin A1; fMLP: N-Formyl-Met-Leu-Phe; IL: interleukin; MPO: Myeloperoxidase; MØ, macrophage; NASH; nonalcoholic steatohepatitis; PMN: polymorphonuclear; NO: nitric oxide; SAA: serum amyloid A; SAnxA1: SuperAnxA1 (proteinase-3 resistant); TGF-β: transforming growth factor-β; TNF-α: tumor necrosis factor alpha.

AnxA1 may also be tightly coupled to the anti-inflammatory properties of other FPR2/ALX agonists such as LXA$_4$ and antiflammin 2 (AF-2) [50]. The nonapeptide AF-2, which corresponds to region 246–254 of AnxA1 [80], is known to interfere with PMN activation, chemotaxis, and adhesion to endothelial cells [60, 61], via FPR2/ALX receptor [81]. Also, LXA$_4$ is a potent regulator of PMN trafficking in experimental inflammation [9, 82]. Interestingly, recent data indicated a crucial role for endogenous AnxA1 in the detachment phenomenon promoted by both compounds [50]. For instance, LXA$_4$ and AF-2 lost their antimigratory effects in AnxA1 KO mice suggesting AnxA1 as a downstream mediator of other proresolving and anti-inflammatory molecules [50].

3.2. AnxA1 Induces Neutrophil Apoptosis. Neutrophils are produced in the bone marrow from myeloid stem cells, which in turn proliferate, differentiate into mature neutrophils, and are delivered into circulation [83]. Although the circulatory half-life of neutrophils is now thought to be longer than previously estimated (days instead of hours) [84], at inflammatory sites the constitutive apoptotic pathway is delayed by the action of local inflammatory mediators, resulting in increased neutrophil half-life [85], an effect that can be opposed by proresolving mediators including AnxA1 and lipoxins [86].

In addition to affecting the migration of leukocytes through FPR activation, strong evidence of the involvement of AnxA1 on neutrophil apoptosis has emerged. Proapoptotic effect of AnxA1 on neutrophils was first described *in vitro* associated with transient calcium fluxes and dephosphorylation of BAD, an intracellular protein whose proapoptotic function is lost upon phosphorylation [57]. Our group [11] demonstrated the *in vivo* proapoptotic functions of endogenous AnxA1 during self-resolving inflammation. In an acute pleurisy model, blockage of the AnxA1 pathway by using a specific anti-AnxA1 antiserum prevented dexamethasone- (dexa-) induced resolution of neutrophilic inflammation, abolishing morphological and biochemical apoptotic events in the pleural cavity. AnxA1 neutralization also hampered

dexa-induced decrease of ERK1/2 and IκB-α phosphorylation and Bax accumulation. In addition, anti-AnxA1 treatment prevented spontaneous resolution of neutrophilic inflammation, suggesting an important role of endogenously produced AnxA1 in the proresolutive program [11]. Furthermore, pharmacological administration of Ac2–26 peptide promoted active resolution and augmented the extent of neutrophil apoptosis. These effects were prevented by the pan-caspase inhibitor zVAD-fmk and linked to activation of the cell death pathways Bax and caspase-3 and inhibition of the survival-controlling pathways Mcl-1, ERK1/2, and NF-κB [11] (Figure 2).

In a skin allograft model, pharmacological treatment with Ac2–26 increased transplantation survival related to inhibition of neutrophil transmigration and induction of apoptosis, thereby reducing the tissue damage compared with control animals [62]. *In vitro*, Ac2–26 counteracted the survival signal in SAA-treated neutrophils, an effect associated with caspase-3 cleavage and prevented by the JNK inhibitor [47]. Dalli and col. (2013) also demonstrated that AnxA1$_{2-50}$ and CR-AnxA1$_{2-50}$ peptides can override the antiapoptotic effect of SAA in human neutrophils *in vitro* [26]. This proapoptotic effect may have contributed to the *in vivo* anti-inflammatory and proresolving actions of the peptides characterized by reduced granulocyte counts and enhanced efferocytosis in peptide-treated mice during peritonitis [26].

AnxA1 has also been described as a mediator of drug-induced apoptosis, supporting its involvement in the induction of cell death. The proapoptotic effect described for the histone deacetylase inhibitor (HDCAI) FK228, in leukemia cells, was linked to the induction of AnxA1 expression, externalization, and cleavage. Neutralization with anti-AnxA1 antibody or gene silencing with AnxA1 siRNA inhibited FK228-induced apoptosis, suggesting the involvement of AnxA1 in apoptotic cell death in response to HDCAI [87]. Recently, the *in vitro* ability of HDACIs to promote apoptosis was also demonstrated in bone-marrow neutrophils from WT but not from AnxA1 knockout mice [88]. *In vivo*, HDACIs significantly reduced neutrophil numbers and

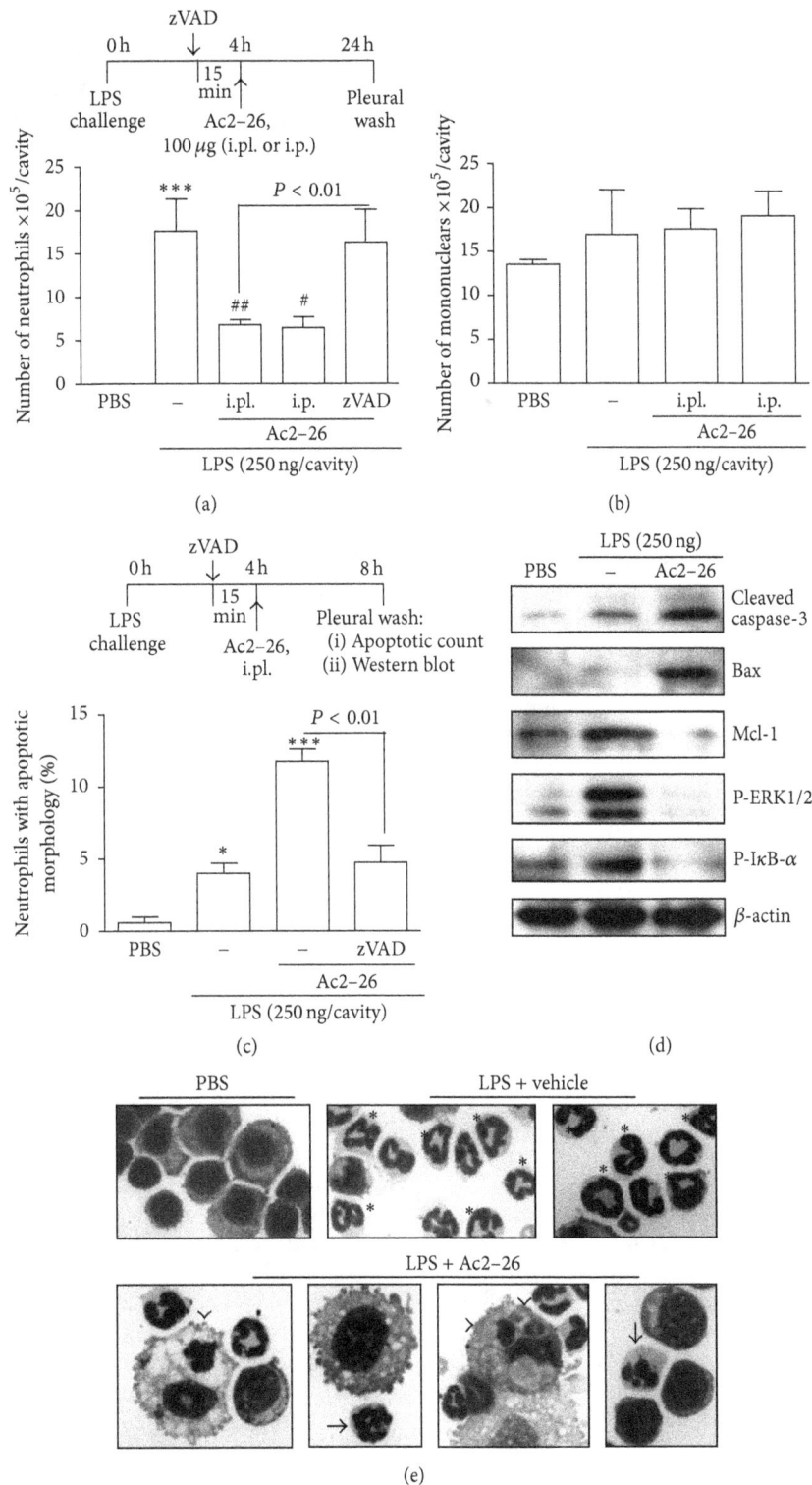

(a)

(b)

(c)

(d)

(e)

FIGURE 2: Effect of exogenous administration of AnxA1 derived peptide Ac2–26 on LPS-induced pleurisy. Mice were injected with LPS (250 ng/cavity, i.pl.) and 4 h later received an injection of Ac2–26 (100 μg/mouse, i.pl. or i.p.). The treatment with the pan-caspase inhibitor zVAD-fmk (1 mg/kg, i.p.) was performed 15 min before the injection of peptide. The numbers of neutrophils (a) and mononuclear cells (b) were evaluated 20 h after drug treatment. Cells with distinctive apoptotic morphology (c and e) and Western blot for detection of cleaved caspase-3, Bax, Mcl-1, P-ERK, and P-IκB-α (d) were evaluated 4 h after the peptide treatment. $^*P < 0.05$ or $^{***}P < 0.001$ when compared with PBS-injected mice and $^\#P < 0.05$ or $^{\#\#}P < 0.01$ when compared with vehicle-treated, LPS-injected mice. (e) Representative figures of nonapoptotic (asterisk) and apoptotic (arrows) neutrophils and apoptotic cells inside macrophages (arrowheads). PBS and vehicle (upper panels) and Ac2–26-treated (lower panels) animals are shown. Original data from Vago et al., 2012 [11].

induced neutrophil apoptosis in a zymosan-induced peritonitis model. Once again, the lack of AnxA1 hampered this *in vivo* proapoptotic effect [88].

It is important to keep in mind that the proapoptotic effect of AnxA1 can be underestimated in dynamic *in vivo* models of inflammation. Regarding other anti-inflammatory drugs, it is documented in a number of diverse experimental and clinical settings that small changes in apoptosis rates can promote dramatic changes in total neutrophil numbers over time. This observation is most likely due to rapid recognition and phagocytosis of apoptotic cells [89–91].

3.3. AnxA1 Induces Monocyte Recruitment and Increases Efferocytosis.
Macrophage phagocytic clearance of apoptotic neutrophils plays an important role in the resolution of inflammation since this process prevents excessive neutrophil activation and the exposure of tissues to noxious neutrophil intracellular contents [92, 93]. For this reason, appropriate (nonphlogistic) monocyte recruitment from the bloodstream to inflammatory sites is a critical step in acute inflammation, enabling the clearance of apoptotic neutrophils and orderly progression towards resolution.

It has long been established that extravasation of PMN to the site of inflammation contributes to the launch of monocyte recruitment, with PMN granule proteins being important monocyte attractors [94]. Recent research from Perretti's group [64] indicates apoptotic neutrophils as the principal reservoir of AnxA1, which acts as important recruiting agent for monocytes to orchestrate the second resolving phase of acute inflammation. Associating *in vitro* and *in vivo* experiments, Professor Mauro Perretti's group filled an important gap in our knowledge by demonstrating the central role of the AnxA1–ALX/FPR2 pathway in modulating monocyte recruitment [64]. The authors demonstrated that intraperitoneal administration of AnxA1 induced monocyte migration, an effect absent in FPR2 null mice. Supporting these findings, both AnxA1 and FPR2/ALX null mice challenged with intraperitoneal zymosan exhibited diminished recruitment of monocytes as compared to WT mice, despite the higher levels of chemoattractants [64].

After initial steps of apoptosis, neutrophils lose their functional properties, such as the ability to move by chemotaxis, generate a respiratory burst, or degranulate [95]. Furthermore, they exhibit alterations on their intracellular pathways and cell surface molecules while some externalized molecules, such as phosphatidylserines (PS), facilitate the recognition and removal of apoptotic neutrophils by macrophages [92, 96].

Recent studies have reported that AnxA1 from apoptotic cells is involved in their phagocytic clearance. The first observation that AnxA1 participates in the engulfment of apoptotic cells was described by Arur and col. (2003) [97]. By using a differential proteomics technology, they showed that AnxA1 is exported to the outer plasma membrane of apoptotic lymphocytes, colocalizes with PS, and is required for efficient clearance of apoptotic cells, suggesting a role for AnxA1 as bridging PS molecules on apoptotic cells to phagocytes [97]. Scannell and col. (2007) [65] subsequently demonstrated that apoptotic neutrophils release AnxA1, which acts on

macrophages, promoting the removal of effete cells [65]. Noteworthily, not only the intact form of AnxA1 released by apoptotic cells but also the cleavage fragments, under 10 kDa, were effective in stimulating efferocytosis [65].

Studies have also documented macrophages as a source of endogenous AnxA1, which in turn facilitates phagocytic uptake of apoptotic cells. Maderna and col. (2005) showed that human macrophages release AnxA1 upon treatment with GC and that this protein acts in autocrine or paracrine manners to increase the engulfment of apoptotic neutrophils [67]. Additional experiments with AnxA1-null mice provided further evidence for a functional role of AnxA1 in efferocytosis, as macrophages derived from their bone marrow were defective in clearance of apoptotic cells [67]. In fact, the authors demonstrated, *in vitro*, the ability of the AnxA1 mimetic peptide Ac2–26 to promote phagocytosis of apoptotic PMN by human macrophages, an effect associated with actin rearrangement in the phagocytic cells and abrogated in the presence of FPR antagonist [67]. Subsequently, it was clearly demonstrated the nonredundant function of FPR2/ALX receptor in Ac2–26 induced efferocytosis since the peptide failed to exert its proefferocytic action on FPR2/ALX deficient macrophages [98]. Furthermore, Yona and coworkers (2006) associated *in vitro* and *in vivo* strategies that indicated reduced phagocytosis of zymosan particles by AnxA1 knockout macrophages [99].

It has been proposed that AnxA1 released by macrophages can opsonize apoptotic cells, probably by interacting with surface-exposed PS, enhancing their uptake by phagocytes [66]. Interestingly, McArthur's group demonstrated that the binding of microglial-derived AnxA1 to PS on the surface of apoptotic neuronal cells is critically required for phagocytosis [69]. Moreover, Dalli and colleagues (2012) reported that AnxA1 expressed by resident macrophages is a critical determinant for the clearance of senescent neutrophils in the bone marrow [100]. Proefferocytic effects were also observed for AnxA1$_{2-50}$ and its cleavage-resistant form (CR- AnxA1$_{2-50}$), which stimulated efferocytosis *in vitro* by human and mice bone-marrow derived macrophages [26]. This effect was confirmed *in vivo* in a zymosan-induced peritonitis model, when the peptides significantly reduced exudate neutrophil counts and increased the number of macrophages containing ingested PMN [26].

Once phagocytic removal of apoptotic cells has failed, neutrophils undergo secondary postapoptotic necrosis, probably leading to the leakage of cytotoxic and antigenic intracellular contents into the surrounding tissue [63]. Blume and col. (2012) revealed, in two complementary studies, the role of externalized AnxA1 as a fail-safe mechanism after neutrophil transition from apoptosis to secondary necrosis. First, they described AnxA1 externalization during secondary necrosis, which in turn promotes the removal of dying cells and prevents proinflammatory cytokine production [66]. In the second study, they demonstrated that *in vitro* AnxA1 proteolysis during secondary necrosis generates a monocytic "find-me" signal, contributing to the recruitment of monocytes and consequently preventing inflammation [63].

The removal of apoptotic cells has dual importance: prevention of potentially toxic content release and induction of macrophage reprogramming toward a resolving phenotype [101–103], another key event to restore tissue homeostasis. Accordingly, AnxA1-induced efferocytosis is coupled with increased release of transforming growth factor- (TGF-) β and lower levels of the proinflammatory cytokine IL-6 [65, 67]. In agreement with this observation, impaired phagocytosis in AnxA1-deficient macrophages is mirrored by increased release of tumor necrosis factor- (TNF-) α and IL-6 [99]. Supporting an immunomodulatory effect of AnxA1 on cytokine production, AnxA1-null mice showed increased mortality in a model of LPS-induced endotoxic shock which was correlated with increased activation of inflammatory cells [104]. The authors detected delayed and more prolonged increase in the levels of TNF-α, IL-1, and IL-6 in the blood of AnxA1-null mice, as well as increased production of these cytokines by AnxA1 KO macrophages [104]. This data is consistent with the increased production of IL-6 and TNF by stimulated AnxA1 KO peritoneal macrophages in comparison to WT cells [105]. Moreover, *in vitro* studies linked AnxA1 to brain homeostasis, demonstrating that exogenous AnxA1 can suppress microglial activation, limiting indiscriminate phagocytosis of healthy neurones and nitric oxide (NO) production during the phagocytic reaction [69]. Recently, the functional role of macrophage-derived AnxA1 in modulating hepatic inflammation and fibrogenesis during nonalcoholic steatohepatitis (NASH) progression was documented [68]. NASH in AnxA1 KO mice was characterized by enhanced lobular inflammation resulting from increased macrophage recruitment and exacerbation of the proinflammatory M1 phenotype [68]. In line with these results, AnxA1 administration to liver macrophages suppressed M1 activation, characterized by reduced expression of iNOS and IL-12p40, and increased IL-10 expression. Interestingly, activation of FPR2 by AnxA1 skewed M1 macrophages to anti-inflammatory M2-like cells, attenuating the expression of IL-6, IL-1β, and TNF-α [44]. Furthermore, Cooray and col. (2013) revealed an AnxA1-specific FPR2/ALX proresolving signal pathway centered in p38, leading to the production of IL-10 by human monocytes, an effect replicated *in vivo* after intraperitoneal AnxA1 injection [47].

Although uptake of secondary necrotic leukocytes was shown to be AnxA1 independent, the protein has an anti-inflammatory action on macrophages, since phagocytosis of AnxA1 knock-down necrotic cells induced increased release of proinflammatory cytokines TNF, IL-6, and IL-1β by phagocytic cells [66]. Pupjalis and col. (2011) added knowledge to the immunosuppressive actions of AnxA1 derived from apoptotic PMN. According to the authors, the treatment of human monocytes with AnxA1-containing supernatant of apoptotic granulocytes or Ac2–26 peptide results in a significantly diminished release of proinflammatory cytokines when the monocytes are subsequently challenged with endotoxin [70].

Taken together, these findings indicate that AnxA1-induced efferocytosis collaborates with the resolution of inflammation by promoting the elimination of effete neutrophils allied to an alternative macrophage activation that downregulates the production of proinflammatory mediators. Such events pave the way to the resolution of inflammation.

4. Concluding Remarks

AnxA1 is a GC-regulated protein that modulates a wide range of cellular and molecular steps of the inflammatory response and is deeply involved in the endogenous mechanisms that are activated to bring about proper resolution. So, it is reasonable to suppose that AnxA1-based pharmacologic strategies could be as effective as steroids, without their metabolic side effects. We have discussed here the ability of AnxA1 and its mimetic peptides to limit neutrophil accumulation in the tissue. Besides limiting neutrophil recruitment and increasing neutrophil apoptosis, AnxA1 promotes apoptotic neutrophil clearance by modulating monocyte recruitment and enhancing efferocytosis. Indeed, AnxA1 contributes to tissue homeostasis by inducing macrophage reprogramming toward a resolving phenotype. The combination of these mechanisms results in an effective resolution of inflammation, pointing to AnxA1 and its mimetic peptides as promising therapeutic agents for treating inflammatory diseases.

The promising findings on the potential therapeutic use of AnxA1 in inflammatory diseases have stimulated the development of pharmaceutical formulations containing AnxA1 mimetic peptides, such as the controlled-release hydrogels for dermal wound repair application [106] and targeted polymeric nanoparticles [107]. The latter demonstrated ability to enhance resolution in zymosan-induced peritonitis [107], promote colonic wounds healing [42], and protect hypercholesterolemic mice against advanced atherosclerosis [108]. These pharmaceutical strategies offer further benefits, overcoming the critical pharmacokinetics of short peptides *in vivo*, protecting them from proteolysis during pharmacological treatment, and facilitating the delivery to injury sites.

Abbreviations

Ac2–26:	Peptide from N-terminal portion of annexin A1 (residues 2–26)
AnxA1:	Annexin A1
FPR2/ALXR:	Formyl peptide receptor 2/lipoxin A4 receptor
Boc-1:	N-t-Boc-Met-Leu-Phe
Dexa:	Dexamethasone
ERK1/2:	Extracellular signal-regulated kinase
FPR:	Formyl peptide receptor
GC:	Glucocorticoid
ICAM-1:	Intercellular adhesion molecule-1
i.pl.:	Intrapleural
IL:	Interleukin
IκB-α:	Inhibitory kappa B alpha
KO:	Knockout
LPS:	Lipopolysaccharide
Mcl-1:	Myeloid cell leukemia-1
NF-κB:	Nuclear factor kappa B
PMN:	Polymorphonuclear
SAnxA1:	SuperAnxA1 or cleavage-resistant AnxA1
TGF-β:	Transforming growth factor-β
TNF:	Tumor necrosis factor

VCAM-1:   Vascular cell adhesion molecule-1
WT: Wild-type
zVAD-fmk: Benzyloxycarbonyl-Val-Ala-Asp-
          fluoromethylketone.

Conflict of Interests

The authors declare that there is no conflict of interests regarding the publication of this paper.

Acknowledgments

The authors would like to acknowledge the funding from Conselho Nacional de Desenvolvimento Científico e Tecnológico (CNPq, Brazil), Comissão de Aperfeiçoamento de Pessoal do Ensino Superior (CAPES, Brazil), Fundação do Amparo a Pesquisa de Minas Gerais (FAPEMIG, Brazil), Instituto Nacional de Ciência e Tecnologia (INCT in Dengue), and the European Community's Seventh Framework Programme (FP7-2007–2013, Timer Consortium) under Grant Agreement HEALTH-F4-2011-281608. The authors apologize to their colleagues if their original contributions could not be included in the list of references due to space limitations.

References

[1] R. Medzhitov, "Inflammation 2010: new adventures of an old flame," *Cell*, vol. 140, no. 6, pp. 771–776, 2010.

[2] M. T. Silva and M. Correia-Neves, "Neutrophils and macrophages: the main partners of phagocyte cell systems," *Frontiers in Immunology*, vol. 3, article 174, 2012.

[3] J. M. Hallett, A. E. Leitch, N. A. Riley, R. Duffin, C. Haslett, and A. G. Rossi, "Novel pharmacological strategies for driving inflammatory cell apoptosis and enhancing the resolution of inflammation," *Trends in Pharmacological Sciences*, vol. 29, no. 5, pp. 250–257, 2008.

[4] S. E. Headland and L. V. Norling, "The resolution of inflammation: principles and challenges," *Seminars in Immunology*, vol. 27, no. 3, pp. 149–160, 2015.

[5] C. Nathan and A. Ding, "Nonresolving inflammation," *Cell*, vol. 140, no. 6, pp. 871–882, 2010.

[6] D. Gilroy and R. De Maeyer, "New insights into the resolution of inflammation," *Seminars in Immunology*, vol. 27, no. 3, pp. 161–168, 2015.

[7] C. N. Serhan and J. Savill, "Resolution of inflammation: the beginning programs the end," *Nature Immunology*, vol. 6, no. 12, pp. 1191–1197, 2005.

[8] L. P. Sousa, A. L. Alessandri, V. Pinho, and M. M. Teixeira, "Pharmacological strategies to resolve acute inflammation," *Current Opinion in Pharmacology*, vol. 13, no. 4, pp. 625–631, 2013.

[9] C. N. Serhan, S. Yacoubian, and R. Yang, "Anti-inflammatory and proresolving lipid mediators," *Annual Review of Pathology: Mechanisms of Disease*, vol. 3, pp. 279–312, 2008.

[10] C. N. Serhan, J. Dalli, R. A. Colas, J. W. Winkler, and N. Chiang, "Protectins and maresins: new pro-resolving families of mediators in acute inflammation and resolution bioactive metabolome," *Biochimica et Biophysica Acta*, vol. 1851, no. 4, pp. 397–413, 2015.

[11] J. P. Vago, C. R. Nogueira, L. P. Tavares et al., "Annexin A1 modulates natural and glucocorticoid-induced resolution of inflammation by enhancing neutrophil apoptosis," *Journal of Leukocyte Biology*, vol. 92, no. 2, pp. 249–258, 2012.

[12] M. Perretti and J. Dalli, "Exploiting the Annexin A1 pathway for the development of novel anti-inflammatory therapeutics," *British Journal of Pharmacology*, vol. 158, no. 4, pp. 936–946, 2009.

[13] P. Raynal and H. B. Pollard, "Annexins: the problem of assessing the biological role for a gene family of multifunctional calcium- and phospholipid-binding proteins," *Biochimica et Biophysica Acta—Biomembranes*, vol. 1197, no. 1, pp. 63–93, 1994.

[14] V. Gerke and S. E. Moss, "Annexins: from structure to function," *Physiological Reviews*, vol. 82, no. 2, pp. 331–371, 2002.

[15] V. Gerke, C. E. Creutz, and S. E. Moss, "Annexins: linking Ca^{2+} signalling to membrane dynamics," *Nature Reviews Molecular Cell Biology*, vol. 6, no. 6, pp. 449–461, 2005.

[16] R. J. Flower and G. J. Blackwell, "Anti-inflammatory steroids induce biosynthesis of a phospholipase A_2 inhibitor which prevents prostaglandin generation," *Nature*, vol. 278, no. 5703, pp. 456–459, 1979.

[17] G. Cirino and R. J. Flower, "Human recombinant lipocortin 1 inhibits prostacyclin production by human umbilical artery in vitro," *Prostaglandins*, vol. 34, no. 1, pp. 59–62, 1987.

[18] G. Cirino, R. J. Flower, J. L. Browning, L. K. Sinclair, and R. B. Pepinsky, "Recombinant human lipocortin 1 inhibits thromboxane release from guinea-pig isolated perfused lung," *Nature*, vol. 328, no. 6127, pp. 270–272, 1987.

[19] F. D'Acquisto, M. Perretti, and R. J. Flower, "Annexin-A1: a pivotal regulator of the innate and adaptive immune systems," *British Journal of Pharmacology*, vol. 155, no. 2, pp. 152–169, 2008.

[20] M. Perretti and F. D'Acquisto, "Annexin A1 and glucocorticoids as effectors of the resolution of inflammation," *Nature Reviews Immunology*, vol. 9, no. 1, pp. 62–70, 2009.

[21] A. Rosengarth, V. Gerke, and H. Luecke, "X-ray structure of full-length annexin 1 and implications for membrane aggregation," *Journal of Molecular Biology*, vol. 306, no. 3, pp. 489–498, 2001.

[22] N.-J. Hu, J. Bradshaw, H. Lauter, J. Buckingham, E. Solito, and A. Hofmann, "Membrane-induced folding and structure of membrane-bound annexin A1 N-terminal peptides: implications for annexin-induced membrane aggregation," *Biophysical Journal*, vol. 94, no. 5, pp. 1773–1781, 2008.

[23] S. M. Oliani, M. J. Paul-Clark, H. C. Christian, R. J. Flower, and M. Perretti, "Neutrophil interaction with inflamed postcapillary venule endothelium alters annexin 1 expression," *American Journal of Pathology*, vol. 158, no. 2, pp. 603–615, 2001.

[24] U. Rescher, V. Goebeler, A. Wilbers, and V. Gerke, "Proteolytic cleavage of annexin 1 by human leukocyte elastase," *Biochimica et Biophysica Acta—Molecular Cell Research*, vol. 1763, no. 11, pp. 1320–1324, 2006.

[25] L. Vong, F. D'Acquisto, M. Pederzoli-Ribeil et al., "Annexin 1 cleavage in activated neutrophils: a pivotal role for proteinase 3," *The Journal of Biological Chemistry*, vol. 282, no. 41, pp. 29998–30004, 2007.

[26] J. Dalli, A. P. Consalvo, V. Ray et al., "Proresolving and tissue-protective actions of annexin A1-based cleavage-resistant peptides are mediated by formyl peptide receptor 2/lipoxin A4 receptor," *Journal of Immunology*, vol. 190, no. 12, pp. 6478–6487, 2013.

[27] M. Pederzoli-Ribeil, F. Maione, D. Cooper et al., "Design and characterization of a cleavage-resistant Annexin A1 mutant to control inflammation in the microvasculature," *Blood*, vol. 116, no. 20, pp. 4288–4296, 2010.

[28] S. F. Smith, T. D. Tetley, A. Guz, and R. J. Flower, "Detection of lipocortin 1 in human lung lavage fluid: lipocortin degradation as a possible proteolytic mechanism in the control of inflammatory mediators and inflammation," *Environmental Health Perspectives*, vol. 85, pp. 135–144, 1990.

[29] F. H. C. Tsao, K. C. Meyer, X. Chen, N. S. Rosenthal, and J. Hu, "Degradation of annexin I in bronchoalveolar lavage fluid from patients with cystic fibrosis," *American Journal of Respiratory Cell and Molecular Biology*, vol. 18, no. 1, pp. 120–128, 1998.

[30] F. H. C. Tsao, Z. Xiang, A. Abbasi, and K. C. Meyer, "Neutrophil necrosis and annexin 1 degradation associated with airway inflammation in lung transplant recipients with cystic fibrosis," *BMC Pulmonary Medicine*, vol. 12, article 44, 2012.

[31] M. Perretti, S. K. Wheller, R. J. Flower, S. Wahid, and C. Pitzalis, "Modulation of cellular annexin I in human leukocytes infiltrating DTH skin reactions," *Journal of Leukocyte Biology*, vol. 65, no. 5, pp. 583–589, 1999.

[32] S. L. Williams, I. R. Milne, C. J. Bagley et al., "A proinflammatory role for proteolytically cleaved annexin A1 in neutrophil transendothelial migration," *Journal of Immunology*, vol. 185, no. 5, pp. 3057–3063, 2010.

[33] R. Hannon, J. D. Croxtall, S. J. Getting et al., "Aberrant inflammation and resistance to glucocorticoids in annexin 1$^{-/-}$ mouse," *The FASEB Journal*, vol. 17, no. 2, pp. 253–255, 2003.

[34] Y. H. Yang, E. F. Morand, S. J. Getting et al., "Modulation of inflammation and response to dexamethasone by Annexin 1 in antigen-induced arthritis," *Arthritis & Rheumatism*, vol. 50, no. 3, pp. 976–984, 2004.

[35] A. S. Damazo, S. Yona, R. J. Flower, M. Perretti, and S. M. Oliani, "Spatial and temporal profiles for anti-inflammatory gene expression in leukocytes during a resolving model of peritonitis," *The Journal of Immunology*, vol. 176, no. 7, pp. 4410–4418, 2006.

[36] F. N. E. Gavins, E. L. Hughes, N. A. P. S. Buss, P. M. Holloway, S. J. Getting, and J. C. Buckingham, "Leukocyte recruitment in the brain in sepsis: involvement of the annexin 1-FPR2/ALX anti-inflammatory system," *FASEB Journal*, vol. 26, no. 12, pp. 4977–4989, 2012.

[37] A. P. Girol, K. K. O. Mimura, C. C. Drewes et al., "Anti-inflammatory mechanisms of the annexin A1 protein and its mimetic peptide Ac2-26 in models of ocular inflammation in vivo and in vitro," *Journal of Immunology*, vol. 190, no. 11, pp. 5689–5701, 2013.

[38] W. Kao, R. Gu, Y. Jia et al., "A formyl peptide receptor agonist suppresses inflammation and bone damage in arthritis," *British Journal of Pharmacology*, vol. 171, no. 17, pp. 4087–4096, 2014.

[39] A. D. Gimenes, T. R. Andrade, C. B. Mello et al., "Beneficial effect of annexin A1 in a model of experimental allergic conjunctivitis," *Experimental Eye Research*, vol. 134, pp. 24–32, 2015.

[40] M. Drechsler, R. de Jong, J. Rossaint et al., "Annexin A1 counteracts chemokine-induced arterial myeloid cell recruitment," *Circulation Research*, vol. 116, no. 5, pp. 827–835, 2015.

[41] D. G. Souza, C. T. Fagundes, F. A. Amaral et al., "The required role of endogenously produced lipoxin A4 and annexin-1 for the production of IL-10 and inflammatory hyporesponsiveness in mice," *Journal of Immunology*, vol. 179, no. 12, pp. 8533–8543, 2007.

[42] G. Leoni, P. Neumann, N. Kamaly et al., "Annexin A1-containing extracellular vesicles and polymeric nanoparticles promote epithelial wound repair," *Journal of Clinical Investigation*, vol. 125, no. 3, pp. 1215–1227, 2015.

[43] R. D. Ye, F. Boulay, M. W. Ji et al., "International union of basic and clinical pharmacology. LXXIII. Nomenclature for the formyl peptide receptor (FPR) family," *Pharmacological Reviews*, vol. 61, no. 2, pp. 119–161, 2009.

[44] Y. Li, L. Cai, H. Wang et al., "Pleiotropic regulation of macrophage polarization and tumorigenesis by formyl peptide receptor-2," *Oncogene*, vol. 30, no. 36, pp. 3887–3899, 2011.

[45] S. Bena, V. Brancaleone, J. M. Wang, M. Perretti, and R. J. Flower, "Annexin A1 interaction with the FPR2/ALX receptor: identification of distinct domains and downstream associated signaling," *The Journal of Biological Chemistry*, vol. 287, no. 29, pp. 24690–24697, 2012.

[46] N. Chiang, I. M. Fierro, K. Gronert, and C. N. Serhan, "Activation of lipoxin A4 receptors by aspirin-triggered lipoxins and select peptides evokes ligand-specific responses in inflammation," *The Journal of Experimental Medicine*, vol. 191, no. 7, pp. 1197–1207, 2000.

[47] S. N. Cooray, T. Gobbetti, T. Montero-Melendez et al., "Ligand-specific conformational change of the G-protein-coupled receptor ALX/FPR2 determines proresolving functional responses," *Proceedings of the National Academy of Sciences of the United States of America*, vol. 110, no. 45, pp. 18232–18237, 2013.

[48] A. Walther, K. Riehemann, and V. Gerke, "A novel ligand of the formyl peptide receptor: annexin I regulates neutrophil extravasation by interacting with FPR," *Molecular Cell*, vol. 5, no. 5, pp. 831–840, 2000.

[49] J. Dalli, T. Montero-Melendez, S. McArthur, and M. Perretti, "Annexin A1 N-terminal derived peptide Ac2-26 exerts chemokinetic effects on human neutrophils," *Frontiers in Pharmacology*, vol. 3, article 28, 2012.

[50] V. Brancaleone, J. Dalli, S. Bena, R. J. Flower, G. Cirino, and M. Perretti, "Evidence for an anti-inflammatory loop centered on polymorphonuclear leukocyte formyl peptide receptor 2/lipoxin A$_4$ receptor and operative in the inflamed microvasculature," *The Journal of Immunology*, vol. 186, no. 8, pp. 4905–4914, 2011.

[51] B. D. Levy, C. B. Clish, B. Schmidt, K. Gronert, and C. N. Serhan, "Lipid mediator class switching during acute inflammation: signals in resolution," *Nature Immunology*, vol. 2, no. 7, pp. 612–619, 2001.

[52] O. Haworth, M. Cernadas, R. Yang, C. N. Serhan, and B. D. Levy, "Resolvin E1 regulates interleukin 23, interferon-γ and lipoxin A4 to promote the resolution of allergic airway inflammation," *Nature Immunology*, vol. 9, no. 8, pp. 873–879, 2008.

[53] C. Nathan, "Neutrophils and immunity: challenges and opportunities," *Nature Reviews Immunology*, vol. 6, no. 3, pp. 173–182, 2006.

[54] R. P. G. Hayhoe, A. M. Kamal, E. Solito, R. J. Flower, D. Cooper, and M. Perretti, "Annexin 1 and its bioactive peptide inhibit neutrophil-endothelium interactions under flow: indication of distinct receptor involvement," *Blood*, vol. 107, no. 5, pp. 2123–2130, 2006.

[55] D. H. Kusters, M. L. Chatrou, B. A. Willems et al., "Pharmacological treatment with annexin A1 reduces atherosclerotic plaque burden in LDLR-/- mice on western type diet," *PLoS ONE*, vol. 10, no. 6, Article ID e0130484, 2015.

[56] L. H. K. Lim, E. Solito, F. Russo-Marie, R. J. Flower, and M. Perretti, "Promoting detachment of neutrophils adherent to

murine postcapillary venules to control inflammation: effect of lipocortin 1," *Proceedings of the National Academy of Sciences of the United States of America*, vol. 95, no. 24, pp. 14535–14539, 1998.

[57] E. Solito, A. Kamal, F. Russo-Marie, J. C. Buckingham, S. Marullo, and M. Perretti, "A novel calcium-dependent proapoptotic effect of annexin 1 on human neutrophils," *The FASEB Journal*, vol. 17, no. 11, pp. 1544–1546, 2003.

[58] H. J. Strausbaugh and S. D. Rosen, "A potential role for annexin 1 as a physiologic mediator of glucocorticoid-induced L-selectin shedding from myeloid cells," *The Journal of Immunology*, vol. 166, no. 10, pp. 6294–6300, 2001.

[59] M. Perretti and R. J. Flower, "Modulation of IL-1-induced neutrophil migration by dexamethasone and lipocortin 1," *The Journal of Immunology*, vol. 150, no. 3, pp. 992–999, 1993.

[60] C. Zouki, S. Ouellet, and J. G. Filep, "The anti-inflammatory peptides, antiflammins, regulate the expression of adhesion molecules on human leukocytes and prevent neutrophil adhesion to endothelial cells," *The FASEB Journal*, vol. 14, no. 3, pp. 572–580, 2000.

[61] J. J. Moreno, "Antiflammin-2 prevents HL-60 adhesion to endothelial cells and prostanoid production induced by lipopolysaccharides," *Journal of Pharmacology and Experimental Therapeutics*, vol. 296, no. 3, pp. 884–889, 2001.

[62] R. A. P. Teixeira, K. K. O. Mimura, L. P. Araujo, K. V. Greco, and S. M. Oliani, "The essential role of annexin A1 mimetic peptide in the skin allograft survival," *Journal of Tissue Engineering and Regenerative Medicine*, 2013.

[63] K. E. Blume, S. Soeroes, H. Keppeler et al., "Cleavage of annexin A1 by ADAM10 during secondary necrosis generates a monocytic 'find-me' signal," *Journal of Immunology*, vol. 188, no. 1, pp. 135–145, 2012.

[64] S. McArthur, T. Gobbetti, D. H. Kusters, C. P. Reutelingsperger, R. J. Flower, and M. Perretti, "Definition of a novel pathway centered on lysophosphatidic acid to recruit monocytes during the resolution phase of tissue inflammation," *The Journal of Immunology*, vol. 195, no. 3, pp. 1139–1151, 2015.

[65] M. Scannell, M. B. Flanagan, A. DeStefani et al., "Annexin-1 and peptide derivatives are released by apoptotic cells and stimulate phagocytosis of apoptotic neutrophils by macrophages," *The Journal of Immunology*, vol. 178, no. 7, pp. 4595–4605, 2007.

[66] K. E. Blume, S. Soeroes, M. Waibel et al., "Cell surface externalization of annexin A1 as a failsafe mechanism preventing inflammatory responses during secondary necrosis," *The Journal of Immunology*, vol. 183, no. 12, pp. 8138–8147, 2009.

[67] P. Maderna, S. Yona, M. Perretti, and C. Godson, "Modulation of phagocytosis of apoptotic neutrophils by supernatant from dexamethasone-treated macrophages and annexin-derived peptide Ac$_{2-26}$," *The Journal of Immunology*, vol. 174, no. 6, pp. 3727–3733, 2005.

[68] I. Locatelli, S. Sutti, A. Jindal et al., "Endogenous annexin A1 is a novel protective determinant in nonalcoholic steatohepatitis in mice," *Hepatology*, vol. 60, no. 2, pp. 531–544, 2014.

[69] S. McArthur, E. Cristante, M. Paterno et al., "Annexin A1: a central player in the anti-inflammatory and neuroprotective role of microglia," *Journal of Immunology*, vol. 185, no. 10, pp. 6317–6328, 2010.

[70] D. Pupjalis, J. Goetsch, D. J. Kottas, V. Gerke, and U. Rescher, "Annexin A1 released from apoptotic cells acts through formyl peptide receptors to dampen inflammatory monocyte activation via JAK/STAT/SOCS signalling," *EMBO Molecular Medicine*, vol. 3, no. 2, pp. 102–114, 2011.

[71] P. Subramanian, I. Mitroulis, G. Hajishengallis, and T. Chavakis, "Regulation of tissue infiltration by neutrophils: role of integrin $\alpha 3\beta 1$ and other factors," *Current Opinion in Hematology*, vol. 23, no. 1, pp. 36–43, 2016.

[72] M. Perretti, J. D. Croxtall, S. K. Wheller, N. J. Goulding, R. Hannon, and R. J. Flower, "Mobilizing lipocortin 1 in adherent human leukocytes downregulates their transmigration," *Nature Medicine*, vol. 2, no. 11, pp. 1259–1262, 1996.

[73] C. D. Gil, M. La, M. Perretti, and S. M. Oliani, "Interaction of human neutrophils with endothelial cells regulates the expression of endogenous proteins annexin 1, galectin-1 and galectin-3," *Cell Biology International*, vol. 30, no. 4, pp. 338–344, 2006.

[74] T. S. Gastardelo, A. S. Damazo, J. Dalli, R. J. Flower, M. Perretti, and S. M. Oliani, "Functional and ultrastructural analysis of annexin A1 and its receptor in extravasating neutrophils during acute inflammation," *The American Journal of Pathology*, vol. 174, no. 1, pp. 177–183, 2009.

[75] J. Dalli, L. V. Norling, D. Renshaw, D. Cooper, K.-Y. Leung, and M. Perretti, "Annexin 1 mediates the rapid anti-inflammatory effects of neutrophil-derived microparticles," *Blood*, vol. 112, no. 6, pp. 2512–2519, 2008.

[76] A. Montresor, L. Toffali, G. Constantin, and C. Laudanna, "Chemokines and the signaling modules regulating integrin affinity," *Frontiers in Immunology*, vol. 3, article 127, 2012.

[77] J. L. Bos, K. de Bruyn, J. Enserink et al., "The role of Rap1 in integrin-mediated cell adhesion," *Biochemical Society Transactions*, vol. 31, no. 1, pp. 83–86, 2003.

[78] B. Stuqui, M. de Paula-Silva, C. P. Carlos et al., "Ac2-26 mimetic peptide of annexin A1 inhibits local and systemic inflammatory processes induced by *Bothrops moojeni* venom and the Lys-49 phospholipase A$_2$ in a rat model," *PLoS ONE*, vol. 10, no. 7, Article ID e0130803, 2015.

[79] B. C. Guido, M. Zanatelli, W. Tavares-De-Lima, S. M. Oliani, and A. S. Damazo, "Annexin-A1 peptide down-regulates the leukocyte recruitment and up-regulates interleukin-10 release into lung after intestinal ischemia-reperfusion in mice," *Journal of Inflammation*, vol. 10, no. 1, article 10, 2013.

[80] L. Miele, E. Cordella-Miele, A. Facchiano, and A. B. Mukherjee, "Novel anti-inflammatory peptides from the region of highest similarity between uteroglobin and lipocortin I," *Nature*, vol. 335, no. 6192, pp. 726–730, 1988.

[81] A. M. Kamal, R. P. G. Hayhoe, A. Paramasivam et al., "Antiflammin-2 activates the human formyl-peptide receptor like 1," *TheScientificWorldJOURNAL*, vol. 6, pp. 1375–1384, 2006.

[82] N. Chiang, C. N. Serhan, S.-E. Dahlén et al., "The lipoxin receptor ALX: potent ligand-specific and stereoselective actions in vivo," *Pharmacological Reviews*, vol. 58, no. 3, pp. 463–487, 2006.

[83] C. Summers, S. M. Rankin, A. M. Condliffe, N. Singh, A. M. Peters, and E. R. Chilvers, "Neutrophil kinetics in health and disease," *Trends in Immunology*, vol. 31, no. 8, pp. 318–324, 2010.

[84] T. Tak, K. Tesselaar, J. Pillay, J. A. M. Borghans, and L. Koenderman, "What's your age again? Determination of human neutrophil half-lives revisited," *Journal of Leukocyte Biology*, vol. 94, no. 4, pp. 595–601, 2013.

[85] J. G. Filep and D. El Kebir, "Neutrophil apoptosis: a target for enhancing the resolution of inflammation," *Journal of Cellular Biochemistry*, vol. 108, no. 5, pp. 1039–1046, 2009.

[86] D. El Kebir, L. József, and J. G. Filep, "Opposing regulation of neutrophil apoptosis through the formyl peptide receptor-like 1/lipoxin A$_4$ receptor: implications for resolution of inflammation," *Journal of Leukocyte Biology*, vol. 84, no. 3, pp. 600–606, 2008.

[87] Y. Tabe, L. Jin, R. Contractor et al., "Novel role of HDAC inhibitors in AML1/ETO AML cells: activation of apoptosis and phagocytosis through induction of annexin A1," *Cell Death and Differentiation*, vol. 14, no. 8, pp. 1443–1456, 2007.

[88] T. Montero-Melendez, J. Dalli, and M. Perretti, "Gene expression signature-based approach identifies a pro-resolving mechanism of action for histone deacetylase inhibitors," *Cell Death and Differentiation*, vol. 20, no. 4, pp. 567–575, 2013.

[89] A. G. Rossi, D. A. Sawatzky, A. Walker et al., "Cyclin-dependent kinase inhibitors enhance the resolution of inflammation by promoting inflammatory cell apoptosis," *Nature Medicine*, vol. 12, no. 9, pp. 1056–1064, 2006.

[90] E. E. McGrath, H. M. Marriott, A. Lawrie et al., "TNF-related apoptosis-inducing ligand (TRAIL) regulates inflammatory neutrophil apoptosis and enhances resolution of inflammation," *Journal of Leukocyte Biology*, vol. 90, no. 5, pp. 855–865, 2011.

[91] C. D. Lucas, D. A. Dorward, M. A. Tait et al., "Downregulation of Mcl-1 has anti-inflammatory pro-resolution effects and enhances bacterial clearance from the lung," *Mucosal Immunology*, vol. 7, no. 4, pp. 857–868, 2014.

[92] I. K. H. Poon, C. D. Lucas, A. G. Rossi, and K. S. Ravichandran, "Apoptotic cell clearance: basic biology and therapeutic potential," *Nature Reviews Immunology*, vol. 14, no. 3, pp. 166–180, 2014.

[93] P. Maderna and C. Godson, "Phagocytosis of apoptotic cells and the resolution of inflammation," *Biochimica et Biophysica Acta (BBA)—Molecular Basis of Disease*, vol. 1639, no. 3, pp. 141–151, 2003.

[94] O. Soehnlein, L. Lindbom, and C. Weber, "Mechanisms underlying neutrophil-mediated monocyte recruitment," *Blood*, vol. 114, no. 21, pp. 4613–4623, 2009.

[95] H. L. Wright, R. J. Moots, R. C. Bucknall, and S. W. Edwards, "Neutrophil function in inflammation and inflammatory diseases," *Rheumatology*, vol. 49, no. 9, pp. 1618–1631, 2010.

[96] K. S. Ravichandran, "Beginnings of a good apoptotic meal: the find-me and eat-me signaling pathways," *Immunity*, vol. 35, no. 4, pp. 445–455, 2011.

[97] S. Arur, U. E. Uche, K. Rezaul et al., "Annexin I is an endogenous ligand that mediates apoptotic cell engulfment," *Developmental Cell*, vol. 4, no. 4, pp. 587–598, 2003.

[98] P. Maderna, D. C. Cottell, T. Toivonen et al., "FPR2/ALX receptor expression and internalization are critical for lipoxin A4 and annexin-derived peptide-stimulated phagocytosis," *The FASEB Journal*, vol. 24, no. 11, pp. 4240–4249, 2010.

[99] S. Yona, S. E. M. Heinsbroek, L. Peiser, S. Gordon, M. Perretti, and R. J. Flower, "Impaired phagocytic mechanism in annexin 1 null macrophages," *British Journal of Pharmacology*, vol. 148, no. 4, pp. 469–477, 2006.

[100] J. Dalli, C. P. Jones, D. M. Cavalcanti, S. H. Farsky, M. Perretti, and S. M. Rankin, "Annexin A1 regulates neutrophil clearance by macrophages in the mouse bone marrow," *The FASEB Journal*, vol. 26, no. 1, pp. 387–396, 2012.

[101] R. E. Voll, M. Herrmann, E. A. Roth, C. Stach, J. R. Kalden, and I. Girkontaite, "Immunosuppressive effects of apoptotic cells," *Nature*, vol. 390, no. 6658, pp. 350–351, 1997.

[102] V. A. Fadok, D. L. Bratton, A. Konowal, P. W. Freed, J. Y. Westcott, and P. M. Henson, "Macrophages that have ingested apoptotic cells in vitro inhibit proinflammatory cytokine production through autocrine/paracrine mechanisms involving TGF-β, PGE2, and PAF," *The Journal of Clinical Investigation*, vol. 101, no. 4, pp. 890–898, 1998.

[103] M.-L. N. Huynh, V. A. Fadok, and P. M. Henson, "Phosphatidylserine-dependent ingestion of apoptotic cells promotes TGF-β1 secretion and the resolution of inflammation," *Journal of Clinical Investigation*, vol. 109, no. 1, pp. 41–50, 2002.

[104] A. S. Damazo, S. Yona, F. D'Acquisto, R. J. Flower, S. M. Oliani, and M. Perretti, "Critical protective role for annexin 1 gene expression in the endotoxemic murine microcirculation," *American Journal of Pathology*, vol. 166, no. 6, pp. 1607–1617, 2005.

[105] Y. H. Yang, D. Aeberli, A. Dacumos, J. R. Xue, and E. F. Morand, "Annexin-1 regulates macrophage IL-6 and TNF via glucocorticoid-induced leucine zipper," *Journal of Immunology*, vol. 183, no. 2, pp. 1435–1445, 2009.

[106] P. Del Gaudio, F. De Cicco, R. P. Aquino et al., "Evaluation of in situ injectable hydrogels as controlled release device for ANXA1 derived peptide in wound healing," *Carbohydrate Polymers*, vol. 115, pp. 629–633, 2015.

[107] N. Kamaly, G. Fredman, M. Subramanian et al., "Development and in vivo efficacy of targeted polymeric inflammation-resolving nanoparticles," *Proceedings of the National Academy of Sciences of the United States of America*, vol. 110, no. 16, pp. 6506–6511, 2013.

[108] G. Fredman, N. Kamaly, S. Spolitu et al., "Targeted nanoparticles containing the proresolving peptide Ac2-26 protect against advanced atherosclerosis in hypercholesterolemic mice," *Science Translational Medicine*, vol. 7, no. 275, Article ID 275ra20, 2015.

15

A Preliminary Comparative Assessment of the Role of CD8+ T Cells in Chronic Fatigue Syndrome/Myalgic Encephalomyelitis and Multiple Sclerosis

Ekua W. Brenu,[1] **Simon Broadley,**[2] **Thao Nguyen,**[1,3] **Samantha Johnston,**[1,3]
Sandra Ramos,[1] **Don Staines,**[1] **and Sonya Marshall-Gradisnik**[1,3]

[1] *The National Centre for Neuroimmunology and Emerging Diseases, Griffith Health Institute, Griffith University, Gold Coast, Australia*
[2] *School of Medicine, Griffith University, Gold Coast, Australia*
[3] *School of Medical Science, Griffith University, Gold Coast, Australia*

Correspondence should be addressed to Sonya Marshall-Gradisnik; s.marshall-gradisnik@griffith.edu.au

Academic Editor: Jacek Tabarkiewicz

Background. CD8+ T cells have putative roles in the regulation of adaptive immune responses during infection. The purpose of this paper is to compare the status of CD8+ T cells in Multiple Sclerosis (MS) and Chronic Fatigue Syndrome/Myalgic Encephalomyelitis (CFS/ME). *Methods.* This preliminary investigation comprised 23 CFS/ME patients, 11 untreated MS patients, and 30 nonfatigued controls. Whole blood samples were collected from participants, stained with monoclonal antibodies, and analysed on the flow cytometer. Using the following CD markers, CD27 and CD45RA (CD45 exon isoform 4), CD8+ T cells were divided into naïve, central memory (CM), effector memory CD45RA− (EM), and effector memory CD45RA+ (EMRA) cells. *Results.* Surface expressions of BTLA, CD127, and CD49/CD29 were increased on subsets of CD8+ T cells from MS patients. In the CFS/ME patients CD127 was significantly decreased on all subsets of CD8+ T cells in comparison to the nonfatigued controls. PSGL-1 was significantly reduced in the CFS/ME patients in comparison to the nonfatigued controls. *Conclusions.* The results suggest significant deficits in the expression of receptors and adhesion molecules on subsets of CD8+ T cells in both MS and CFS/ME patients. These deficits reported may contribute to the pathogenesis of these diseases. However, larger sample size is warranted to confirm and support these encouraging preliminary findings.

1. Background

Chronic Fatigue Syndrome/Myalgic Encephalomyelitis (CFS/ME) is characterised by significant impairments in physical activity as a consequence of severe fatigue and other flu like symptoms. CFS/ME remains an unexplained disorder with substantial physiological impairments where diagnosis is based on self-report measures. Fatigue is present in other disorders, including Multiple Sclerosis (MS), where 70% of patients are plagued with fatigue and this can be disabling in a minority of patients [1–3]. This fatigue can be severe and has consequences on normal daily activity [4, 5]. CFS/ME has been reported in some MS patients where patients demonstrate classic CFS/ME symptoms such as intermittent headaches, malaise, and joint and muscle

pain [6]. Nonetheless, diagnosis of MS also relies upon the demonstration of dissemination in time and space of central nervous system (CNS) lesions clinically or radiographically, often supported by biochemical and electrophysiological tests [7]. MS patients may be classified as relapsing remitting (RR-MS), primary-progressive (PP-MS), secondary-progressive (SP-MS), or clinically isolated syndrome [8].

MS is a neurological disorder characterised by inflammatory demyelination in the CNS while CFS/ME patients may experience nervous system manifestations of lack of concentration and autonomic symptoms [9–12]. Neuroimaging studies have suggested the presence of neuroinflammation in the midbrain of CFS/ME patients [11]. Despite some relative ambiguities in CFS/ME symptomatology, immune dysregulation is a common occurrence in CFS/ME as well as in MS. It has previously been postulated that symptom similarities between CFS/ME and MS may be explained by shared neuroimmune pathways [13]. The most common immune abnormality in both CFS/ME and MS is related to Natural Killer (NK) cell cytotoxic activity. Dysfunctional NK cell activity has been reported in patients with MS and CFS/ME. In MS patients, alterations in NK cell function and receptor expression contribute significantly to the pathogenesis of the disease [14, 15]. In CFS/ME, NK cell dysfunction involves decreased cytotoxic activity [16–18]. T cells have also been implicated in MS. Importantly, regulatory T cells (Tregs) are dysregulated and levels of these cells are related to the phase of the disease [19, 20].

Expansion of autoreactive lymphocytes in MS results in inflammatory and active immune responses in the CNS as these lymphocytes are able to migrate to the CNS and induce damage [21]. Reducing the activities of these autoreactive lymphocytes is the fundamental goal of many therapeutic interventions in MS [22]. CD8+ T cells have been extensively studied in MS owing to their presence in the CNS lesions of MS patients. In MS, pathogenic CD8+ T cells may induce proinflammatory reactions via interleukin- (IL-) 17 and interferon- (IFN-) γ and eliminate oligodendrocytes while regulatory CD8+ T cells suppress autoreactive CD4+ T cells reactions and promote anti-inflammatory reactions [23]. In CFS/ME patients CD8+ T cells may display diminished levels of activation, reduced cytotoxicity, and low numbers of effector memory cells [18, 24].

It is apparent that CD8+ T cells are involved in the pathogenesis of CFS/ME and MS; hence, the aim of this study was to determine whether dysregulation in cytotoxic CD8+ T cells follows a similar pattern in CFS/ME and MS.

2. Methods

2.1. Subjects. CFS/ME participants were defined according to the International Consensus Criteria (ICC) [25]. Disability in the CFS/ME patients was measured using Dr. Bell's Disability Adjustment scale [26]. MS cases were clinically diagnosed as having MS according to the revised McDonald criteria [7]. MS disease progression and responsiveness were assessed using the Expanded Disability Status Scale (EDSS) [27] and disease severity was measured using the MS Severity Scale (MSSS) [7]. Nonfatigued controls had no incidence of CFS/ME or MS and were in good health without evidence of fatigue. Excluded from the study were smokers, pregnant woman, breastfeeding, or having been clinically diagnosed with any other major diseases. All subjects gave informed written consent to participate in the study and the study received ethical approval from the Griffith University Human Ethics Committee (MSC/18/13/HREC) prior to commencement.

2.2. Assessment of CD8+ T Cell Phenotypes. Whole blood (10 mL) was collected from all participants and analysed within 12 hours of collection. To identify subsets of CD8+ T cells at different stages of differentiation, samples were labelled with fluorochrome conjugated monoclonal antibodies, including CD3, CD8, CD27, and CD45RA (CD45 exon

isoform 4). Cells were analysed on the Fortessa 2.0 (Becton Dickenson (BD) Biosciences, San Jose). For each CD8+ T cell assessment, forward and side scatter plots were used to determine the lymphocyte population. Cells of interest were identified from the lymphocyte population as cells expressing CD3+ and CD8+. The expression of cytokines, chemokine receptors, adhesion molecules, and migratory molecules on CD8+ T cells were also examined using the following markers: CCR5, CCR7, CXCR3, CD49d, CD29, CD18, CD11a, PSGL-1, and CD127. Glycoprotein, CD44, was also examined.

2.3. Assessment of CD8+ T Cell Receptors. Inhibitory receptors were measured in whole blood cells stained with monoclonal antibodies including KLRG1, LAG3, CTLA4, and BTLA. The expression patterns of these inhibitory receptors were examined on the CD8+ T cell phenotypes. Coexpression of these receptors was also assessed on subsets of CD8+ T cells.

2.4. Statistical Analysis. Statistical analyses were executed using SPSS (version 18.0, SPSS Inc., Chicago, USA) and Graph Pad Prism (version 6.0, Graph Pad Software, Inc., San Diego, USA). A test for normality was performed using the Kolmogorov-Smirnov tests. ANOVA was used to determine significance for normally distributed data while the independent sample Kruskal Wallis test was used as the nonparametric. Bonferroni analysis was used to assess significant parameter differences post hoc. Pearson chi square test was used to determine significant gender differences. P values less than or equal to 0.05 were considered significant. The data is expressed as either median or mean ± standard error of the mean (SEM).

3. Results

3.1. Subject Characteristics. The characteristics of the participants recruited in the study are outlined in Table 1. A number of the CFS/ME patients were taking a combination of different medications at the time of the study. These medications include anticholinergic ($n = 1$), antihistamine ($n = 1$), antidepressant ($n = 10$), blood pressure medication ($n = 1$), steroids ($n = 2$), anticonvulsants ($n = 4$), Benodiazepines ($n = 1$), opioid receptor antagonist ($n = 1$), asthma ($n = 3$), cardiotonic agent ($n = 2$), anti-inflammatory ($n = 3$), opioids ($n = 2$), opioid analgesics ($n = 4$), triptans ($n = 1$), proton pump inhibitors ($n = 3$), vitamins and supplements ($n = 5$), anticoagulants ($n = 2$), and laxatives ($n = 1$). Nine of the CFS/ME patients were on no medications at the time of the study. Mean disability in the CFS/ME cases was 47.14% ± 2.20 (SD) using Dr. Bell's Disability score and classifying CFS/ME as moderate CFS/ME patients as described [28] (Table 2).

MS patients were not on any immunomodulatory therapies during this study, nor had they taken these previously. Of the 11 MS patients, there were relapsing-remitting ($n = 4$), secondary-progressive ($n = 2$), primary-progressive ($n = 2$), and clinically isolated syndrome ($n = 3$) cases. The average number of relapses (ever) rate among the MS cases

TABLE 1: Characteristics of participants and blood parameters.

	CFS/ME	MS	Controls	Overall	P value MS versus CFS/ME	P value MS versus control	P value CFS/ME versus control
Participants (n)	23	11	30				
Age (years)	49.0 ± 2.5	56.0 ± 4.9	53.5 ± 2.2	0.72	>0.99	>0.99	>0.99
Females, n (%)	17 (73.9)	10 (90.9)	19 (63.3)	0.44			
Haemoglobin (g/L)	135.0 ± 2.25	136.0 ± 2.90	139.0 ± 2.35	0.24	>0.99	0.89	0.32
White cell count ($\times 10^9$/L)	5.60 ± 0.32	6.80 ± 0.64	6.00 ± 0.25	**0.04***	**0.04***	0.52	0.28
Platelets	228.0 ± 13.34	264.0 ± 15.80	249.50 ± 10.69	0.76	>0.99	>0.99	>0.99
Haematocrit (%)	0.41 ± 0.01	0.40 ± 0.01	0.41 ± 0.01	0.35	>0.99	>0.99	0.49
Red cell count ($\times 10^{12}$/L)	4.49 ± 0.07	4.55 ± 0.13	4.61 ± 0.07	0.53	>0.99	>0.99	0.79
MCV (fL)	89.17 ± 0.69	89.20 ± 0.85	89.53 ± 0.68	0.72	>0.99	>0.99	>0.99
Neutrophils ($\times 10^9$/L)	3.38 ± 0.25	4.20 ± 0.49	3.53 ± 0.17	0.39	0.53	0.82	>0.99
Lymphocytes ($\times 10^9$/L)	1.63 ± 0.09	2.30 ± 0.23	1.95 ± 0.10	**0.001***	**0.001***	0.13	0.11
Monocytes ($\times 10^9$/L)	0.31 ± 0.02	0.45 ± 0.03	0.33 ± 0.02	**0.0004***	**0.002***	**0.0004***	>0.99
Eosinophils ($\times 10^9$/L)	0.14 ± 0.015	0.21 ± 0.03	0.12 ± 0.01	**0.02***	0.13	**0.01***	0.91
Basophils ($\times 10^9$/L)	0.02 ± 0.004	0.03 ± 0.004	0.02 ± 0.003	0.41	0.56	>0.99	>0.99
ESR (mm/Hr)	10.50 ± 2.59	13.00 ± 5.29	10.00 ± 1.91	0.21	>0.99	0.89	0.26

Data is represented as mean ± SEM, where * represents $P < 0.05$.

TABLE 2: Clinical characteristics of CFS/ME and MS.

	CFS/ME (n = 23, mean ± SD)	MS (n = 11, mean ± SD)
Dr. Bell's Disability	47.14% ± 2.20	
Expanded Disability Status Scale		2.41 ± 0.79
Multiple Sclerosis Severity Scale		2.85 ± 0.89
Courses		
(i) Relapsing-remitting		n = 4
(ii) Secondary-progressive		n = 2
(iii) Primary-progressive		n = 2
(iv) Clinically isolated syndrome		n = 3
Age of onset (years)	35.28 ± 4.63	6.11 ± 2.45
Duration (years)	14.96 ± 8.87	13.76 ± 3.83
Relapses rate		2.4 ± 0.55

was 2.4±0.55. MS mean age was 56.0±4.9 (SD) years reported illness onset of an average of 6.11 years ± 2.45 (SD) for a duration of 13.76 years ± 3.83 (SD). The mean EDSS and MSSS scores for the MS patients were 2.41±0.79 (SD) and 2.85±0.89 (SD), respectively, which classifies MS patients as moderately disabled (Table 2).

In each group there were a large percentage of females in comparison to males but there was no significant difference in gender. Full blood count analyses were performed on all samples to determine the distribution of the different blood cells (Table 1). White blood cells, lymphocytes, monocytes, and eosinophils were significantly higher in the MS group compared to the other groups. CD8+ T cell phenotypes CD27 and CD45RA surface markers were used to determine lineage differentiation (naïve and memory phenotypes) of the CD8+ T cells. Four different subsets of CD8+ T cells were characterized including CD8+CD3+CD27+CD45RA+ cells (naïve), CD8+CD3+CD27+CD45RA− cells (central memory [2]), CD8+CD3+CD27−CD45RA− cells (effector memory [EM]), and CD8+CD3+CD27−CD45RA+ cells (CD45RA+ effector memory [EMRA]). There were no significant differences in total CD8+ T cells, naïve, CM, EM, and EMRA CD8+ T cells among the three groups (Table 3).

3.1.1. Quantitation of Inhibitory Receptors on CD8+ T Cells. Surface expression of the following inhibitory receptors was examined on the CD8+ T cells, KLRG1, LAG3, CTLA4, and BTLA. These receptors were measured on total CD8+ T cells and subsets of CD8+ T cells at different stages of differentiation as previously described. Only BTLA was significantly elevated in the naïve and CM CD8+ T cells from the MS patients compared with the CFS/ME patients and the nonfatigued controls (Figure 1).

TABLE 3: Distribution of total and subsets of CD8+ T cells in CFS/ME patients, MS patients, and nonfatigued controls.

CD8+ T cells (%)	CFS/ME	MS	Nonfatigued controls	P value			
				Overall	MS versus CFS/ME	CFS/ME versus control	MS versus control
Total CD8+ T cells	13.25 ± 0.86	12.36 ± 1.89	13.24 ± 0.88	0.84	>0.99	>0.99	>0.99
Naïve CD8+ T cells	33.86 ± 3.89	36.76 ± 5.76	24.20 ± 2.19	0.07	>0.99	0.12	0.29
CM CD8+ T cells	31.88 ± 2.63	38.50 ± 2.36	32.93 ± 2.75	0.51	0.81	>0.99	0.88
EM CD8+ T cells	12.52 ± 2.15	15.83 ± 2.77	18.64 ± 2.13	0.07	>0.99	0.08	0.51
EMRA CD8+ T cells	10.18 ± 2.21	6.86 ± 2.22	13.38 ± 2.13	0.06	0.82	0.43	0.08

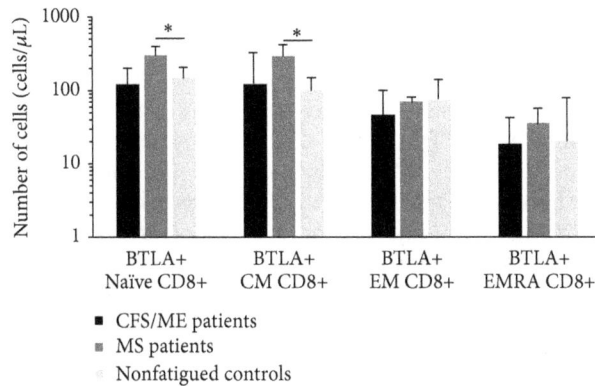

FIGURE 1: Expression of BTLA on CD8+ T cells in CFS/ME, MS, and nonfatigued controls. BTLA was increased on naïve and CM CD8+ T cells in the MS compared with controls. Data is represented as median ± SEM, where * represents $P < 0.05$ (EM: effector memory, EMRA: effector memory RA, and CM: central memory).

3.1.2. Expression Pattern of Cytokine and Chemokine Receptors. Expression of cytokine receptors including CCR7, CCR5, and CD127 was measured on total CD8+ T cells and subsets of CD8+ T cells at different stages of differentiation. CD49/CD29 was significantly reduced on the EM CD8+ T cells of the CFS/ME patients in comparison to the nonfatigued controls, while in the MS patients, CD49d/CD29 was significantly elevated in the naïve and EMRA CD8+ T cells in comparison to the nonfatigued controls (Figure 2(a)). When the expressions of these receptors were examined, significant decrease in the expression of CD127+ was observed on most subsets of CD8+ T cells from the CFS/ME patients while in the MS patients, CD127 expression was reduced on naïve, EM, and EMRA subsets of CD8+ T cells in the CFS/ME patients (Figure 2(b)). Differential levels of integrins and selectins and cell surface glycoproteins PSGL, KLRG1, CD11a/CD18, and CD44 were measured on total and subsets of CD8+ T cells at different stages of differentiation. PSGL-1 was significantly reduced on EMRA CD8+ T cells in the CFS/ME patients in comparison to the nonfatigued controls (Figure 3).

4. Discussion

This preliminary study has identified significant impairments in subsets of CD8+ T cells in CFS/ME and MS patients. Overall the MS patients showed significant differences in the expression of receptors and adhesion molecules in comparison to the CFS/ME patients. These results demonstrate CD8+ T cells might play a role in the pathogenesis of MS compared with CFS/ME. PSGL-1 is elevated on CD4+ T cells in RR-MS patients and this may suggest an important role in the transmigration of lymphocytes to the CNS [29]. However, total CD8+ T cells in these patients have stable levels of PSGL-1 [29]. Therefore, the expression of PSGL-1 on CD8+ T cells may to some extent be dependent on the stage and type of disease. Nonetheless, it is possible that these cells have high affinity to transmigrate the blood brain barrier (BBB) and this may be specific to naïve CD8+ T cells in MS. In MS, PSGL-1 is important for the adhesion and recruitment of CD8+ T cells to the inflamed CNS [30]. CD49d/CD29 represents the $\alpha 4\beta 1$ integrin, adhesion molecules which are important during inflammation. CD49d/CD29 has been shown to be significantly elevated on PBMCs in demyelinated lesions in the CNS [31]. An increase in the expression of $\alpha 4\beta 1$ on the cell surface may suggest increased migration of CD8+ T cells to the CNS. High levels of $\alpha 4\beta 1$ on the CD8+ T cells in particular, in the naïve and EMRA subsets may indicate a reduced prevalence of soluble VCAM-1, IFN-γ, and TNF [32]. Soluble VCAM-1 is known to suppress the function of $\alpha 4\beta 1$ under normal physiological concentration, while in the CFS/ME patients decreased expression of CD49d/CD29 on EM CD8+ T cells may indicate reduced migration of effector cells to sites of inflammation. CD127 is the receptor for IL-7 and is an important marker for T cell maturation and function. Binding of IL-7 to this receptor is a vital component in the release of granzymes resulting in demyelination [33]. In MS polymorphism in the CD127 gene sequence is an associated risk factor [34]. CD127 has four different haplotypes. Haplotype 1 results in the production of enormous amounts of sCD127; haplotype 2 is associated with a less soluble form of sCD127 due to low levels of exon 6 splicing and is associated with a lower risk of MS [35]. Homozygosity for haplotype

(a)

(b)

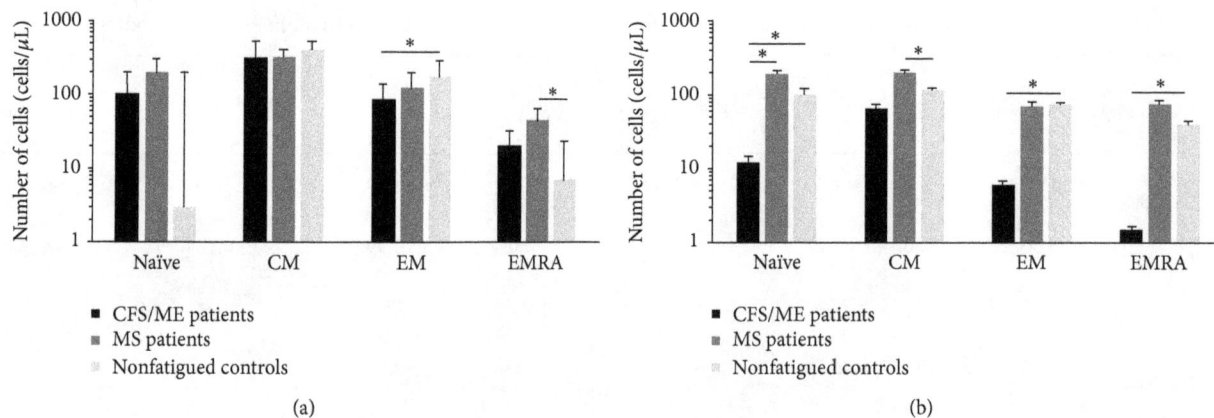

FIGURE 2: Expression of receptors in CFS/ME, MS, and nonfatigued controls. (a) CD49d/CD29 was reduced in EM subsets of CD8+ T cells in the CFS/ME patients but elevated in EMRA subsets of CD8+ T cells in MS patients compared to controls. (b) CD127 expression was reduced on naïve, EM, and EMRA subsets of CD8+ T cells in the CFS/ME patients but not CM subsets as CD127+ CD8+ T cells were evaluated in MS patients compared with controls. MS patients also demonstrated elevated naïve CD8 T cells compared with controls. Data is represented as median ± SEM, where * represents $P < 0.05$ (EM: effector memory, EMRA: effector memory RA, and CM: central memory).

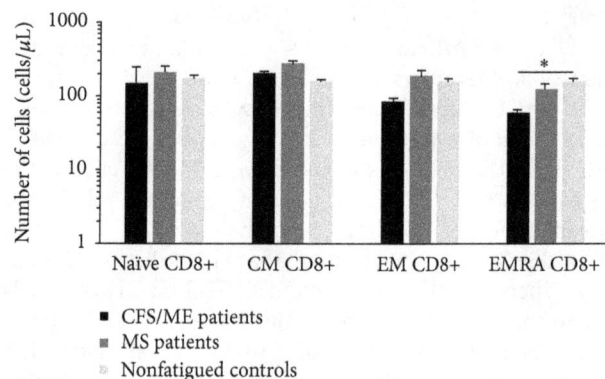

FIGURE 3: Expression of adhesion molecules on subsets of CD8+ T cells in CFS/ME, MS, and nonfatigued controls. Expression levels of PSGL-1 were reduced on EMRA CD8+ T cells in the CFS/ME patients compared with the nonfatigued controls. Data is represented as ± SEM, where * represents $P < 0.05$ (EM: effector memory, EMRA: effector memory RA, and CM: central memory).

4 increases the likelihood of MS [36]. It has been suggested that polymorphisms in CD127 and its cytokine IL-7 may be correlated with susceptibility to MS [37]. The MS group in this study demonstrated heightened levels of CD127+ on all subsets of CD8+ T cells in comparison to the CFS/ME patients but this was only significant in the EMRA CD8+ T cells. Interestingly, IL-7 may inhibit the function of VCAM-1 by binding to it and thus allowing the dominance of $\alpha 4\beta 1$ integrin which facilitates the movement of T cells to the CNS. In the CNS, CD8+ T cell cytotoxic activity may be further enhanced by IL-7 resulting in an overabundance of granzymes and consequently increasing demyelination in the CNS [38, 39]. The expression of CD127+ was decreased on most CD8+ T cell subsets in the CFS/ME patients compared with both MS and controls. Reduced CD127 in the CFS/ME patients was corroborated with reduced $\alpha 4\beta 1$

integrin confirming significant alterations in the migratory potential of the CD8+ T cells in CFS/ME patients. The exact role of CD127 on CD8+ T cells in CFS/ME is unclear though it has been suggested that reduced CD127 on exhausted CD8+ T cells might be responsible for the inability for CD8+ T cells to suppress viral persistence [40]. CD8+ T cell exhaustion has been previously suggested in CFS/ME owing to the overwhelming levels of other exhaustion markers including PD1 and CD95 [24]. BTLA is another inhibitory coreceptor expressed on CD8+ T cell; similar to CD127, BTLA expression was increased in the MS patients compared to the CFS/ME patients. BTLA is known to bind to TNF receptor family member herpesvirus entry mediator (HVEM). This initiates a sequence of events involving phosphorylation of ITIM motifs and induction of phosphatases SHP-1 and SHP-2 [41]. BTLA and HVEM interact in either cis or trans configuration and this inhibits or activates NF-κB, respectively [42]. Increased expression of BTLA on naïve and CM CD8+ T cells may indicate suppression of T cell receptor signalling via CD3 and/or CD28 [43]. Additionally, BTLA interaction with HVEM promotes cell survival and memory generation of effector CD8+ T cells [44].

Previous research has indicated decreases in total CD8+ T cells in particularly EM and EMRA CD8+ T cells [45, 46]. However, in the present study although total CD8+ EM and EMRA T cells were reduced in MS patients this was not statistically significant.

5. Conclusions

In summary, these preliminary findings provide new insight into the possibility of hyper activated inflammatory CD8+ T cell profile in untreated MS patients while CFS/ME patients may display an exhausted profile which permits viral prevalence and persistence. The above data may suggest that the differential expressions of receptors and adhesion molecules in MS patients are in response to imbalances in neuroimmune homeostasis. In comparison to CFS/ME patients, MS patients may have more severe immune dysregulation. Nevertheless it is likely that impairments in CD8+ T cells in CFS/ME patients relate to abnormal levels of adhesion and migratory molecules and these abnormalities may contribute to the persistent immune dysregulation observed and warrant further validation in a larger sample size.

Abbreviations

CD: Cluster of differentiation
MS: Multiple Sclerosis
CFS/ME: Chronic Fatigue Syndrome/Myalgic Encephalomyelitis
CM: Central memory
EM: Effector memory
EMRA: Effector memory cells expressing CD45RA
BTLA: B- and T-lymphocyte attenuator
KLRG1: Killer cell lectin-like receptor subfamily G member 1
LAG3:   Lymphocyte-activation protein 3
CTLA-4: Cytotoxic T-lymphocyte-associated protein 4
CCR7:   Chemokine receptor type 7
CCR5:   Chemokine receptor type 5
VCAM-1: Vascular cell adhesion protein 1
IFN-γ: Interferon gamma
TNF: Tumor necrosis factor
IL-7:   Interleukin-7
CNS: Central Nervous System
PD1:   Programmed cell death protein 1
HVEM: Herpes virus entry mediator
NF-κB: Nuclear factor kappa-light-chain enhancer of activated B cells.

Disclaimer

The authors alone are responsible for the content and writing of the paper.

Conflict of Interests

The authors report no conflict of interests.

Authors' Contribution

Ekua W. Brenu, Thao Nguyen, and Samantha Johnston wrote the paper, Simon Broadley provided the MS patients and reviewed the paper, and Sonya Marshall-Gradisnik and Don Staines provided supervision and assisted with the writing of the paper.

Acknowledgments

The authors would like to acknowledge the National Centre for Neuroimmunology and Emerging Diseases, Alison Hunter Memorial Foundation, Mason Foundation (Grant no. MA43120), and Queensland Government Science, Information Technology, Innovation and the Arts Smart Futures Fund (Grant no. 216702MRE) for their support.

References

[1] P. J. Jongen, D. Lehnick, J. Koeman et al., "Fatigue and health-related quality of life in relapsing-remitting multiple sclerosis after 2 years glatiramer acetate treatment are predicted by changes at 6 months: an observational multi-center study," *Journal of Neurology*, vol. 261, no. 8, pp. 1469–1476, 2014.

[2] M. H. Cameron, V. Peterson, E. A. Boudreau et al., "Fatigue is associated with poor sleep in people with multiple sclerosis and cognitive impairment," *Multiple Sclerosis International*, vol. 2014, Article ID 872732, 5 pages, 2014.

[3] A. A. Holland, D. Graves, B. M. Greenberg, and L. L. Harder, "Fatigue, emotional functioning, and executive dysfunction in pediatric multiple sclerosis," *Child Neuropsychology*, vol. 20, no. 1, pp. 71–85, 2014.

[4] H. Hildebrandt and P. Eling, "A longitudinal study on fatigue, depression, and their relation to neurocognition in multiple sclerosis," *Journal of Clinical and Experimental Neuropsychology*, vol. 36, no. 4, pp. 410–417, 2014.

[5] N. Razazian, N. Shokrian, A. Bostani, N. Moradian, and S. Tahmasebi, "Study of fatigue frequency and its association with sociodemographic and clinical variables in patients with multiple sclerosis," *Neurosciences*, vol. 19, no. 1, pp. 38–42, 2014.

[6] T. A.-Z. K. Gaber, W. W. Oo, and H. Ringrose, "Multiple sclerosis/chronic fatigue syndrome overlap: when two common disorders collide," *NeuroRehabilitation*, vol. 35, no. 3, pp. 529–534, 2014.

[7] C. H. Polman, S. C. Reingold, B. Banwell et al., "Diagnostic criteria for multiple sclerosis: 2010 revisions to the McDonald criteria," *Annals of Neurology*, vol. 69, no. 2, pp. 292–302, 2011.

[8] W. I. McDonald, A. Compston, G. Edan et al., "Recommended diagnostic criteria for multiple sclerosis: guidelines from the International Panel on the diagnosis of multiple sclerosis," *Annals of Neurology*, vol. 50, no. 1, pp. 121–127, 2001.

[9] L. R. Barnden, B. Crouch, R. Kwiatek et al., "A brain MRI study of chronic fatigue syndrome: evidence of brainstem dysfunction and altered homeostasis," *NMR in Biomedicine*, vol. 24, no. 10, pp. 1302–1312, 2011.

[10] D. B. Cook, G. Lange, J. Deluca, and B. H. Natelson, "Relationship of brain MRI abnormalities and physical functional status in chronic fatigue syndrome," *International Journal of Neuroscience*, vol. 107, no. 1-2, pp. 1–6, 2001.

[11] Y. Nakatomi, K. Mizuno, A. Ishii et al., "Neuroinflammation in patients with chronic fatigue syndrome/myalgic encephalomyelitis: An11C-(R)-PK11195 PET study," *Journal of Nuclear Medicine*, vol. 55, no. 6, pp. 945–950, 2014.

[12] B. K. Puri, P. M. Jakeman, M. Agour et al., "Regional grey and white matter volumetric changes in myalgic encephalomyelitis (chronic fatigue syndrome): a voxel-based morphometry 3 T MRI study," *British Journal of Radiology*, vol. 85, no. 1015, pp. e270–e273, 2012.

[13] G. Morris and M. Maes, "Myalgic encephalomyelitis/chronic fatigue syndrome and encephalomyelitis disseminata/multiple sclerosis show remarkable levels of similarity in phenomenology and neuroimmune characteristics," *BMC Medicine*, vol. 11, no. 1, article 205, 2013.

[14] C. Chanvillard, R. F. Jacolik, C. Infante-Duarte, and R. C. Nayak, "The role of natural killer cells in multiple sclerosis and their therapeutic implications," *Frontiers in Immunology*, vol. 4, article 63, 2013.

[15] G. Kaur, J. Trowsdale, and L. Fugger, "Natural killer cells and their receptors in multiple sclerosis," *Brain*, vol. 136, no. 9, pp. 2657–2676, 2013.

[16] E. W. Brenu, T. K. Huth, S. L. Hardcastle et al., "Role of adaptive and innate immune cells in chronic fatigue syndrome/myalgic encephalomyelitis," *International Immunology*, vol. 26, no. 4, Article ID dxt068, pp. 233–242, 2014.

[17] E. W. Brenu, M. L. van Driel, D. R. Staines et al., "Longitudinal investigation of natural killer cells and cytokines in chronic fatigue syndrome/myalgic encephalomyelitis," *Journal of Translational Medicine*, vol. 10, no. 1, article 88, 2012.

[18] E. W. Brenu, M. L. van Driel, D. R. Staines et al., "Immunological abnormalities as potential biomarkers in Chronic Fatigue Syndrome/Myalgic Encephalomyelitis," *Journal of Translational Medicine*, vol. 9, article 81, 2011.

[19] D. E. Lowther and D. A. Hafler, "Regulatory T cells in the central nervous system," *Immunological Reviews*, vol. 248, no. 1, pp. 156–169, 2012.

[20] L. Cervantes-Barragán, S. Firner, I. Bechmann et al., "Regulatory T cells selectively preserve immune privilege of self-antigens during viral central nervous system infection," *The Journal of Immunology*, vol. 188, no. 8, pp. 3678–3685, 2012.

[21] S. Markovic-Plese, C. Pinilla, and R. Martin, "The initiation of the autoimmune response in multiple sclerosis," *Clinical Neurology and Neurosurgery*, vol. 106, no. 3, pp. 218–222, 2004.

[22] R. S. Lopez-Diego and H. L. Weiner, "Novel therapeutic strategies for multiple sclerosis—a multifaceted adversary," *Nature Reviews Drug Discovery*, vol. 7, no. 11, pp. 909–925, 2008.

[23] S. Sinha, F. R. Itani, and N. J. Karandikar, "Immune regulation of multiple sclerosis by CD8+ T cells," *Immunologic Research*, vol. 59, no. 1–3, pp. 254–265, 2014.

[24] M. Curriu, J. Carrillo, M. Massanella et al., "Screening NK-, B- and T-cell phenotype and function in patients suffering from Chronic Fatigue Syndrome," *Journal of Translational Medicine*, vol. 11, article 68, 2013.

[25] B. M. Carruthers, M. I. Van de Sande, K. L. De Meirleir et al., "Myalgic encephalomyelitis: International Consensus Criteria," *Journal of Internal Medicine*, vol. 270, no. 4, pp. 327–338, 2011.

[26] M. M. Brown, D. S. Bell, L. A. Jason, C. Christos, and D. E. Bell, "Understanding long-term outcomes of chronic fatigue syndrome," *Journal of Clinical Psychology*, vol. 68, no. 9, pp. 1028–1035, 2012.

[27] I. Kister, E. Chamot, A. R. Salter, G. R. Cutter, T. E. Bacon, and J. Herbert, "Disability in multiple sclerosis: a reference for patients and clinicians," *Neurology*, vol. 80, no. 11, pp. 1018–1024, 2013.

[28] S. L. Hardcastle, E. Brenu, S. Johnston et al., "Analysis of the relationship between immune dysfunction and symptom severity in patients with chronic fatigue syndrome/myalgic encephalomyelitis (CFS/ME)," *Journal of Clinical & Cellular Immunology*, vol. 5, article 190, 2014.

[29] B. Bahbouhi, L. Berthelot, S. Pettré et al., "Peripheral blood CD4+ T lymphocytes from multiple sclerosis patients are characterized by higher PSGL-1 expression and transmigration capacity across a human blood-brain barrier-derived endothelial cell line," *Journal of Leukocyte Biology*, vol. 86, no. 5, pp. 1049–1063, 2009.

[30] L. Battistini, L. Piccio, B. Rossi et al., "CD8+ T cells from patients with acute multiple sclerosis display selective increase of adhesiveness in brain venules: a critical role for P-selectin glycoprotein ligand-1," *Blood*, vol. 101, no. 12, pp. 4775–4782, 2003.

[31] L. Bö, J. W. Peterson, S. Mørk et al., "Distribution of immunoglobulin superfamily members ICAM-1, -2, -3, and the $\beta2$ integrin LFA-1 in multiple sclerosis lesions," *Journal of Neuropathology and Experimental Neurology*, vol. 55, no. 10, pp. 1060–1072, 1996.

[32] B. A. Kallmann, V. Hummel, T. Lindenlaub, K. Ruprecht, K. V. Toyka, and P. Rieckmann, "Cytokine-induced modulation of cellular adhesion to human cerebral endothelial cells is mediated by soluble vascular cell adhesion molecule-1," *Brain*, vol. 123, no. 4, pp. 687–697, 2000.

[33] R. Mazzucchelli and S. K. Durum, "Interleukin-7 receptor expression: intelligent design," *Nature Reviews Immunology*, vol. 7, no. 2, pp. 144–154, 2007.

[34] S. G. Gregory, S. Schmidt, P. Seth et al., "Interleukin 7 receptor α chain (IL7R) shows allelic and functional association with multiple sclerosis," *Nature Genetics*, vol. 39, no. 9, pp. 1083–1091, 2007.

[35] F. C. McKay, L. I. Swain, S. D. Schibeci et al., "Haplotypes of the interleukin 7 receptor alpha gene are correlated with altered expression in whole blood cells in multiple sclerosis," *Genes and Immunity*, vol. 9, no. 1, pp. 1–6, 2008.

[36] E. Hoe, F. C. McKay, S. D. Schibeci et al., "Functionally significant differences in expression of disease-associated IL-7 receptor α haplotypes in CD4 T cells and dendritic cells," *The Journal of Immunology*, vol. 184, no. 5, pp. 2512–2517, 2010.

[37] K. L. Kreft, E. Verbraak, A. F. Wierenga-Wolf et al., "Decreased systemic IL-7 and soluble IL-7Ralpha in multiple sclerosis patients," *Genes and Immunity*, vol. 13, no. 7, pp. 587–592, 2012.

[38] C. Malmeström, J. Lycke, S. Haghighi et al., "Relapses in multiple sclerosis are associated with increased CD8+ T-cell mediated cytotoxicity in CSF," *Journal of Neuroimmunology*, vol. 196, no. 1-2, pp. 159–165, 2008.

[39] K. L. Kreft, E. Verbraak, A. F. Wierenga-Wolf et al., "The IL-7Rα pathway is quantitatively and functionally altered in CD8 T cells in multiple sclerosis," *The Journal of Immunology*, vol. 188, no. 4, pp. 1874–1883, 2012.

[40] M. Paiardini, B. Cervasi, H. Albrecht et al., "Loss of CD127 expression defines an expansion of effector CD8+ T cells in HIV-infected individuals," *Journal of Immunology*, vol. 174, no. 5, pp. 2900–2909, 2005.

[41] J. R. Sedy, M. Gavrieli, K. G. Potter et al., "B and T lymphocyte attenuator regulates T cell activation through interaction with herpesvirus entry mediator," *Nature Immunology*, vol. 6, no. 1, pp. 90–98, 2005.

[42] T. C. Cheung, L. M. Oborne, M. W. Steinberg et al., "T cell intrinsic heterodimeric complexes between HVEM and BTLA determine receptivity to the surrounding microenvironment," *The Journal of Immunology*, vol. 183, no. 11, pp. 7286–7296, 2009.

[43] A. C. Vendel, J. Calemine-Fenaux, A. Izrael-Tomasevic, V. Chauhan, D. Arnott, and D. L. Eaton, "B and T lymphocyte attenuator regulates B cell receptor signaling by targeting Syk and BLNK," *The Journal of Immunology*, vol. 182, no. 3, pp. 1509–1517, 2009.

[44] M. W. Steinberg, Y. Huang, Y. Wang-Zhu, C. F. Ware, H. Cheroutre, and M. Kronenberg, "BTLA interaction with HVEM expressed on CD8+ T cells promotes survival and memory

generation in response to a bacterial infection," *PLoS ONE*, vol. 8, no. 10, Article ID e77992, 2013.

[45] M. P. Pender, P. A. Csurhes, C. M. Pfluger, and S. R. Burrows, "Deficiency of CD8+ effector memory T cells is an early and persistent feature of multiple sclerosis," *Multiple Sclerosis Journal*, vol. 20, no. 14, pp. 1825–1832, 2014.

[46] M. P. Pender, P. A. Csurhes, C. M. M. Pfluger, and S. R. Burrows, "CD8 T cell deficiency impairs control of Epsteine-Barr virus and worsens with age in multiple sclerosis," *Journal of Neurology, Neurosurgery and Psychiatry*, vol. 83, no. 3, pp. 353–354, 2012.

16

The Role of Aggregates of Therapeutic Protein Products in Immunogenicity: An Evaluation by Mathematical Modeling

Liusong Yin,[1] Xiaoying Chen,[2] Abhinav Tiwari,[2] Paolo Vicini,[3] and Timothy P. Hickling[1]

[1]*Pharmacokinetics, Dynamics and Metabolism-New Biological Entities, Pfizer, Andover, MA 01810, USA*
[2]*Pharmacokinetics, Dynamics and Metabolism-New Biological Entities, Pfizer, Cambridge, MA 02138, USA*
[3]*Pharmacokinetics, Dynamics and Metabolism-New Biological Entities, Pfizer, San Diego, CA 92121, USA*

Correspondence should be addressed to Timothy P. Hickling; timothy.hickling@pfizer.com

Academic Editor: Marzio Pennisi

Therapeutic protein products (TPP) have been widely used to treat a variety of human diseases, including cancer, hemophilia, and autoimmune diseases. However, TPP can induce unwanted immune responses that can impact both drug efficacy and patient safety. The presence of aggregates is of particular concern as they have been implicated in inducing both T cell-independent and T cell-dependent immune responses. We used mathematical modeling to evaluate several mechanisms through which aggregates of TPP could contribute to the development of immunogenicity. Modeling interactions between aggregates and B cell receptors demonstrated that aggregates are unlikely to induce T cell-independent immune responses by cross-linking B cell receptors because the amount of signal transducing complex that can form under physiologically relevant conditions is limited. We systematically evaluate the role of aggregates in inducing T cell-dependent immune responses using a recently developed multiscale mechanistic mathematical model. Our analysis indicates that aggregates could contribute to T cell-dependent immune response by inducing high affinity epitopes which may not be present in the nonaggregated TPP and/or by enhancing danger signals to break tolerance. In summary, our computational analysis is suggestive of novel insights into the mechanisms underlying aggregate-induced immunogenicity, which could be used to develop mitigation strategies.

1. Introduction

Therapeutic protein products (TPP) from nonhuman, humanized, and human origins include monoclonal antibodies (mAbs), Fc fusion proteins, blood factors, hormones, cytokines, chemokines, and engineered protein scaffolds [1]. They have been widely used to treat a variety of human diseases, including cancer, anemia, hemophilia, rheumatoid arthritis, multiple sclerosis, and inflammatory bowel diseases [1, 2]. Their large success is mainly due to increased target specificity, decreased intrinsic toxicity, and longer half-lives compared with small molecule drugs [3]. These advantages have led to the expansion of TPP in the drug market, with annual revenues of over 100 billion US dollars [1, 2]. However, unwanted immune responses against TPP, such as generation of anti-drug antibodies (ADA), have raised concerns on both drug efficacy and patient safety [4–8]. The effect of ADA on clinical outcomes ranges from no obvious

impact to severe loss of efficacy and adverse effects such as infusion reactions [7]. The mechanisms leading to the generation of immunogenicity are yet to be established, but several risk factors have been proposed [9–12], which can be classified as follows: (i) patient-related: genetic background, immunological status, and prior exposure [10], (ii) treatment-related: route, dose, and frequency of administration [7, 13], and (iii) product-related: drug origins, characteristics such as protein structures and aggregates, and formulations [10].

Among these risk factors, aggregates of TPP are of particular concern due to their potential role in inducing both T cell-independent and T cell-dependent immune responses [14–17] (Figure 1). It has been previously found that aggregated recombinant human interferon alpha2b generated by thermal stress, low pH, or oxidization stress is more immunogenic in mice compared with nonaggregated product [18–20]. High immunogenicity in mice has also been observed for aggregates of other TPP, such as human mAbs [21–23],

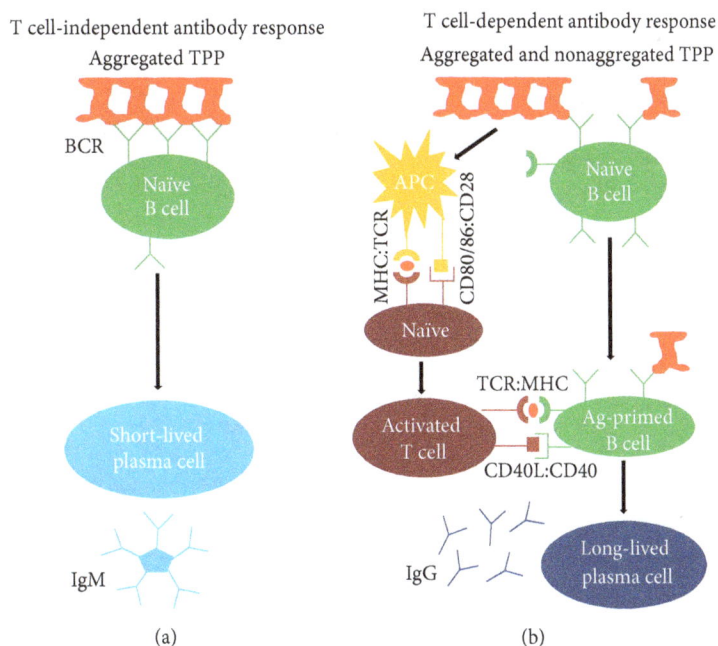

FIGURE 1: Schematic overview of aggregate-induced T cell-independent and T cell-dependent antibody responses. (a) In the T cell-independent pathway aggregates of TPP cross-link BCRs and activate B cells, which differentiate into short-lived plasma cells that generate antigen-specific IgM pentamers. (b) In the T cell-dependent pathway both aggregated and nonaggregated TPP can be captured by B cells or by APC which present TPP-derived epitopes to activate T cells, which in turn activate antigen-primed B cells. The activated B cells differentiate into long-lived plasma cells that generate isotype-switched IgG.

human epoetin alfa [24], human factor VIII [25, 26], human interferon beta [27], and murine growth hormone [28]. In the clinic, the different ADA incidence rates for several recombinant human interferon beta drugs have been attributed to the differences in aggregation levels [29]. However, the detailed mechanism by which aggregates increase immunogenicity, especially in humans, is yet to be established. For example, it is unknown whether aggregates increase immunogenicity through a T cell-dependent or T cell-independent pathway; and which processes of ADA production could be altered by aggregates is also unknown. In the case of TPP, immunogenicity could be induced through both T cell-dependent and T cell-independent pathways [9, 12]. In the T cell-dependent pathway, antigenic peptides derived from TPP could be presented by major histocompatibility complex class II molecules (MHC II) on antigen-presenting cells (APC) that have been matured by danger signal to stimulate antigen-specific CD4+ T cells. Activated CD4+ T cells would then stimulate antigen-specific B cells that will be responsible for the production of ADA, which are usually affinity matured IgG. It has been found that, in comparison with the nonaggregated form, aggregated mAb results in an increase in the amount of total peptides and the number of epitopes eluted from MHC II [30]. This suggests that aggregates may increase immunogenicity by enhancing antigen processing and presentation in the T cell-dependent pathway. Aggregates could also contribute to T cell-dependent immunogenicity by increasing the danger signal for dendritic cell maturation. Consistent with this, a recent study suggested that aggregated mAb induces significantly higher dendritic cell maturation compared with unstressed mAb [30]. Lastly, aggregates could

form repetitively arranged B cell epitopes in a paracrystalline manner to cross-link B cell receptors (BCRs), which in turn will activate antigen-specific B cells to generate ADA, mostly IgM, via the T cell-independent pathway [14]. However, the scarcity of clinical data and the difficulty to isolate the impact of aggregates from other immunogenicity risk factors are major impediments to understand the mechanisms of aggregate-induced immunogenicity.

Mathematical modeling offers the advantage of fast and cost-effective assessment and so it can be used in complement with experimental analysis to study immune responses [31–34]. It also provides quantitative means to dissect each component of a complex response for a deeper understanding of the mechanisms underlying aggregate-induced immunogenicity. Multiple mechanistic mathematical models have been previously developed to study immune responses against various pathogens. For example, antigen processing and presentation by APC and the activation of T helper cells by interactions between T cell receptors and MHC II-peptide complexes have been modeled and the simulation results agree with a variety of experimental data [35]. A mathematical model was also developed for predicting the clonal selection of B cells and antibody production by plasma cells [36]. The role of activation threshold and infections in the dynamics of autoimmune diseases has been studied mathematically as well [37, 38]. Mathematical models have been proposed and experimentally validated for T cell-dependent antibody responses to a wide range of antigens, including *Haemophilus influenzae* type b, hepatitis B virus, cancer antigens, and influenza A virus [39–43]. The T cell-independent activation of B cells by multivalent hapten-polymer has been modeled, where fitting to experimental data revealed that a minimum number of BCRs, in the range of 7 to 15, need to be cross-linked by a single multivalent ligand to stimulate a B cell [44, 45]. With regards to TPP-induced immunogenicity, several pharmacokinetics (PK) models have been developed to study the impact of ADA on mAb therapy [32]. For example, by incorporating ADA-drug interactions into empirical PK modeling, we developed a PK/ADA model to quantitatively assess the extent and timing of ADA generation, affinity maturation, and ADA-mediated TPP elimination [46]. More recently, we built a mechanistic, multiscale mathematical model of TPP-induced immunogenicity, recapitulating the key processes underlying T cell-dependent generation of ADA, such as antigen presentation, activation of immune cells, and production of ADA as well as *in vivo* disposition of ADA and TPP [47, 48]. This system-level model consists of a subcellular module for antigen presentation, a cellular module for immune system activation and antibody production, and a whole-body module for drug disposition. The model is able to reproduce key immunological phenomena such as antibody affinity maturation and enhanced secondary response [47, 48]. More importantly, a case study on immune response against adalimumab (a fully human anti-TNF alpha IgG1 mAb) showed reasonable agreement between model simulations and experimental observations [47, 48]. Owing to its flexibility and comprehensiveness this system-level model provides us with an ideal platform to probe mechanisms through which aggregates could generate immunogenicity.

In this study, we evaluate whether aggregates could induce T cell-independent or T cell-dependent immune response. In the former case, we model the interactions between multivalent aggregates and BCRs and examine the formation of signal-transducing complex (STC) under physiologically relevant conditions. For the latter case, we use our previously developed system-level model to investigate the impact of antigen processing and presentation, number and affinity of epitopes, and danger signal on ADA production due to aggregates.

2. Materials and Methods

2.1. Aggregates in the T Cell-Independent Pathway: Interactions between Multivalent Aggregates and BCRs. An aggregate (Ag_a) is assumed to be a homogeneous product formed by the combination of n monomers, which gives it a valency of n. The binding of Ag_a to BCR is assumed to be sequential (see Figure 2(a) for an example with $n = 4$) and can be represented by the following second-order reactions:

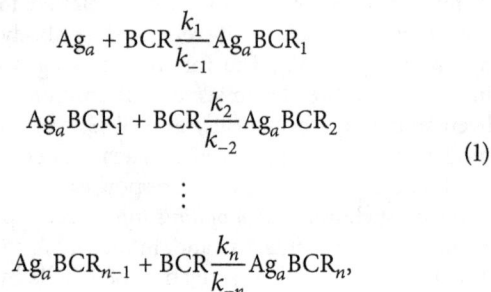

$$Ag_a + BCR \underset{k_{-1}}{\overset{k_1}{\rightleftharpoons}} Ag_a BCR_1$$

$$Ag_a BCR_1 + BCR \underset{k_{-2}}{\overset{k_2}{\rightleftharpoons}} Ag_a BCR_2$$

$$\vdots$$

$$Ag_a BCR_{n-1} + BCR \underset{k_{-n}}{\overset{k_n}{\rightleftharpoons}} Ag_a BCR_n, \tag{1}$$

where k_i and k_{-i} are the ith reaction's binding and dissociation rates, respectively, and $Ag_a BCR_i$ is the complex formed by binding of Ag_a to i BCRs. It is assumed that a BCR could bind to any free site on Ag_a and dissociate from any bound site on $Ag_a BCR_i$. The above reactions can be described by the following ordinary differential equations that govern the time evolution of $Ag_a BCR_i$, Ag_a, and BCR:

$$\frac{dAg_a BCR_1}{dt} = n \cdot k_1 \cdot BCR \cdot Ag_a + 2 \cdot k_{-2} \cdot Ag_a BCR_2$$
$$- [k_{-1} + (n-1) \cdot k_2 \cdot BCR] \cdot Ag_a BCR_1$$

$$\frac{dAg_a BCR_i}{dt} = (n - i + 1) \cdot k_i \cdot BCR \cdot Ag_a BCR_{i-1} + (i + 1) \cdot k_{-(i+1)} \cdot Ag_a BCR_{i+1} - [ik_{-i} + (n-i) \cdot k_{(i+1)} \cdot BCR] \cdot Ag_a BCR_i, \quad 1 \le i \le n-1$$

$$\frac{dAg_a BCR_n}{dt} = k_n \cdot BCR \cdot Ag_a BCR_{n-1} - n \cdot k_{-n} \cdot Ag_a BCR_n \tag{2}$$

$$\frac{dAg_a}{dt} = -k_1 \cdot n \cdot BCR \cdot Ag_a + k_{-1} \cdot Ag_a BCR_1$$

$$\frac{dBCR}{dt} = -k_1 \cdot n \cdot BCR \cdot Ag_a + k_{-1} \cdot Ag_a BCR_1$$
$$- \sum_{j=2}^{n} \left(k_j \cdot (n - j + 1) \cdot BCR \cdot Ag_a BCR_{j-1} + k_{-j} \cdot j \cdot Ag_a BCR_j \right).$$

We selected three (low, medium, and high) physiologically relevant levels for input parameters association constant ($K_a = k_1/k_{-1}$) and initial Ag_a concentration ($[Ag_a^0]$). $[Ag_a^0]$ is Ag_a concentration at $t = 0$, as an initial condition for ordinary differential equations, which is estimated using the following equation:

$$\left[Ag_a^0\right] = [Ag] \cdot \frac{p}{n}, \tag{3}$$

where $[Ag]$ is the total TPP concentration, p is the aggregation percentage in TPP, and n is the valency of aggregates. $[Ag]$ ranges from 500 to 10^5 pM based on 30 μg dose of interferon beta 1b and 40 mg dose of anti-TNF mAb adalimumab, respectively [29, 47–49]; p spans from 2 to 15% based on a previous report on the characterization and quantitation of aggregates in recombinant human interferon beta drug products [29]; and n varies from 10 to 100 based on the sizes of nonaggregated and aggregated TPP [18, 23, 29, 50, 51]. Taken together, the low and high levels of Ag_a^0 are 0.1 and 1500 pM, respectively. The association constant K_a has been previously reported to be 10^{-7} pM^{-1} for antibodies with low intrinsic affinities and 10^{-3} pM^{-1} for affinity matured antibodies, and hence these were selected as low and high levels [52]. The middle levels for total Ag_a^0 (12 pM) and K_a (10^{-5} pM^{-1}) are the geometric means of corresponding low and high levels.

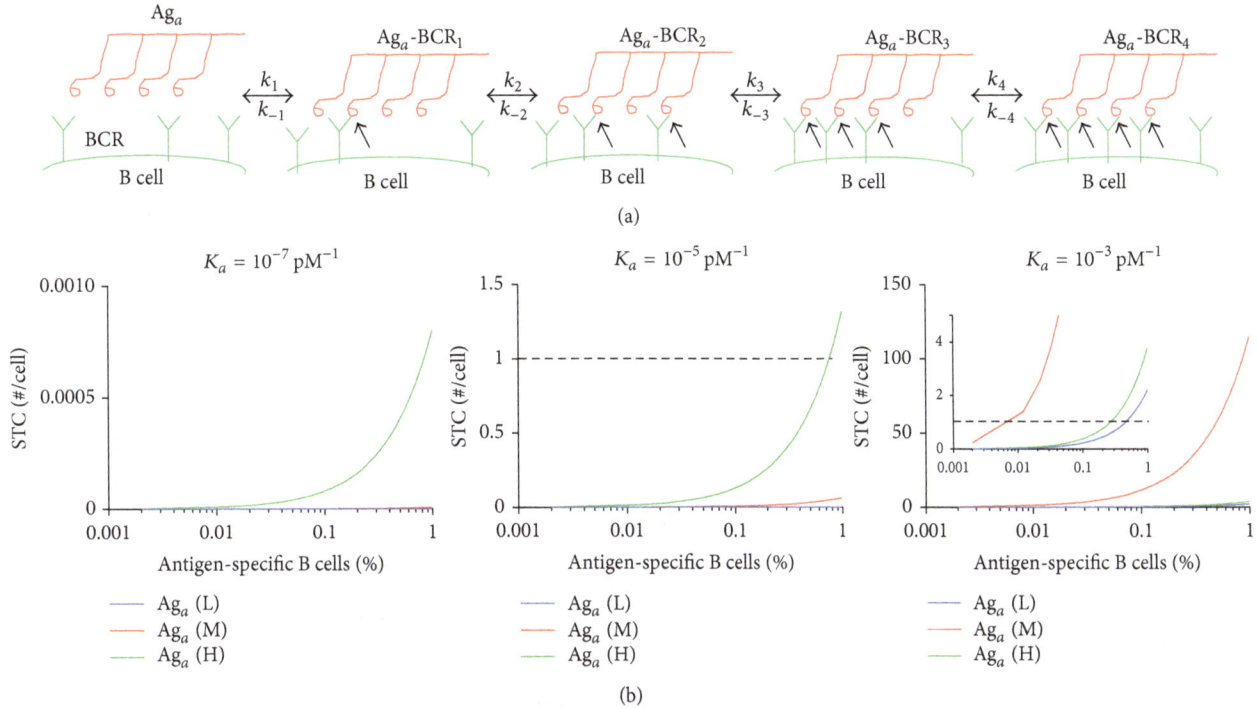

FIGURE 2: Significant number of STC per cell only forms under limited conditions. (a) Schematic representation of a tetravalent aggregate (Ag_a) binding to BCRs to form Ag_aBCR_i, where i denotes the number of BCRs bound to Ag_a. Black arrow points out the binding of Ag_a to a BCR. Each binding step i is governed by its binding (k_i) and dissociation (k_{-i}) rates. (b) Simulated levels of STC formed per cell are plotted against percentage of antigen-specific B cells under low (L, 0.1 pM), medium (M, 12 pM), and high (H, 1500 pM) levels of total Ag_a, for binding affinity $K_a = 10^{-7}$ pM^{-1} (left panel), 10^{-5} pM^{-1} (middle panel), and 10^{-3} pM^{-1} (right panel). Inset in the right panel is the zoomed-in version of the plot. STC per B cell is defined as the number of aggregates that cross-link a minimum number (s) of BCRs. Here $s = 2$ and valency $n = 100$. The horizontal dashed line denotes one STC.

The rate of binding of an antigen to its corresponding BCR, k_i, is relatively constant [52, 53], so we fixed it to 8.64 × 10^{-3} pM^{-1} day^{-1}. By contrast, the rate of dissociation (k_{-i}) is expected to increase with i because the resistance of Ag_a against torsion and bending grows due to the steric hindrance from progressive binding of BCRs [45]. For simplicity we assume that k_{-i} decreases exponentially with i and the base for exponential decay is 0.5 as previously identified while modeling interactions between multivalent hapten-polymer and BCRs [45]. The initial BCR concentration is the product of number of BCRs per cell, B cell concentration, and percentage of antigen-specific B cells. The number of BCRs per cell and B cell concentration have been previously reported as ~10^5 and ~10^8 L^{-1}, respectively [41, 44, 45, 47, 48]. Studies on the percentage of antigen-specific B cells are limited, but it has been reported to be <0.002% for vaccinia virus [54] and <1% for individual antigens [55]. The above estimates were used to define the input range of BCR concentration at $t = 0$ as an initial condition for the ordinary differential equations in the simulation.

In the model, the STC is the number of Ag_a that cross-links at least s BCRs as defined in [44, 45]:

$$STC = \sum_{s}^{n} Ag_a BCR_s. \tag{4}$$

The model was simulated using the ordinary differential equation solver *ode15s* in MATLAB (The MathWorks, Inc., Natick, MA).

2.2. Aggregates in the T Cell-Dependent Pathway: Impact on Antigen Processing and Presentation and Danger Signal. For this analysis, we use our previously developed mechanistic, multiscale mathematical model for T cell-dependent ADA production [47, 48]. In this system-level model aggregates could contribute to increased ADA production by enhancing either the antigen processing and presentation or the danger signal for dendritic cell maturation (denoted by red arrows in Figure 3). We simulate the impact of aggregates by increasing (i) the rate of internalization of TPP into the endosome, (ii) the rate of degradation/processing of TPP into antigenic peptides, (iii) the number of epitopes generated, (iv) the affinity of epitopes to MHC II, and (v) the level of danger signal. Subsequently, for each of these conditions, we examine the endosomal levels of aggregates and epitope, the number of MHC II-peptide complexes on APC, and the levels of ADA production. To simulate B cell clonal selection and antibody affinity maturation, B cells and ADA are divided into 17 subgroups based on the binding affinity to antigen [36, 47, 48]. In our analysis, we define ADA production as the sum of the 17 subgroups.

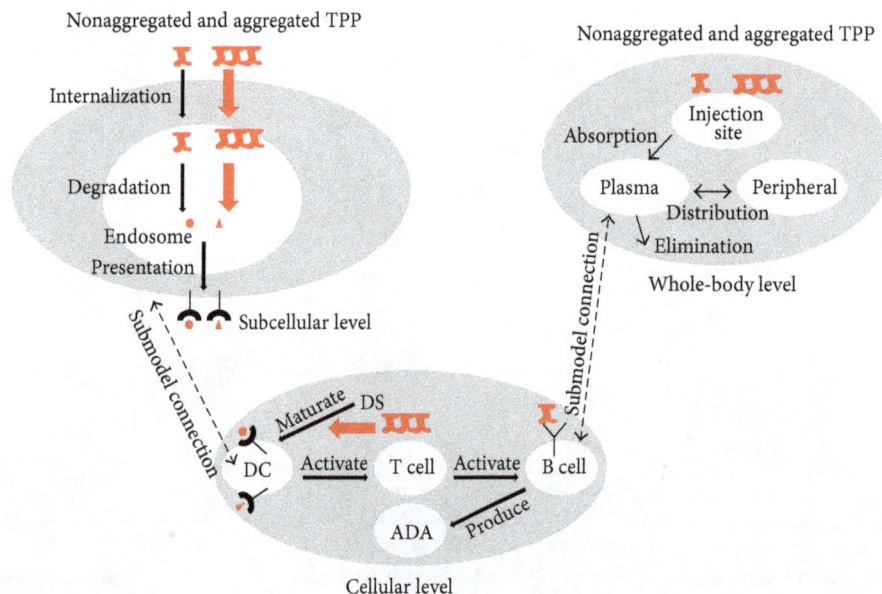

FIGURE 3: Schematic highlighting of the potential role of aggregates in T cell-dependent ADA production. A recapitulation of our system-level model for T cell-dependent ADA production [47, 48]. At the subcellular level, TPP are internalized into endosome of APC, such as dendritic cells (DC), and then degraded into antigenic peptides. Epitopes derived from TPP could be loaded onto MHC II and presented on the surface of APC. Aggregates could contribute to enhanced ADA production by having increased internalization or degradation rate or number and affinity of epitopes generated (indicated by thick red arrows). At the cellular level, danger signal (DS) maturated DC activate T cells which in turn activate B cells to generate ADA. Aggregates could enhance the DS to maturate DC (see red arrow). At the whole-body level, aggregated and nonaggregated TPP are absorbed from the injection site into plasma and will be distributed into periphery, eliminated, or captured by B cells through BCR binding.

3. Results

3.1. Aggregates Are Unlikely to Induce T Cell-Independent Immune Response because the Number of STC Formed Is Limited. To evaluate whether aggregates could induce T cell-independent antibody responses through BCR cross-linking, we examine the number of STC formed per B cell for different parameter combinations (see Section 2 for details). The model output for interactions between aggregates and BCR is the STC formed per B cell, which was previously defined as the number of Ag_a which cross-links a minimum number of BCRs [44, 45]. It has been reported that a multivalent ligand stimulates B cell activation only if it cross-links a minimum number (s) of BCRs, which is usually between 7 and 15 [44, 45]. We calculated the number of STC for $s =$ 2, 5, and 10 under different total Ag_a, K_a, and BCR levels. Surprisingly, our computer simulation analysis showed that if $s = 10$ or 5, no more than one STC per cell could be observed under physiological levels of total Ag_a, BCR, and K_a (data not shown). Even if s is lowered to 2, more than one STC per cell can form only under limited conditions, when the sensitive parameters are near the upper limits of the physiologically plausible ranges (Figure 2(b)). In the case of $K_a = 10^{-7}$ pM^{-1}, no more than one STC could form (Figure 2(b), left panel). For $K_a = 10^{-5}$ pM^{-1}, more than one STC could form at high levels of total Ag_a (1.5×10^{-3} pM) but only near the upper limit of antigen-specific B cells percentage (1%) (Figure 2(b), middle panel). Finally, when $K_a = 10^{-3}$ pM^{-1}, more than one

STC could form at all total Ag_a levels but only with antigen-specific B cell percentage >0.006% (Figure 2(b), right panel). These results from our computer simulation showed that STC per cell is very sensitive to K_a and total concentrations of Ag_a and BCRs (but not to binding rate k_i, data not shown). Overall, this analysis suggests that aggregates are unlikely to induce T cell-independent activation of B cells and consequent ADA production under physiologically plausible conditions. Therefore, aggregates may only contribute to ADA production through a T cell-dependent pathway, which we explore next.

3.2. Aggregates Could Enhance ADA Production by Increasing the Danger Signal to Maturate Dendritic Cells. To evaluate the T cell-dependent effect of aggregates on ADA production, we modulated those parameters in our system-level immunogenicity model [47, 48] that may be impacted by aggregation. This model consists of a subcellular module for antigen presentation in APC, a cellular module for immune cell activation and ADA production, and a whole-body module for drug and ADA disposition (Figure 3). Aggregates have been previously shown to increase danger signal for dendritic cell maturation and T cell activation [12, 22, 30, 56]. Specifically, aggregated mAb upregulated the dendritic cell maturation marker CD83 and CD4+ T cell costimulatory molecules CD80 and CD86 as well as cytokines produced by CD4+ T cells, such as IL-2 and IL-10 [30, 56]. Due to the complexity of dendritic cell maturation by danger signal and

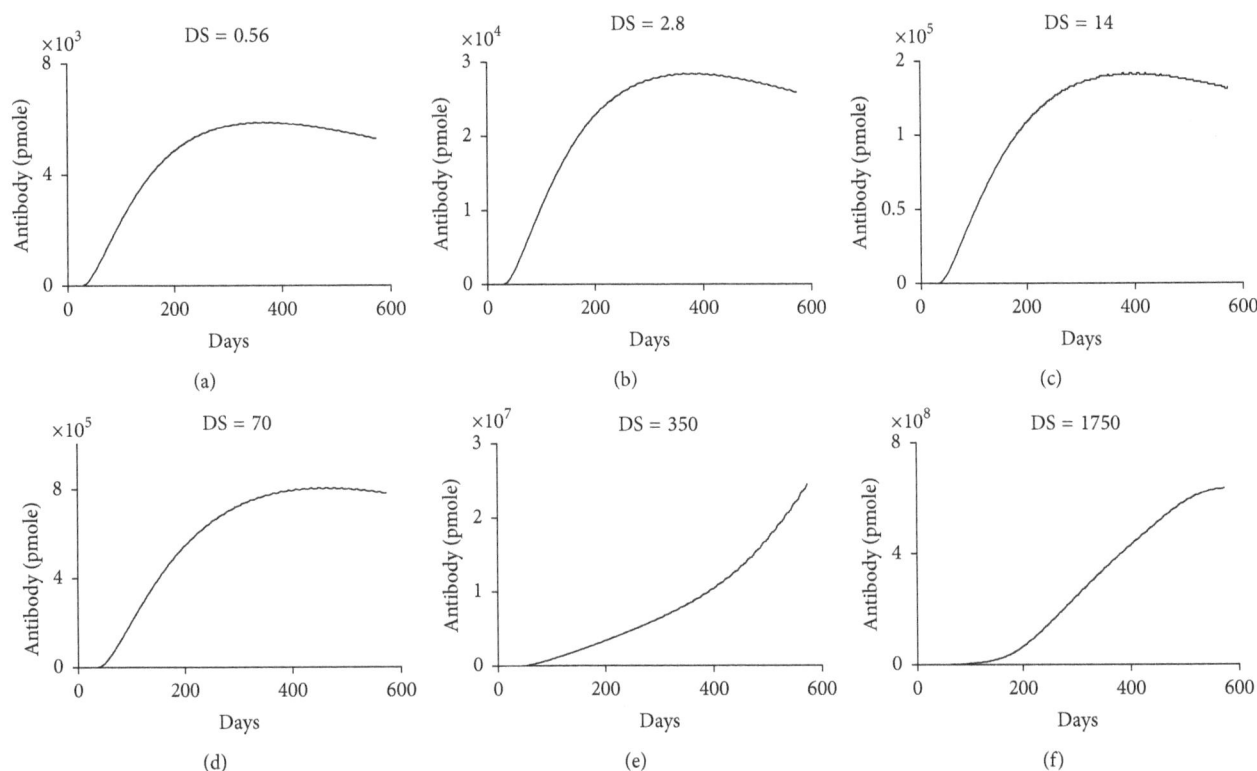

FIGURE 4: Aggregates could contribute to ADA production by increasing danger signal to maturate dendritic cells. ((a)–(f)) Simulated ADA production is shown at various levels of danger signal (DS) which is modeled as the amount of LPS in ng. Remaining parameter values are the same as in the original simulation for nonaggregated adalimumab [47, 48]. DS = 350 ng LPS shows the original simulation for nonaggregated adalimumab [47, 48]. ADA production is shown as the sum of the 17 subgroups. Dose = 40 mg administered biweekly.

the unavailability of many parameters associated with this process, it is simply modeled as being driven by endotoxin lipopolysaccharide (LPS) [47, 48]. LPS is widely used in immunological studies for dendritic cell maturation [57–61] and is present in many TPP [62]. The cytokine profiles induced by LPS and aggregates of mAb are very similar [22, 63]. Using our system-level model, we previously simulated ADA production induced by adalimumab, a fully anti-TNF alpha IgG1 mAb used to treat various inflammatory and autoimmune diseases, with a danger signal of 350 ng LPS [47] (Figure 4(e)). If aggregates increase the danger signal by 5-fold, ADA production is increased by 20-fold (Figure 4(f)). We also simulated ADA production for low danger signal levels (Figures 4(a)–4(d)) as the actual amount induced by nonaggregated TPP is unknown. In essence, ADA production depends on the level of danger signal (Figures 4(a)–4(f)). Therefore, our simulations suggest aggregates could enhance ADA production by increasing danger signal to enhance maturation of dendritic cells and subsequently activate T cells.

3.3. Aggregates Could Not Enhance ADA Production by Increasing Antigen Processing and Presentation If High Affinity Epitopes Are Already Present in Nonaggregated TPP. Antigen processing and presentation are the key events in T cell-dependent immunogenicity of TPP [12]. Previous studies have demonstrated that aggregation enhances antigen's

uptake, processing, and presentation by APC [12, 22, 30, 56, 64]. More recently, a study showed that aggregated mAb could directly increase the total number of different peptides and the number of epitopes presented by MHC II compared with nonaggregated mAb [30]. To evaluate whether aggregation-enhanced antigen processing and presentation could increase ADA production, we simulated these effects of aggregates in our model by changing its internalization or degradation rate or the number and affinity of epitopes generated and assessing their impact on final ADA production.

We previously simulated ADA production induced by adalimumab with an internalization rate of 14.4 day^{-1} (IR$_0$), a degradation rate of 17.28 day^{-1} (DR$_0$), and two predicted adalimumab epitopes with high binding affinities of 123 and 85 nM to common MHC II allele DRB1*04:01 [47]. To model the aggregates' effect on antigen processing, we increased either internalization or degradation rate by 16.6-fold based on a previous study which reported that aggregated mAb resulted in a 16.6-fold increase in total peptides associated with MHC II [30] and then assessed the levels of endosomal aggregates and epitopes, MHC II-peptide complexes on cell surface, and ADA production. As expected, conditional on the parameters and structure of the model simulation, increasing internalization rate by 16.6-fold resulted in a similar fold increase in aggregates internalized into endosome and epitopes generated by its degradation (Figures 5(a)-5(b) and 5(e)-5(f)). Increasing degradation rate by 16.6-fold resulted

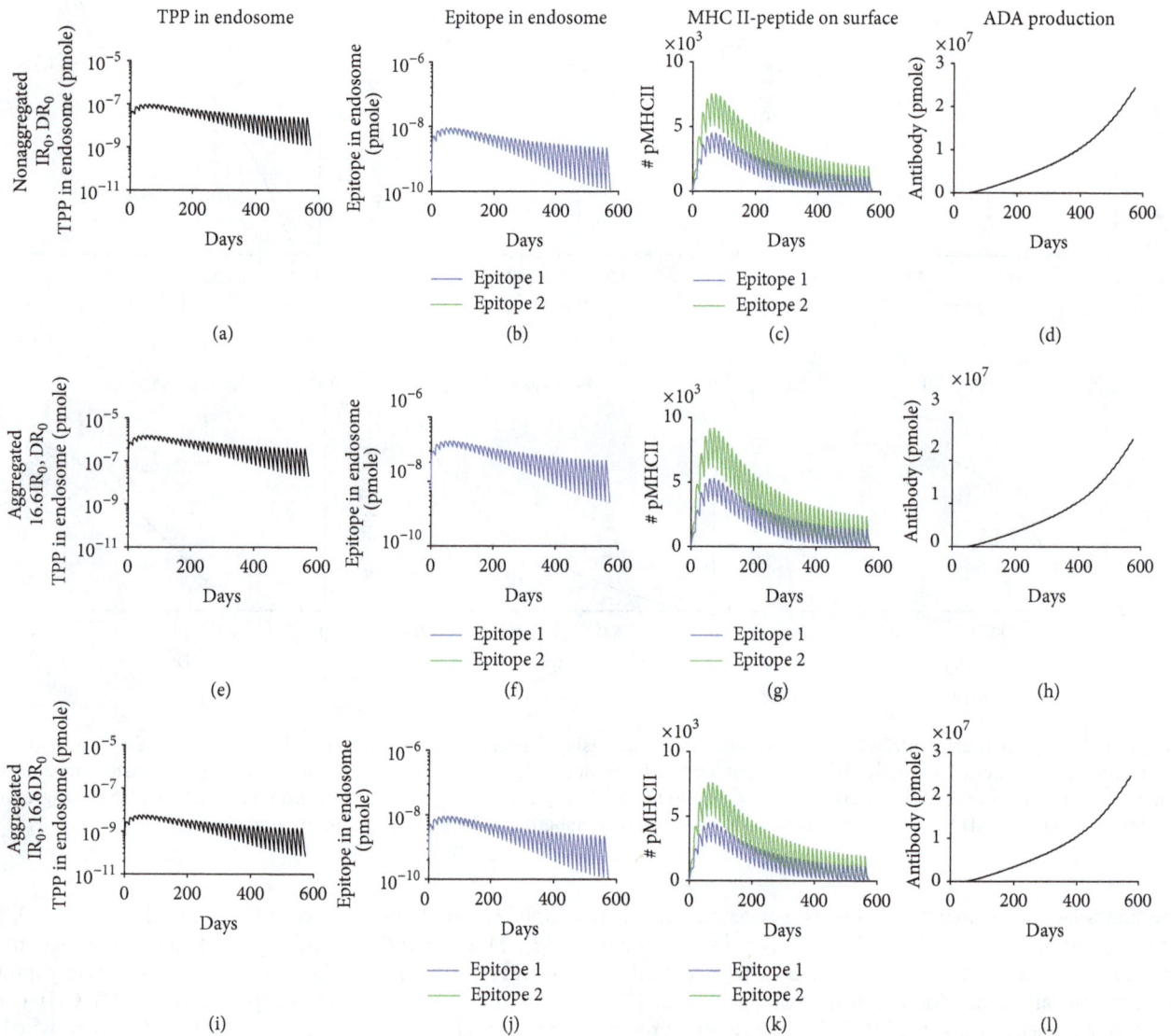

FIGURE 5: Aggregates could not enhance ADA production through faster antigen internalization or degradation if high affinity epitopes are already present in nonaggregated TPP. Simulated levels of nonaggregated and aggregated TPP in endosome, epitopes in endosome, MHC II-peptide complex on cell surface, and ADA production are shown for ((a)–(d)) original internalization ($IR_0 = 14.4$ day^{-1}) and degradation ($DR_0 = 17.28$ day^{-1}) rate for nonaggregated adalimumab [47, 48], ((e)–(h)) $16.6IR_0$ and DR_0 for hypothetical aggregated form, and ((i)–(l)) IR_0 and $16.6DR_0$ for hypothetical aggregated form. ADA production has the same definition and dose has the same value as in Figure 4.

in the same fold decrease in endosomal aggregates, but the levels of epitopes were unchanged, which suggested that epitope generation was limited by the amount of aggregates internalized and not by the degradation rate (Figures 5(a)-5(b) and 5(i)-5(j)). Moreover, increasing internalization or degradation rate by 16.6-fold did not significantly change the number of MHC II-peptide complexes presented on the surface of APC (Figures 5(c), 5(g), and 5(k)). Aggregates could also impact the FcR binding and potentially affect the antigen uptake [44]. We therefore evaluated a larger range of internalization and degradation rate. Our conclusions were unaffected by larger increases (200-fold) in internalization or degradation rate (data not shown). Consistent with MHC

II-peptide complex presentation levels, increasing internalization or degradation rate by 16.6-fold had little impact on final ADA production (Figures 5(d), 5(h), and 5(l)). We next modeled the effect of aggregates on the number of epitopes presented. As expected, including aggregate-induced generation of new epitopes led to the surface presentation of corresponding MHC II-peptide complexes whose levels depend on the binding affinity of epitope to MHC II (Figures 6(a)–6(c), 6(e)–6(g), and 6(i)–6(k)). Surprisingly, if two high affinity epitopes are already present, then the inclusion of new epitopes did not increase ADA production (Figures 6(d), 6(h), and 6(l)). Taken together, these analyses suggest that aggregate-induced high antigen processing and presentation

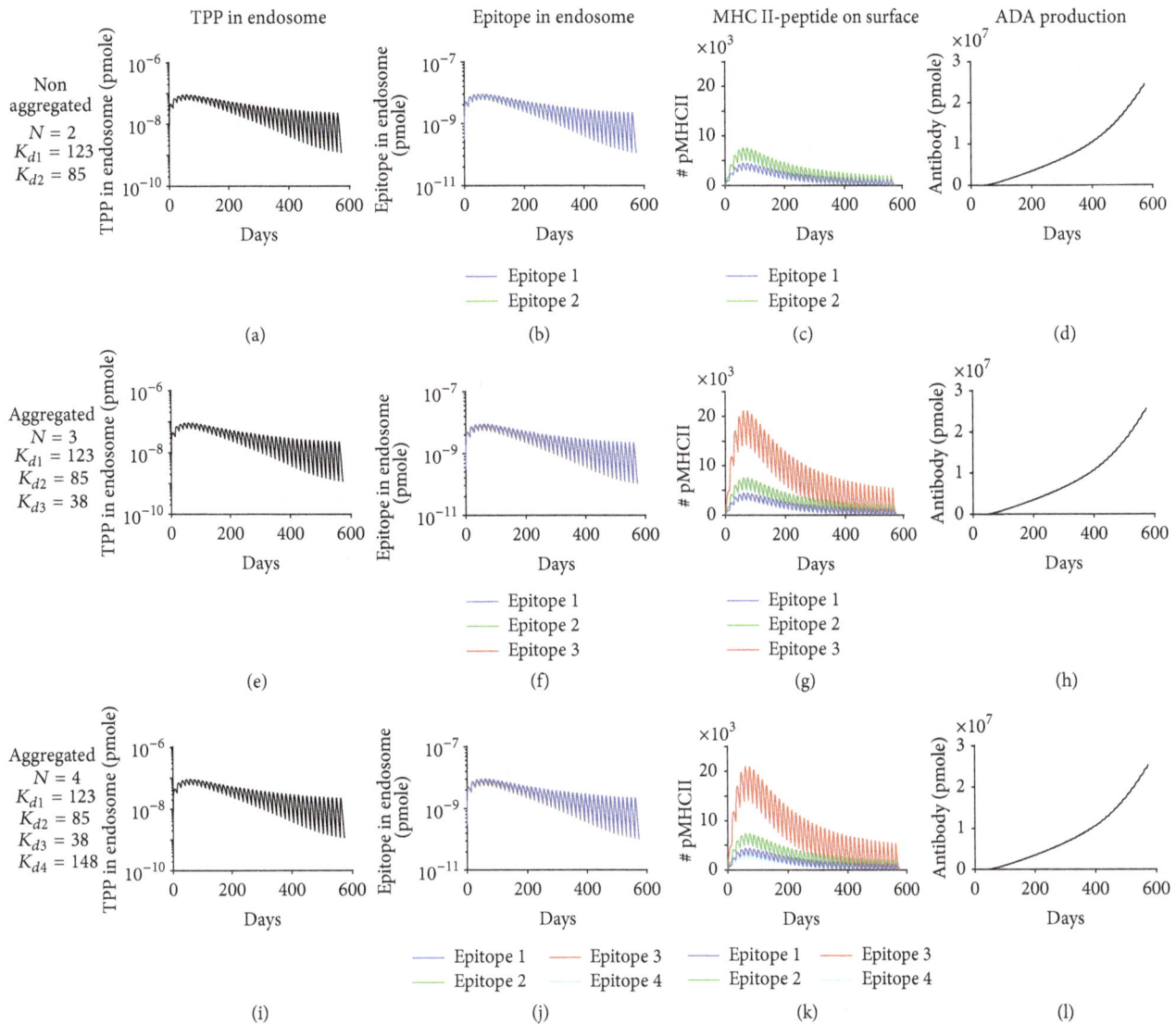

FIGURE 6: Aggregates could not enhance ADA production by increasing number of epitopes if high affinity epitopes are already present in nonaggregated TPP. Simulated levels of TPP in endosome, epitope in endosome, MHC II-peptide complex on cell surface, and ADA production are shown for ((a)–(d)) original two predicted epitopes for nonaggregated adalimumab [47, 48], ((e)–(h)) three epitopes for hypothetical aggregated form, and ((i)–(l)) four epitopes for hypothetical aggregated form. The predicted dissociation constant (K_d, unit: nM) for binding of each epitope to MHC II is indicated. ADA production has the same definition and dose has the same value as in Figure 4.

cannot enhance ADA production if high affinity epitopes are already present.

3.4. Aggregates Could Enhance ADA Production by Inducing the Presentation of Epitopes with Higher Affinities than Those from Nonaggregated TPP.

MHC II-restricted epitopes are generated with μM to nM affinity range [65]. We next evaluated whether aggregate-induced high antigen processing and presentation could increase immunogenicity when nonaggregated TPP present low affinity (μM range) epitopes. We started with 40 mg dose of nonaggregated TPP administered biweekly and two epitopes with K_d of 1230 and 850 nM representing low affinity epitopes of μM range [65, 66] and monitored the number of MHC II-peptide complexes on

surface of APC and ADA production (Figures 7(a)–7(d)). We next increased the internalization rate by 16.6-fold to mimic the effect of aggregates and again saw no increase in antigen presentation and ADA production (Figures 7(e)–7(h)). Notably, when aggregates induced the presentation of a high affinity epitope ($K_d = 38$ nM), ADA production increased by >4-fold (Figure 7(l)) due to enhanced antigen presentation (Figures 7(i)–7(k)). We further evaluated the effect of aggregate-induced high affinity epitopes on ADA production under different dose levels, all of which demonstrated that induction of a high affinity epitope could significantly increase ADA production (compare top and bottom rows in Figure 8), whereas increase in internalization rate had no effect (compare top and middle rows in Figure 8).

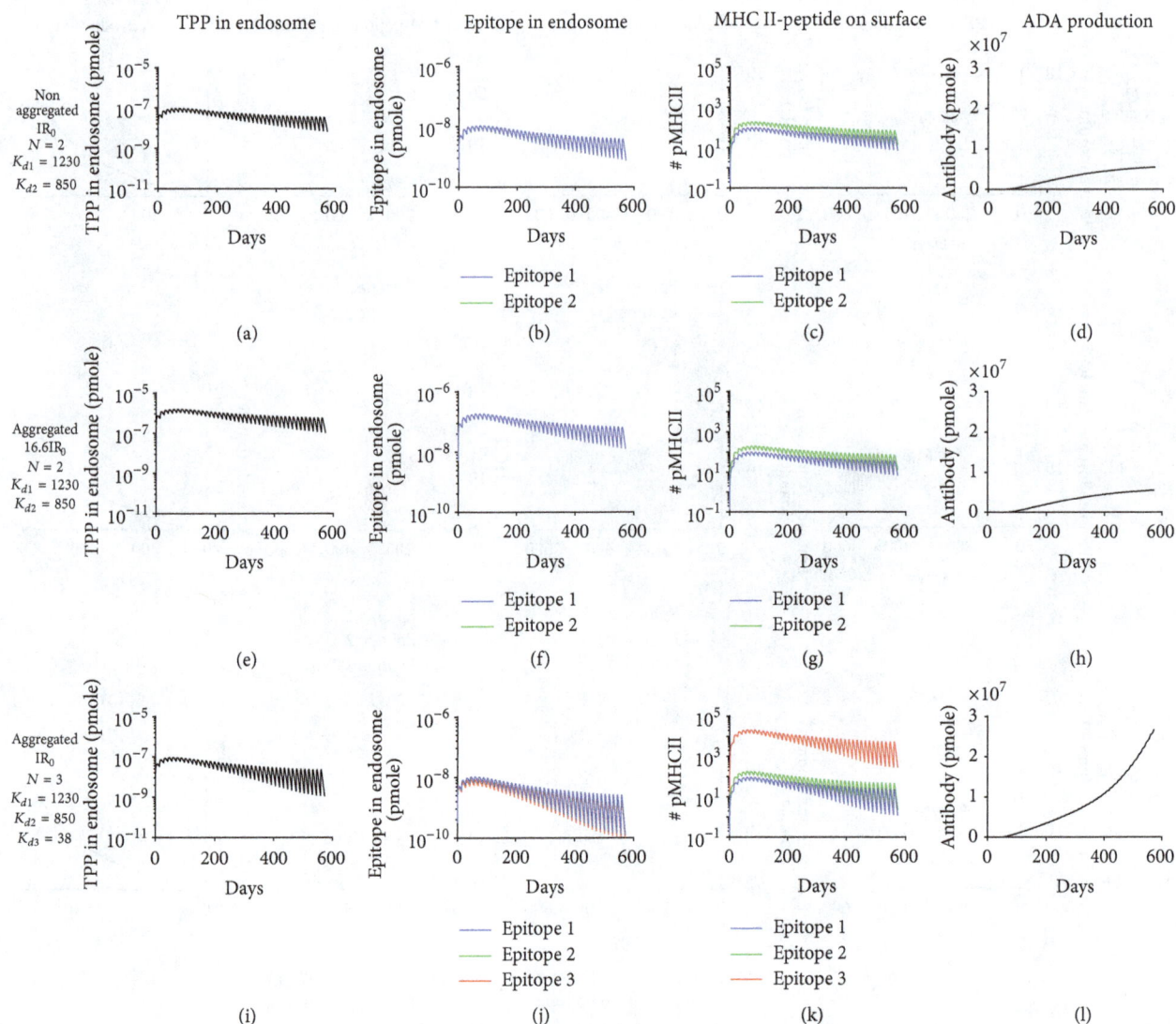

FIGURE 7: Aggregation could contribute to ADA production by inducing the presentation of high affinity epitopes that may not be present in nonaggregated TPP. Simulated levels of TPP in endosome, epitope in endosome, MHC II-peptide complex on cell surface, and ADA production are shown for ((a)–(d)) original internalization rate (IR_0) and two low affinity epitopes for hypothetical nonaggregated TPP, ((e)–(h)) $16.6IR_0$ and two low affinity epitopes for hypothetical aggregated form, and ((i)–(l)) IR_0 and inclusion of a high affinity third epitope for hypothetical aggregated form. The predicted dissociation constant (K_d, unit: nM) for binding of each epitope to MHC II is indicated. ADA production has the same definition and dose and IR_0 have the same values as in Figure 4.

These computational modeling results indicate that aggregates could contribute to ADA production by inducing the presentation of high affinity epitopes that may not be present in nonaggregated TPP.

4. Discussion

In this study, we used mathematical modeling to comprehensively evaluate mechanisms through which aggregates of TPP could contribute to immunogenicity. By modeling the interactions between aggregates and BCRs, we find that aggregates are unlikely to induce T cell-independent antibody responses through BCR cross-linking due to the limited number of STC that could form under physiologically

plausible conditions. Thereafter, using our previously developed multiscale, mechanistic mathematical model for the T cell-dependent induction of ADA by TPP, we systematically evaluated the potential roles of aggregates in ADA generation by dissecting the individual steps leading to it. Our analyses indicate that aggregates could contribute to immunogenicity by increasing the danger signal to mature dendritic cells and activate T cells and/or by inducing the presentation of high affinity epitopes that may not be present in nonaggregated TPP.

TPP could aggregate during manufacturing, storage, handling, or delivery to patients due to agitation, light exposure, temperature elevation, oxidation, pH change, and leaching [12, 17, 23, 24, 29, 30, 56, 67]. Aggregation has been proposed

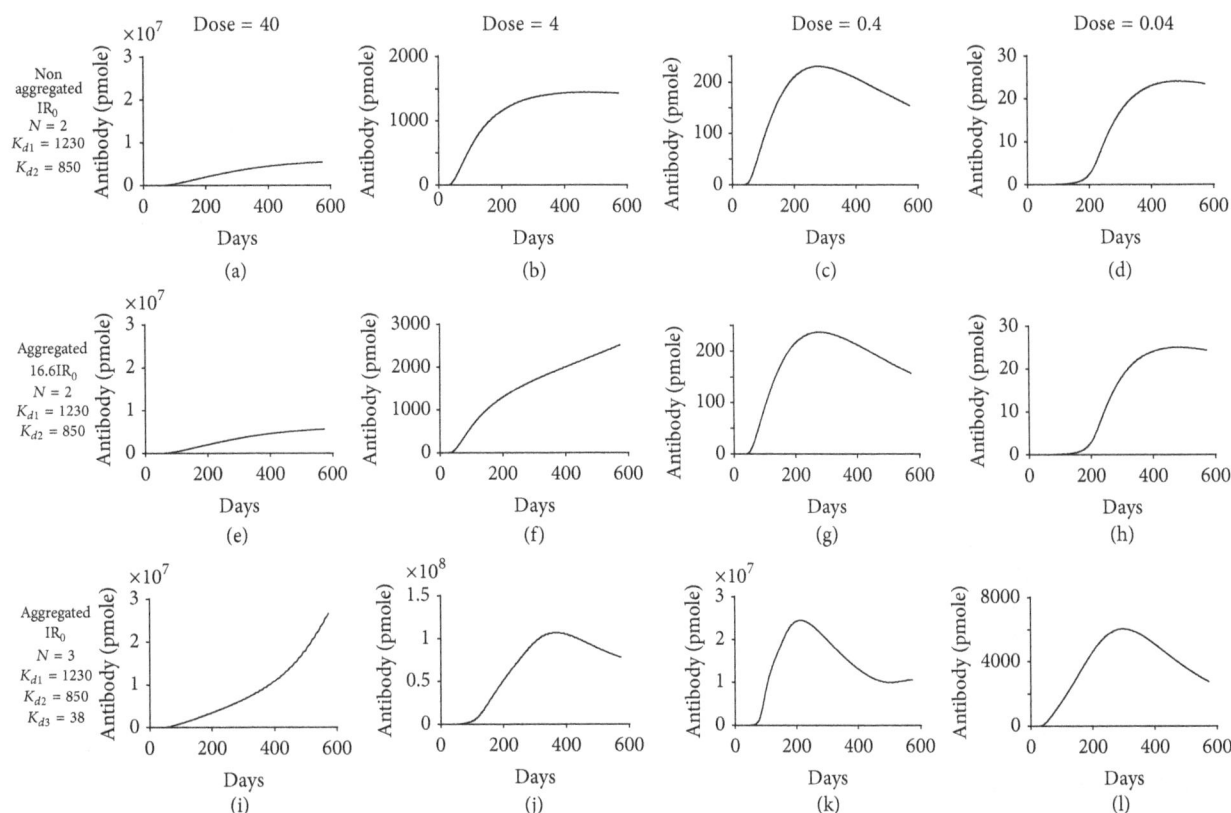

FIGURE 8: Aggregation could contribute to immunogenicity by inducing the presentation of high affinity epitopes that may not be present in nonaggregated TPP under a variety of drug doses. Simulated ADA production is shown for the same conditions as in Figure 7 for biweekly administered dose of 40 mg ((a), (e), and (i)), 4 mg ((b), (f), and (j)), 0.4 mg ((c), (g), and (k)), and 0.04 mg ((d), (h), and (l)). ADA production has the same definition as in Figure 4.

as a strong risk factor for TPP-induced immunogenicity due to its potential role in both T cell-independent and T cell-dependent antibody responses [10, 12, 14, 16, 17]. Several previous studies in mice have demonstrated that for different TPP aggregates induced a stronger ADA production compared with nonaggregated forms [18–21, 25, 27, 28]. However, the mechanisms underlying aggregate-induced ADA production are not clear. A recent study in mice transgenic for human IgG demonstrated that only light-induced oligomers of IgG induced an immune response, which was ablated by the depletion of CD4+ cells [66]. The data from this mouse model are in agreement with the mathematical model in which aggregates induce immune responses in a T cell-dependent manner.

Repetitively arranged epitopes in a paracrystalline structure of viral particles could cross-link BCRs to induce T cell-independent IgM or in some cases IgG3 responses [68–72]. It is expected that aggregates of TPP, potentially resembling the structure of highly repetitive epitopes, could induce T cell-independent antibody responses in a similar way [12, 16, 17]. The model does not directly consider the nature of a polyclonal B cell response, but it is consistent with that. Specifically, multiple epitopes from the aggregates being bound by the BCR can be represented by the differential binding rate constants in the model, and the different number of B cell epitopes on aggregates can be captured by the complex forming between aggregates and various number of BCRs. Surprisingly, by modeling the interactions between aggregates and BCRs, we find that aggregates are unlikely to induce T cell-independent antibody responses because only a few STC can form under physiologically plausible conditions for antigen-specific B cells, antigen dose, and binding affinity (Figure 2(b), left and center panels). This is consistent with previous studies in mice that showed no significant T cell-independent IgG3 antibody response against aggregated recombinant murine growth hormone [28] or anti-TNFα murine mAb [23], although IgM production was not evaluated in either case. However, it should be noted that, under conditions of high binding affinity and BCR concentration and appropriate antigen concentrations, significant number of STC could form, with a potential to induce T cell-independent antibody response (Figure 2(b), right panel). High BCR concentration can be achieved through high percentage of antigen-specific B cells for particular TPP or through B cell proliferation due to lowering of activation threshold by cytokines [73], second messenger diacylglycerol [74], costimulatory signal [75], or Bruton's tyrosine kinase [76]. Appropriate antigen concentration can result from specific dosing strategies. Therefore, particular attention should be given while administering TPP to patients in those conditions. Future experiments directly investigating the downstream signaling of BCR cross-linking in the presence of aggregated and nonaggregated TPP and studies evaluating whether T cell-independent IgM is induced in response to aggregates can further elucidate the role of aggregates in T cell-independent ADA production.

T cell-dependent ADA production is thought to be the major pathway through which TPP induce immunogenicity as in the case of IgG1 and IgG4 generated against anti-TNFα mAb to treat a variety of inflammatory and autoimmune diseases [7]. Antigen processing and presentation by professional APC, such as dendritic cells, macrophages, and B cells, play a key role in T cell-dependent antibody responses [12]. It has been shown that aggregates could enhance antigen uptake by APC thereby increasing peptides associated with MHC II and could induce dendritic cell maturation and T cell activation [22, 30, 56]. However, human data directly ascribing ADA levels to aggregates are still lacking. In this study, we systematically evaluated whether aggregate-enhanced antigen processing and presentation could increase ADA production. Our computer simulation suggests that the amount of antigenic peptides in endosome is limited by antigen internalization rate, not degradation rate, and the number of MHC II-peptide complexes presented on cell surface is mainly restricted by the binding affinity of epitopes. Our modeling analyses indicate that induction of high affinity epitopes by aggregates that may not be present in nonaggregated TPP and increased danger signal by aggregates to maturate dendritic cells could result in increased ADA production (Figures 4–8). A specifically designed experimental study that examines the binding affinities of peptides to MHC II derived from dendritic cells treated with aggregated or nonaggregated TPP would verify whether aggregates can induce the presentation of high affinity epitopes not present in nonaggregated TPP. In this work, we modeled aggregates-induced danger signal as LPS. However, it should be noted that aggregates have the potential to bind to a variety of pattern recognition receptors as well as FcR. Therefore the kinetics, activation thresholds, and receptors engaged by aggregates are more diverse and complicated than those of LPS and need further investigation.

This work improves our understanding of aggregate-induced immunogenicity and could be utilized to develop prediction and mitigation strategies. Overall, this modeling study suggests that aggregates could enhance immunogenicity; therefore enough attention should be given to reduce aggregation during manufacturing, storage, handling, and administration. In particular, potential high affinity CD4+ T cell epitopes are of great concern because their presentation in nonaggregated TPP will result in high levels of immunogenicity regardless of aggregation. On the other hand, even if they are not presented in nonaggregated TPP, an aggregation-induced presentation will also result in enhanced immunogenicity. Thus, efforts should be made towards experimental identification or *in silico* prediction of high affinity epitopes during immunogenicity assessment, and potential high affinity epitopes should be avoided while designing novel TPP as they carry a strong risk for ADA generation.

Our recently developed mechanistic system-level mathematical model for ADA production is a useful tool to evaluate human immunogenicity against TPP as it incorporates protein-specific antigenic properties and host-specific immunological characteristics, although further experimental validation is needed to increase confidence in ADA predictions [47, 48]. Multiple product- and patient-related risk factors have been proposed to impact immunogenicity of TPP [7, 8, 10–14, 77, 78]. As confidence in its properties increases, this system-level model could potentially be used to design new hypotheses and study other risk factors besides aggregation. For example, though the model is developed for healthy subjects, it can be easily modified to account for the effect of different disease statuses. For example, the profile of ADA generation observed in autoimmune patients [79, 80] can be simulated by including either a lower activation threshold for immune cells [37, 38] or preexisting immunity against TPP [79, 80]. Also, peptide editor HLA-DM plays a key role in MHC II antigen presentation and CD4+ T cell epitope selection by favoring the presentation of peptides with higher kinetic stabilities [65, 81–84]. To evaluate the effect of HLA-DM-mediated epitope selection on ADA production, it could be included in the subcellular module of antigen processing and presentation to select the epitopes presented based on peptide susceptibility to HLA-DM-mediated peptide exchange [84]. Other ADA production impact factors that could be evaluated by this system-level model include time delays between administration, immune cell activation and migration from tissue to lymphoid compartments [42], contraction of effector B cells and T cells [85, 86], effect of immunomodulators through comedication [87], and different antibody isotypes generated by short- and long-lived plasma cells [42, 88, 89]. Therefore, this model could generate new hypotheses about immunogenicity and could be used with experiments to decipher the mechanisms underlying immunogenicity of TPP and develop corresponding mitigation strategies.

5. Conclusion

In summary, our computational analyses suggest that aggregates are unlikely to induce T cell-independent antibody responses through BCR cross-linking due to limited formation of STC under physiologically plausible conditions. In contrast, aggregates could contribute to immunogenicity via the T cell-dependent pathway by inducing the presentation of high affinity epitopes that may not be present in nonaggregated TPP and/or by enhancing danger signal to maturate dendritic cells and activate T cells. This study provides novel insights into how aggregates could contribute to overall immunogenicity and suggests novel mechanistic hypotheses eventually suitable for experimental testing.

Disclosure

Paolo Vicini is currently working at Clinical Pharmacology and DMPK, MedImmune, Cambridge CB21 6GH, UK.

Conflict of Interests

All authors are current or former employees of Pfizer Inc.

Authors' Contribution

Xiaoying Chen and Abhinav Tiwari contributed to the work equally.

Acknowledgments

This work was supported by a Pfizer Worldwide Research and Development Postdoctoral Fellowship.

References

[1] D. S. Dimitrov, "Therapeutic proteins," in *Therapeutic Proteins*, vol. 899 of *Methods in Molecular Biology*, pp. 1–26, Humana Press, 2012.

[2] G. Walsh, "Biopharmaceutical benchmarks 2014," *Nature Biotechnology*, vol. 32, no. 10, pp. 992–1000, 2014.

[3] V. Brinks, D. Weinbuch, M. Baker et al., "Preclinical models used for immunogenicity prediction of therapeutic proteins," *Pharmaceutical Research*, vol. 30, no. 7, pp. 1719–1728, 2013.

[4] R. T. Purcell and R. F. Lockey, "Immunologic responses to therapeutic biologic agents," *Journal of Investigational Allergology & Clinical Immunology*, vol. 18, no. 5, pp. 335–342, 2008.

[5] V. Jawa, L. P. Cousens, M. Awwad, E. Wakshull, H. Kropshofer, and A. S. De Groot, "T-cell dependent immunogenicity of protein therapeutics: preclinical assessment and mitigation," *Clinical Immunology*, vol. 149, no. 3, pp. 534–555, 2013.

[6] J. R. Maneiro, E. Salgado, and J. J. Gomez-Reino, "Immunogenicity of monoclonal antibodies against tumor necrosis factor used in chronic immune-mediated inflammatory conditions: systematic review and meta-analysis," *JAMA Internal Medicine*, vol. 173, no. 15, pp. 1416–1428, 2013.

[7] P. A. van Schouwenburg, T. Rispens, and G. J. Wolbink, "Immunogenicity of anti-TNF biologic therapies for rheumatoid arthritis," *Nature Reviews Rheumatology*, vol. 9, no. 3, pp. 164–172, 2013.

[8] G. Shankar, S. Arkin, L. Cocea et al., "Assessment and reporting of the clinical immunogenicity of therapeutic proteins and peptides—harmonized terminology and tactical recommendations," *The AAPS Journal*, vol. 16, no. 4, pp. 658–673, 2014.

[9] A. S. De Groot and D. W. Scott, "Immunogenicity of protein therapeutics," *Trends in Immunology*, vol. 28, no. 11, pp. 482–490, 2007.

[10] S. K. Singh, "Impact of product-related factors on immunogenicity of biotherapeutics," *Journal of Pharmaceutical Sciences*, vol. 100, no. 2, pp. 354–387, 2011.

[11] C. Krieckaert, T. Rispens, and G. Wolbink, "Immunogenicity of biological therapeutics: from assay to patient," *Current Opinion in Rheumatology*, vol. 24, no. 3, pp. 306–311, 2012.

[12] S. Sethu, K. Govindappa, M. Alhaidari, M. Pirmohamed, K. Park, and J. Sathish, "Immunogenicity to biologics: mechanisms, prediction and reduction," *Archivum Immunologiae et Therapiae Experimentalis*, vol. 60, no. 5, pp. 331–344, 2012.

[13] A. C. Moss, V. Brinks, and J. F. Carpenter, "Review article: immunogenicity of anti-TNF biologics in IBD—the role of patient, product and prescriber factors," *Alimentary Pharmacology & Therapeutics*, vol. 38, no. 10, pp. 1188–1197, 2013.

[14] S. Kumar, S. K. Singh, X. Wang, B. Rup, and D. Gill, "Coupling of aggregation and immunogenicity in biotherapeutics: T- and B-cell immune epitopes may contain aggregation-prone regions," *Pharmaceutical Research*, vol. 28, no. 5, pp. 949–961, 2011.

[15] S. Kumar, M. A. Mitchell, B. Rup, and S. K. Singh, "Relationship between potential aggregation-prone regions and HLA-DR-binding T-cell immune epitopes: implications for rational design of novel and follow-on therapeutic antibodies," *Journal of Pharmaceutical Sciences*, vol. 101, no. 8, pp. 2686–2701, 2012.

[16] K. D. Ratanji, J. P. Derrick, R. J. Dearman, and I. Kimber, "Immunogenicity of therapeutic proteins: influence of aggregation," *Journal of Immunotoxicology*, vol. 11, no. 2, pp. 99–109, 2014.

[17] M. Sauerborn, V. Brinks, W. Jiskoot, and H. Schellekens, "Immunological mechanism underlying the immune response to recombinant human protein therapeutics," *Trends in Pharmacological Sciences*, vol. 31, no. 2, pp. 53–59, 2010.

[18] S. Hermeling, L. Aranha, J. M. A. Damen et al., "Structural characterization and immunogenicity in wild-type and immune tolerant mice of degraded recombinant human interferon alpha2b," *Pharmaceutical Research*, vol. 22, no. 12, pp. 1997–2006, 2005.

[19] S. Hermeling, H. Schellekens, C. Maas, M. F. B. G. Gebbink, D. J. A. Crommelin, and W. Jiskoot, "Antibody response to aggregated human interferon alpha2b in wild-type and transgenic immune tolerant mice depends on type and level of aggregation," *Journal of Pharmaceutical Sciences*, vol. 95, no. 5, pp. 1084–1096, 2006.

[20] P. Human, H. Ilsley, C. Roberson et al., "Assessment of the immunogenicity of mechanically induced interferon aggregates in a transgenic mouse model," *Journal of Pharmaceutical Sciences*, vol. 104, no. 2, pp. 722–730, 2015.

[21] V. Filipe, W. Jiskoot, A. H. Basmeleh, A. Halim, H. Schellekens, and V. Brinks, "Immunogenicity of different stressed IgG monoclonal antibody formulations in immune tolerant transgenic mice," *mAbs*, vol. 4, no. 6, pp. 740–752, 2012.

[22] M. K. Joubert, M. Hokom, C. Eakin et al., "Highly aggregated antibody therapeutics can enhance the in vitro innate and late-stage T-cell immune responses," *The Journal of Biological Chemistry*, vol. 287, no. 30, pp. 25266–25279, 2012.

[23] A. J. Freitag, M. Shomali, S. Michalakis et al., "Investigation of the immunogenicity of different types of aggregates of a murine monoclonal antibody in mice," *Pharmaceutical Research*, vol. 32, no. 2, pp. 430–444, 2015.

[24] A. Seidl, O. Hainzl, M. Richter et al., "Tungsten-induced denaturation and aggregation of epoetin alfa during primary packaging as a cause of immunogenicity," *Pharmaceutical Research*, vol. 29, no. 6, pp. 1454–1467, 2012.

[25] V. S. Purohit, C. R. Middaugh, and S. V. Balasubramanian, "Influence of aggregation on immunogenicity of recombinant human factor VIII in hemophilia A mice," *Journal of Pharmaceutical Sciences*, vol. 95, no. 2, pp. 358–371, 2006.

[26] D. S. Pisal, M. P. Kosloski, C. R. Middaugh, R. B. Bankert, and S. V. Balu-Iyer, "Native-like aggregates of factor VIII are immunogenic in von Willebrand factor deficient and hemophilia a mice," *Journal of Pharmaceutical Sciences*, vol. 101, no. 6, pp. 2055–2065, 2012.

[27] M. M. C. van Beers, M. Sauerborn, F. Gilli, V. Brinks, H. Schellekens, and W. Jiskoot, "Aggregated recombinant human interferon beta induces antibodies but no memory in immune-tolerant transgenic mice," *Pharmaceutical Research*, vol. 27, no. 9, pp. 1812–1824, 2010.

[28] A. H. Fradkin, J. F. Carpenter, and T. W. Randolph, "Glass particles as an adjuvant: a model for adverse immunogenicity of therapeutic proteins," *Journal of Pharmaceutical Sciences*, vol. 100, no. 11, pp. 4953–4964, 2011.

[29] J. G. Barnard, K. Babcock, and J. F. Carpenter, "Characterization and quantitation of aggregates and particles in interferon-β products: potential links between product quality attributes and immunogenicity," *Journal of Pharmaceutical Sciences*, vol. 102, no. 3, pp. 915–928, 2013.

[30] V. Rombach-Riegraf, A. C. Karle, B. Wolf et al., "Aggregation of human recombinant monoclonal antibodies influences the capacity of dendritic cells to stimulate adaptive T-cell responses in vitro," *PLoS ONE*, vol. 9, no. 1, Article ID e86322, 2014.

[31] C. Lundegaard, O. Lund, C. Keşmir, S. Brunak, and M. Nielsen, "Modeling the adaptive immune system: predictions and simulations," *Bioinformatics*, vol. 23, no. 24, pp. 3265–3275, 2007.

[32] J. D. Gómez-Mantilla, I. F. Trocóniz, Z. Parra-Guillén, and M. J. Garrido, "Review on modeling anti-antibody responses to monoclonal antibodies," *Journal of Pharmacokinetics and Pharmacodynamics*, vol. 41, no. 5, pp. 523–536, 2014.

[33] T. P. Hickling, X. Chen, P. Vicini, and S. Nayak, "A review of quantitative modeling of B cell responses to antigenic challenge," *Journal of Pharmacokinetics and Pharmacodynamics*, vol. 41, no. 5, pp. 445–459, 2014.

[34] S. Palsson, T. P. Hickling, E. L. Bradshaw-Pierce et al., "The development of a fully-integrated immune response model (FIRM) simulator of the immune response through integration of multiple subset models," *BMC Systems Biology*, vol. 7, article 95, 2013.

[35] N. G. B. Agrawal and J. J. Linderman, "Mathematical modeling of helper T lymphocyte/antigen-presenting cell interactions: analysis of methods for modifying antigen processing and presentation," *Journal of Theoretical Biology*, vol. 182, no. 4, pp. 487–504, 1996.

[36] G. I. Bell, "Mathematical model of clonal selection and antibody production," *Journal of Theoretical Biology*, vol. 29, no. 2, pp. 191–232, 1970.

[37] K. B. Blyuss and L. B. Nicholson, "The role of tunable activation thresholds in the dynamics of autoimmunity," *Journal of Theoretical Biology*, vol. 308, pp. 45–55, 2012.

[38] K. B. Blyuss and L. B. Nicholson, "Understanding the roles of activation threshold and infections in the dynamics of autoimmune disease," *Journal of Theoretical Biology*, vol. 375, pp. 13–20, 2015.

[39] M. Oprea and A. S. Perelson, "Exploring the mechanisms of primary antibody responses to T cell-dependent antigens," *Journal of Theoretical Biology*, vol. 181, no. 3, pp. 215–236, 1996.

[40] A. Rundell, R. DeCarlo, H. HogenEsch, and P. Doerschuk, "The humoral immune response to *Haemophilus influenzae* type b: a mathematical model based on T-zone and germinal center B-cell dynamics," *Journal of Theoretical Biology*, vol. 194, no. 3, pp. 341–381, 1998.

[41] F. Castiglione, F. Toschi, M. Bernaschi et al., "Computational modeling of the immune response to tumor antigens," *Journal of Theoretical Biology*, vol. 237, no. 4, pp. 390–400, 2005.

[42] H. Y. Lee, D. J. Topham, S. Y. Park et al., "Simulation and prediction of the adaptive immune response to influenza A virus infection," *Journal of Virology*, vol. 83, no. 14, pp. 7151–7165, 2009.

[43] S. M. Ciupe, R. M. Ribeiro, and A. S. Perelson, "Antibody responses during hepatitis B viral infection," *PLoS Computational Biology*, vol. 10, no. 7, Article ID e1003730, 2014.

[44] B. Sulzer and A. S. Perelson, "Equilibrium binding of multivalent ligands to cells: effects of cell and receptor density," *Mathematical Biosciences*, vol. 135, no. 2, pp. 147–185, 1996.

[45] B. Sulzer and A. S. Perelson, "Immunons revisited: binding of multivalent antigens to b cells," *Molecular Immunology*, vol. 34, no. 1, pp. 63–74, 1997.

[46] X. Chen, T. Hickling, E. Kraynov, B. Kuang, C. Parng, and P. Vicini, "A mathematical model of the effect of immunogenicity on therapeutic protein pharmacokinetics," *The AAPS Journal*, vol. 15, no. 4, pp. 1141–1154, 2013.

[47] X. Chen, T. P. Hickling, and P. Vicini, "A mechanistic, multiscale mathematical model of immunogenicity for therapeutic proteins: part 2—model applications," *CPT: Pharmacometrics & Systems Pharmacology*, vol. 3, no. 9, article e134, 10 pages, 2014.

[48] X. Chen, T. P. Hickling, and P. Vicini, "A mechanistic, multiscale mathematical model of immunogenicity for therapeutic proteins: part 1—theoretical model," *CPT: Pharmacometrics & Systems Pharmacology*, vol. 3, no. 9, pp. 1–9, 2014.

[49] S. E. Grossberg, J. Oger, L. D. Grossberg, A. Gehchan, and J. P. Klein, "Frequency and magnitude of interferon beta neutralizing antibodies in the evaluation of interferon beta immunogenicity in patients with multiple sclerosis," *Journal of Interferon & Cytokine Research*, vol. 31, no. 3, pp. 337–344, 2011.

[50] L. O. Narhi, J. Schmit, K. Bechtold-Peters, and D. Sharma, "Classification of protein aggregates," *Journal of Pharmaceutical Sciences*, vol. 101, no. 2, pp. 493–498, 2012.

[51] M. Reth, "Matching cellular dimensions with molecular sizes," *Nature Immunology*, vol. 14, no. 8, pp. 765–767, 2013.

[52] J. Foote and H. N. Eisen, "Kinetic and affinity limits on antibodies produced during immune responses," *Proceedings of the National Academy of Sciences of the United States of America*, vol. 92, no. 5, pp. 1254–1256, 1995.

[53] J. Foote and C. Milstein, "Kinetic maturation of an immune response," *Nature*, vol. 352, no. 6335, pp. 530–532, 1991.

[54] S. Crotty, P. Felgner, H. Davies, J. Glidewell, L. Villarreal, and R. Ahmed, "Cutting edge: long-term B cell memory in humans after smallpox vaccination," *The Journal of Immunology*, vol. 171, no. 10, pp. 4969–4973, 2003.

[55] A. P. Kodituwakku, C. Jessup, H. Zola, and D. M. Roberton, "Isolation of antigen-specific B cells," *Immunology and Cell Biology*, vol. 81, no. 3, pp. 163–170, 2003.

[56] M. Ahmadi, C. J. Bryson, E. A. Cloake et al., "Small amounts of sub-visible aggregates enhance the immunogenic potential of monoclonal antibody therapeutics," *Pharmaceutical Research*, vol. 32, no. 4, pp. 1383–1394, 2015.

[57] C. Buelens, V. Verhasselt, D. De Groote, K. Thielemans, M. Goldman, and F. Willems, "Human dendritic cell responses to lipopolysaccharide and CD40 ligation are differentially regulated by interleukin-10," *European Journal of Immunology*, vol. 27, no. 8, pp. 1848–1852, 1997.

[58] F. Granucci, E. Ferrero, M. Foti, D. Aggujaro, K. Vettoretto, and P. Ricciardi-Castagnoli, "Early events in dendritic cell maturation induced by LPS," *Microbes and Infection*, vol. 1, no. 13, pp. 1079–1084, 1999.

[59] R. M. Cisco, Z. Abdel-Wahab, J. Dannull et al., "Induction of human dendritic cell maturation using transfection with RNA encoding a dominant positive toll-like receptor 4," *Journal of Immunology*, vol. 172, no. 11, pp. 7162–7168, 2004.

[60] K. Kawamura, K. Iyonaga, H. Ichiyasu, J. Nagano, M. Suga, and Y. Sasaki, "Differentiation, maturation, and survival of dendritic cells by osteopontin regulation," *Clinical and Diagnostic Laboratory Immunology*, vol. 12, no. 1, pp. 206–212, 2005.

[61] Y.-C. Wang, X.-B. Hu, F. He et al., "Lipopolysaccharide-induced maturation of bone marrow-derived dendritic cells is regulated by notch signaling through the up-regulation of CXCR4," *The Journal of Biological Chemistry*, vol. 284, no. 23, pp. 15993–16003, 2009.

[62] D. Verthelyi and V. Wang, "Trace levels of innate immune response modulating impurities (IIRMIs) synergize to break tolerance to therapeutic proteins," *PLoS ONE*, vol. 5, no. 12, Article ID e15252, 2010.

[63] M. Rossol, H. Heine, U. Meusch et al., "LPS-induced cytokine production in human monocytes and macrophages," *Critical Reviews in Immunology*, vol. 31, no. 5, pp. 379–446, 2011.

[64] J. C. Jones, E. W. Settles, C. R. Brandt, and S. Schultz-Cherry, "Virus aggregating peptide enhances the cell-mediated response to influenza virus vaccine," *Vaccine*, vol. 29, no. 44, pp. 7696–7703, 2011.

[65] L. Yin, J. M. Calvo-Calle, O. Dominguez-Amorocho, and L. J. Ster, "HLA-DM constrains epitope selection in the human CD4 T cell response to vaccinia virus by favoring the presentation of peptides with longer HLA-DM-mediated half-lives," *Journal of Immunology*, vol. 189, no. 8, pp. 3983–3994, 2012.

[66] J. Bessa, S. Boeckle, H. Beck et al., "The immunogenicity of antibody aggregates in a novel transgenic mouse model," *Pharmaceutical Research*, vol. 32, no. 7, pp. 2344–2359, 2015.

[67] W. Wang, "Protein aggregation and its inhibition in biopharmaceutics," *International Journal of Pharmaceutics*, vol. 289, no. 1-2, pp. 1–30, 2005.

[68] M. F. Bachmann and R. M. Zinkernagel, "Neutralizing antiviral B cell responses," *Annual Review of Immunology*, vol. 15, pp. 235–270, 1997.

[69] E. Szomolanyi-Tsuda and R. M. Welsh, "T-cell-independent antiviral antibody responses," *Current Opinion in Immunology*, vol. 10, no. 4, pp. 431–435, 1998.

[70] C. Babin, N. Majeau, and D. Leclerc, "Engineering of papaya mosaic virus (PapMV) nanoparticles with a CTL epitope derived from influenza NP," *Journal of Nanobiotechnology*, vol. 11, article 10, 2013.

[71] C. M. Snapper, T. M. McIntyre, R. Mandler et al., "Induction of IgG3 secretion by interferon γ: a model for T cell-independent class switching in response to T cell-independent type 2 antigens," *The Journal of Experimental Medicine*, vol. 175, no. 5, pp. 1367–1371, 1992.

[72] T. Fehr, M. F. Bachmann, E. Bucher et al., "Role of repetitive antigen patterns for induction of antibodies against antibodies," *The Journal of Experimental Medicine*, vol. 185, no. 10, pp. 1785–1792, 1997.

[73] P. K. A. Mongini, P. F. Highet, and J. K. Inman, "Human B cell activation: effect of T cell cytokines on the physicochemical binding requirements for achieving cell cycle progression via the membrane IgM signaling pathway," *Journal of Immunology*, vol. 155, no. 7, pp. 3385–3400, 1995.

[74] M. L. Wheeler, M. B. Dong, R. Brink, X.-P. Zhong, and A. L. DeFranco, "Diacylglycerol kinase zeta limits B cell antigen receptor-dependent activation of ERK Signaling to inhibit early antibody responses," *Science Signaling*, vol. 6, no. 297, article ra91, 2013.

[75] G. G. B. Klaus, M. Holman, C. Johnson-Léger, J. R. Christenson, and M. R. Kehry, "Interaction of B cells with activated T cells reduces the threshold for CD40-mediated B cell activation," *International Immunology*, vol. 11, no. 1, pp. 71–79, 1999.

[76] L. P. Kil, M. J. W. de Bruijn, M. van Nimwegen et al., "Btk levels set the threshold for B-cell activation and negative selection of autoreactive B cells in mice," *Blood*, vol. 119, no. 16, pp. 3744–3756, 2012.

[77] D. W. Scott and A. S. De Groot, "Can we prevent immunogenicity of human protein drugs?" *Annals of the Rheumatic Diseases*, vol. 69, supplement 1, pp. i72–i76, 2010.

[78] V. Brinks, W. Jiskoot, and H. Schellekens, "Immunogenicity of therapeutic proteins: the use of animal models," *Pharmaceutical Research*, vol. 28, no. 10, pp. 2379–2385, 2011.

[79] L. Xue, M. Fiscella, M. Rajadhyaksha et al., "Pre-existing biotherapeutic-reactive antibodies: survey results within the american association of pharmaceutical scientists," *The AAPS Journal*, vol. 15, no. 3, pp. 852–855, 2013.

[80] L. Xue and B. Rup, "Evaluation of pre-existing antibody presence as a risk factor for posttreatment anti-drug antibody induction: analysis of human clinical study data for multiple biotherapeutics," *The AAPS Journal*, vol. 15, no. 3, pp. 893–896, 2013.

[81] V. S. Sloan, P. Cameron, G. Porter et al., "Mediation by HLA-DM of dissociation of peptides from HLA-DR," *Nature*, vol. 375, no. 6534, pp. 802–806, 1995.

[82] N. K. Nanda and A. J. Sant, "DM determines the cryptic and immunodominant fate of T cell epitopes," *The Journal of Experimental Medicine*, vol. 192, no. 6, pp. 781–788, 2000.

[83] A. J. Sant, F. A. Chaves, S. A. Jenks et al., "The relationship between immunodominance, DM editing, and the kinetic stability of MHC class II:peptide complexes," *Immunological Reviews*, vol. 207, pp. 261–278, 2005.

[84] L. Yin, P. Trenh, A. Guce et al., "Susceptibility to HLA-DM protein is determined by a dynamic conformation of major histocompatibility complex class II molecule bound with peptide," *The Journal of Biological Chemistry*, vol. 289, no. 34, pp. 23449–23464, 2014.

[85] K. R. Garrod, H. D. Moreau, Z. Garcia et al., "Dissecting T cell contraction in vivo using a genetically encoded reporter of apoptosis," *Cell Reports*, vol. 2, no. 5, pp. 1438–1447, 2012.

[86] H. Lee, S. Haque, J. Nieto et al., "A p53 axis regulates B cell receptor-triggered, innate immune system-driven B cell clonal expansion," *Journal of Immunology*, vol. 188, no. 12, pp. 6093–6108, 2012.

[87] C. L. M. Krieckaert, G. M. Bartelds, W. F. Lems, and G. J. Wolbink, "The effect of immunomodulators on the immunogenicity of TNF-blocking therapeutic monoclonal antibodies: a review," *Arthritis Research & Therapy*, vol. 12, no. 5, article 217, 2010.

[88] A. Radbruch, G. Muehlinghaus, E. O. Luger et al., "Competence and competition: the challenge of becoming a long-lived plasma cell," *Nature Reviews Immunology*, vol. 6, no. 10, pp. 741–750, 2006.

[89] C. H. Rozanski, R. Arens, L. M. Carlson et al., "Sustained antibody responses depend on CD28 function in bone marrow-resident plasma cells," *The Journal of Experimental Medicine*, vol. 208, no. 7, pp. 1435–1446, 2011.

17

Genetic Factors in Systemic Lupus Erythematosus: Contribution to Disease Phenotype

Fulvia Ceccarelli,[1] Carlo Perricone,[1] Paola Borgiani,[2] Cinzia Ciccacci,[2] Sara Rufini,[2] Enrica Cipriano,[1] Cristiano Alessandri,[1] Francesca Romana Spinelli,[1] Antonio Sili Scavalli,[1] Giuseppe Novelli,[2] Guido Valesini,[1] and Fabrizio Conti[1]

[1]Reumatologia, Dipartimento di Medicina Interna e Specialità Mediche, Sapienza Università di Roma, 00161 Rome, Italy
[2]Department of Biomedicine and Prevention, Section of Genetics, School of Medicine, University of Rome "Tor Vergata", 00133 Rome, Italy

Correspondence should be addressed to Fulvia Ceccarelli; fulviaceccarelli@gmail.com

Academic Editor: Nejat K. Egilmez

Genetic factors exert an important role in determining Systemic Lupus Erythematosus (SLE) susceptibility, interplaying with environmental factors. Several genetic studies in various SLE populations have identified numerous susceptibility loci. From a clinical point of view, SLE is characterized by a great heterogeneity in terms of clinical and laboratory manifestations. As widely demonstrated, specific laboratory features are associated with clinical disease subset, with different severity degree. Similarly, in the last years, an association between specific phenotypes and genetic variants has been identified, allowing the possibility to elucidate different mechanisms and pathways accountable for disease manifestations. However, except for Lupus Nephritis (LN), no studies have been designed to identify the genetic variants associated with the development of different phenotypes. In this review, we will report data currently known about this specific association.

1. Introduction

Systemic Lupus Erythematosus (SLE) is an autoimmune disease with multifactorial etiology, in which genetic and environmental factors interplay determining disease susceptibility [1].

Starting from 1970, several genetic studies in various SLE populations have identified numerous susceptibility loci. However, the genetic variability so far identified accounts for less than half of the SLE heritability, with modest overall effect sizes (OR ~ 1.5 to 1.2) (Figure 1) [2–7]. It is well established that some specific genetic factors are not shared between all SLE patients, excluding a role in the disease susceptibility and suggesting an association with specific phenotypes (Table 1) [6, 8]. However, this discrepancy could be related to multiple mechanisms that can lead to SLE development.

As widely demonstrated, specific autoantibodies resulted in being associated with different disease-related manifestations, identifying distinctive subset in terms of morbidity and

mortality and suggesting different underlying etiologies [9]. Similarly, in the last years, some studies have evaluated the relationships between SLE risk genes and disease phenotypes, in order to elucidate different mechanisms and pathways accountable for disease manifestations. However, except for Lupus Nephritis (LN), no studies have been specifically designed to evaluate the genetic risk factors associated with different manifestations. Therefore, these data could be extrapolated from studies evaluating disease susceptibility, which include a genotype-phenotype analysis.

2. Renal Involvement

Renal involvement could affect up to 60% of SLE patients, as initial manifestation or during disease course. Despite the improvement in terms of diagnostic accuracy and management, LN patients showed higher morbidity and mortality compared with those without this manifestation [10].

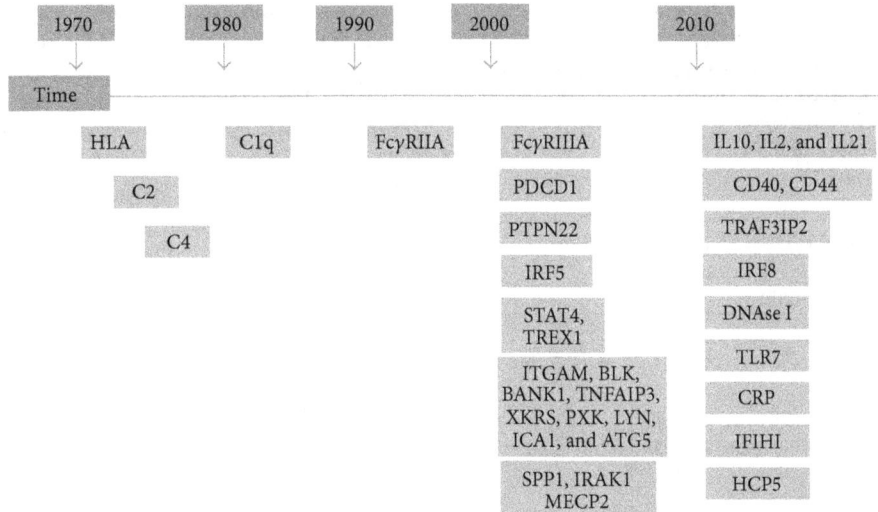

FIGURE 1: Schematic representation of genetic variants associated with SLE susceptibility identified from 1970.

Accordingly, the identification of markers able to identify most severe disease and to predict the end-stage renal disease (ESRD) development is a crucial topic. In particular, during the last years, numerous attempts have been made in order to identify serological and urinary biomarkers able to discriminate the different severity degree and to monitor response to treatment in LN patients, obtaining contrasting results [11]. Moreover, the use of resistive index (RI) as a severity marker in LN patients has been suggested in a recent study published by Conti et al. The authors identified a significant association between a pathologic RI (>0.7) and class IV glomerulonephritis, widely identified as the most severe [12].

In the context of biomarkers, genetic factors could have an important role in SLE patients with renal involvement in order to identify subject at risk to develop most severe and rapidly progressive forms. Moving from the genetic variants previously associated with disease susceptibility, several studies have verified the association of the same alleles with the presence of renal involvement.

The first genetic association described for SLE based on the case-control methodology was with the human leucocyte antigen (HLA) region at chromosome 6p21.3, encoding more than 200 genes, many of them with a specific immunological role. Seven HLA Class II alleles were demonstrated to be significantly associated with SLE and LN [13]. The HLA-DR2 and DR3 alleles resulted in being the most strongly associated with SLE susceptibility in African, Asian, European, and North, Central, and South American populations, even though HLA-DR3 tends to be more associated in European-derived populations [8]. In particular, the association between the disease susceptibility and highly conserved HLA-DRB1*03:01 and HLA-DRB1*15:01 haplotypes has been well established in European populations [8]. The punctual mechanism by which HLA-DR alleles determine an increased risk to develop SLE is not completely defined.

The most reliable hypothesis suggests the influence of HLA-DR on the selection and enrichment of autoreactive T cells through the presentation of molecular mimics [14].

Moving from these premises, the association with renal involvement has been investigated, showing the primary role exerted by HLA-DR3 and DR-2 [15]. In particular, the results obtained from the study conducted by Taylor and colleagues in 2011 and by Bolin in 2013 showed the association between HLA-DR3 and LN (OR = 1.37 and $P < 1 \times 10^{-4}$, resp.) [16, 17]. Particularly, Bolin et al. found an association between HLA-DR3 allele and proliferative nephritis ($P < 0.001$) [17].

Numerous evidences identified an association between *signal transducer and activator of transcription 4* (STAT4) genetic variants and increased risk to develop SLE, suggesting a role of these genetic variants in influencing disease phenotype.

In 2008, Taylor and colleagues analyzed a large SLE population, obtained from four sources (UCSF Lupus Genetics Project; Autoimmune Biomarkers Collaborative Network; Multiple Autoimmune Disease Genetics Consortium; Pittsburgh Lupus Registry) in order to evaluate the association between SNP rs7574865 of STAT4 and the different SLE-related manifestations. The phenotype case-only analysis identified a significant association with the presence of severe nephritis, defined as ESRD, or histopathologic evidence of severe, progressive renal disease (OR = 1.50) [18]. Simultaneously, the study conducted by Kawasaki et al. in a Japanese population confirmed the association between this STAT4 risk allele and renal involvement. In particular, the authors identified the association with rs7574865 both in SLE patients with nephritis (OR = 1.85) and in those without (OR = 1.55), which was stronger in nephritis cases [19].

More recently, Bolin and colleagues evaluated a cohort constituted by 567 Swedish Caucasian SLE patients and 512 healthy controls to elucidate the genetic components of LN [17]. By performing a LN case/controls analysis, a significant association between the SNPs rs11889341, rs7574865,

TABLE 1: Genetic variants associated with disease manifestations.

Disease phenotypes	Genetic variants associated with related SNPs
Skin involvement	ITGAM rs1143679 FCGR2A rs1801274 IL-6 174G/C VDR rs1168268
Serositis	TRAF3IP2 rs33980500, rs13190932, and rs13196377 PTPN2 rs2542151
Kidney involvement	HLADR2, HLADR3 rs2187668 STAT4 rs7574865, rs11889341, rs7568275, and rs7582694 ITGAM rs1143683, rs1143679 IRF5 rs2004640, rs2079197, and rs10488631 IRF7 rs4963128 TNFS4 rs2205960 DNAse I Q222R
Neurologic disorder	TREX1 rs922075, rs6776700, rs6442123, rs2242150, and rs11797
Joint involvement	ITGAM rs1143679 FGCR2A, FCGR3A VDR rs3890733 Mir146a rs2910164
Hematological features	IL-21 rs907715 STK17A haplotype TAGTC

Immunologic disorders	Anti-dsDNA
	  HLADR2, HLADR3 rs2187668
	  STAT4 rs7582694, rs7574865
	  ITGAM rs1143679, rs9888739
	  IRF5 rsrs10488631
	SSA/SSB
	  ITGAM rs1143679
	  IRF7 rs4963128
	  HCP5 rs3099855
	  HLADR3 rs2187668
	RNP
	  ITGAM rs1143679
	Sm
	  ITGAM rs7574865
	aCL
	  HCP5 rs3099844
	C3 reduction
	  Mir146a rs2910164
	C4 reduction
	  TRAF3IP2 rs33980500

rs7568275, and rs7582694 of STAT4 gene and the development of LN (r^2 = 0.98) was identified. In particular, the rs7582694 allele resulted in being associated with the presence of a proliferative nephritis (OR = 2.27) and with the development of a severe renal insufficiency (defined as a GRF < 30 mL/min/1.73 m^2 at follow-up) (OR = 3.61) [17]. This association was not always confirmed. In the study conducted by Li and colleagues in 2011 on a Northern Han Chinese SLE population, the SNP rs7574865 of STAT4 did not show any correlation with clinical manifestations [20].

Several hypothesis have been suggested to understand the mechanisms by which STAT4 could contribute to LN development. Interleukin-12 (IL-12), the main STAT4 activating cytokine, is able to induce the Th1 and Th17 differentiation with consequent production of IFN-γ and IL-17. These specific pathways seem to be crucial for the LN pathogenic mechanism: in particular, IL-17 could exert a direct role, as demonstrated by the identification of Th17 cells in kidney tissue and by the association between high IL-17 levels and less favorable outcome [21]. Moreover, SLE patients carrying the STAT4 risk allele rs7574865 showed an increased sensitivity to IFN-α signaling, as demonstrated by the overexpression of IFN-α regulated gene. Among these, TNFSF13B codifies the B lymphocyte stimulator (BLyS), which is able to promote B cell differentiation and autoantibody production [22].

The influence of ITGAM genetic variants on SLE susceptibility has been demonstrated in populations with different ethnicity: in particular, convincing data derived from European ancestry, but also from Hispanic, African-Americans, Mexicans, and Colombians cohorts [23]. Moving from these results, the association with specific clinical manifestations has been investigated. In 2009, Yang and colleagues identified a significant association between renal involvement and the ITGAM risk alleles rs1143683 and rs1143679 (OR = 3.35, OR = 2.05, resp.) in a Hong Kong SLE cohort [24]. Moreover, this association was confirmed in an analysis conducted on Finnish and Swedish population of patients affected by SLE. The authors observed increased risk in SLE patients with renal involvement, with an OR = 2.49 for the rs1143679 SNP [25].

The study conducted by Kim-Howard and colleagues in 2010 on a very large population, constituted by 2366 SLE patients and 2931 unaffected controls with European ancestry, confirmed the link between the genetic variant rs1143679 of ITGAM and renal disorders as defined by the American College of Rheumatology (ACR) criteria (OR = 1.39) [26]. To better assess the magnitude of this association, a comparison between patients with the specific ACR-criteria renal manifestations and healthy controls was performed. This statistical approach allowed the identification of a strong effect concerning the association with renal criteria (OR = 2.15) [26].

More recently, in 2011 Sanchez et al. confirmed this association (OR = 1.25) by evaluating a population constituted by 4001 European-derived, 1547 Hispanic, 1590 African-American, and 1191 Asian patients. This association seems to be driven prevalently by the European-derived cohort, as demonstrated by a higher OR in this specific subset (OR = 1.39) and by the lack of a significant association with African-American or Asian individuals [27].

ITGAM encodes the CD11b chain of the Mac-1 (alphaM-beta2; CD11b/CD18; complement receptor-3) integrin, a surface receptor protein implicated in the interaction of monocytes, macrophages, and granulocytes. The genetic variants of this molecule, resulting in amino acid substitution in the extracellular portion, could determine a dysfunctional integrin, not able to mediate cell adhesion to integrin ligands and phagocytosis. Moreover, this defective integrin does not seem to be able to restrict the production of inflammatory cytokines in macrophages [28].

Under physiological conditions, ITGAM is expressed by endothelial cells of glomerular and peritubular capillaries of Bowman's capsule. It has been suggested that an increased expression of a defective molecule, due to the presence of a genetic variant, could be associated with a loss of clearance of glomerular deposits, with inflammatory process development [26]. Similarly, defective handling of immune complexes could be the mechanism explaining the association between genetic variants of FCGR3A and kidney involvement in SLE patients. A meta-analysis conducted by Karassa and colleagues in 2003 evaluated the study examining the association of the FCGR3A V/F158 polymorphism and LN, published until August 2002 [29]. Data deriving from the analysis on 16 studies demonstrated a significant overrepresentation of the low-binding F158 allele in patients with renal disease compared with those without (P = 0.003). Moreover, the presence of this allele seems to confer a 1.2-fold greater risk for renal disease development, irrespective of the ethnicity [29]. More recently, the PROFILE cohort, constituted by 1008 SLE patients, with renal involvement in 43.4% of the cases (438 patients), was evaluated in order to identify the association with FCGR3A polymorphism. The authors identified an overrepresentation of FCGR3A*GG in SLE patient developing ESRD (21.9%) compared with those who did not develop it (7.5%) (P = 0.0175) [30]. Interestingly, the evaluation of FCGR3A variants demonstrated different genetic association for the global lupus phenotype and for the renal involvement (FCGR3A*T and FCGR3A*GG, resp.). This observation confirms the hypothesis of different genetic background for susceptibility and disease phenotype, leading to different pathogenic mechanisms associated with the corresponding molecule [30].

FCGR plays a pivotal role in removing antigen-antibody complexes at the tissue and organ level. Allelic variants could alter this function, causing an inflammatory response with damage development. In particular, as widely demonstrated, a homozygosity condition for this FCGR3A SNP could lead to impaired handling of immune complexes, causing a proinflammatory status [29, 30]. This could justify the impact of genetic variants of FCGR3A in the determination of a specific phenotype, such as renal involvement.

In the last 20 years, the role of Interferon (IFN) signature in the SLE pathogenesis has been recognized, as demonstrated by the dysregulation in the expression of genes in the IFN pathway in more than half of SLE patients [31]. IFN pathway is involved in several pathologic mechanisms, involving Th1 and B cells activation and survival. Moreover, IFN acts as a bridge between innate and adaptive immune systems. Interferon Regulatory Factors (IRF) ensure the regulation of this complex pathway, by acting on signaling and immune cell development [31]. Genetic variants of IRF5, IRF7, and IRF8 genes have been associated with SLE susceptibility (OR = 1.88, OR = 0.78, and OR = 1.17, resp.) since they associated with increased levels of protein expression [32]. Starting from these evidences, the association with renal involvement in SLE patients has been investigated. The study conducted on 190 LN patients and 182 healthy Chinese blood donors demonstrated a significantly higher frequency of the T allele of IRF5 rs2004640 SNP in LN patients (OR = 1.60) [33].

The abovementioned study conducted by Bolin and colleagues in 2013 identified a strong association between LN and two nearly perfectly linked SNPs in IRF5 (rs2070197 and rs10488631, r^2 1.0). In particular, the risk allele C of rs10488631 was associated with proliferative nephritis (OR = 2.61) and severe renal insufficiency (OR = 3.03) [17]. More recently, an association between IRF7 rs4963128 and LN (OR = 2.69) has been identified in the study conducted by Li and colleagues in 2011 in a Northern Han Chinese population [34].

In 2011, for the first time, Sanchez and colleagues suggested a new interesting genetic factor related to renal disorders in SLE patients by identifying a significant association with rs2205960 TNFSF4 risk allele (OR = 1.14) [27]. TNFSF4, also called OX40L, is a member of the TNF superfamily, expressed prevalently on antigen-presenting cells; activated T cells express the receptor of this molecule (TNFSFR4 or OX40) [35]. The expression of TNFSF4 at the epithelial level of the glomerular capillary has been demonstrated in LN patients [36]. More recently, Zhou and colleagues demonstrated a modification of cytokine production in PBMC in LN patients after treatment with anti-CD134 monoclonal antibody [37]. Finally, significantly higher TNFSF4 serum levels have been demonstrated in SLE patients with renal involvement, compared with patients without nephritis, suggesting the role of this molecule as a marker. Moreover, the increased expression on CD4 positive T cells seems to be associated with LN and disease activity [38]. Taken together, these evidences could justify the link between a genetic variant in the TNFSF4 gene and renal involvement.

Several other genetic variants have been associated with kidney manifestations in SLE patients. Panneer and colleagues suggested the role of polymorphism in the gene codifying the DNAse I, an endonuclease involved in the cleavage and clearance of chromatin during apoptotic processes [39]. The reduction of the DNAse I function, related to the genetic modification, could alter this cleavage and the clearance of immune-complexes and NETs, resulting in the persistence of apoptotic debris [40]. By evaluating 300 South Indian Tamil SLE patients, the authors identified a significantly higher frequency of heterozygous genotype of Q222R polymorphism in patients with nephritis than in those without (67% versus 53%, OR = 1.93) [39]. Some interesting data concerning the association between LN development and polymorphism on the gene codifying C1q have been recently published [41, 42]. However, due to the small cohorts evaluated in these studies, their results should be confirmed in large populations.

3. Neuropsychiatric Manifestations

Neuropsychiatric SLE is a major disease manifestation, characterized by a wide heterogeneity in terms of clinical features, degrees of morbidity, and severity between patients [43]. A percentage of SLE patients ranging from 14 to 75% may refer to neurological symptoms: this wide variability is probably related to the great heterogeneity of this disease manifestation. Despite the relevance of this involvement, studies focusing on genetic variants specifically associated with NPSLE have been rarely conducted. Nonetheless, Koga and colleagues in 2011 evaluated 282 Japanese SLE patients and 222 healthy controls in order to assess the cumulative number of risk alleles associated with SNPs of HLA-DRB1, IRF5, STAT4, BLK, TNFAIP3, TNIP1, FCGR2B, and TNFSF13 genes. SLE patients registered a significantly higher number of risk alleles compared with controls (8.07 ± 1.60 versus 7.02 ± 1.64, $P = 1.63 \times 10^{-12}$). Interestingly, when considering SLE patients carrying more than 10 risk alleles, the proportion of patients with neurological involvement was significantly higher compared with subjects with a number of risk alleles lower than 10 (OR = 2.30). This result could suggest that a higher number of risk alleles could determine most severe disease manifestations [44].

Genetic variants in TREX1 gene, codifying a threeprime repair exonuclease 1 (also known as DNAse III), have been considered a good candidate for NPSLE. de Vries and colleagues scanned genomic DNA of 60 NPSLE patients for exonic TREX1 mutations using direct sequencing. This study identified a novel heterozygous p.Arg128His mutation in one NPSLE patient, admitted to the hospital because of lethargy and progressive migraine-like headache [45]. The authors suggested that the p.Arg128His mutation is responsible for neurological manifestations at the light of the absence of this mutation in 400 control chromosomes and in 1712 healthy individuals, previously screened by Lee-Kirsch et al. [46]. More recently, this association has been confirmed in the study conducted by Namjou and colleagues in 2011. By evaluating the European population enrolled in the analysis, the authors identified a significant association between the presence of neurological manifestations (as defined by ACR criteria), especially seizure, and specific variants in TREX1 gene. In particular, the rs922075 (OR = 1.644); rs6776700 (OR = 1.689); rs6442123 (OR = 1.747); rs2242150 (OR = 1.638); rs11797 (OR = 1.714) SNPs resulted in being significantly associated [47].

4. Joint Involvement

Joint involvement is a frequent manifestation in patients with SLE and could affect up to 90% of patients. A wide heterogeneity, varying from arthralgia to erosive arthritis similar to rheumatoid arthritis, characterizes this manifestation [48]. Nevertheless, the number of reports is relatively scarce. Concerning the identification of specific genetic variants, few studies have evaluated the association with joint involvement.

ITGAM gene risk variants have been associated with arthritis in SLE patients. The study conducted by Warchoł et al. in 2011 in a Polish SLE population demonstrated an association between the rs1143679 genetic variant and occurrence of arthritis (OR = 3.486) [49].

A strong association with arthritis and Vitamin D Receptor (VDR) polymorphism was identified in the study conducted by de Azevêdo Silva and colleagues in 2013 [50]. Through the Vitamin D Receptor (VDR), Vitamin D exerts an immune-modulatory effect. In particular, it intervenes in downregulation of Th1 immune response, modulation of dendritic cells differentiation, depressing activated B cell proliferation, upregulation of regulatory T cells, and preserving immune response [50]. A number of evidences showed that patients with SLE often present reduced levels of Vitamin D suggesting an involvement of this molecule in disease pathogenesis [51]. There is still a debate concerning the precise role of VDR in SLE [52]. The study conducted by de Azevêdo Silva in 2013 did not identify any association between VDR polymorphism and SLE susceptibility. Conversely, the T/T genotype (rs3890733) resulted in being significantly associated with the presence of joint involvement (OR = 17.05). The authors underlined that this association should be interpreted with caution because the frequencies observed for this VDR polymorphism were not in Hardy-Weinberg equilibrium [50].

Other associations between genetic variants and joint involvement have been suggested: some data identified an association with C4 and ACP5 genetic variants, but no replication studies are available [53, 54]. Moreover, Ciccacci and colleagues identified an association between joint involvement and rs2910164 of mir146a gene (OR = 1.93) [55].

The association between arthritis and the FCGR2A and FCGR3A low copy number genotype has been identified in a cohort of Taiwan SLE patients [56, 57]. In particular, in the most recent study, the FCGR3A low copy number genotype was significantly enriched in SLE patients with arthritis ($P = 0.001$; OR = 1.56) [57].

Finally, the study conducted by Fonseca et al. in 2013 identified an association between arthritis and the SNP rs15866 of STK17A gene (OR = 2.92), encoding serine/threonine-protein kinase 17A [58]. The mechanism explaining this association is not clarified and replication studies are needed to confirm these results.

5. Skin Manifestations

Skin involvement represents a frequent manifestation in SLE patients (up to 75%), characterized by a great heterogeneity, including acute and chronic phenotypes. Some genetic variants have been associated with different skin manifestations in SLE cohorts.

ITGAM genetic polymorphisms are to date the most frequently associated variants with skin involvement. In 2010, Kim-Howard et al. have identified an association between malar rash and the polymorphism rs1143679 of ITGAM (OR = 1.27) [26]. Moreover, the presence of discoid rash resulted in being associated with ITGAM rs1143679 (OR = 1.20) in the study conducted by Sanchez et al. in 2011 [27].

Järvinen and colleagues conducted an analysis specifically designed to address the role of ITGAM genetic variants in a cohort of Finnish and Swedish patients with discoid LE, without signs of systemic disease. The analysis demonstrated a strong association between the allele rs1143679 and DLE (OR = 3.2). The authors identified a significant association also in SLE patients with discoid rash (OR = 3.76). Moreover, other variants in ITGAM resulted in being associated with these manifestations, but the authors hypothesized that the strong linkage disequilibrium with rs1143679 could explain this result [25].

The link between ITGAM and photosensitivity, frequently identified in patients with discoid LE, could explain this association. Ultraviolet- (UV-) B irradiation determines the activation of several proinflammatory events at the skin level, involving prevalently macrophages ITGAM-expressing and dendritic cells. Genetic-determined modification in the function of ITGAM could modify the processes regulating the dendritic cell differentiation, inducing inflammatory reactions in discoid LE patients [25]. On the other hand, the absence of CD11b seems to enhance the differentiation of naive T cells to IL-17 producing Th17 cells, determining the increase of IL-17 serum levels, identified in discoid LE and SLE patients with skin involvement [59].

Moreover, genetic variants of FCGR2A seem to be associated with skin manifestations. In particular, Sanchez and colleagues identified an association between malar rash and FCGR2A rs1801274 (OR = 1.11) [27].

The abovementioned study conducted by de Azevêdo Silva et al. in 2013 identified an association between the SNP rs11168268 of VDR and cutaneous alterations in a cohort of Brazilian SLE patients [50]. Photosensitivity, one of the most common cutaneous alterations described in SLE patients derives from the exposure to UV light, causing a macular or erythematous rash. After UV exposure, keratinocytes begin apoptotic process due to DNA damage with release of nuclear material. A defective clearance of apoptotic body could trigger an immune response. Vitamin D has proved to be able to reduce the UV-induced DNA damage and suppress cutaneous immunity, playing an important role in the maintenance of cell integrity after UV light exposure [60]. The presence of genetic variants in VDR, expressed in the skin epithelial cells, could modify this Vitamin D ability, promoting cutaneous alterations in SLE patients [61].

A recent meta-analysis identified a significant association between the IL-6-174 G/C polymorphism and discoid skin lesions by the evaluation of 15 studies (OR = 2.271). These results support the role of IL-6 in the pathogenesis discoid skin lesions [62].

6. Serositis

Few data are available in the literature about the genetic risk for the serositis development. The study published by Perricone et al. in 2013 identified an interesting correlation between the TRAF3IP2 SNPs and the development of pericarditis. The authors identified a significant association with the three TRAF3IP2 SNPs evaluated (rs33980500: OR = 2.59; rs13190932: OR = 2.38; rs13196377: OR = 2.44). Moreover, the authors analyzed the contribution of SLE antibody to the development of this specific manifestation, showing a significant association between the risk to develop pericarditis and anti-La/SSB positivity (OR = 2.65). A binary logistic regression analysis demonstrated that both TRAF3IP2 rs33980500 and anti-La/SSB could be independently associated with the development of pericarditis (P = 0.006 and P = 0.032, resp.) [63]. In this study, for the first time, the role of TRAF3IP2 genetic variants on SLE susceptibility has been ascertained. Interestingly, TRAF3IP2 polymorphism resulted also in being

associated with a specific disease manifestation. TRAF3IP2 codifies the molecule Act1, which from one side is involved in the IL-17 pathways, but it is also a negative regulator of the CD40-mediated signaling pathway [64, 65].

The study conducted by Ciccacci and colleagues in 2014 identified a new association between the occurrence of pericarditis and the genetic variant rs2542151 of PTPN2 gene (OR = 2.49) [55]. PTPN2 codifies the enzyme tyrosine-protein phosphatase nonreceptor type 2, a member of the protein tyrosine kinases (PTP) superfamily. PTPN2 genetic variants have been previously associated with susceptibility to both Crohn's disease and ulcerative colitis and with an earlier onset of type 1 diabetes [66, 67]. The abovementioned study by Ciccacci and colleagues analyzed for the first time the role of PTPN2 genetic variants in the SLE susceptibility, without identifying significant differences between patients and healthy controls. Conversely, the SNP rs2542151 of PTPN2 resulted in being associated with serositis, and specifically with pericarditis [55]. The relevance of this association should be clarified by larger studies.

7. Hematological Manifestations

Similarly to the other SLE-related manifestations, few studies focusing on the association between genetic variants and hematological features have been conducted to date. The extrapolation from genotype-phenotype studies identified some associations. Among these, Sanchez and colleagues in 2011 identified an association between hematological features and IL-21 rs907715 (OR = 1.13). When the different ACR hematological criteria were analyzed, an association with leucopenia was confirmed (OR = 1.14). IL-21, primarily produced by activated CD4+ T cells, is involved in differentiation and functional activity of T and B cells [68–70]. This evidence could justify this association, by hypothesizing that a genetic variant of IL-21 could be related to a modification of this activity on B and T cells, influencing disease phenotype.

More recently, Fonseca et al. in 2013 described a significant association between hematological features and haplotype TAGTC of STK17A gene (OR = 0.03). The patients stratification according to ethnicity and gender suggested a protective role of this haplotype on hematological manifestations development (OR 0.37) [58]. Similarly to the association with arthritis, the mechanism explaining this association is not identified and other replication studies are needed to confirm these results.

8. Immunological Abnormalities

The production of a wide range of autoantibodies, resulting from polyclonal B cells activation, impaired apoptotic pathways, or idiotypic network dysregulation, characterizes SLE [1, 71]. Among these, the anti-double-stranded DNA antibodies (anti-dsDNA) are considered the most specific marker for SLE, due to their high frequency (ranging from 70% to 98%) and sensitivity and specificity (57.3% and 97.4%, resp.) [72, 73].

Several evidences suggested a role of genetic factors in autoantibodies determination [74]. The same genetic variants, previously described as associated with renal involvement, have been investigated in order to identify a link with anti-dsDNA production. Since 1998, Podrebarac and colleagues described the association between anti-dsDNA production and the presence of HLA-DRB1*1501 (DR2) allele [75]. More recently, the association between HLA-DR2 and DR3 with the presence of anti-dsDNA has been confirmed by several analysis [16, 76].

Starting from 2008, the association between the STAT4-risk allele of the SNP rs7582694 and positivity for anti-dsDNA has been identified by different studies [16, 18, 77]. Finally, ITGAM polymorphism has been also associated with the presence of anti-dsDNA. In particular, the study conducted by Kim-Howard and colleagues in 2010 identified an association with rs1143679 (OR 1.65) in a case-only analysis performed by comparing SLE patients positive and negative for anti-dsDNA [26].

Four years ago, Chung and colleagues conducted the first genome wide study focused to identify genetic factors associated with anti-dsDNA autoantibody production, by analyzing 1278 SLE cases and 3334 healthy controls of European descent [78]. Genetic variants STAT4 (rs7574865), IRF5 (rs10488631), ITGAM (rs9888739), and MHC (HLA-DR3, rs2187668) resulted in being strongly associated with anti-dsDNA positivity (OR = 1.77, OR = 1.92, OR = 1.80, and OR = 2.23, resp.). Moreover, the authors assessed the relationship between the anti-dsDNA autoantibody production and the cumulative genetic risk, calculated by counting the total number of risk alleles identified in a single subject. The mean SLE genetic risk was higher in SLE patients positive for anti-dsDNA (15.5 ± 3.1) compared with anti-dsDNA negative patients (14.5 ± 3.0) and healthy controls (13.1 ± 2.8), even though this difference was not significant [78]. The results of this study suggest that some genetic variants are more strongly associated with anti-dsDNA autoantibody production than with SLE susceptibility, and they could be described as "autoantibody propensity genes" [78].

Even though the majority of the studies have focused on the anti-dsDNA antibodies, some evidences demonstrated an association between genetic variants and production of other autoantibodies in patients affected by SLE.

Järvinen and colleagues in 2010 identified an association between the polymorphism rs1143679 in ITGAM gene and the presence of Ro/SSA autoantibodies in the Finnish (OR = 2.65) and Swedish (OR 1.62) populations [25]. The involvement of both Ro-autoantibodies and the ITGAM protein product in the same biological pathways of apoptosis and phagocytosis could explain this association, which remains mostly unknown [25].

The study conducted by Li and colleagues in 2011 suggested a new association between IRF7 rs4963128 polymorphism and anti-SSA/SSB (OR = 0.61) [20]. Moreover, the study conducted by Ciccacci and colleagues in 2014 identified for the first time an association between anti-Ro/SSA and HCP5 rs3099855 polymorphism (OR = 2.28) [55]. This SNP has been previously associated not only with Steven Johnson syndrome and toxic epidermal necrolysis susceptibility, but

also with primary sclerosing cholangitis, another autoimmune condition [79, 80]. More interestingly, as demonstrated by a genome-wide association study, the same polymorphism resulted in being associated with cardiac manifestations of SLE, a clinical condition frequently associated with the presence of anti-Ro/SSA antibodies [81]. These data suggest a pathological link between anti-Ro/SSA antibodies and this HCP5 polymorphism, requiring further studies to clarify the specific underlying mechanisms. Moreover, both anti-Ro/SSA and anti-La/SSB autoantibodies resulted in being significantly associated with HLA-DRB1*03:01 (OR = 1.60, OR = 2.57, resp.), as demonstrated by the largest SLE subphenotype genetic association study conducted so far [82].

A recent study published by Niewold et al. in 2012 evaluated the association between IFR5 haplotype and different SLE-related manifestations. Interestingly, the authors identified a strong and strikingly distinct association between different autoantibodies and different IRF5 haplotypes. In particular, TACA haplotype was associated with anti-dsDNA and anti-Ro/SSA (OR = 1.5, OR = 1.51, resp.), TATA haplotype with anti-dsDNA (OR = 1.68), and TCTA haplotype with anti-La/SSB (OR = 3.51) [83]. These results suggest the possible role of IRF5 genotype to predispose the antibodies formation: IRF5 haplotypes could influence susceptibility to form particular antibodies. Immune complexes containing these antibodies are internalized into cells, and the nucleic acid component could trigger endosomal TLR7 and TLR9. The presence of IRF5 SLE-risk variants could increase IFN-α production in the setting of different antibodies, resulting in high serum IFN-α and subsequent SLE risk [83].

The studies published until now have suggested other associations between specific autoantibodies and genetic variants, among which are the associations between anti-RNP and rs1143679 of ITGAM (OR = 1.89), anti-RNP and rs56203834 of TREX1 in European populations (OR = 5.2), anti-Sm and rs7574865 of ITGAM (OR = 0.65), and anti-cardiolipin and rs3099844 of HCP5 (OR = 0.34) [20, 26, 47, 55]. However, all these associations should be confirmed in larger populations and the mechanisms explaining must be identified.

The reduction of C3 and/or C4 serum levels represents a frequent manifestation in patients affected by SLE and could correlate with disease activity [84]. A strong association was well established between homozygous hereditary deficiency of each of the early proteins of the classical pathway of complement activation and SLE development. The deficiency of the C1 complex proteins and of total C4 is recognized as the most prevalent and most severe disease. Indeed, more than 75% of all individuals with deficiency of one of these proteins develop SLE [84]. Conversely, the deficiency of C2 protein seems to be associated with lower prevalence of disease (10%), while C3 deficiency is rarely associated with SLE development, probably due to the rarity of homozygous C3 deficiency [84]. Even though the association between complement proteins deficiency and SLE development has been largely clarified, very few data are available concerning genetic variants associated with C3 and C4 levels reduction, extrapolated by studies not focusing on this specific aspect.

A correlation between C4 reduction and the SNP rs33980500 of TRAF3IP2 has been identified in the study conducted by Perricone et al. (OR = 1.96) [63]. Conversely, the reduction of C3 serum level was associated with the genetic variant mir146a rs2910164 (OR = 1.91) [55].

9. Age at Disease Diagnosis

The evaluation of the studies published so far identified interesting data concerning the influence of STAT4 genetic variants on age at diagnosis. The SNP rs7574865 of STAT4 resulted in being associated with age at diagnosis lower than 30 years (OR = 1.22) [16, 18]. The frequency of the same genetic variant resulted in being slightly higher in SLE Japanese patients with an age of onset lower than 20 years as compared with patients with age ≥ 20 years, although this difference was not statistically significant [19].

Moreover, rs2233945 of PSORS1C1 resulted in being associated with age at diagnosis. Ciccacci and colleagues observed that patients carrying the variant allele present a lower mean age at disease onset compared with those not carrying the variant (28.6 ± 11.57 years *versus* 32.2 ± 11.46 years, *P* = 0.042) [55].

10. Chronic Damage

The increase of survival of SLE patients determined the accrual of cumulative organ damage: adverse events of treatment, disease activity, and comorbidities seem to be the major risk factors. The prevention of damage development is a critical issue in the management of SLE patients, as underlined by the recent treat-to-target recommendations [85]. Consequently, the identification of specific biomarkers, able to identify SLE patients with a major risk to develop chronic damage, is an attractive topic. Among the different biomarkers, genetic variants could play a role. The study conducted by Carvalho and colleagues in 2015 suggested a role of VDR polymorphism [86]. The evaluation of 170 Portuguese SLE patients and 192 healthy controls demonstrated an association between different genetic variants and accrual damage. In particular, the frequency of VDR genotypes TaqI TT (rs731236) and Fok I CT (rs2228570) was higher in SLE patients with damage, evaluated by using the SLICC Damage Index (SDI) [86, 87].

The development of osteoporosis with fractures is considered chronic damage in SLE patients and is inserted in the SDI [87]. Bonfá and colleagues performed a case-control study by evaluating 211 premenopausal SLE patients and 154 healthy women, in order to evaluate the association between the RANKL, OPG, and RANK gene polymorphisms and bone parameters. A significantly lower frequency of the RANKL 290 G allele (AG/GG) was identified in the patients with vertebral fractures compared with those without (*P* = 0.011). In the logistic regression analysis, in addition to the age, only RANKL 290A>G remained as an independent risk factor for vertebral fractures in SLE patients [88]. The authors hypothesized that the protection against vertebral fractures that is associated with the AG/GG genotype could be a consequence of decreased osteoclast activation due to

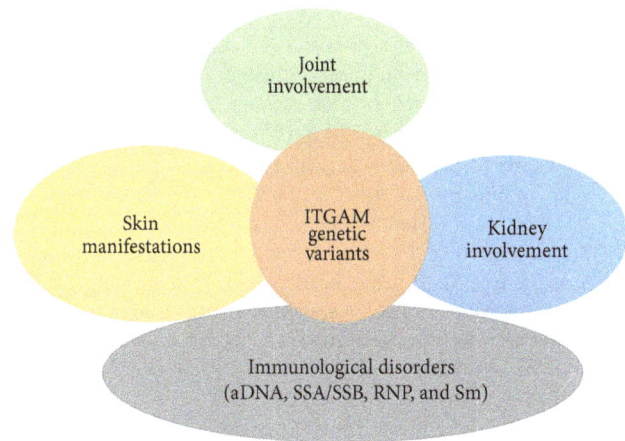

FIGURE 2: Disease manifestations associated with ITGAM genetic variants.

RANKL dysfunction or to a local reduction of this molecule in the bone [88].

11. Conclusion

As widely demonstrated, genetic factors play a pivotal role in SLE pathogenesis. Moreover, in the last years several evidences suggested the role of genetic factors not only in disease susceptibility, but also in the development of specific disease phenotype. Several data are available to date concerning genetic variants involved in renal involvement, while fewer studies have been focused on SLE clinical and immunological manifestations. Interestingly, some genetic variants seem to be involved in the determination of different disease-related manifestations, suggesting a common pathogenetic mechanism, able to identify specific subset of patients. An example of this concept is represented by ITGAM genetic variants that resulted in being simultaneously associated with different disease manifestations (Figure 2). The recent progress leading to the discovery of novel methods to perform genetic studies will definitely allow clearly defining the associations between genes variability and SLE susceptibility and phenotype. Possibly, risk algorithms will be developed permitting a more personalized management of the disease.

However, small populations and lack of all clinical data characterize the studies evaluating the association between genetic and different disease phenotypes, not allowing a sufficient statistical power. Further studies specifically designed to evaluate this issue are needed to clarify the strongest associations.

Conflict of Interests

The authors declare that there is no conflict of interests regarding the publication of this paper.

Authors' Contribution

Fulvia Ceccarelli and Carlo Perricone equally contributed.

References

[1] G. C. Tsokos, "Systemic lupus erythematosus," *The New England Journal of Medicine*, vol. 365, no. 22, pp. 2110–2121, 2011.

[2] R. R. Graham, S. V. Kozyrev, E. C. Baechler et al., "A common haplotype of interferon regulatory factor 5 (IRF5) regulates splicing and expression and is associated with increased risk of systemic lupus erythematosus," *Nature Genetics*, vol. 38, no. 5, pp. 550–555, 2006.

[3] J. B. Harley, M. E. Alarcón-Riquelme, L. A. Criswell et al., "Genome-wide association scan in women with systemic lupus erythematosus identifies susceptibility variants in *ITGAM*, *PXK*, *KIAA1542* and other loci," *Nature Genetics*, vol. 40, no. 2, pp. 204–210, 2008.

[4] E. F. Remmers, R. M. Plenge, A. T. Lee et al., "STAT4 and the risk of rheumatoid arthritis and systemic lupus erythematosus," *The New England Journal of Medicine*, vol. 357, no. 10, pp. 977–986, 2007.

[5] V. Gateva, J. K. Sandling, G. Hom et al., "A large-scale replication study identifies TNIP1, PRDM1, JAZF1, UHRF1BP1 and IL10 as risk loci for systemic lupus erythematosus," *Nature Genetics*, vol. 41, no. 11, pp. 1228–1233, 2009.

[6] O. J. Rullo and B. P. Tsao, "Recent insights into the genetic basis of systemic lupus erythematosus," *Annals of the Rheumatic Diseases*, vol. 72, no. 2, pp. ii56–ii61, 2013.

[7] Y. Ghodke-Puranik and T. B. Niewold, "Genetics of the type I interferon pathway in systemic lupus erythematosus," *International Journal of Clinical Rheumatology*, vol. 8, no. 6, pp. 657–669, 2013.

[8] J. B. Harley, J. A. Kelly, and K. M. Kaufman, "Unraveling the genetics of systemic lupus erythematosus," *Springer Seminars in Immunopathology*, vol. 28, no. 2, pp. 119–130, 2006.

[9] G. Yaniv, G. Twig, D. B. E.-A. Shor et al., "A volcanic explosion of autoantibodies in systemic lupus erythematosus: a diversity of 180 different antibodies found in SLE patients," *Autoimmunity Reviews*, vol. 14, no. 1, pp. 75–79, 2015.

[10] R. Cervera, M. A. Khamashta, J. Font, G. D. Sebastiani, A. Gil, P. Lavilla et al., "Morbidity and mortality in systemic lupus erythematosus during a 5-year period. A multicenter prospective study of 1,000 patients. Morbidity and mortality in systemic lupus erythematosus during a 5-year period. A multicenter prospective study of 1,000 patients. European Working Party on Systemic Lupus Erythematosus," *Medicine*, vol. 78, no. 3, pp. 167–175, 1999.

[11] Y. Li, X. Fang, and Q.-Z. Li, "Biomarker profiling for lupus nephritis," *Genomics, Proteomics and Bioinformatics*, vol. 11, no. 3, pp. 158–165, 2013.

[12] F. Conti, F. Ceccarelli, A. Gigante et al., "Ultrasonographic evaluation of renal resistive index in patients with lupus nephritis: correlation with histologic findings," *Ultrasound in Medicine and Biology*, vol. 40, no. 11, pp. 2573–2580, 2014.

[13] Z. Niu, P. Zhang, and Y. Tong, "Value of HLA-DR genotype in systemic lupus erythematosus and lupus nephritis: a meta-analysis," *International Journal of Rheumatic Diseases*, vol. 18, no. 1, pp. 17–28, 2015.

[14] U. S. Deshmukh, D. L. Sim, C. Dai et al., "HLA-DR3 restricted T cell epitope mimicry in induction of autoimmune response to lupus-associated antigen SmD," *Journal of Autoimmunity*, vol. 37, no. 3, pp. 254–262, 2011.

[15] S. A. Chung, E. E. Brown, A. H. Williams et al., "Lupus nephritis susceptibility loci in women with systemic lupus erythematosus," *Journal of the American Society of Nephrology*, vol. 25, no. 12, pp. 2859–2870, 2014.

[16] K. E. Taylor, S. A. Chung, R. R. Graham et al., "Risk alleles for systemic lupus erythematosus in a large case-control collection and associations with clinical subphenotypes," *PLoS Genetics*, vol. 7, no. 2, Article ID e1001311, 2011.

[17] K. Bolin, J. K. Sandling, A. Zickert et al., "Association of STAT4 polymorphism with severe renal insufficiency in lupus nephritis," *PLoS ONE*, vol. 8, no. 12, Article ID e84450, 2013.

[18] K. E. Taylor, E. F. Remmers, A. T. Lee et al., "Specificity of the STAT4 genetic association for severe disease manifestations of systemic lupus erythematosus," *PLoS Genetics*, vol. 4, no. 5, Article ID e1000084, 2008.

[19] A. Kawasaki, I. Ito, K. Hikami et al., "Role of STAT4 polymorphisms in systemic lupus erythematosus in a Japanese population: a case-control association study of the STAT1-STAT4 region," *Arthritis Research and Therapy*, vol. 10, article R113, 2008.

[20] P. Li, C. Cao, H. Luan et al., "Association of genetic variations in the STAT4 and IRF7/KIAA1542 regions with systemic lupus erythematosus in a Northern Han Chinese population," *Human Immunology*, vol. 72, no. 3, pp. 249–255, 2011.

[21] J. C. Crispín, M. Oukka, G. Bayliss et al., "Expanded double negative T cells in patients with systemic lupus erythematosus produce IL-17 and infiltrate the kidneys," *The Journal of Immunology*, vol. 181, no. 12, pp. 8761–8766, 2008.

[22] S. Morimoto, S. Nakano, T. Watanabe et al., "Expression of B-cell activating factor of the tumour necrosis factor family (BAFF) in T cells in active systemic lupus erythematosus: the role of (BAFF) in T cell-dependent B cell pathogenic autoantibody production," *Rheumatology*, vol. 46, no. 7, pp. 1083–1086, 2007.

[23] Y. Deng and B. P. Tsao, "Genetic susceptibility to systemic lupus erythematosus in the genomic era," *Nature Reviews Rheumatology*, vol. 6, no. 12, pp. 683–692, 2010.

[24] W. Yang, M. Zhao, N. Hirankarn et al., "ITGAM is associated with disease susceptibility and renal nephritis of systemic lupus erythematosus in Hong Kong Chinese and Thai," *Human Molecular Genetics*, vol. 18, no. 11, pp. 2063–2070, 2009.

[25] T. M. Järvinen, A. Hellquist, S. Koskenmies et al., "Polymorphisms of the ITGAM gene confer higher risk of discoid cutaneous than of systemic lupus erythematosus," *PLoS ONE*, vol. 5, no. 12, Article ID e14212, 2010.

[26] X. Kim-Howard, A. K. Maiti, J.-M. Anaya et al., "ITGAM coding variant (rs1143679) influences the risk of renal disease, discoid rash and immunological manifestations in patients with systemic lupus erythematosus with European ancestry," *Annals of the Rheumatic Diseases*, vol. 69, no. 7, pp. 1329–1332, 2010.

[27] E. Sanchez, A. Nadig, B. C. Richardson et al., "Phenotypic associations of genetic susceptibility loci in systemic lupus erythematosus," *Annals of the Rheumatic Diseases*, vol. 70, no. 10, pp. 1752–1757, 2011.

[28] S. C. Fagerholm, M. Macpherson, M. J. James, C. Sevier-Guy, and C. S. Lau, "The CD11b-integrin (ITGAM) and systemic lupus erythematosus," *Lupus*, vol. 22, no. 7, pp. 657–663, 2013.

[29] F. B. Karassa, T. A. Trikalinos, and J. P. A. Ioannidis, "The FcγRIIIA-F158 allele is a risk factor for the development of lupus nephritis: a meta-analysis," *Kidney International*, vol. 63, no. 4, pp. 1475–1482, 2003.

[30] G. S. Alarcón, G. McGwin Jr., M. Petri et al., "Time to renal disease and end-stage renal disease in PROFILE: a multiethnic lupus cohort," *PLoS Medicine*, vol. 3, article e396, 2006.

[31] R. Salloum and T. B. Niewold, "Interferon regulatory factors in human lupus pathogenesis," *Translational Research*, vol. 157, no. 6, pp. 326–331, 2011.

[32] S. G. Guerra, T. J. Vyse, and D. S. Cunninghame Graham, "The genetics of lupus: a functional perspective," *Arthritis Research & Therapy*, vol. 14, article 211, 2012.

[33] L. Qin, X. Lv, X. Zhou, P. Hou, H. Yang, and H. Zhang, "Association of IRF5 gene polymorphisms and lupus nephritis in a Chinese population," *Nephrology*, vol. 15, no. 7, pp. 710–713, 2010.

[34] P. Li, C. Cao, H. Luan et al., "Association of genetic variations in the STAT4 and IRF7/KIAA1542 regions with systemic lupus erythematosus in a Northern Han Chinese population," *Human Immunology*, vol. 72, no. 3, pp. 249–255, 2011.

[35] E. Stüber and W. Strober, "The T cell-B cell interaction via OX40-OX40L is necessary for the T cell-dependent humoral immune response," *The Journal of Experimental Medicine*, vol. 183, no. 3, pp. 979–989, 1996.

[36] J. Aten, A. Roos, N. Claessen, E. J. M. Schilder-Tol, I. J. M. Ten Berge, and J. J. Weening, "Strong and selective glomerular localization of CD134 ligand and TNF receptor-1 in proliferative lupus nephritis," *Journal of the American Society of Nephrology*, vol. 11, no. 8, pp. 1426–1438, 2000.

[37] Y.-B. Zhou, R.-G. Ye, Y.-J. Li, and C.-M. Xie, "Targeting the CD134-CD134L interaction using anti-CD134 and/or rhCD134 fusion protein as a possible strategy to prevent lupus nephritis," *Rheumatology International*, vol. 29, no. 4, pp. 417–425, 2009.

[38] M. N. Farres, D. S. Al-Zifzaf, A. A. Aly, and N. M. Abd Raboh, "OX40/OX40L in systemic lupus erythematosus: association with disease activity and lupus nephritis," *Annals of Saudi Medicine*, vol. 31, no. 1, pp. 29–34, 2011.

[39] D. Panneer, P. T. Antony, and V. S. Negi, "Q222R polymorphism in DNAse I gene is a risk factor for nephritis in South Indian SLE patients," *Lupus*, vol. 22, no. 10, pp. 996–1000, 2013.

[40] A. Hakkim, B. G. Fürnrohr, K. Amann et al., "Impairment of neutrophil extracellular trap degradation is associated with lupus nephritis," *Proceedings of the National Academy of Sciences of the United States of America*, vol. 107, no. 21, pp. 9813–9818, 2010.

[41] Y. M. Mosaad, A. Hammad, Z. Fawzy et al., "C1q rs292001 polymorphism and C1q antibodies in juvenile lupus and their relation to lupus nephritis," *Clinical & Experimental Immunology*, vol. 182, no. 1, pp. 23–34, 2015.

[42] M. Radanova, V. Vasilev, T. Dimitrov, B. Deliyska, V. Ikonomov, and D. Ivanova, "Association of rs172378 C1q gene cluster polymorphism with lupus nephritis in Bulgarian patients," *Lupus*, vol. 24, no. 3, pp. 280–289, 2015.

[43] H. Jeltsch-David and S. Muller, "Neuropsychiatric systemic lupus erythematosus: pathogenesis and biomarkers," *Nature Reviews Neurology*, vol. 10, pp. 579–596, 2014.

[44] M. Koga, A. Kawasaki, I. Ito et al., "Cumulative association of eight susceptibility genes with systemic lupus erythematosus in a Japanese female population," *Journal of Human Genetics*, vol. 56, no. 7, pp. 503–507, 2011.

[45] B. de Vries, G. M. Steup-Beekman, J. Haan et al., "TREX1 gene variant in neuropsychiatric systemic lupus erythematosus," *Annals of the Rheumatic Diseases*, vol. 69, no. 10, pp. 1886–1887, 2010.

[46] M. A. Lee-Kirsch, M. Gong, D. Chowdhury et al., "Mutations in the gene encoding the 3′-5′ DNA exonuclease TREX1 are associated with systemic lupus erythematosus," *Nature Genetics*, vol. 39, no. 9, pp. 1065–1067, 2007.

[47] B. Namjou, P. H. Kothari, J. A. Kelly et al., "Evaluation of the TREX1 gene in a large multi-ancestral lupus cohort," *Genes and Immunity*, vol. 12, no. 4, pp. 270–279, 2011.

[48] E. M. A. Ball and A. L. Bell, "Lupus arthritis—do we have a clinically useful classification?" *Rheumatology*, vol. 51, no. 5, Article ID ker381, pp. 771–779, 2012.

[49] T. Warchoł, M. Lianeri, J. K. Łącki, M. Olesińska, and P. P. Jagodziński, "ITGAM Arg77His is associated with disease susceptibility, arthritis, and renal symptoms in systemic lupus erythematosus patients from a sample of the polish population," *DNA and Cell Biology*, vol. 30, no. 1, pp. 33–38, 2011.

[50] J. de Azevêdo Silva, K. Monteiro Fernandes, J. A. Trés Pancotto et al., "Vitamin D receptor (VDR) gene polymorphisms and susceptibility to systemic lupus erythematosus clinical manifestations," *Lupus*, vol. 22, no. 11, pp. 1110–1117, 2013.

[51] A. Singh and D. L. Kamen, "Potential benefits of vitamin D for patients with systemic lupus erythematosus," *Dermato-Endocrinology*, vol. 4, no. 2, pp. 146–151, 2012.

[52] M. Abbasi, Z. Rezaieyazdi, J. T. Afshari, M. Hatef, M. Sahebari, and N. Saadati, "Lack of association of vitamin D receptor gene BsmI polymorphisms in patients with systemic lupus erythematosus," *Rheumatology International*, vol. 30, no. 11, pp. 1537–1539, 2010.

[53] T. A. Briggs, G. I. Rice, S. Daly et al., "Tartrate-resistant acid phosphatase deficiency causes a bone dysplasia with autoimmunity and a type I interferon expression signature," *Nature Genetics*, vol. 43, no. 2, pp. 127–131, 2011.

[54] A. Jönsen, I. Gunnarsson, B. Gullstrand et al., "Association between SLE nephritis and polymorphic variants of the CRP and FcγRIIIa genes," *Rheumatology*, vol. 46, no. 9, pp. 1417–1421, 2007.

[55] C. Ciccacci, C. Perricone, F. Ceccarelli et al., "A multilocus genetic study in a cohort of Italian SLE patients confirms the association with STAT4 gene and describes a new association with HCP5 gene," *PLoS ONE*, vol. 9, no. 11, Article ID e111991, 2014.

[56] J.-Y. Chen, C. M. Wang, C.-C. Ma et al., "Association of a transmembrane polymorphism of Fcγ receptor IIb (FCGR2B) with systemic lupus erythematosus in Taiwanese patients," *Arthritis and Rheumatism*, vol. 54, no. 12, pp. 3908–3917, 2006.

[57] J. Y. Chen, C. M. Wang, S. W. Chang et al., "Association of FCGR3A and FCGR3B copy number variations with systemic lupus erythematosus and rheumatoid arthritis in Taiwanese patients," *Arthritis & Rheumatology*, vol. 66, pp. 3113–3121, 2014.

[58] A. M. D. S. Fonseca, J. D. A. Silva, J. A. T. Pancotto et al., "Polymorphisms in STK17A gene are associated with systemic lupus erythematosus and its clinical manifestations," *Gene*, vol. 527, no. 2, pp. 435–439, 2013.

[59] C. Tanasescu, E. Balanescu, P. Balanescu et al., "IL-17 in cutaneous lupus erythematosus," *European Journal of Internal Medicine*, vol. 21, no. 3, pp. 202–207, 2010.

[60] D. L. Damian, Y. J. Kim, K. M. Dixon, G. M. Halliday, A. Javeri, and R. S. Mason, "Topical calcitriol protects from UV-induced genetic damage but suppresses cutaneous immunity in humans," *Experimental Dermatology*, vol. 19, no. 8, pp. 23–30, 2010.

[61] D. Wang, R. Liu, H. Zhu, D. Zhou, Q. Mei, and G. Xu, "Vitamin D receptor Fok I polymorphism is associated with low bone mineral density in postmenopausal women: a meta-analysis focused on populations in Asian countries," *European Journal of Obstetrics Gynecology and Reproductive Biology*, vol. 169, no. 2, pp. 380–386, 2013.

[62] Y. X. Cui, C. W. Fu, F. Jiang, L. X. Ye, and W. Meng, "Association of the interleukin-6 polymorphisms with systemic lupus erythematosus: a meta-analysis," *Lupus*, vol. 24, no. 12, pp. 1308–1317, 2015.

[63] C. Perricone, C. Ciccacci, F. Ceccarelli et al., "TRAF3IP2 gene and systemic lupus erythematosus: association with disease susceptibility and pericarditis development," *Immunogenetics*, vol. 65, no. 10, pp. 703–709, 2013.

[64] L. Wu, C. Wang, B. Boisson et al., "The differential regulation of human ACT1 isoforms by Hsp90 in IL-17 signaling," *Journal of Immunology*, vol. 193, no. 4, pp. 1590–1599, 2014.

[65] X. Li, "Act1 modulates autoimmunity through its dual functions in CD40L/BAFF and IL-17 signaling," *Cytokine*, vol. 41, no. 2, pp. 105–113, 2008.

[66] A. Strange, F. Capon, C. C. Spencer, J. Knight, M. E. Weale, M. H. Allen et al., "A genome-wide association study identifies new psoriasis susceptibility loci and an interaction between *HLA-C* and *ERAP1*," *Nature Genetics*, vol. 42, no. 11, pp. 985–990, 2010.

[67] L. Espino-Paisan, H. de la Calle, M. Fernández-Arquero et al., "A polymorphism in PTPN2 gene is associated with an earlier onset of type 1 diabetes," *Immunogenetics*, vol. 63, no. 4, pp. 255–258, 2011.

[68] R. Spolski and W. J. Leonard, "The Yin and Yang of interleukin-21 in allergy, autoimmunity and cancer," *Current Opinion in Immunology*, vol. 20, no. 3, pp. 295–301, 2008.

[69] G. Monteleone, F. Pallone, and T. T. MacDonald, "Interleukin-21: a critical regulator of the balance between effector and regulatory T-cell responses," *Trends in Immunology*, vol. 29, no. 6, pp. 290–294, 2008.

[70] I. Peluso, M. C. Fantini, D. Fina et al., "IL-21 counteracts the regulatory T cell-mediated suppression of human CD4$^+$ T lymphocytes," *The Journal of Immunology*, vol. 178, no. 2, pp. 732–739, 2007.

[71] Y. Sherer, A. Gorstein, M. J. Fritzler, and Y. Shoenfeld, "Autoantibody explosion in systemic lupus erythematosus: more than 100 different antibodies found in SLE patients," *Seminars in Arthritis and Rheumatism*, vol. 34, no. 2, pp. 501–537, 2004.

[72] C. Fabrizio, C. Fulvia, P. Carlo et al., "Systemic lupus erythematosus with and without anti-dsDNA antibodies: analysis from a large monocentric cohort," *Mediators of Inflammation*, vol. 2015, Article ID 328078, 6 pages, 2015.

[73] M. R. Arbuckle, M. T. McClain, M. V. Rubertone et al., "Development of autoantibodies before the clinical onset of systemic lupus erythematosus," *The New England Journal of Medicine*, vol. 349, no. 16, pp. 1526–1533, 2003.

[74] C. Perricone, N. Agmon-Levin, F. Ceccarelli, G. Valesini, J.-M. Anaya, and Y. Shoenfeld, "Genetics and autoantibodies," *Immunologic Research*, vol. 56, no. 2-3, pp. 206–219, 2013.

[75] T. A. Podrebarac, D. M. Boisert, and R. Goldstein, "Clinical correlates, serum autoantibodies and the role of the major histocompatibility complex in French Canadian and non-French Canadian Caucasians with SLE," *Lupus*, vol. 7, no. 3, pp. 183–191, 1998.

[76] C. Vasconcelos, C. Carvalho, B. Leal et al., "HLA in Portuguese systemic lupus erythematosus patients and their relation to clinical features," *Annals of the New York Academy of Sciences*, vol. 1173, pp. 575–580, 2009.

[77] S. Sigurdsson, G. Nordmark, S. Garnier et al., "A risk haplotype of STAT4 for systemic lupus erythematosus is over-expressed, correlates with anti-dsDNA and shows additive effects with two risk alleles of IRF5," *Human Molecular Genetics*, vol. 17, no. 18, pp. 2868–2876, 2008.

[78] S. A. Chung, K. E. Taylor, R. R. Graham et al., "Differential genetic associations for systemic lupus erythematosus based on anti-dsDNA autoantibody production," *PLoS Genetics*, vol. 7, no. 3, Article ID e1001323, 2011.

[79] E. Génin, M. Schumacher, J.-C. Rouäeau et al., "Genome-wide association study of Stevens-Johnson Syndrome and Toxic Epidermal Necrolysis in Europe," *Orphanet Journal of Rare Diseases*, vol. 6, article 52, 2011.

[80] T. H. Karlsen, A. Franke, E. Melum et al., "Genome-wide association analysis in primary sclerosing cholangitis," *Gastroenterology*, vol. 138, no. 3, pp. 1102–1111, 2010.

[81] R. M. Clancy, M. C. Marion, K. M. Kaufman et al., "Identification of candidate loci at 6p21 and 21q22 in a genome-wide association study of cardiac manifestations of neonatal lupus," *Arthritis & Rheumatism*, vol. 62, no. 11, pp. 3415–3424, 2010.

[82] D. L. Morris, M. M. A. Fernando, K. E. Taylor et al., "MHC associations with clinical and autoantibody manifestations in European SLE," *Genes and Immunity*, vol. 15, no. 4, pp. 210–217, 2014.

[83] T. B. Niewold, J. A. Kelly, S. N. Kariuki et al., "IRF5 haplotypes demonstrate diverse serological associations which predict serum interferon alpha activity and explain the majority of the genetic association with systemic lupus erythematosus," *Annals of the Rheumatic Diseases*, vol. 71, no. 3, pp. 463–468, 2012.

[84] M. J. Walport and P. J. Lachmann, "Complement deficiencies and abnormalities of the complement system in systemic lupus erythematosus and related disorders," *Current Opinion in Rheumatology*, vol. 2, no. 4, pp. 661–663, 1990.

[85] R. F. van Vollenhoven, M. Mosca, G. Bertsias et al., "Treat-to-target in systemic lupus erythematosus: recommendations from an international task force," *Annals of the Rheumatic Diseases*, vol. 73, no. 6, pp. 958–967, 2014.

[86] C. Carvalho, A. Marinho, B. Leal et al., "Association between vitamin D receptor (VDR) gene polymorphisms and systemic lupus erythematosus in Portuguese patients," *Lupus*, vol. 24, no. 8, pp. 846–853, 2015.

[87] D. Gladman, E. Ginzler, C. Goldsmith et al., "The development and initial validation of the systemic lupus international collaborating clinics/American college of rheumatology damage index for systemic lupus erythematosus," *Arthritis & Rheumatism*, vol. 39, no. 3, pp. 363–369, 1996.

[88] A. C. Bonfá, L. P. C. Seguro, V. Caparbo, E. Bonfá, and R. M. R. Pereira, "RANKL and OPG gene polymorphisms: associations with vertebral fractures and bone mineral density in premenopausal systemic lupus erythematosus," *Osteoporosis International*, vol. 26, no. 5, pp. 1563–1571, 2015.

18

Neutrophil Leukocyte: Combustive Microbicidal Action and Chemiluminescence

Robert C. Allen

Department of Pathology, Creighton University School of Medicine, Omaha, NE 68131, USA

Correspondence should be addressed to Robert C. Allen; robertallen@creighton.edu

Academic Editor: Carlos Rosales

Neutrophil leukocytes protect against a varied and complex array of microbes by providing microbicidal action that is simple, potent, and focused. Neutrophils provide such action via redox reactions that change the frontier orbitals of oxygen (O_2) facilitating combustion. The spin conservation rules define the symmetry barrier that prevents direct reaction of diradical O_2 with nonradical molecules, explaining why combustion is not spontaneous. In burning, the spin barrier is overcome when energy causes homolytic bond cleavage producing radicals capable of reacting with diradical O_2 to yield oxygenated radical products that further participate in reactive propagation. Neutrophil mediated combustion is by a different pathway. Changing the spin quantum state of O_2 removes the symmetry restriction to reaction. Electronically excited singlet molecular oxygen ($^1O_2^*$) is a potent electrophilic reactant with a finite lifetime that restricts its radius of reactivity and focuses combustive action on the target microbe. The resulting exergonic dioxygenation reactions produce electronically excited carbonyls that relax by light emission, that is, chemiluminescence. This overview of neutrophil combustive microbicidal action takes the perspectives of spin conservation and bosonic-fermionic frontier orbital considerations. The necessary principles of particle physics and quantum mechanics are developed and integrated into a fundamental explanation of neutrophil microbicidal metabolism.

Respectfully dedicated to my deceased mentor Dr. Richard H. Steele and to my friend and colleague Dr. Randolph M. Howes

1. Introduction

Considered as an organ, the collective mass of hematopoietic bone marrow in a healthy adult is greater than that of the liver. The major proportion of this hematopoietic activity is directed to producing neutrophil leukocytes. Each day a healthy human adult releases about a hundred billion neutrophils into the circulating blood [1]. This baseline production is greatly expanded in inflammatory states and by treatment with a granulocyte-colony stimulating factor (G-CSF) such as filgrastim [2]. In addition to stimulating neutrophil hyperplasia, that is, increased production, G-CSF treatment also results in hypertrophic changes, that is, larger neutrophils with severalfold greater azurophilic granule content and proportionally increased myeloperoxidase (MPO) [3].

The neutrophil serves as the principal leukocyte of the acute inflammatory response and is the primary microbicidal phagocyte of the innate and acquired immune defense systems. Accomplishing such function starts in the circulation with intricate neutrophil-endothelial contact. When stimulated by microbial products, complement activation peptides, cytokines, *et cetera*, neutrophils fuse their specific (a.k.a., secondary) granules with their cytoplasmic membrane (i.e., specific degranulation), thus providing the increased surface-to-volume ratio necessary for locomotion and exposing the cytokine receptors and opsonin receptors required for close endothelial contact and diapedesis (i.e., transit) from the vascular space through the endothelial lining into the tissue interstitial space. Chemotactic locomotion to the site of infection is directed by concentration gradients of bacterial products, anaphylatoxin, cytokines, *et cetera*.

Contact and receptor-mediated recognition of an opsonified (e.g., complement-, immunoglobulin-labeled) microbe results in phagocytosis, formation of a phagosome, and

Cytoplasmic milieu   Phagolysosome milieu

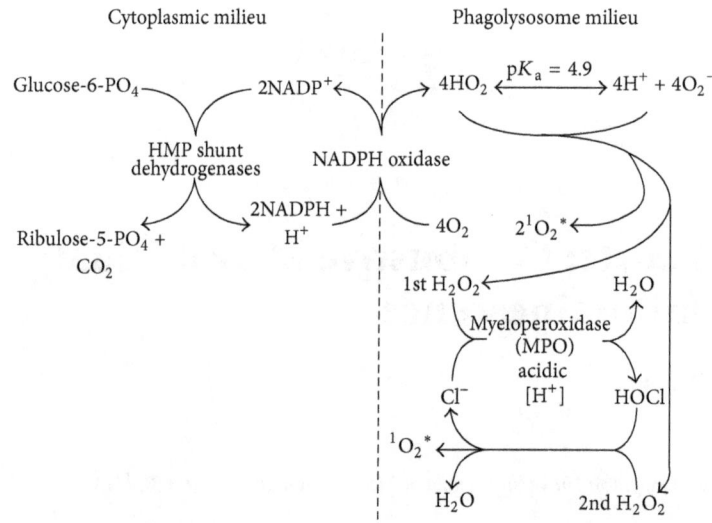

FIGURE 1: Schematic depiction of neutrophil HOCl and $^1O_2^*$ generation.

fusion with azurophilic (a.k.a. primary) granules containing myeloperoxidase to produce the phagolysosome [4].

2. Respiratory Burst Metabolism

The morphologic changes of phagocytosis are associated with magnitudinal increase in hexose monophosphate shunt metabolism of glucose and with proportionally increased molecular oxygen (O_2) consumption, that is, the respiratory burst. This mitochondria-independent metabolic activity is required for effective microbicidal action [5, 6]. The resulting microbicidal oxygenation reactions have exergonicities sufficient to produce electronic excited products yielding light emission in the visible spectrum, that is, chemiluminescence or luminescence [7].

Phagocytosis is linked to activation of NADPH oxidase. This complex flavocytochrome oxidase drives the respiratory burst [6, 8]. Two reducing equivalents (i.e., two electrons (e^-) plus two protons (H^+)) are transferred from NADPH to the oxidase where they distribute in a manner allowing for univalent (one equivalent) reduction of O_2, yielding hydrodioxylic acid (HO_2; a.k.a. hydroperoxyl radical) [9, 10]. HO_2 is an acid with a pK_a of 4.9 and, as such, dissociates yielding a proton and its conjugate base, the superoxide anion (O_2^-). Production of HO_2 within the neutrophil phagosome or phagolysosome dynamically acidifies the confined space. As the pH of the space approaches the pK_a (i.e., 4.9), the ratio of HO_2 to O_2^- approaches unity, removing the anionic barrier to direct radical-radical disproportionation [10, 11]. In such acidic milieu, HO_2 reacts directly with O_2^- to produce hydrogen peroxide (H_2O_2) and singlet molecular oxygen ($^1O_2^*$) [10–12].

NADPH oxidase dynamically acidifies the phagolysosome and produces H_2O_2. These activities provide the optimal milieu and H_2O_2 substrate for myeloperoxidase (MPO) oxidation of chloride (Cl^-) to the chloronium (Cl^+) state yielding hypochlorous acid (HOCl) [13]. Spontaneous

reaction of HOCl with an additional H_2O_2 yields Cl^-, H_2O, and $^1O_2^*$ [14]. Both HOCl and $^1O_2^*$ are potent microbicidal reactants. The metabolic generation of these reactants is depicted in Figure 1.

3. Oxygen Reactivity

With regard to electronegativity, oxygen is second only to fluorine. The order of electronegativity values for fluorine (F), oxygen (O), and chorine (Cl) is 4.0, 3.5, and 3.0, respectively [15]. The energy difference separating O_2 from water (H_2O) is large, that is, a difference of 1.23 volts (V) or 96.5 kilocalories per mole (kcal mol^{-1}), and provides the driving force of life on earth.

The Merriam-Webster Dictionary defines combustion as a chemical reaction that occurs when oxygen combines with other substances to produce heat and usually light. As such, neutrophil microbicidal action is combustive. Dioxygenation reactions are among the most exergonic in biology. The heat of reaction calculations for the reaction of O_2 with ethylene liberates 93 kcal mol^{-1} (i.e., 389 kilojoules per mole (kJ mol^{-1})) or the energy equivalent to an einstein (i.e., one mole) of ultraviolet photons [16]. The electronegativity of oxygen predicts the high exergonicity of oxygenation reactions, but such reactions are not spontaneous. Placed together in a chamber, O_2 does not react with ethylene. For reaction to occur, a photon or spark with energy sufficient to initiate ethylene bond homolytic cleavage must be applied.

This presentation addresses the questions: why does not oxygen spontaneously react with organic material? Why is oxygen reduction, a process that decreases its thermodynamic potential, required as a first step for neutrophil combustive microbicidal action? And what is the best viewpoint for considering oxygen reactivity? The review provides the background physics and chemistry for a fundamental perspective with regard to oxygen reactivity in particular, neutrophil combustive microbicidal action with its associated luminescence, and reaction chemistry in general. Hopefully, it will encourage interested researchers out of their comfort zone and broaden their scientific outlook.

4. Particle Physics, Quantum Mechanics, and Reaction Symmetry

Particles are of two symmetry types, each with unique statistical mechanical properties [17, 18]. They are either Bose-Einstein particles (bosons) or Fermi-Dirac particles (fermions). According to the exchange principle, a pair of particles, that is, a and b, can be described by a wave function, $\Psi(a, b)$, representing the space and spin coordinates of the particles. Exchanging the particles generates a new wave function, $\Psi(b, a)$. Even if the particles are indistinguishable (e.g., electrons), the particle sites are distinguishable. Each site is unique with regard to its spin-state, that is, spin-up ($\uparrow$) or spin-down ($\downarrow$). Each combination is distinct. For indistinguishable particles, the result of exchange can differ by no more than a quantum phase factor. There are only two symmetry possibilities. Exchange can be symmetric: $\Psi(a, b) = \Psi(b, a)$; or exchange can be antisymmetric: $\Psi(a, b) = -\Psi(b, a)$ [19].

4.1. Bosons. The wave functions of bosons are symmetric to exchange of a pair of particles; that is, $\Psi(a, b) = \Psi(b, a)$. Bosons obey ordinary commutation; $a \times b = b \times a$. Rotating a boson through 360 degrees, $\Psi - 360° \rightarrow \Psi$, returns it to its original state. Bosons are symmetric particles with integral spin. Photons, the force carrier particles of electromagnetic energy, are bosons and are described by the Planck equation: $E = h\nu$, where E is energy, h is Planck's constant, and ν is frequency.

Two antisymmetric fermions can also couple to produce a symmetric bosonic product. Such products include large bosons with mass, such as alpha (α) particles. The character of atomic and molecular orbitals can likewise be considered as bosonic or fermionic [20]. As will be developed subsequently, the frontier orbital of an atom or molecule is bosonic if composed of paired antisymmetric electrons. As such, the highest fully occupied atomic or molecular orbital (HO(A)MO) has bosonic character. Such atoms and molecules are nonradical and diamagnetic.

4.2. Fermions. The wave functions of fermions are antisymmetric to exchange of particles; that is, $\Psi(a, b) = -\Psi(b, a)$. Spin is an intrinsic property of the particle and is quantized. Fermions are characterized as having half-integer spin and appear as multiples of the basic unit $(1/2)\hbar$, where $\hbar$ (h-bar) equals Planck's constant (h) divided by 2π. Fermions anticommute; that is, $a \times b \neq b \times a$. Rotating a fermion through 360 degrees, $\Psi - 360° \rightarrow -\Psi$, changes the phase but does not return the fermion to its original state. An additional 360 degrees' rotation, $-\Psi - 360° \rightarrow \Psi$, is required to return the antisymmetric particle to its original state.

Fermions compose the solid stuff of the universe and are subject to time. Electrons, protons, and neutrons are fermions. The frontier orbitals of atoms, such as hydrogen (H), nitrogen (N), and oxygen (O), and molecules, such as O_2 and nitrous oxide (NO), have singly occupied atomic or molecular orbitals (SO(A)MO). An orbital with a single electron has fermionic character. Atoms and molecules with fermionic orbitals are radical and paramagnetic.

4.3. Principal, Radial, and Angular Quantum Numbers. Atomic hydrogen (H) is composed of a positively charged nuclear proton (H^+) and a negatively charged electron (e^-). Both H^+ and e^- are fermions. H^+ is thousandfold more massive than e^-, and, as such, the kinetic and potential energies of e^- are described as its "orbit" relative to the massive H^+. The orbital wave function describes the energy possibilities. Using polar coordinates, the position of e^- can be described as its distance, r, from its nucleus and two angles, θ and φ. The total wave function is isolated into 3 separate contributions, $\Psi(r, \theta, \varphi) = R(r)\Theta(\theta)\Phi(\varphi)$, where $R(r)$ is the radial component and $\Theta(\theta)$ and $\Phi(\varphi)$ are the angular components. Solution of each component yields a quantum number. The radial component yields the principal quantum number, n. The angular components yield the azimuthal quantum number, l, and the magnetic quantum number, m_l.

The principal quantum number, n, describes the energy of the orbital. The degree of orbital degeneracy is the square of the principal quantum number, n^2. When $n = 1$, the degeneracy is $1^2 = 1$, yielding the 1s orbital. When $n = 2$, the degeneracy is $2^2 = 4$, yielding the 2s, $2p_x$, $2p_y$, and $2p_z$ orbitals. The azimuthal quantum number, l, describes the shape of the orbit and the orbital angular momentum of e^-. The magnetic quantum number, m_l, describes the number of orbitals with a given value of l. The value of the total orbital angular momentum, L, is $L = \sqrt{[l(l + 1)]}\hbar$.

4.4. Spin Quantum Number. Electrons and other fermions possess intrinsic angular momentum that is independent of orbital motion. This intrinsic quantum mechanical property, that is, spin, is described by the spin quantum number, s. The magnitude of s is restricted to a value of $1/2$. The total spin angular momentum, S, of a system is expressed by the equation $S = \sqrt{[s(s + 1)]}\hbar$. The intrinsic spin with its value of $(1/2)\hbar$ (abbreviated to $1/2$) is a quality of fermions without analogy in classical physics. Just as l gives rise to m_l, s gives rise to the spin quantum number m_s. Only two values are allowed for m_s. When $m_s = 1/2$, e^- is described as spin-up ($\uparrow$); when $m_s = -1/2$, e^- is described as spin-down ($\downarrow$).

4.5. Pauli Exclusion Principle. Each e^- of an atom or molecule is defined by its five quantum numbers: n, l, m_l, s, and m_s. The Pauli exclusion principle states that no two electrons of a given atom can have identical quantum numbers; that is, the total wave function for a system must be antisymmetric to the exchange of any pair of electrons. For an orbit to accommodate two electrons, the electrons must have opposite spins. If one orbital e^- has $m_s = 1/2$ ($\uparrow$), the other orbital e^- must have $m_s = -1/2$ ($\downarrow$). As such, the total spin quantum number, S, for an orbital electron-couple is $1/2 + -1/2 = 0$ ($\uparrow\downarrow$). Orbital coupling of the fermionic electrons results in spin-neutralization. In effect, the antisymmetric fermions combine

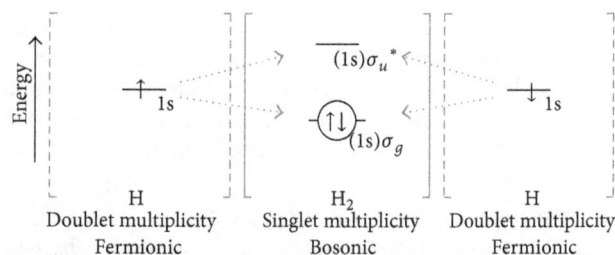

FIGURE 2: Combination of two doublet multiplicity hydrogen atoms (H, shown on the left and right of the graphic) yields singlet multiplicity molecular hydrogen (H_2, shown in the center of the graphic). Multiplicity is defined as $|2(S)| + 1$, where S is the total spin number. Constructive overlap of the two antisymmetric 1s SOAOs of the H atoms yields the HOMO σ of H_2. The (1s) notation before σ indicates the atomic source of the molecular orbital. σ^* is the LUMO antibonding orbital (* indicates antibonding) of H_2. The energy differences in the figures are for illustration and not drawn to scale.

TABLE 1: Spin conservation rules. Multiplicity states from the perspective of the bosonic-fermionic orbital character of reactants and products.

Reactants	Product(s)
Singlet + singlet	Singlet
Bosonic + bosonic	*Bosonic*
Singlet + doublet	Doublet
Bosonic + fermionic	*Fermionic*
Singlet + triplet	Triplet
Bosonic + bifermionic	*Bifermionic*
Doublet + doublet	Singlet (triplet)*
Fermionic + fermionic	*Bosonic (bifermionic)**
Doublet + triplet	Doublet (quartet)*
Fermionic + bifermionic	*Fermionic (trifermionic)**
Doublet + quartet	Triplet
Fermionic + trifermionic	*Bifermionic*
Triplet + triplet	Singlet
Bifermionic + bifermionic	*Bosonic*
Triplet + quartet	Doublet
Bifermionic + trifermionic	*Fermionic*
Quartet + quartet	Singlet
Trifermionic + trifermionic	*Bosonic*

*The products in parentheses are symmetrically possible but improbable.

into a symmetric boson. This concept is illustrated in Figure 2 by the reaction of two H atoms to generate molecular H_2.

4.6. Multiplicity. Multiplicity is defined as $|2(S)| + 1$, where S is the total spin number. Multiplicity is a spectroscopic term and indicates the number of wave functions possible for the system; that is, singlet indicates 1, doublet indicates 2, triplet indicates 3, *et cetera*. In its ground (lowest energy) electronic state, atomic H has a single e^- in the 1s orbital and has an S value of $1/2$ or $-1/2$; thus $|2(1/2$ or $-1/2)| + 1 = 2$; the multiplicity is doublet. For molecular H_2 the value of S is 0; thus, $|2(0)| + 1 = 1$; the multiplicity is singlet. In Figure 2, the orbital possibilities are depicted by a horizontal bar (—). The spin quantum number of each e^- is represented as spin-up ($m_s = 1/2 = \uparrow$) or spin-down ($m_s = -1/2 = \downarrow$). The circle surrounding the σ orbital electron-couple of the HOMO of H_2 symbolizes the bosonic character of the filled orbital.

Orbital overlap of the two H atoms can be constructive or destructive. When the electrons are antisymmetric, that is, $\uparrow$ and $\downarrow$, overlap is constructive resulting in chemical bonding; that is, there is an increased probability of finding electrons in the internuclear region between the two H nuclei. Combining the two atomic 1s orbitals yields the bonding sigma molecular orbital, σ. Note that bonding lowers the energy of the system. When the electrons are $\uparrow$ and $\uparrow$ or $\downarrow$ and $\downarrow$, the overlap is destructive and no bonding occurs.

5. Frontier Orbital Theory

Chemical reaction involves frontier orbital interaction. Frontier orbital theory focuses on the initial orbital conditions of the reactants and on reactive transition with special emphasis on the highest occupied and lowest unoccupied orbitals [21, 22]. The frontier orbitals, that is, the highest occupied atomic or molecular orbital (HO(A)MO) and the lowest unoccupied molecular orbital (LUMO), define the reactive possibilities. As depicted in Figure 2, the electrons of the singly occupied atomic orbital (SOAO) of the two H atoms constructively

overlap in a radical-radical (i.e., doublet-doublet) annihilation producing the σ bonding HOMO orbital of singlet multiplicity, diamagnetic molecular hydrogen (H_2).

For the H atoms, the electrons of the 1s orbitals have identical energies, but with covalent bonding to form H_2, the wave functions overlap and split producing two molecular orbitals, one with lower and one with higher energy than the original 1s atomic orbitals. The bonding orbital (σ) is lower in energy and stable, thus promoting bonding. The antibonding orbital (σ^*) is of higher energy. Populating the antibonding orbital promotes bond breaking [23]. Consequently, if a photon of sufficient frequency is captured by a σ electron, its electronic excitation to the σ^* orbital results in H_2 bond cleavage.

6. Wigner-Witmer Spin Conservation and Boson-Fermion Orbital Symmetry

The Wigner-Witmer spin conservation rules describe reaction symmetry possibilities in terms of reactant and product multiplicities [24, 25]. The spin conservation rules state that the overall spin angular momentum of a system must be conserved. The symmetries of reactants and products must correlate. Reactant and product state possibilities can also be considered in terms of fermionic and bosonic frontier orbital character [20].

In Table 1 reactants and products are presented in terms of multiplicity and also in terms of bosonic or fermionic orbital character. As depicted in Figure 2, combining two doublet multiplicity H atoms produces singlet multiplicity

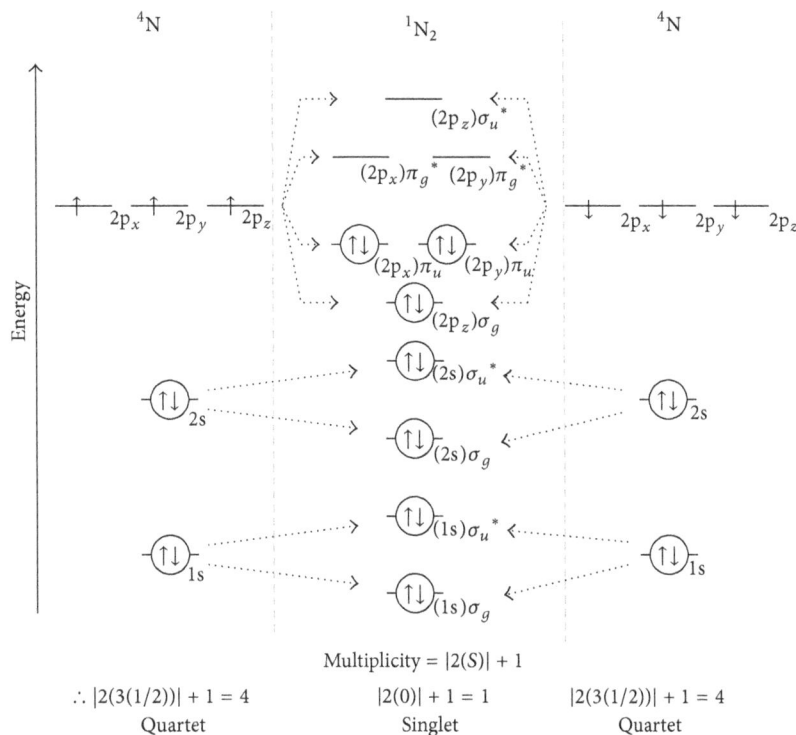

FIGURE 3: Combination of two quartet multiplicity nitrogen atoms (^{4}N; the superscript 4 indicates multiplicity) to yield singlet multiplicity molecular nitrogen (^{1}N$_2$).

H_2. With regard to orbital spin character, the two antisymmetric fermionic electrons of the atomic orbitals are coupled (condensed or combined) resulting in the bosonic electron pair of the σ orbital of H_2. Since the Pauli principle requires the total wave function for any system of electrons to be antisymmetric to exchange an orbital pair of electrons, only phase-opposite electrons can occupy a given orbital state. Orbital coupling of such fermionic electrons imposes bosonic character.

6.1. *Hund's Maximum Multiplicity Rule.* Hund's maximum multiplicity rule states that the electronic configuration with highest multiplicity has the lowest energy. The greater the number of wave functions possible for a system, the lower the energy. Figure 3 depicts the combination of two nitrogen atoms (N) to yield molecular nitrogen (N_2). Ground state atomic N is a paramagnetic triradical with one electron in each of its three 2p orbitals. Note that each electron has the same m_s value resulting in quartet multiplicity; that is, $|2(3(1/2 \text{ or } -1/2))|+1 = 4$. The orbitals of higher multiplicity states are more contracted than those of lower multiplicity. Higher multiplicity states produce greater nuclear-electron attraction and are of lower energy [26].

Combining the atomic orbitals of the two quartet multiplicity nitrogen atoms (N) generates the filled (bosonic) (1s and 2s) σ and σ^* orbitals; constructive overlap of the phase-opposite electrons of the three 2p orbitals of the two N atoms generates one σ and two π bonds of triple-bonded ground state singlet multiplicity N_2. The triradical N atoms combine to produce nonradical N_2. From the fermion-boson frontier

orbital perspective, each N presents a complex of trifermionic SOAOs, that is, Ψ (i.e., $S = 3(1/2)$) or $-\Psi$ (i.e., $S = 3(-1/2)$). Consistent with Table 1, antisymmetric coupling produces triple-bonded bosonic (i.e., $S = 0$) N_2.

6.2. *Oxygen Chemistry.* Frontier orbital overlap of two oxygen atoms with antisymmetric SOMO is constructive producing $^1O_2^*$ as depicted in Figure 4. As per Table 1, combining two ground state triplet multiplicity paramagnetic, diradical oxygen atoms (O) produces an electronically excited singlet multiplicity, diamagnetic, nonradical $^1O_2^*$. Note the product $^1O_2^*$ obeys the spin symmetry rules but violates Hund's maximum multiplicity rule. As such, $^1O_2^*$ is electronically excited (indicated by $*$) with an energy of 22.5 kcal mol^{-1} greater than that of triplet multiplicity ground state O_2 [14].

The spin conservation rules predict that the change in spin multiplicity, that is, a singlet-to-triplet transition, is of low probability. As such, electronically excited $^1O_2^*$ is metastable with a relatively long half-life. The estimated four-microsecond lifetime of $^1O_2^*$ is sufficient to allow its participation as an electrophilic reactant in dioxygenation reactions. However, such reactions are restricted to within a radius of about 0.2 microns (μm) from its point of generation [27, 28]. As depicted in Figure 5, unreacted $^1O_2^*$ relaxes to its triplet multiplicity ground state ($^3O_2$) by emitting a 1270 nm (near infrared) photon.

As per the maximum multiplicity rule, ground state molecular oxygen is a triplet multiplicity, paramagnetic diradical with one e$^-$ occupying each of its two π^* SOMOs;

^3O $^1O_2$ ^3O

Energy

$(2p)\sigma_u{}^*$

$(2p)\pi_g{}^*$ $(2p)\pi_g{}^*$

$2p_x$ $2p_y$ $2p_z$ $(2p)\pi_u$ $(2p)\pi_u$ $2p_x$ $2p_y$ $2p_z$

$(2p)\sigma_g$

$(2s)\sigma_u{}^*$

$2s$ $(2s)\sigma_g$ $2s$

$(1s)\sigma_u{}^*$

$1s$ $(1s)\sigma_g$ $1s$

Multiplicity $= |2(S)| + 1$

$\therefore |2(2(1/2))| + 1 = 3$ $|2(0)| + 1 = 1$ $|2(2(1/2))| + 1 = 3$
Triplet   Singlet   Triplet

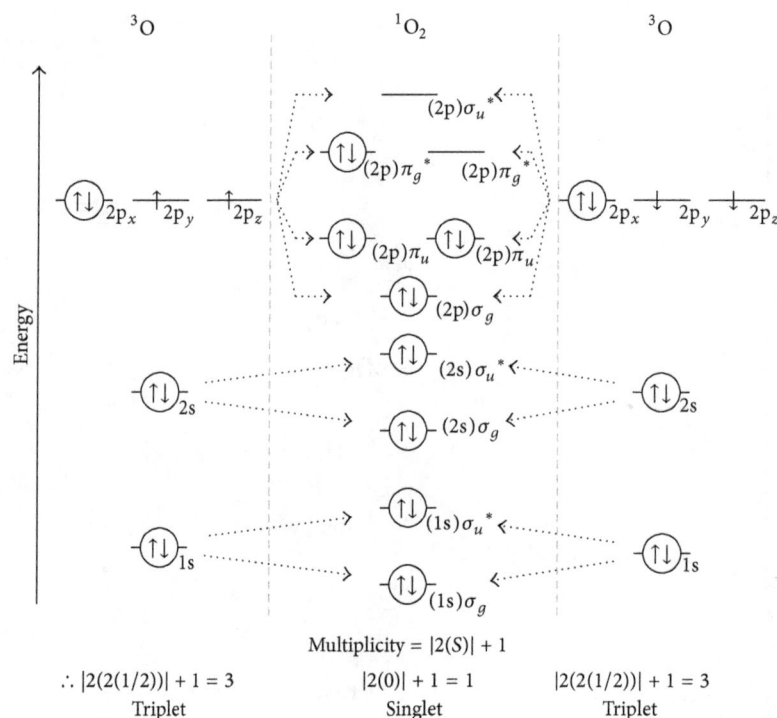

FIGURE 4: Combination of two triplet multiplicity oxygen atoms (^3O) to yield electronically excited singlet multiplicity molecular hydrogen ($^1O_2{}^*$).

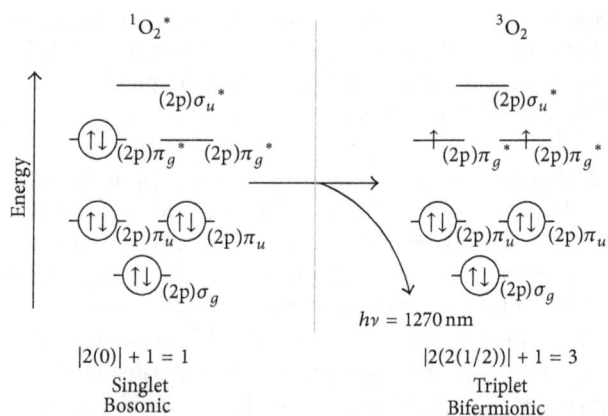

$^1O_2{}^*$ $^3O_2$

Energy

$(2p)\sigma_u{}^*$ $(2p)\sigma_u{}^*$

$(2p)\pi_g{}^*$ $(2p)\pi_g{}^*$ $(2p)\pi_g{}^*$ $(2p)\pi_g{}^*$

$(2p)\pi_u$ $(2p)\pi_u$ $(2p)\pi_u$ $(2p)\pi_u$

$(2p)\sigma_g$ $(2p)\sigma_g$

$h\nu = 1270\,nm$

$|2(0)| + 1 = 1$ $|2(2(1/2))| + 1 = 3$
Singlet   Triplet
Bosonic   Bifermionic

FIGURE 5: Relaxation of singlet molecular oxygen to its triplet ground state by infrared photon emission. For simplicity, only the $(2p)$ σ, π, π^*, and σ^* orbitals of O_2 are shown.

it is bifermionic. Ground state O_2 can be in either the Ψ (i.e., $S = 1/2 + 1/2 = 2(1/2) = 1$) or the $-\Psi$ (i.e., $S = -1/2 - 1/2 = 2(-1/2) = -1$) state; thus, the multiplicity is $|2(1) + 1| = 3$, that is, triplet.

The vast majority of biological molecules are singlet multiplicity—that is, $S = 0$—and, as such, present bosonic frontier orbitals. For such molecules, chemistry is confined to bosonic HOMO-LUMO exchange of a composite orbital electron-couple. The fermionic orbital character of radicals is atypical and favors radicals-radical reaction. Antisymmetric fermionic frontier orbital overlap is constructive resulting in

covalent bonding of the bosonic singlet product. As described in Table 1, constructive SOMO-SOMO overlap of a doublet reactant and a triplet reactant produces a doublet product; that is, the fermionic character is preserved.

Direct reaction of ground state triplet multiplicity O_2 with singlet multiplicity organic molecules violates the spin conservation rules, and, as such, combustion is not spontaneous. Overlap of the bifermionic π^* (the 2 SOMO) frontier orbitals of triplet multiplicity O_2 with the empty LUMO or bosonic HOMO of singlet multiplicity organic molecules is not constructive. Such reactions are symmetry-restricted, and the only product possible would also be a bifermionic triplet. O_2 with its triplet multiplicity ground state is relatively exotic. The triplet multiplicity states of most molecules are electronically excited. The relaxation of such excited triplet multiplicity molecules to their singlet ground state, that is, triplet-to-singlet transition, violates the conservation rules and is of low probability. The delayed relaxation of an excited triplet to its singlet ground state by photon emission is responsible for the phenomenon of phosphorescence [29].

6.3. Neutrophils Change the Spin Number of O_2. Considering the complexity and variety of potentially pathogenic organisms, neutrophil microbicidal action must be simple, potent, and focused so as to maximize microbicidal action and minimize collateral damage. Microbicidal combustion is realized by changing the frontier orbitals of oxygen from bifermionic to bosonic. Neutrophil combustive action is expected to produce light. Oxygenation reactions yield electronically excited products that relax to ground state by emission of light in the visible spectral range. Bioluminescence and chemiluminescence reactions are essentially limited to such oxygenation reactions. Neutrophil luminescence is energetic proof of such combustive activity.

Respiratory burst metabolism mobilizes the reducing equivalents required for changing the frontier orbitals of O_2. One equivalent (radical) reduction is unusual in cytoplasmic metabolism. When it does occur, the semiquinone of a riboflavin prosthetic group is typically involved. Such flavoenzymes mark the departure from two equivalent cytoplasmic transfers to one equivalent cytochrome transfer. One equivalent reduction of O_2 changes its multiplicity from triplet to doublet, thus reducing its overall fermionic orbital character. The flavocytochrome enzyme NADPH oxidase catalyzes the reduction of bifermionic triplet multiplicity O_2 to fermionic doublet multiplicity HO_2 [9, 10]. Acidic dissociation of HO_2 yields its conjugate base, doublet multiplicity superoxide anion (O_2^-) [11]. As per Figure 1 and Table 1, direct SOMO-SOMO orbital overlap of HO_2 with O_2^- produces singlet multiplicity ground state H_2O_2 plus $^1O_2{}^*$ [10, 12].

The H_2O_2 produced serves as substrate for myeloperoxidase (MPO) oxidation of chloride producing hypochlorous acid; that is, $H_2O_2 + Cl^- \rightarrow H_2O + HOCl$. Note that all reactants and products are exclusively singlet multiplicity (bosonic). The hypochlorous acid (HOCl) produced reacts directly with additional H_2O_2. This reaction involves the bosonic HOMO of H_2O_2 and the bosonic LUMO of HOCl producing the intermediate singlet multiplicity chloroperoxy acid (HOOCl) and singlet multiplicity H_2O [14]. Disintegration of the chloroperoxy intermediate yields ground state singlet multiplicity chloride and electronically excited singlet multiplicity oxygen. The net reaction is $H_2O_2 + HOCl \rightarrow {}^1O_2{}^* + H_2O + Cl^- + H^+$. The bosonic orbital symmetry of $^1O_2{}^*$ allows direct constructive spin-allowed overlap with the bosonic frontier orbitals of biological substrates producing singlet multiplicity dioxygenated products of bosonic symmetry.

In conventional combustive burning, sufficient energy must be applied to a nonradical (singlet) substrate to produce homolytic bond cleavage yielding two radical (doublet) products. The fermionic SOMO of these doublet multiplicity radical products can now constructively overlap with one of the fermionic SOMOs of triplet multiplicity ground state O_2. As described in Table 1, the product of doublet-triplet reaction will have doublet multiplicity. Such radical-diradical reactions yield heat plus additional radical products that can further participate in the radical propagation process of burning.

Neutrophil microbicidal action is combustion by a different pathway. Instead of radicalizing a substrate to facilitate reaction with diradical O_2, the bifermionic orbitals of ground state triplet O_2 are converted to the bosonic orbitals of $^1O_2{}^*$. In its electronically excited singlet multiplicity state, the bosonic frontier orbitals of oxygen can participate in spin-allowed electrophilic oxygenation reactions with a broad spectrum of singlet multiplicity biological molecules. As per spin conservation, the products of these reactions are singlet multiplicity. Such products are nonradical, diamagnetic, and

unable to participate in the radical propagation reactions that are characteristic of burning.

The potent electrophilic reactivity of $^1O_2{}^*$ is restricted to its metastable lifetime. The microsecond lifetime range of $^1O_2{}^*$ confines reactions to within about a $0.2\,\mu m$ radius from its point of origin [27, 28]. Thus, phagolysosomal generation of $^1O_2{}^*$ in close proximity to the target microbe guarantees that combustive action is focused on the microbe with minimal collateral damage to the host. By changing the spin quantum number of oxygen, the neutrophil not only realizes its potent electrophilic microbicidal action, but also limits such combustive action to the target microbe.

6.4. Neutrophil Luminescence. The endoperoxide and dioxetane products of dioxygenation are of relatively high energy. These dioxygenated products are typically unstable and of singlet multiplicity. Disintegration of such products yields two carbonyl functions. One carbonyl is in the ground singlet multiplicity state, and the other carbonyl is in the electronically excited $n\pi^*$ singlet multiplicity state. As depicted in Figure 6, the $n\pi^*$ description indicates that an electron from the ground state nonbonding (n) orbital of the atomic oxygen (O) component occupies the π^* orbital of the electronically excited carbonyl function. When the spin of the excited π^* electron is antisymmetric to that of the ground state n electron of O, the electronically excited carbonyl is singlet multiplicity. Thus, π^*-to-n relaxation to ground state is spin-allowed and yields a photon with energy proportional to the difference between the two orbital states.

In bioluminescence and chemiluminescence processes, dioxygenated products disintegrate by oxygen-oxygen bond cleavage producing the singlet multiplicity $n\pi^*$ electronically excited carbonyl. This electronically excited state is chemically generated. In fluorescence, electronic excitation to the $n\pi^*$ state can occur when a photon of proper energy is captured by an electron in the nonbonding (n) orbital of the O component of the carbonyl.

As depicted in Figure 6, relaxation of the electron from π^* of the singlet excited carbonyl back to the n orbital of O results in photon ($h\nu$) emission and returns the carbonyl function to its ground singlet state. The frequency of the emitted photon is the energy difference that separates the n orbital from the π^* orbital. Photons are symmetric bosons; their absorbance or emission does not affect the electron spin.

In fluorescence, photon capture promotes an electron of an orbital to an appropriately higher energy orbital. Such photon excitation results in transient antibonding and fermionic character, but the overall spin symmetry is retained; that is, singlet character is retained. Relaxation of an $n\pi^*$ electronically excited singlet multiplicity carbonyl to its singlet ground state by fluorescence or chemiluminescence is spin-allowed, and, as such, the lifetime of the excited state is very short-lived, typically in the nanosecond range. Consequently the excited carbonyl is unable to participate in reaction chemistry.

6.5. Native and Substrate Specific Chemiluminescence. The chemiluminescence produced by neutrophils is an energy byproduct of microbicidal combustion and varies with the

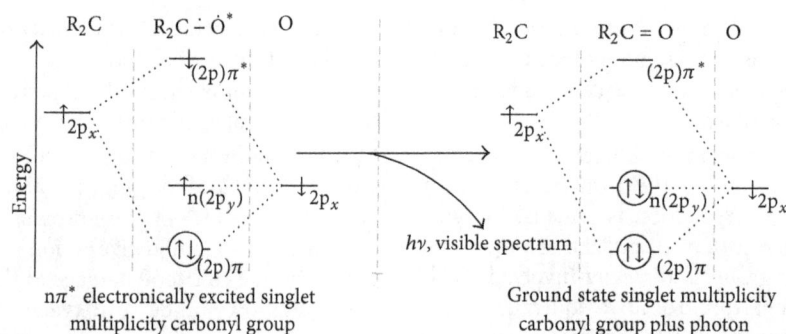

FIGURE 6: Relaxation (pi antibonding to nonbonding ($\pi^* \rightarrow$ n) electronic orbital transition) of a singlet electronically excited carbonyl product of dioxygenation to its singlet ground state by photon emission.

molecular composition of the microbe. Different microbes present substrates that vary with regard to dioxygenation susceptibility and combustion quantum efficiencies, that is, the photon yield per dioxygenation reaction. Native luminescence is easily measured using a luminometer, but the photon yield is insufficient for measurement of less than a hundred thousand neutrophils. In order to increase photon yield and impose reaction specificity, chemiluminigenic substrates can be introduced to the milieu. Chemiluminigenic substrates are susceptible to dioxygenation producing endoperoxides or dioxetanes ultimately yielding $n\pi^*$ electronically excited carbonyl products. Such substrates increase the sensitivity for detecting dioxygenation activity by several orders of magnitude [30]. In addition to increasing sensitivity, chemiluminigenic substrates can be selected for specificity with regard to the type of oxygenation activity measured [31].

The state of the circulating neutrophil reflects the state of inflammatory immune defense [32]. The sensitivity and specificity obtained using selective chemiluminigenic probe in combination with phagocytic and chemical stimuli allow simultaneous quantification of multiple neutrophil metrics using a microliter or less of unseparated whole blood. When subjected to discriminant function analysis, such neutrophil luminescence measurements allow assessment of host inflammatory state and hematopoietic marrow stress [32–35].

7. Neutrophil Myeloperoxidase and Lactic Acid Bacteria (LAB)

Neutrophil leukocytes respond to cytokines and other agents by fusing specific granules with the cytoplasmic membrane, that is, specific degranulation. Such fusion effectively increases the surface-to-volume ratio of the neutrophil, as is required for locomotion and phagocytosis, and for upregulated membrane expression of cytokine and opsonin receptors, as is required for effective recognition and phagocytosis. Microbicidal effectiveness is optimized by coordinating phagocytosis with activation of NADPH oxidase, resulting in dynamic acidification and H_2O_2 production. Fusion of the lysosomal azurophilic granules with the microbe-containing phagosome produces a phagolysosome with a relatively high MPO concentration in an acidic milieu replete with

H_2O_2. The phagolysosomal milieu is optimal for combustive microbicidal action.

The neutrophils of patients with chronic granulomatous disease (CGD) have defective NADPH oxidase function and consequently have defective microbicidal combustion and do not chemiluminesce [36]. These CGD neutrophils phagocytose microbes and release MPO into the phagolysosomal space, but the neutrophil respiratory burst is defective and microbicidal action is poor. Consequently, CGD patients have an increased susceptibility to infection. Interestingly, the incidence of pneumococcal and other streptococcal infections is not increased in CGD patients; that is, infection rates for these microbes are about equivalent to those for healthy subjects [37]. Pneumococci and streptococci are cytochrome-deficient lactic acid bacteria (LAB) that produce lactic acid and H_2O_2 as metabolic products [38, 39]. Phagocytosis of live LAB by CGD neutrophils does result in microbicidal action. In the case of CGD neutrophils, the phagocytosed LAB provides the acid and H_2O_2 necessary for effective MPO-mediated microbicidal combustion and chemiluminescence [36].

Human neutrophils contain a relatively high concentration of MPO (about 5% of the dry weight of the neutrophil) in their azurophilic granules [40]. Following departure of the neutrophil leukocyte from the hematopoietic marrow and a relatively short transit time in the circulating blood, the neutrophil leaves the circulating and enters the tissue pool [1]. Neutrophils characteristically migrate to sites of injury and infection and accumulate in high concentrations. However, even in the absence of inflammation and infection, healthy humans have significant concentrations of neutrophils present in tissue fluids. The oral and vaginal cavities have neutrophil concentrations in proportion to blood neutrophil concentrations [41, 42].

When neutrophils transit from the blood to tissue and body spaces, they carry MPO into these spaces. Each neutrophil carries about four femtograms of MPO. As such, neutrophils deliver relatively large quantities of MPO into body spaces on a routine basis. The oral and vaginal cavities have acidic pH. The normal florae of these spaces are cytochrome-negative LAB that generate lactic acid and H_2O_2 as metabolic products. The transit of neutrophils into such spaces delivers MPO into milieux that are rich in LAB.

MPO selectively binds to Gram-negative and many Gram-positive bacteria. However, LAB show relatively poor MPO binding [43]. When small concentrations of neutrophil-free MPO are added to bacterial suspensions containing viridans streptococci with other competing bacteria, a potent synergistic microbicidal action is directed against MPO-binding Gram-positive, for example, *Staphylococcus aureus*, and Gram-negative, for example, *Pseudomonas aeruginosa* and *Escherichia coli*, microbes [44]. Damage to the LAB is only observed at significantly higher MPO concentrations. This LAB-MPO synergistic action may explain the dominance of streptococci and lactobacilli in healthy oral and vaginal cavities [45].

Selective binding of MPO to a microbe guarantees that $^1O_2{}^*$ is generated in close proximity to the target microbe, resulting in selective, focused combustive microbicidal action. The $^1O_2{}^*$ lifetime of a few microseconds limits damage to within about a $0.2\ \mu m$ radius of its point of generation [27, 28]. Thus, combustion is focused on potential pathogens with minimal collateral damage to the host cells and the normal LAB flora [44].

8. Conclusions and Perspectives

There are no restrictions on biologic evolution other than those imposed by physical reality. The spin conservation rules describe fundamental symmetry restrictions that define reactive possibilities. These rules forbid the direct reaction of triplet oxygen with singlet organic molecules, and, as such, combustion is not spontaneous. Chemical reactions involve frontier orbitals. Changing the multiplicity of oxygen changes its frontier orbitals, eliminating the symmetry barrier to its electrophilic reactive potential.

Neutrophils kill microbes by a unique, focused combustive action. The redox reactions of neutrophil respiratory burst metabolism change triplet ground state (diradical) O_2 to singlet electronically excited (nonradical) $^1O_2{}^*$. In addition, other singlet multiplicity (nonradical) microbicidal reactants, for example, H_2O_2 and HOCl, are generated. These agents are uniformly singlet multiplicity (nonradical) reactants with bosonic frontier orbitals. Their reactions with microbes are consistent with the spin conservation rules. $^1O_2{}^*$ has one empty (LUMO) π^* orbital and one full (HOMO) π^* orbital with bosonic character. This highly electrophilic LUMO can participate in spin-allowed bosonic LUMO-HOMO reactions with biological molecules. The dioxygenated products of such combustions yield the electronically excited carbonyl functions that relax by photon emission, that is, luminescence or chemiluminescence.

Considering frontier orbital reactivity in the bosonic-fermionic terms of particle physics broadens the perspective for explaining oxygen chemistry in particular and for appreciating reaction chemistry in general. Biological reactions typically involve constructive frontier HOMO-LUMO overlap. Radical reactions involving singly occupied atomic or molecular orbitals (SO(A)MO) are uncommon in biology under normal conditions, that is, in the absence of high energy radiation or heat producing homolytic bond cleavage. Biological reactions involving one electron transfer are typically restricted to flavoenzymes and to highly ordered cytochrome electron transport systems such as those found in mitochondria. Cytoplasmic redox reactions typically involve two equivalent transfers and are nonradical. Orbital pairing of antisymmetric fermionic electrons imposes a bosonic (nonradical) character.

Chemical reactions can be generalized as constructive bosonic transfers (i.e., HOMO-LUMO) or constructive fermionic annihilations. Both reactions produce bosonic products. Radical-radical (i.e., SO(A)MO-SO(A)MO) orbital overlap is typically constructive; that is, fermionic radicals react with fermionic radicals. Overlap of a bosonic HOMO with a fermionic SO(A)MO is not constructive. As illustrated in Figure 1, the first steps of the hexose monophosphate metabolic pathway involve dehydrogenation of glucose-6-phosphate and reduction of $NADP^+$ yielding NADPH; these redox reactions involve balanced two equivalent bosonic transfers. Bosonic orbital pair transfers are the norm in biochemistry. The bosonic nature of the antisymmetric orbital electron-couple may be essential for such biologic redox transfer. Any fermionic electron transfer would open the possibility for reaction with bifermionic oxygen.

There are advantages to transferring electrons as a bosonic orbital-couple. As stated by Dirac, "If a state has zero total angular momentum, the dynamical system is equally likely to have any orientation, and hence spherical symmetry occurs" [19]. A bosonic orbital electron-couple has $S = 0$. This has significance with regard to the Heisenberg uncertainty principle which states that the uncertainty of momentum (Δp) multiplied by the uncertainty of position (Δx) is always equal to or greater than $(1/2)\hbar$; that is, $\Delta p \Delta x \geq (1/2)\hbar$ [46]. The spin momentum of the bosonic orbital electron-couple is known, that is, zero. Consequently, the positional uncertainty of the electron-couple must be proportionally large. Thus, the intermolecular redox transfer of a bosonic orbital electron-couple may proceed by a quantum tunneling mechanism analogous to the emission of a bosonic alpha particle from an atomic nucleus in alpha radiation decay [20]. Such a quantum tunneling mechanism explains the facility for electron-couple transfer in biologic redox reactions.

Conflict of Interests

The author declares no conflict of interests regarding the publication of this paper.

References

[1] D. F. Bainton, "Developmental biology of neutrophils and eosinophils," in *Inflammation: Basic Principles and Clinical Correlates*, J. I. Gallin and R. S. Snyderman, Eds., pp. 13–34, Lippincott Williams & Wilkins, Philadelphia, Pa, USA, 3rd edition, 1999.

[2] D. C. Dale, L. Boxer, and W. C. Liles, "The phagocytes: neutrophils and monocytes," *Blood*, vol. 112, no. 4, pp. 935–945, 2008.

[3] R. C. Allen, P. R. Stevens, T. H. Price, G. S. Chatta, and D. C. Dale, "In vivo effects of recombinant human granulocyte colony-stimulating factor on neutrophil oxidative functions in

normal human volunteers," *Journal of Infectious Diseases*, vol. 175, no. 5, pp. 1184–1192, 1997.

[4] S. J. Klebanoff and R. A. Clark, *The Neutrophil: Function and Clinical Disorders*, North-Holland, New York, NY, USA, 1978.

[5] A. J. Sbarra and M. L. Karnovsky, "The biochemical basis of phagocytosis. I. Metabolic changes during the ingestion of particles by polymorphonuclear leukocytes," *The Journal of Biological Chemistry*, vol. 234, no. 6, pp. 1355–1362, 1959.

[6] C. C. Winterbourn and A. J. Kettle, "Redox reactions and microbial killing in the neutrophil phagosome," *Antioxidants and Redox Signaling*, vol. 18, no. 6, pp. 642–660, 2013.

[7] R. C. Allen, R. L. Stjernholm, and R. H. Steele, "Evidence for the generation of an electronic excitation state(s) in human polymorphonuclear leukocytes and its participation in bactericidal activity," *Biochemical and Biophysical Research Communications*, vol. 47, no. 4, pp. 679–684, 1972.

[8] F. Rossi, D. Romeo, and P. Patriarca, "Mechanism of phagocytosis associated oxidative metabolism in polymorphonuclear leukocytes and macrophages," *Journal of the Reticuloendothelial Society*, vol. 12, no. 2, pp. 127–149, 1972.

[9] R. C. Allen, S. J. Yevich, R. W. Orth, and R. H. Steele, "The superoxide anion and singlet molecular oxygen: their role in the microbicidal activity of the polymorphonuclear leukocyte," *Biochemical and Biophysical Research Communications*, vol. 60, no. 3, pp. 909–917, 1974.

[10] R. C. Allen, "Reduced, radical, and excited state oxygen in leukocyte microbicidal activity," *Frontiers of Biology*, vol. 48, article 197, 1979.

[11] D. Behar, G. Czapski, J. Rabani, L. M. Dorfman, and H. A. Schwarz, "The acid dissociation constant and decay kinetics of the perhydroxyl radical," *Journal of Physical Chemistry*, vol. 74, no. 17, pp. 3209–3213, 1970.

[12] A. U. Khan, "Singlet molecular oxygen from superoxide anion and sensitized fluorescence of organic molecules," *Science*, vol. 168, no. 3930, pp. 476–477, 1970.

[13] R. C. Allen, "Halide dependence of the myeloperoxidase-mediated antimicrobial system of the polymorphonuclear leukocyte in the phenomenon of electronic excitation," *Biochemical and Biophysical Research Communications*, vol. 63, no. 3, pp. 675–683, 1975.

[14] M. Kasha and A. Khan, "The physics, chemistry, and biology of singlet molecular oxygen," *Annals of the New York Academy of Sciences*, vol. 171, pp. 1–33, 1970.

[15] L. Pauling, *The Nature of the Chemical Bond*, Cornell University Press, New York, NY, USA, 1960.

[16] R. C. Allen, "Role of oxygen in phagocyte microbicidal action," *Environmental Health Perspectives*, vol. 102, no. 10, pp. 201–208, 1994.

[17] J. R. Waldram, *The Theory of Thermodynamics*, Cambridge University Press, Cambridge, UK, 1985.

[18] A. Sudbery, *Quantum Mechanics and the Particles of Nature*, Cambridge University Press, Cambridge, Cambridge, UK, 1986.

[19] P. A. M. Dirac, *The Principles of Quantum Mechanics*, Oxford, Oxford, UK, 4th edition, 1958.

[20] R. C. Allen, "Molecular oxygen (O_2): reactivity and luminescence," in *Bioluminescence and Chemiluminescence. Progress & Current Applications*, P. E. Stanley and L. J. Kricka, Eds., pp. 223–232, World Scientific, Cambridge, UK, 2002.

[21] K. Fukui, T. Yonezawa, and H. Shingu, "A molecular orbital theory of reactivity in aromatic hydrocarbons," *The Journal of Chemical Physics*, vol. 20, no. 4, pp. 722–725, 1952.

[22] I. Fleming, *Frontier Orbitals and Organic Chemical Reactions*, John Wiley & Sons, Chichester, UK, 1978.

[23] M. Orchin and H. H. Jaffe, *The Importance of Antibonding Orbitals*, Houghton Mifflin, 1967.

[24] G. Herzberg, *Molecular Spectra and Molecular Structure. Spectra of Diatomic Molecules*, Van Nostrand Reinhold, New York, NY, USA, 1950.

[25] M. Hargittai and I. Hargittai, *Symmetry through the Eyes of a Chemist*, Springer, New York, NY, USA, 2010.

[26] J. Katriel and R. Pauncz, "Theoretical interpretation of Hund's rule," *Advances in Quantum Chemistry*, vol. 10, pp. 143–185, 1977.

[27] E. Skovsen, J. W. Snyder, J. D. C. Lambert, and P. R. Ogilby, "Lifetime and diffusion of singlet oxygen in a cell," *The Journal of Physical Chemistry B*, vol. 109, no. 18, pp. 8570–8573, 2005.

[28] R. W. Redmond and I. E. Kochevar, "Spatially resolved cellular responses to singlet oxygen," *Photochemistry and Photobiology*, vol. 82, no. 5, pp. 1178–1186, 2006.

[29] N. J. Turro, V. Ramamurthy, and J. C. Scaiano, *Principles of Molecular Photochemistry*, University Science Books, Sausalito, Calif, USA, 2009.

[30] R. C. Allen, "Biochemiexcitation: chemiluminescence and the study of biological oxygenation," in *Chemical and Biological Generation of Excited States*, pp. 310–344, Academic Press, New York, NY, USA, 1982.

[31] R. C. Allen, "Phagocytic leukocyte oxygenation activities and chemiluminescence: a kinetic approach to analysis," *Methods in Enzymology*, vol. 133, pp. 449–493, 1986.

[32] D. L. Stevens, A. E. Bryant, J. Huffman, K. Thompson, and R. C. Allen, "Analysis of circulating phagocyte activity measured by whole blood luminescence: correlations with clinical status," *Journal of Infectious Diseases*, vol. 170, no. 6, pp. 1463–1472, 1994.

[33] R. C. Allen and D. L. Stevens, "The circulating phagocyte reflects the in vivo state of immune defense," *Current Opinion in Infectious Diseases*, vol. 5, no. 3, pp. 389–398, 1992.

[34] R. C. Allen, D. C. Dale, and F. B. Taylor Jr., "Blood phagocyte luminescence: gauging systemic immune activation," *Methods in Enzymology*, vol. 305, pp. 591–629, 2000.

[35] F. Taylor Jr., P. A. Haddad, G. Kinasewitz, A. Chang, G. Peer, and R. C. Allen, "Luminescence studies of the phagocyte response to endotoxin infusion into normal human subjects: multiple discriminant analysis of luminescence response and correlation with phagocyte morphologic changes and release of elastase," *Journal of Endotoxin Research*, vol. 6, no. 1, pp. 3–15, 2000.

[36] R. C. Allen, E. L. Mills, T. R. McNitt, and P. G. Quie, "Role of myeloperoxidase and bacterial metabolism in chemiluminescence of granulocytes from patients with chronic granulomatous disease," *Journal of Infectious Diseases*, vol. 144, no. 4, pp. 344–348, 1981.

[37] E. L. Kaplan, T. Laxdal, and P. G. Quie, "Studies of polymorphonuclear leukocytes from patients with chronic granulomatous disease of childhood: bactericidal capacity for streptococci," *Pediatrics*, vol. 41, no. 3, pp. 591–599, 1968.

[38] W. H. Holzapfel, P. Haberer, R. Geisen, J. Björkroth, and U. Schillinger, "Taxonomy and important features of probiotic microorganisms in food and nutrition," *The American Journal of Clinical Nutrition*, vol. 73, no. 2, pp. 365S–373S, 2001.

[39] J. W. McLeod and J. Gordon, "Production of hydrogen peroxide by bacteria," *Biochemical Journal*, vol. 16, pp. 499–504, 1922.

[40] J. Schultz and K. Kaminker, "Myeloperoxidase of the leucocyte of normal human blood. I. Content and localization," *Archives of Biochemistry and Biophysics*, vol. 96, no. 3, pp. 465–467, 1962.

[41] D. G. Wright, A. I. Meierovics, and J. M. Foxley, "Assessing the delivery of neutrophils to tissues in neutropenia," *Blood*, vol. 67, no. 4, pp. 1023–1030, 1986.

[42] S. Cauci, S. Guaschino, D. De Aloysio et al., "Interrelationships of interleukin-8 with interleukin-1β and neutrophils in vaginal fluid of healthy and bacterial vaginosis positive women," *Molecular Human Reproduction*, vol. 9, no. 1, pp. 53–58, 2003.

[43] R. C. Allen and J. T. Stephens Jr., "Reduced-oxidized difference spectral analysis and chemiluminescence-based Scatchard analysis demonstrate selective binding of myeloperoxidase to microbes," *Luminescence*, vol. 26, no. 3, pp. 208–213, 2011.

[44] R. C. Allen and J. T. Stephens Jr., "Myeloperoxidase selectively binds and selectively kills microbes," *Infection and Immunity*, vol. 79, no. 1, pp. 474–485, 2011.

[45] R. C. Allen and J. T. Stephens Jr., "Role of lactic acid bacteria-myeloperoxidase synergy in establishing and maintaining the normal flora in man," *Food and Nutrition Sciences*, vol. 4, no. 11, pp. 67–72, 2013.

[46] P. S. C. Matthews, *Quantum Chemistry of Atoms and Molecules*, Cambridge University Press, Cambridge, UK, 1986.

19

Differential Use of Human Neutrophil Fcγ Receptors for Inducing Neutrophil Extracellular Trap Formation

Omar Rafael Alemán,[1] Nancy Mora,[1] Ricarda Cortes-Vieyra,[1]
Eileen Uribe-Querol,[2] and Carlos Rosales[1]

[1]*Departamento de Inmunología, Instituto de Investigaciones Biomédicas, Universidad Nacional Autónoma de México,*
  04510 México, DF, Mexico
[2]*División de Estudios de Posgrado e Investigación, Facultad de Odontología, Universidad Nacional Autónoma de México,*
  04510 México, DF, Mexico

Correspondence should be addressed to Carlos Rosales; carosal@biomedicas.unam.mx

Academic Editor: Kurt Blaser

Neutrophils (PMN) are the most abundant leukocytes in the blood. PMN migrate from the circulation to sites of infection, where they are responsible for antimicrobial functions. PMN use phagocytosis, degranulation, and formation of neutrophil extracellular traps (NETs) to kill microbes. NETs are fibers composed of chromatin and neutrophil-granule proteins. Several pathogens, including bacteria, fungi, and parasites, and also some pharmacological stimuli such as phorbol 12-myristate 13-acetate (PMA) are efficient inducers of NETs. Antigen-antibody complexes are also capable of inducing NET formation. However the particular Fcγ receptor involved in triggering this function is a matter of controversy. In order to provide some insight into what Fcγ receptor is responsible for NET formation, each of the two human Fcγ receptors was stimulated individually by specific monoclonal antibodies and NET formation was evaluated. FcγRIIa cross-linking did not promote NET formation. Cross-linking other receptors such as integrins also did not promote NET formation. In contrast FcγRIIIb cross-linking induced NET formation similarly to PMA stimulation. NET formation was dependent on NADPH-oxidase, PKC, and ERK activation. These data show that cross-linking FcγRIIIb is responsible for NET formation by the human neutrophil.

1. Introduction

Neutrophils (PMN) are the most abundant leukocytes in the blood. PMN are innate immune cells that migrate from the circulation to sites of infection, where they are responsible for antimicrobial functions [1]. PMN use phagocytosis, degranulation, and formation of neutrophil extracellular traps (NETs) to kill microbes [2, 3]. NETs are formed through a unique cell death program named "NETosis" that involves activation in most cases of nicotinamide adenine dinucleotide phosphate- (NADPH-) oxidase, which produces reactive oxygen species (ROS) [4–6]. During NETosis, the characteristic lobular nucleus of neutrophils disappears, and the chromatin expands in the cytosol, while the cell membrane remains intact. Three or four hours after stimulation, the cell membrane breaks and the chromatin fibers get released forming a netlike structure outside the cell. NET fibers are composed of chromatin covered with histones [7] and antimicrobial proteins derived from the neutrophil granules, such as the bactericidal/permeability-increasing protein (BPI), elastase, myeloperoxidase, lactoferrin, and metalloprotease 9 [2, 4]. The requirements for NADPH-oxidase and myeloperoxidase in NET formation differ depending on the stimulus [8, 9]. Besides their antimicrobial capacity, NETs seem to act as a physical barrier where microorganisms get trapped and consequently prevent further spread of pathogens. Thus, NETs bind, block, and kill microorganisms extracellularly and independently of phagocytosis [10].

Binding of receptors for the Fc portion of antibodies (Fc receptors) to opsonized microorganisms is one of the most important mechanisms for pathogen recognition and activation of neutrophils [11]. Human neutrophils express constitutively two antibody receptors that are members of the Fc receptor family for IgG molecules, namely, FcγRIIa (CD32a) and FcγRIIIb (CD16b) [12]. These receptors are exclusive human receptors. FcγRIIa is composed of a single polypeptide chain bearing an ITAM on its cytoplasmic domain [11]. This ITAM confers on FcγRIIa the ability to initiate signaling events that regulate cell responses, including phagocytosis, cytokine production, antibody-dependent cell-mediated cytotoxicity, and the respiratory burst [13]. FcγRIIIb is present exclusively on neutrophils and it is a glycophosphatidylinositol- (GPI-) linked receptor, lacking transmembrane and cytoplasmic domains [14]. Although signaling molecules associated with FcγRIIIb are still unknown and its signaling mechanism remains unidentified, several reports show that FcγRIIIb can initiate signaling events leading to calcium transients [15], actin polymerization [16], activation of integrins [17], and NF-κB activation [18].

Several pathogens, including virus, bacteria, fungi, and parasites, have all been reported to be inducers of NET formation [10]. In addition, proinflammatory stimuli such as lipopolysaccharide (LPS) [19], interleukin- (IL-) 8, and tumor necrosis factor (TNF) [20, 21] and also some pharmacological stimuli such as phorbol 12-myristate 13-acetate (PMA), an activator of protein kinase C (PKC), are efficient inducers of NETs [2]. Some reports indicate that NET formation was increased when microorganisms were opsonized with autologous serum [3]. This suggested a possible role for FcγR in NET formation.

Recent reports indicated that antigen-antibody complexes seem capable of inducing NET formation [22, 23]. In one report, a B cell-deficient mouse was used to show NETs could not be formed, thus suggesting a direct role for Fc receptors in this function [23]. In this study, however no particular receptor was identified. In another report, soluble immune complexes were used to activate neutrophils and induce NET formation. It was determined that FcγRIIIb promoted endocytosis of soluble immune complexes and that FcγRIIa promoted NET formation in vivo [22]. However, more recently, it was reported that FcγRIIIb is the receptor responsible for NET formation in response to immobilized immune complexes [24]. Thus, in order to provide some insight into this controversy, each of the two human Fcγ receptors was stimulated individually by specific monoclonal antibodies and NET formation was evaluated.

FcγRIIa cross-linking did not promote NET formation. Cross-linking other receptors such as integrins also did not promote NET formation. In contrast FcγRIIIb cross-linking induced efficient NET formation similarly to PMA stimulation. NET formation was dependent on NADPH-oxidase, PKC, and extracellular signal-regulated kinase (ERK) activation. These data support the idea that different Fc receptors promote independent cell functions.

2. Materials and Methods

2.1. Neutrophils. Neutrophils (PMN) were purified from blood collected from adult healthy volunteers exactly as previously described [25]. All volunteers provided a written informed consent for their participation in this study. The informed consent form and all experimental procedures were approved by the Bioethics Committee at Instituto de Investigaciones Biomédicas, UNAM.

2.2. Reagents. Bovine serum albumin (BSA) was from F. Hoffmann-La Roche Ltd. (Mannheim, Germany). Piceatannol, a spleen tyrosine kinase (Syk) inhibitor, was from Acros Organics (New Jersey, USA). Wortmannin, a phosphatidylinositol 3-kinase (PI-3K) inhibitor; GÖ6976, a protein kinase C (PKC) inhibitor; GÖ6983, another PKC inhibitor; 3-(1-methyl-1H-indol-3-yl-methylene)-2-oxo-2,3-dihydro-1H-indole-5-sulfonamide (iSyk), another Syk inhibitor (catalog number 574711); and the antibleaching mounting medium FluorSave (catalog number 345789) were from Calbiochem/EMD Millipore (Billerica, MA). UO126, a MEK (ERK kinase) inhibitor, was from Promega (Madison, WI, USA). Diphenyleneiodonium (DPI), an NADPH-oxidase inhibitor; (E)-3-[4-methylphenylsulfonyl]-2-propenenitrile (BAY 117082), an NF-κB inhibitor; phorbol 12-myristate 13-acetate (PMA); and all other chemicals were from Sigma Aldrich (St. Louis, MO). The following antibodies were used: anti-human FcγRIIa (CD32) mAb IV.3 [26] (ATCC HB-217) was from American Type Culture Collection (Manassas, VA). Anti-β1 integrin mAb TS2/16 was donated by Martin Hemler (Dana Farber Cancer Research Institute, Boston, MA). Anti-β2 integrin (CD18) mAb IB4 and anti-human FcγRIIIb (CD16) mAb 3G8 [27] were donated by Dr. Eric J. Brown (University of California in San Francisco, San Francisco, CA). Mouse monoclonal anti-neutrophil elastase (D-7; catalog number sc-365950), rabbit polyclonal anti-histone H2B (FL-126; catalog number sc-10808), rabbit polyclonal anti-ERK 1 (catalog number sc-94), and mouse monoclonal anti-phospho-ERK 1 (pTyr204) (catalog number sc-7383) were from Santa Cruz Biotechnology (Santa Cruz, CA). Alexa Fluor 555-conjugated donkey anti-rabbit IgG (catalog number A-31572), Alexa Fluor 488-conjugated donkey anti-mouse IgG (catalog number A-21202), and FITC-conjugated F(ab′)₂ goat anti-mouse IgG (catalog number A-10683) were from Invitrogen Molecular Probes (Eugene, OR). F(ab′)₂ goat anti-mouse IgG (catalog number 0855468), HRP-conjugated F(ab′)₂ goat anti-mouse IgG (catalog number 0855572), and HRP-conjugated F(ab′)₂ goat anti-rabbit IgG (catalog number 0855686) were from MP Biomedicals (Santa Ana, CA).

2.3. Preparation of Specific Monoclonal Antibodies. Hybridoma cells were grown in DMEM (Gibco; Grand Island, NY) containing 10% fetal bovine serum (FBS) also from Gibco (Grand Island, NY). Antibodies were purified from saturated (8-day-old) tissue culture supernatants with Protein-G Sepharose 4 Fast Flow from GE Healthcare Bio-Sciences AB (Uppsala, Sweden). After elution from the Sepharose with 0.1 M glycine-HCl, pH 2.7, antibodies were dialyzed against PBS, adjusted to 1 mg/mL, and filter-sterilized. Finally, antibodies were stored in small aliquots at −80°C. The functionality of antibodies was confirmed by their binding to neutrophil receptors (Supplemental Figure 1S in Supplementary Material available online at http://dx.doi.org/10.1155/2016/2908034).

2.4. Labeling of Neutrophil Receptors with Specific Monoclonal Antibodies. For receptor stimulation, PMN were treated with specific anti-receptor monoclonal antibodies as follows. PMN (1×10^6) in 500 μL PBS were placed into a 1.5 mL Eppendorf tube, and 10 μg/mL of the corresponding anti-receptor monoclonal antibody was added. Cells were incubated at 4°C for 20 minutes and then washed twice with 1 mL of cold PBS (4°C) centrifuged at 1,743 ×g, 1 minute each time. This centrifugation protocol did not preactivate cells as long as they were maintained cold. Next, PMN were resuspended in 500 μL cold (4°C) RPMI-1640 medium (Gibco; Grand Island, NY) containing 5% fetal bovine serum (FBS) also from Gibco (Grand Island, NY).

2.5. NET Formation Assay. Neutrophils were left untreated for PMA stimulation or previously treated with anti-receptor antibodies (as described above) for receptor stimulation. Neutrophils (1×10^6) in 500 μL RPMI-1640 medium were added to each well of a 24-well plate, containing a 12 mm coverslip, and then incubated in a humidified incubator with 5% CO_2 at 37°C for 30 minutes. Then 100 μL of 120 nM PMA in PBS or 100 μL of 450 μg/mL F(ab')$_2$ goat anti-mouse IgG (for receptor stimulation) was added to each well. Plates were incubated in 5% CO_2 at 37°C for 4 hours. Next, 600 μL of 2% paraformaldehyde in PBS was added to each well, and the plates were incubated overnight in 5% CO_2 at 37°C.

In selected experiments, PMN were incubated for 30 minutes before stimulation, with the inhibitors piceatannol (50 μM), wortmannin (50 nM), UO126 (50 μM), GÖ6983 (1 μM), GÖ6976 (1 μM), DPI (10 μM), BAY 117082 (2.5 μM), or the vehicle dimethyl sulfoxide (DMSO) alone.

2.6. NET Visualization and Immunofluorescence. All washes and incubations were done at room temperature by placing the coverslip upside down over a 250 μL drop of each solution formed on a well of Parafilm placed on a tube rack, exactly as previously described [28]. Coverslips were taken out of the 24-well plate one at a time and washed four times with water for 5 minutes each. Next, they were placed over 0.1% Triton X-100 in 4% paraformaldehyde for 10 minutes, then on PBS for 5 minutes, and then on 10 μg/mL of the corresponding primary antibody (anti-neutrophil elastase or anti-histone) in 5% BSA in PBS for 60 minutes. Coverslips were then washed four times with PBS for 5 minutes each and placed on 8 μg/mL of the corresponding secondary antibody (Alexa Fluor-conjugated anti-rabbit IgG or anti-mouse IgG) in 5% BSA in PBS containing 300 nM DAPI. Coverslips were incubated in the dark for 60 minutes. Finally, coverslips were mounted on a microscope slide with one drop of FluorSave. Slides were observed with a fluorescence inverted microscope model IX-70 from Olympus (Center Valley, PA). Images were captured with an Evolution-VF Cooled Color camera from Media Cybernetics (Rockville, MD) and the computer program QCapture Pro 6.0 from QImaging, Surrey (British Columbia, Canada). Images were processed with the computer program ImageJ 1.47v from the National Institutes of Health (Bethesda, MD).

2.7. NET Formation with Opsonized Particles. Opsonization of 4.8 μm fluorescent (catalog number 16592) or nonfluorescent (catalog number 17135) latex particles from Polysciences, Inc. (Warrington, PA), was performed exactly as described [29]. These particles were used in phagocytosis assays as described [30] or in NET formation assays as follows. PMN (1×10^6 cells) in 500 μL were centrifuged in a 1.5 mL Eppendorf tube at 1,743 ×g for 1 min. After removing the supernatant, the cell pellet was disaggregated by tapping the tube against a rack, and 80 μL of opsonized latex particles (1.25×10^8 particles/mL) resuspended in RPMI-1640 medium with 5% FBS was added. The PMN-particle mixture was incubated at 4°C for 20 min. Then, 1 mL of cold PBS was added, the tube was centrifuged at 1,743 ×g for 1 min, and the cell pellet was resuspended in 500 μL RPMI-1640 medium with 5% FBS. Cell suspension was transferred into a well of a 24-well plate, containing a 12 mm coverslip, and then incubated in a humidified incubator with 5% CO_2 at 37°C for 4 h. Then 500 μL of 2% paraformaldehyde in PBS was added to each well, and the plate was kept in the incubator overnight. Finally, the coverslip was used for NET visualization as described above.

2.8. Quantification of NETs. A 96-well plate was previously covered with 25 μg/mL poly-D-lysine for three hours at room temperature. Each well was then washed three times with 50 μL PBS for 5 minutes each time, and the plate was allowed to air dry inside a flow laminar hood for two hours. Neutrophils were resuspended at 1.25×10^6 cells/mL in RPMI-1640 medium, containing 500 nM SYTOX Green (Molecular Probes, Inc.; Eugene, OR), and 80 μL of this cell suspension (1×10^5 PMN) was added to each well of the 96-well plate. Next, the plate was incubated at 37°C in a 5% CO_2 incubator for 20 minutes. For FcγR stimulation, the supernatant was removed gently with a micropippetor and 50 μL of 10 μg/mL of the corresponding anti-Fc receptor antibody was added to each well. The plate was placed in a 35°C prewarmed microplate reader model Synergy HT from BioTek Instruments (Winooski, VT) and incubated there for 20 minutes. Next, the supernatant was removed gently with a micropippetor and 100 μL of 75 μg/mL of F(ab')$_2$ goat anti-mouse IgG containing 500 nM SYTOX Green was added to each corresponding well. At this time, for PMA stimulation 20 μL of 100 nM PMA was added to each corresponding well. The plate was then incubated for up to 4 hours. For this assay, cells were not fixed. Finally the fluorescence from the bottom of the plate was read, using the 485 nm excitation and 528 emission filters.

For NET formation induced with opsonized latex particles, PMN (1×10^6 cells) in 500 μL RPMI-1640 medium with 5% FBS and 500 nM SYTOX Green were mixed with 80 μL of opsonized latex particles (1.25×10^8 particles/mL). Then 100 μL of the PMN-particle mixture was transferred into a well of a 96-well plate and incubated in a 35°C prewarmed microplate reader for 4 hours. Fluorescence from the bottom of the plate was read using the 485 nm excitation and 528 emission filters.

2.9. Western Blotting. Western blots were performed exactly as previously described [31]. Cells were lysed in RIPA buffer (150 mM NaCl, 5 mM EDTA, 50 mM HEPES, 0.5% sodium deoxycholate, 1% Nonidet P-40, and 10 mM 2-mercaptoethanol, pH 7.5) containing cOmplete protease inhibitor cocktail from Roche (Basel, Switzerland), for 15 minutes at 4°C. Cell lysates were then cleared by centrifugation and proteins resolved on SDS 12% PAGE. Proteins were then electrotransferred onto polyvinylidene fluoride (PVDF) membranes (Immobilon-P; Millipore, Bedford, MA). Membranes were incubated in blocking buffer (1% BSA and 5% nonfat dry milk (Carnation; Nestle, Glendale, CA) and 0.1% Tween 20 in PBS) overnight at 4°C. Membranes were subsequently probed with the corresponding antibody in blocking buffer, for 1 hour at room temperature, anti-ERK 1 (1/1000 dilution) or anti-phospho-ERK 1 (1/500 dilution). Membranes were washed with PBS six times and incubated with a 1/3000 dilution of HRP-conjugated $F(ab')_2$ goat anti-rabbit IgG or HRP-conjugated $F(ab')_2$ goat anti-mouse IgG for 1 hour at room temperature. After washing six more times, the membrane was developed with a chemiluminescence substrate (SuperSignal; Pierce, Rockford, IL) according to the manufacturer's instructions.

2.10. Determination of Apoptosis. Apoptosis was assayed with the FITC annexin V and propidium iodide (PI) dead cell apoptosis kit for flow cytometry (catalog number V13242) from Molecular Probes, Inc. (Eugene, OR), following the manufacturer's instructions. Briefly, PMN were treated with nothing, PMA, or the antibodies against each of the Fcγ receptors as described above. After a two-hour incubation at 37°C, PMN (1×10^5) were washed in PBS and resuspended in annexin-binding buffer (10 mM HEPES, 140 mM NaCl, and 2.5 mM Ca^{2+}, pH 7.4), and 2 μL of FITC annexin V and 1 μL of 1.5 mM PI were added. Cells were incubated for 15 min at room temperature and then 400 μL of annexin-binding buffer was added. Cells were immediately analyzed by flow cytometry. PMN apoptosis (positive control) was induced by UV-light irradiation as previously described [32].

2.11. Reactive Oxygen Species (ROS). ROS production was assessed with the DCFDA-Cellular Reactive Oxygen Species Detection Assay Kit (catalog number ab113851) from Abcam, Inc. (Cambridge, MA), following the manufacturer's instructions. Briefly, PMN were treated with mAb IV.3 or mAb 3G8 at 10 μg/mL for 20 minutes on ice. PMN were washed with 1x buffer and then incubated with 15 μM DCFDA in 1x buffer for 30 minutes at 37°C. After one wash in 1x buffer, 5 × 10^4 PMN were placed in each well of a 96-well clear-bottom black plate from Corning Inc. (New York, NY) and incubated for 20 minutes at 35°C in a plate reader, model Synergy HT from BioTek Instruments (Winooski, VT). Then, for antibody treatment 50 μL of goat anti-mouse IgG (150 μg/mL) was added and for PMA treatment, 50 μL of PMA (40 nM) was added. Fluorescence was read for two hours at excitation 485 nm and emission 535 nm.

2.12. Phagocytosis Assays. Neutrophil phagocytosis was determined as previously described [29]. Briefly, PMN

(1×10^5 cells) were resuspended in 100 μL cold phagocytosis buffer (2 mM calcium chloride, 1.5 mM magnesium chloride, and 1% human serum albumin in PBS) and mixed with 3.5 μL of a suspension (1×10^8 beads/mL) of IV.3-opsonized, or 3G8-opsonized or control-opsonized (no antibody) fluorescent latex beads. PMN and beads were incubated at 37°C for 30 min, centrifuged at 6000 rpm for 1 min, and resuspended in 100 μL of ice-cold trypsin-EDTA solution (0.05% trypsin, 1 mM EDTA in PBS) to detach uninternalized beads from the cells. After a 15 min incubation on ice, PMN were washed with 1 mL cold PBS plus 0.5% BSA plus 2 mM EDTA and resuspended in 500 μL cold 1% paraformaldehyde in PBS. To analyze phagocytosis by flow cytometry, latex particles were gated out during sample acquisition and 10,000 cells were acquired per sample. Phagocytosis was reported as percent of fluorescence-positive cells (cells internalizing at least one fluorescent particle). Phagocytosis was also analyzed by microscopy and reported as phagocytic index, the number of beads internalized by 100 cells.

2.13. Statistical Analysis. Quantitative data were expressed as mean ± standard error of mean (SEM). Single variable data were compared by unpaired-sample Student's t-tests using the computer program KaleidaGraph version 3.6.2 for Mac (Synergy Software; Reading, PA). Also, variance homogeneity was checked by using Levene's test, and multiple pair-comparisons were performed using Tukey's test after ordinary one-way analysis of variance (ANOVA) [33]. Post hoc differences were considered statistically different at a value $p < 0.05$. Analyses were done using the SAS software version 9.0 (2012) from SAS Institute Inc. (Cary, NC).

3. Results

Several types of pathogens have been reported to induce NET formation, but there are not reports on particular receptors used by neutrophils to recognize these pathogens and to induce NETosis. Most studies on NETs have used PMA, a potent activator of PKC, and efficient inducer of NETs [2]. In this case, no receptor is involved since PMA directly activates intracellular signaling. Some reports indicated that NET formation was increased when microorganisms were opsonized with autologous serum and also that antigen-antibody complexes seemed to be capable of inducing NET formation. These studies suggested a possible role for IgG Fc receptors (FcγR) in NET formation. However the particular Fcγ receptor involved in triggering this function is a matter of controversy. Thus, in order to explore what particular Fc receptor could induce NET formation, PMN were stimulated by cross-linking individual receptors with specific monoclonal antibodies.

When PMN were stained with DAPI, the typical lobular nuclei were clearly seen (Figure 1(a)). Immunolabeling of histones also showed the localization of these proteins within the PMN nucleus (Figure 1(b)). When PMN were treated with PMA, nuclei lost their typical morphology and long NETs were formed (Figure 1(d)). Also, the cell morphology was altered; PMN appeared larger and diffuse (Supplemental

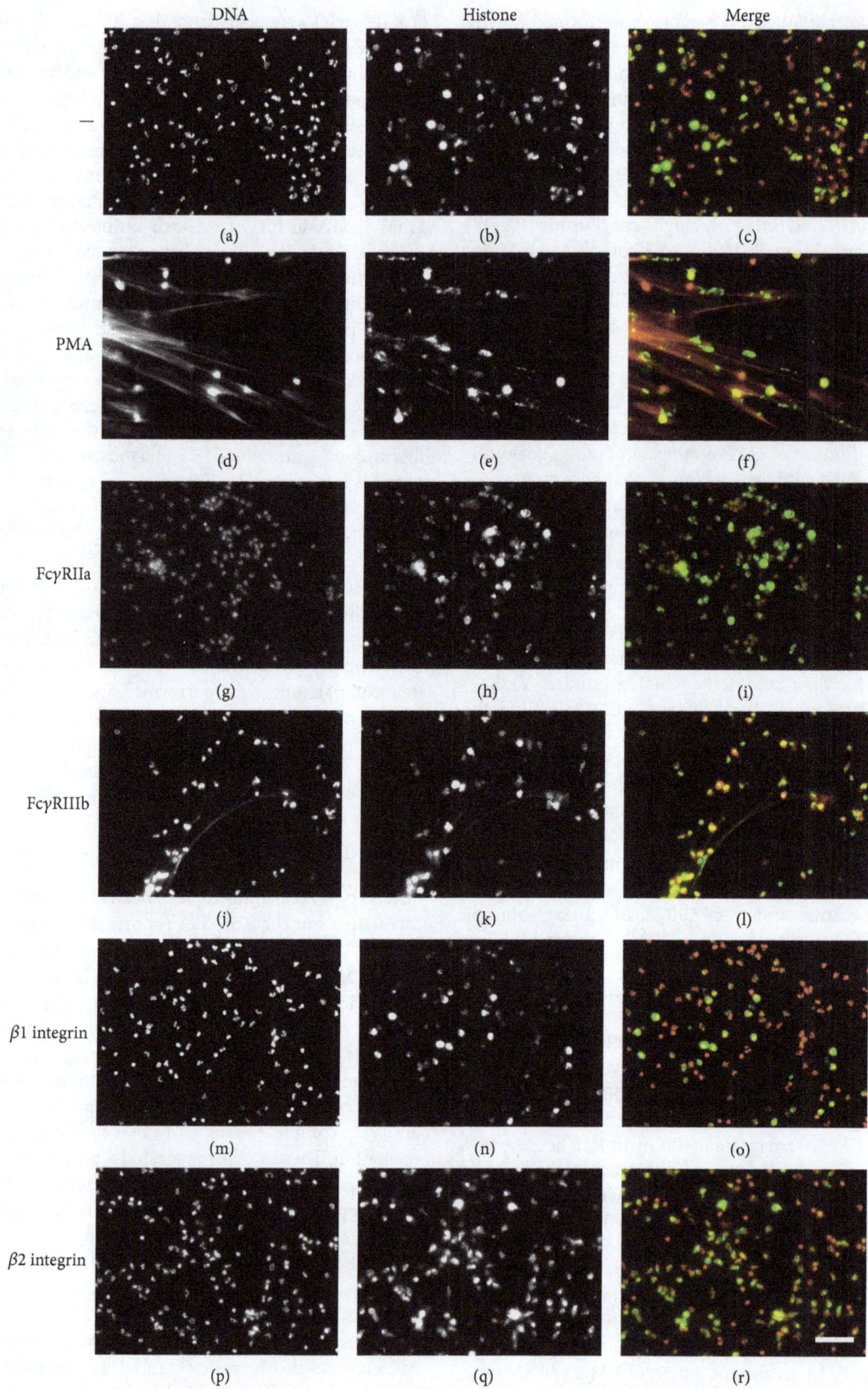

FIGURE 1: FcγRIIIb induces NET formation. (a) Human neutrophils (PMN) were left untreated (—) or were stimulated with 20 nM phorbol 12-myristate 13-acetate (PMA), by cross-linking FcγRIIa with mAb IV.3, by cross-linking FcγRIIIb with mAb 3G8, by cross-linking β1 integrins with mAb TS2/16, or by cross-linking β1 integrins with mAb IB4. After four hours, PMN were fixed and stained for DNA (DAPI, red) and for histone (green). Microphotographs were taken at 200x magnification and are representative of more than 10 experiments. Bar is 50 μm.

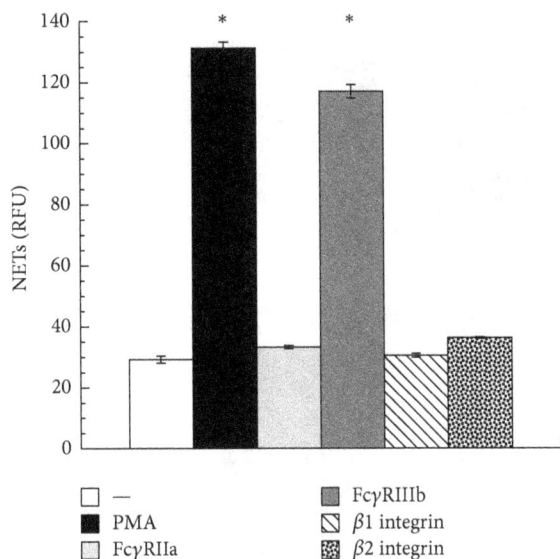

FIGURE 2: NETs are induced by PMA and FcγRIIIb cross-linking. Human neutrophils (PMN) were left untreated (—) or were stimulated with 20 nM phorbol 12-myristate 13-acetate (PMA), by cross-linking FcγRIIa with mAb IV.3, by cross-linking FcγRIIIb with mAb 3G8, by cross-linking β1 integrins with mAb TS2/16, or by cross-linking β2 integrins with mAb IB4. The relative amount of NETs, as extracellular DNA of nonfixed cells, was estimated from SYTOX Green fluorescence in relative fluorescent units (RFU) at 4 hours after stimulation, as described in Materials and Methods. Data are mean ± SEM of 4 experiments. Asterisks denote conditions that are statistically different from control ($p < 0.05$).

Figure 2S). Histones were also present along the extracellular DNA fibers (Figure 1(e)). Cross-linking FcγRIIa with the specific mAb IV.3 did not induce NET formation and PMN retained intact nuclei with typical lobular morphology (Figures 1(g) and 1(h)). Similarly, cross-linking β1 integrins (Figures 1(m) and 1(n)) or β2 integrins (Figures 1(p) and 1(q)) did not induce any NET formation (Supplemental Figure 2S). In contrast, cross-linking FcγRIIIb with the specific mAb 3G8 induced strong NET formation (Figure 1(j)) similar to the one induced by PMA (Figure 2). These FcγRIIIb-induced extracellular DNA fibers were also covered with histones (Figure 1(k) and Supplemental Figure 3S). Cross-linking of FcγRIIa together with FcγRIIIb or β2 integrins together with FcγRIIIb did not induce changes in the amount of NET formation induced by FcγRIIIb alone (not shown). An important characteristic of NETs is that they are covered with antimicrobial proteins from the PMN granules. The presence of neutrophil elastase on NETs was confirmed for NETs induced both by PMA and by FcγRIIIb (Figure 3 and Supplemental Figure 4S). These data indicated that cross-linking FcγRIIIb is an efficient stimulus for NET formation. NETosis [4] is a form of cell death different from apoptosis [34]. In neutrophils, apoptosis appears spontaneously when these cells get older or after they have activated their proinflammatory functions [35]. Because the NET quantification method is related to detection of extracellular DNA, it was important to determine whether PMN were in apoptosis

after stimulation of Fcγ receptors. After PMA stimulation or Fcγ receptor cross-linking, PMN did not have an increase in annexin V-binding, indicating that PMN were not in apoptosis [34, 36] (Supplemental Figure 5S).

Because PMA is an activator of PKC, the involvement of this kinase in NET formation induced by FcγRIIIb was tested with two specific PKC inhibitors. PMN treated with PMA formed NETs as expected (Figure 4). However, when PMN were treated previously with GÖ6983, an inhibitor of PKCα, PKCβ, and PKCγ isozymes (Figure 4), or with GÖ6976, a conventional PKC inhibitor (Figure 4), NETs were not formed after PMA stimulation. Similarly, NET formation after FcγRIIIb cross-linking (Figure 4) was inhibited by these PKC inhibitors (Figure 4). In addition, downstream of PKC, the MEK, ERK pathway has been reported to participate in NET formation after PMA stimulation [37]. When PMN were treated with UO126, a potent specific MEK inhibitor, NETs were not formed after PMA stimulation (Figure 5). Also, UO126 treatment blocked NET formation after FcγRIIIb stimulation (Figure 5). These data suggested that FcγRIIIb stimulation led to NET formation using PKC and ERK. To confirm that ERK 1 was activated after PMA or Fc receptor stimulation as previously reported [38], PMN were stimulated in the presence or absence of the MEK inhibitor and ERK 1 activation was detected by Western blotting. PMA induced ERK phosphorylation in PMN (Figure 6(a)), and this ERK activation was completely blocked by the MEK inhibitor UO126 (Figure 6(a)). Similarly, FcγRIIa cross-linking (Figure 6(b)) or FcγRIIIb cross-linking (Figure 6(c)) resulted in efficient ERK 1 phosphorylation. This ERK 1 activation was completely blocked in both cases by the MEK inhibitor (Figures 6(b) and 6(c)). These data suggested that both Fcγ receptors can induce ERK activation, but this enzyme is not sufficient for NET formation, since only FcγRIIIb led to release of NETs.

Other signaling molecules that are important for Fc receptor signaling via ITAM are Syk and PI-3K. Although, FcγRIIIb does not have an ITAM, it has been suggested that FcγRIIIb might signal in cooperation with FcγRIIa [39]. Thus, to explore the possible involvement of these molecules in FcγRIIIb-induced NET formation, PMN were treated with piceatannol (Figure 7) or iSyk (Supplemental Figure 6S), selective inhibitors of Syk, or with wortmannin (Figure 7), a selective inhibitor of PI-3K, before stimulation. These inhibitors prevented NET formation when PMN were stimulated by PMA (Figure 7). Similarly, NET formation was inhibited after cross-linking of FcγRIIIb in the presence of piceatannol (Figure 7) but proceeded normally in the presence of wortmannin (Figure 7). Interestingly, iSyk only caused small but statistically significant inhibition of NET formation after PMA stimulation, while it did not block FcγRIIIb-induced NET formation (Supplemental Figure 6S). These data suggested that FcγRIIIb-induced NET formation involves Syk, but it is independent of PI-3K.

NETs formed after PMA stimulation require activation of NADPH-oxidase and formation of ROS [40] and also activation of NF-κB [41]. Thus, we explored the involvement of these molecules in FcγRIIIb-induced NET formation.

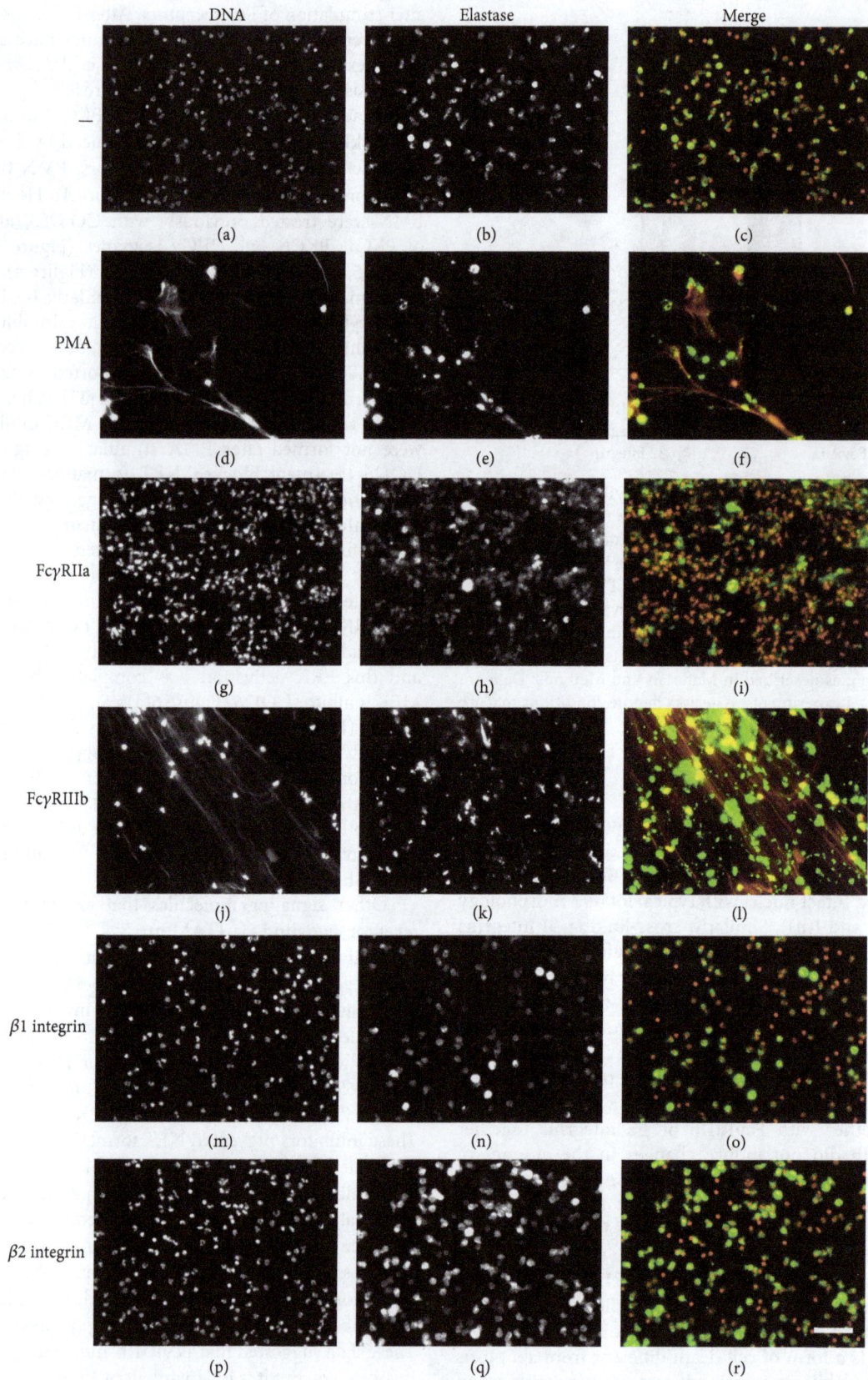

FIGURE 3: NETs are decorated with neutrophil elastase. Human neutrophils (PMN) were stimulated with 20 nM phorbol 12-myristate 13-acetate (PMA), by cross-linking FcγRIIa with mAb IV.3, by cross-linking FcγRIIIb with mAb 3G8, by cross-linking β1 integrins with mAb TS2/16, or by cross-linking β1 integrins with mAb IB4. After four hours, PMN were fixed and stained for DNA (DAPI, red) or for elastase (green). Microphotographs were taken at 200x magnification and are representative of five experiments. Bar is 50 μm.

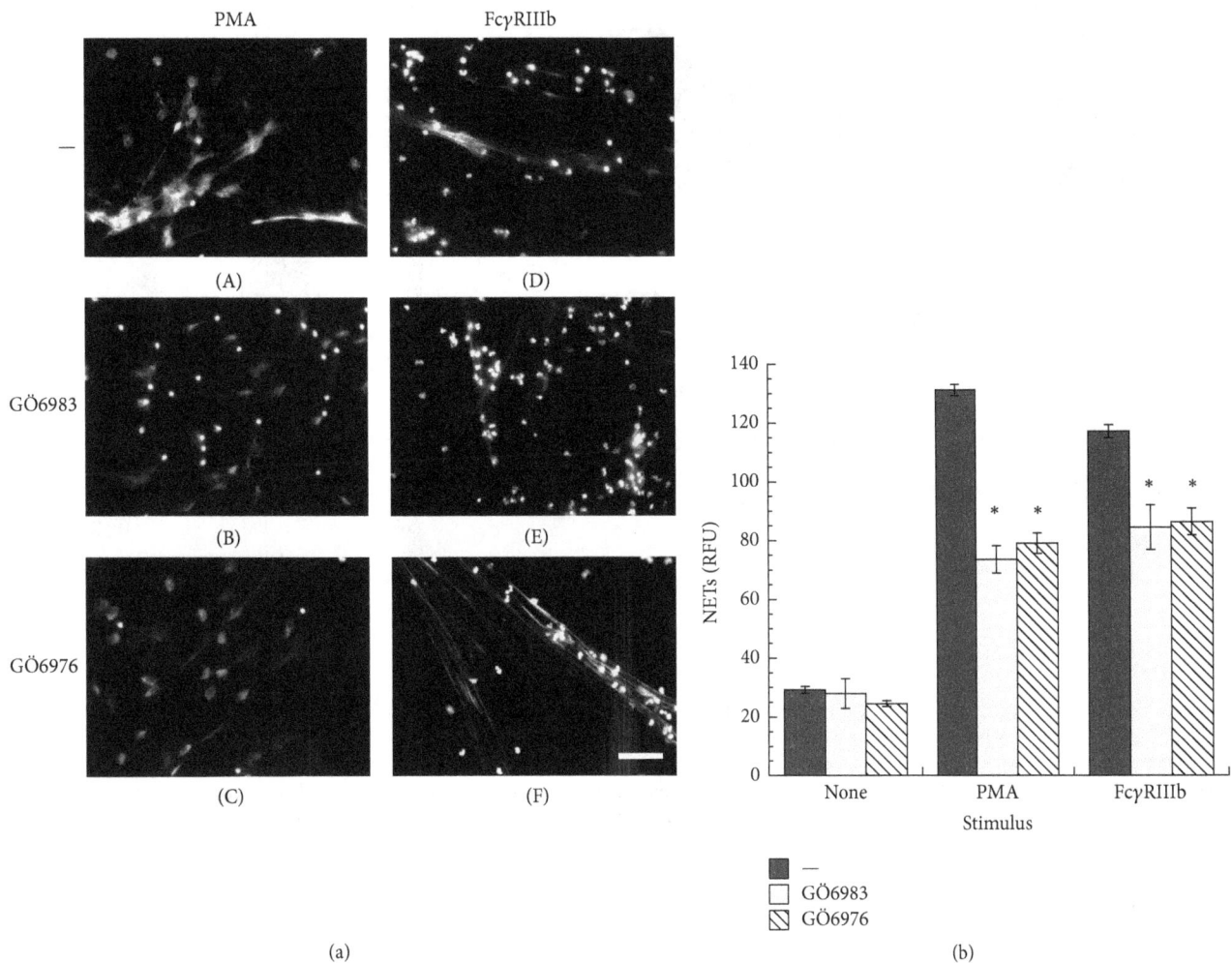

FIGURE 4: FcγRIIIb-induced NET formation is dependent on PKC. (a) Human neutrophils (PMN) were stimulated with 20 nM phorbol 12-myristate 13-acetate (PMA) or by cross-linking FcγRIIIb with mAb 3G8. PMN were previously treated with solvent alone (—) or with the PKC inhibitors GÖ6983 (1 μM) or GÖ6976 (1 μM). After four hours, PMN were fixed and stained for DNA (DAPI). Microphotographs were taken at 200x magnification and are representative of five experiments. Bar is 50 μm. (b) The relative amount of NETs was estimated from SYTOX Green fluorescence in relative fluorescent units (RFU) at 4 hours after stimulation. Data are mean ± SEM of 11 experiments. Asterisks denote conditions that are statistically different from control ($p < 0.001$).

PMN treated with diphenyleneiodonium (DPI), an NADPH-oxidase inhibitor, were not able to form NETs after PMA stimulation (Figure 8). Similarly, DPI-treated PMN could not form NETs after cross-linking of FcγRIIIb (Figure 8). PMA treatment, as well as cross-linking of both FcγRIIa and FcγRIIIb, indeed induced ROS production that was completely blocked by DPI (Supplemental Figure 7S). In addition, PMN treated with BAY 117082, an NF-κB inhibitor, were not able to form NETs after PMA stimulation (Figure 9). In contrast, PMN treated with BAY 117082 at two different concentrations formed NETs efficiently after cross-linking of FcγRIIIb (Figure 9). These data suggested that FcγRIIIb could indeed induce the formation of NETs via NADPH-oxidase activation, but independently of NF-κB activation.

Clearly, selective activation of FcγRIIIb on the PMN membrane was enough to induce the formation of NETs. In order to explore whether cross-linking of Fc receptors by a more natural stimulus could also induce NET formation, PMN were mixed with opsonized latex particles. These particles covered with Protein A and then opsonized with selective anti-Fc receptor antibodies can be recognized by only one or the other of the Fc receptors. As shown previously [30], PMN were capable of efficient phagocytosis of latex beads opsonized with mAb IV.3 (anti-FcγRIIa) and of very poor phagocytosis of latex beads opsonized with mAb 3G8 (anti-FcγRIIIb) (Figure 10). These beads were opsonized at similar levels with both anti-Fcγ receptor antibodies (Supplemental Figure 8S). PMN and fluorescent beads can be easily separated as two distinct populations in a flow cytometer. Thus, by gating on cells an increase in fluorescence indicates efficient phagocytosis (Supplemental Figure 9S). The efficient FcγRIIa-mediated phagocytosis was dependent on ERK activation [30], since the MEK inhibitor UO126 prevented it (Figure 10), and it was independent of NF-κB activation,

(a)

(b)

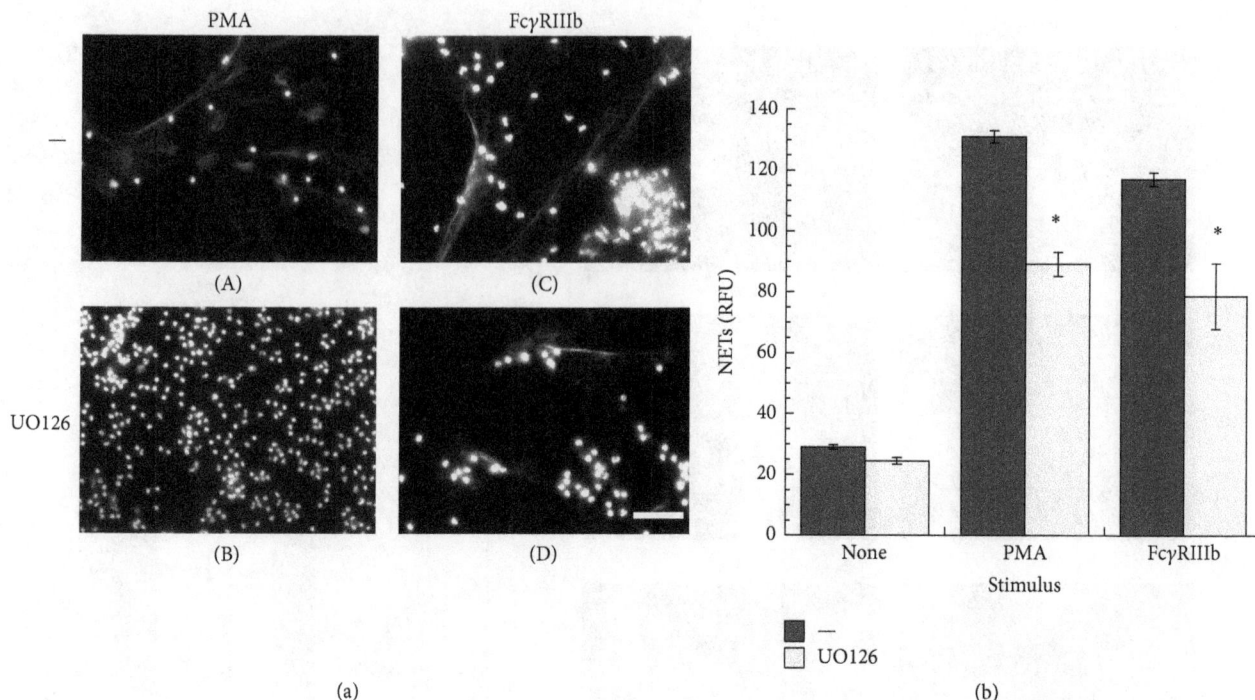

FIGURE 5: FcγRIIIb-induced NET formation is dependent on MEK. (a) Human neutrophils (PMN) were not stimulated (None) or were stimulated with 20 nM phorbol 12-myristate 13-acetate (PMA) or by cross-linking FcγRIIIb with mAb 3G8. PMN were previously treated with solvent alone (—) or with the MEK inhibitor UO126 (50 μM). After four hours, PMN were fixed and stained for DNA (DAPI). Microphotographs were taken at 200x magnification and are representative of five experiments. Bar is 50 μm. (b) The relative amount of NETs was estimated from SYTOX Green fluorescence in relative fluorescent units (RFU) at 4 hours after stimulation. Data are mean ± SEM of 8 experiments. Asterisks denote conditions that are statistically different from control ($p < 0.001$).

since the inhibitor BAY 117082 did not affect it (Figure 10). These data were also confirmed by evaluating phagocytosis by microscopy (Supplemental Figure 10S). In contrast, the poor phagocytic response of FcγRIIIb was independent of both MEK and NF-κB (Figure 11). These beads when not opsonized (Figure 11(a)(A)) or when opsonized with anti-FcγRIIa antibodies (Figure 11(a)(B)) could not induce the formation of NETs. However, beads opsonized with anti-FcγRIIIb antibodies efficiently induced the formation of NETs (Figure 11(a)(C and D)). In addition, a mixture of beads opsonized with either anti-FcγRIIa antibodies or anti-FcγRIIIb antibodies also induced NET formation to the same level as anti-FcγRIIIb beads alone (Figure 11(b)). These data strongly suggested that FcγRIIa can efficiently promote phagocytosis, while it cannot induce the formation of NETs. In contrast, FcγRIIIb poorly promotes phagocytosis, but it can efficiently induce the formation of NETs.

4. Discussion

Neutrophils are the most abundant circulating leukocytes in mammals and they are rapidly recruited to sites of infection, where they act as the first line of defense against invading pathogens [42]. Neutrophil activation, through various membrane receptors, is also required for the initiation of the several defense mechanisms displayed by these cells [43],

including phagocytosis, respiratory burst, release of various microbicidal molecules by degranulation [44], and the recently described formation of neutrophil extracellular traps (NETs) [3]. NETs are extracellular fibers formed by chromatin covered with histones [7] and antimicrobial proteins derived from neutrophil granules [2]. NETs seem to act as a physical barrier where microorganisms get trapped [10] and display antimicrobial activity that is independent of phagocytosis [45]. Despite the fact that many pathogens, including virus, bacteria, fungi, and parasites [10], have all been reported to induce NET formation, no particular receptors on the neutrophil membrane leading to release of NETs have been identified until very recently. IgA-opsonized bacteria or IgA-opsonized beads activated the FcαRI (CD89) leading to release of NETs [46]. Other previous reports indicated that NET formation was increased when microorganisms were opsonized with autologous serum [3], and also antigen-antibody complexes seemed capable of inducing NET formation [22, 23]. These reports thus suggested a role for IgG Fc receptors (FcγRs) in NET formation.

In the neutrophil two types of FcγR are constitutively expressed, namely, FcγRIIa and FcγRIIIb [12, 13]. This fact has made it difficult to establish which functions are initiated by each of these two FcγRs. For phagocytosis, there is no doubt that FcγRIIa is an important receptor [30]. In contrast, FcγRIIIb is an important receptor for signaling to the

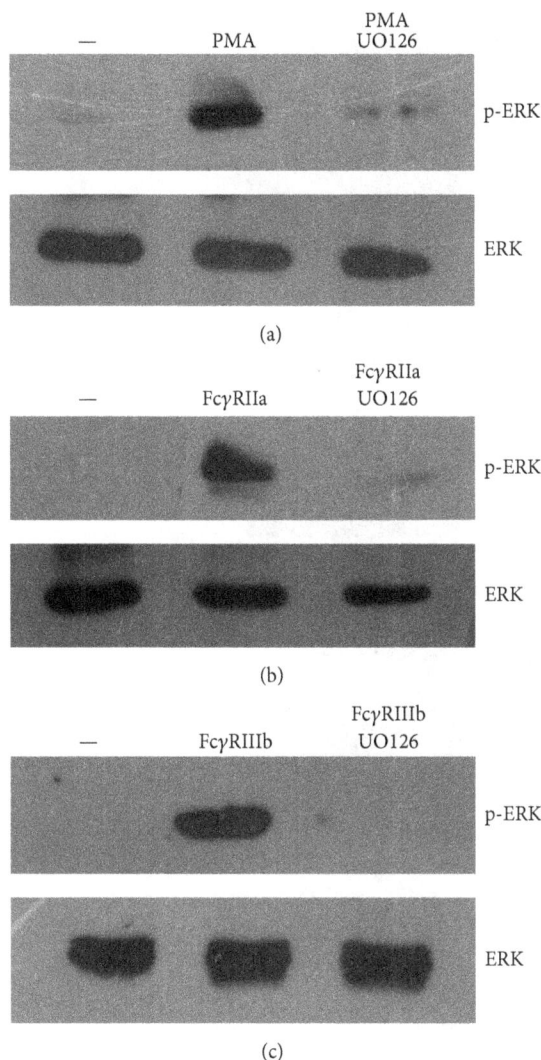

FIGURE 6: FcγR-cross-linking induces activation of ERK. Human neutrophils (PMN) were left untreated (—) or were stimulated (a) with 20 nM phorbol 12-myristate 13-acetate (PMA) or (b) by cross-linking FcγRIIa with mAb IV.3 or (c) by cross-linking FcγRIIIb with mAb 3G8. PMN were also stimulated in the presence of the MEK inhibitor UO126 (50 μM). PMN cell lysates were prepared after 30 min stimulation. Proteins were resolved by SDS-PAGE and then Western blotted for phosphorylated-ERK (p-ERK) (upper panel) or for total ERK (lower panel). Data are representative of three separate experiments.

nucleus [38]. In the case of NET formation, it is not clear which FcγR is preferentially responsible for this function. It was previously reported that FcγRIIIb promoted endocytosis of soluble immune complexes and that FcγRIIa promoted NET formation in vivo [22]. However, more recently, it was reported that FcγRIIIb is the receptor responsible for NET formation in response to immobilized immune complexes [24]. In addition, neutrophil stimulation by IgG antineutrophil cytoplasmic antibodies (ANCA) led to degranulation and neutrophil extracellular trap formation in an FcγRIIIb allele-specific manner [47]. Here, we have found that indeed

FcγRIIIb, but not FcγRIIa, induced significant amounts of NETs.

Selective FcγRIIIb cross-linking with specific monoclonal antibodies on human neutrophils induced NET formation. The release of these NETs was detected 3-4 hours after stimulation and was dependent on ROS, since the NADPH-oxidase inhibitor DPI abrogated trap release. This NET release was similar to the one induced by cross-linking FcαRI [46] or by phorbol 12-myristate 13-acetate (PMA) stimulation [2] but different from the rapid, oxidant-independent NET release recently described [48]. FcγRIIIb-induced NETs consisted of long DNA fibers decorated with histones and neutrophil elastase showing a bona fide neutrophil extracellular trap structure. Although both FcγRIIa and FcγRIIIb induced a strong respiratory burst as shown by activated ROS production, cross-linking of FcγRIIa alone did not induce NET formation. ROS are required for NET formation in most cases [2, 4, 8], but they are not sufficient, since ROS production induced by phagocytosis cannot initiate NET formation [9].

FcγRIIIb-induced NETs are similar in shape and molecular structure to those induced by PMA [9], and the molecular mechanism leading to their release seems to be also similar. Most studies on NET formation have been conducted with PMA stimulation [2]. PMA is a direct activator of protein kinase C (PKC); thus any possible receptor involved in NET formation is bypassed. Several inhibitors of PKC have been shown to block NET formation [49]. In agreement with those reports, we found that two different inhibitors of PKC indeed blocked NET formation after PMA and FcγRIIIb stimulation. In addition, inhibition of Syk with piceatannol blocked the release of NETs induced either by PMA or by FcγRIIIb (Figure 7). However, inhibition of Syk with iSyk slightly reduced only PMA-induced NETosis (Figure 6S). The differential inhibition of NET formation with two reported Syk inhibitors suggests that some of the discrepancies in the literature regarding signaling pathways regulating NETosis may be due to the use of various pharmacological inhibitors. It is necessary to revise these pathways more carefully in future studies. Despite this caveat, inhibition of Syk with piceatannol points to an important role for this kinase in NET formation induced by specific cross-linking of FcγRIIIb. Syk was also found to participate in NET formation induced by soluble immune complexes [22, 50], by insoluble immune complexes [24], and by PMA [24]. Syk is normally associated with initial signaling events at the level of cell surface receptors, but PMA can bypass these receptors to directly activate PKC [51]. Yet activation of Syk by PMA has been previously described in neutrophils. PMA induced PKC-dependent phosphorylation of Syk [52], and piceatannol reduced ROS production in response to PMA [53]. Together these reports and our data support the idea that Syk activation is involved in both PMA- and also FcγRIIIb-induced ROS-dependent NETosis.

Downstream of PKC, a role for the MEK, ERK pathway [54] and for NF-κB [41] in PMA-induced NET formation has been suggested. MEK inhibition blocked PMA- and FcγRIIIb-induced NETosis indicating that ERK activation is required in this process. ERK was also found to be required for NET formation in response to soluble immune

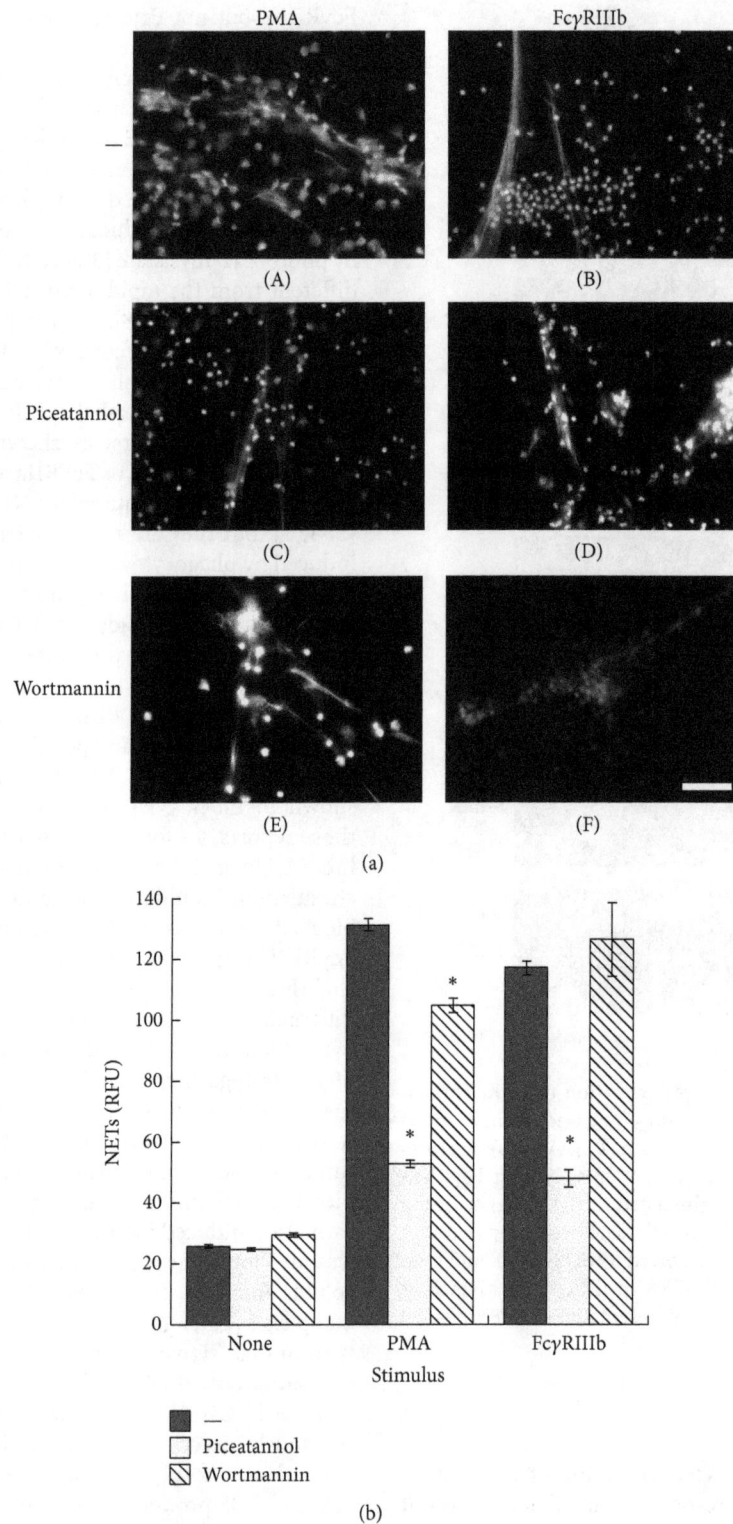

FIGURE 7: FcγRIIIb-induced NET formation requires Syk but is independent of PI-3K. (a) Human neutrophils (PMN) were not stimulated (None) or were restimulated with 20 nM phorbol 12-myristate 13-acetate (PMA) or by cross-linking FcγRIIIb with mAb 3G8. PMN were previously treated with solvent alone (—) or with the Syk inhibitor piceatannol (50 μM) or with the PI-3K inhibitor wortmannin (50 nM). After four hours, PMN were fixed and stained for DNA (DAPI). Microphotographs were taken at 200x magnification and are representative of three experiments. Bar is 50 μm. (b) The relative amount of NETs was estimated from SYTOX Green fluorescence in relative fluorescent units (RFU) at 4 hours after stimulation. Data are mean ± SEM of 5 experiments. Asterisks denote conditions that are statistically different from control ($p < 0.05$).

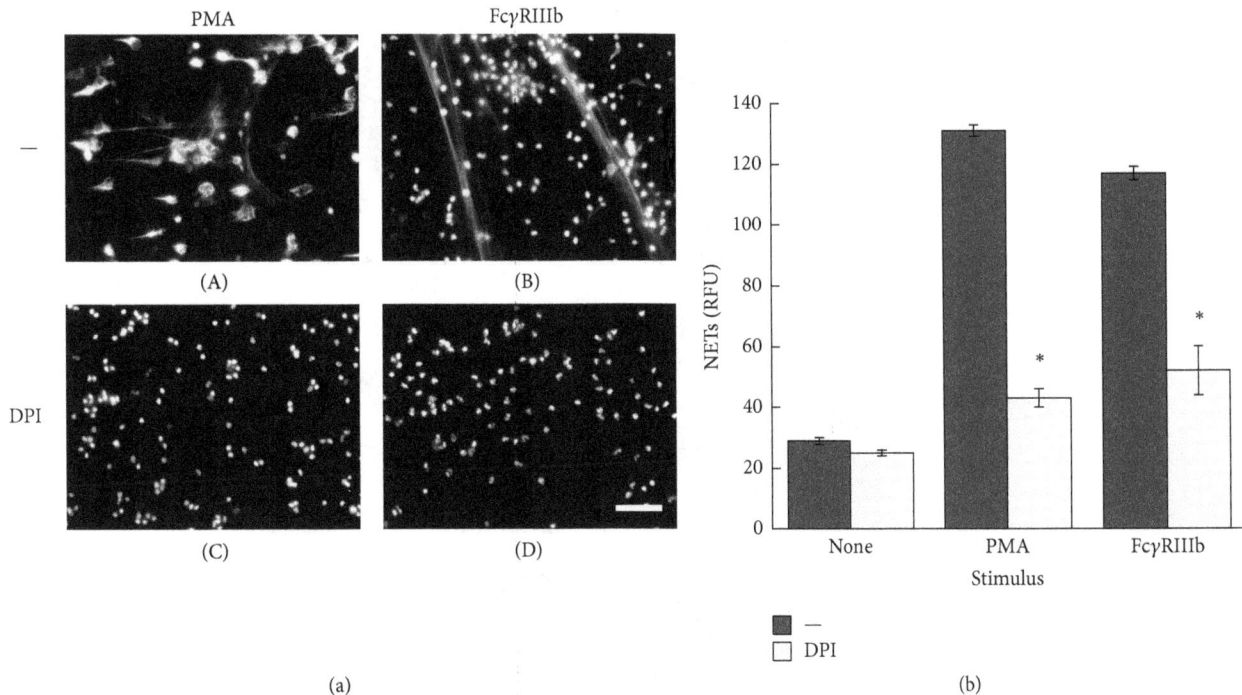

(a)

(b)

FIGURE 8: FcγRIIIb-induced NET formation is dependent on NADPH-oxidase. (a) Human neutrophils (PMN) were not stimulated (None) or were stimulated with 20 nM phorbol 12-myristate 13-acetate (PMA) or by cross-linking FcγRIIIb with mAb 3G8. PMN were previously treated with solvent alone (—) or with the NADPH-oxidase inhibitor diphenyleneiodonium (DPI) (10 μM). After four hours, PMN were fixed and stained for DNA (DAPI). Microphotographs were taken at 200x magnification and are representative of three experiments. Bar is 50 μm. (b) The relative amount of NETs was estimated from SYTOX Green fluorescence in relative fluorescent units (RFU) at 4 hours after stimulation. Data are mean ± SEM of 5 experiments. Asterisks denote conditions that are statistically different from control ($p < 0.001$).

complexes [22] and immobilized immune complexes [24]. However, the role of ERK in NET formation remains unclear. A previous report indicated that ERK is required for NADPH-oxidase activation [37], placing ERK upstream of ROS production, while another report suggested that ROS are downstream of ERK activation [54]. Therefore, it seems that NADPH-oxidase activation for NET formation may proceed not only through an ERK pathway, but also independently of ERK activation, depending on the stimulus [19, 20]. As previously reported, NF-κB inhibition reduced PMA-induced NET formation [41]. However, FcγRIIIb-induced NETosis was unaffected when neutrophils were treated with the same inhibitor for NF-κB (Figure 9). Similarly, inhibition of PI-3K by wortmannin reduced NET formation by PMA but had no effect on FcγRIIIb-induced NET formation (Figure 7). A possible role for PI-3K involvement in NET formation induced by immobilized immune complexes was also found using the inhibitor LY29004 [24]. We did not find the same result, but as mentioned above for Syk the particular inhibitor used may be responsible for these different results. It was proposed that PI-3K could influence NF-κB activation via phosphatidylinositol-trisphosphate and in turn NF-κB activate genes important for signaling to NET formation [41]. These ideas, however, have not been proven experimentally and the role of PI-3K and NF-κB in FcγRIIIb-mediated NETosis needs further exploration.

FcγRIIIb has been suggested to signal in cooperation with other molecules such as integrin Mac-1 (CD11b/CD18), also known as complement receptor 3 [55]. However, complement receptor ligands are not sufficient to induce NET formation in isolated neutrophils [9]. Similarly, in our case selective cross-linking of β2 integrins with mAb IB4 also did not induce any NET formation. In contrast, blocking Mac-1 with antibodies against both CD11b and CD18 chains prevented NET formation by LPS [19], by β-glucan [56], and by immobilized immune complexes [24]. These reports and our data suggest that β2 integrins cooperate with other receptors to induce NETosis, but they cannot by themselves cause NET formation. The involvement of β2 integrins in NET formation might be more related to the adhesion requirement of neutrophils to form NETs [28] than to a signaling capacity of the integrin. Along the same line of thought, cross-linking of other receptors such as β1 integrins also did not promote any NET formation (Figure 1), although the same procedure was capable of activating NF-κB in neutrophils [25]. Recently, it was also reported that NET formation in response to Candida albicans required fibronectin via β1 integrins. However, β1 integrin engagement alone was not sufficient to activate NETosis [56]. Similarly, the adhesive protein invasin from Yersinia pseudotuberculosis promotes bacteria crossing the intestine epithelium by binding to β1 integrins on M-cells. Invasin was also shown to induce

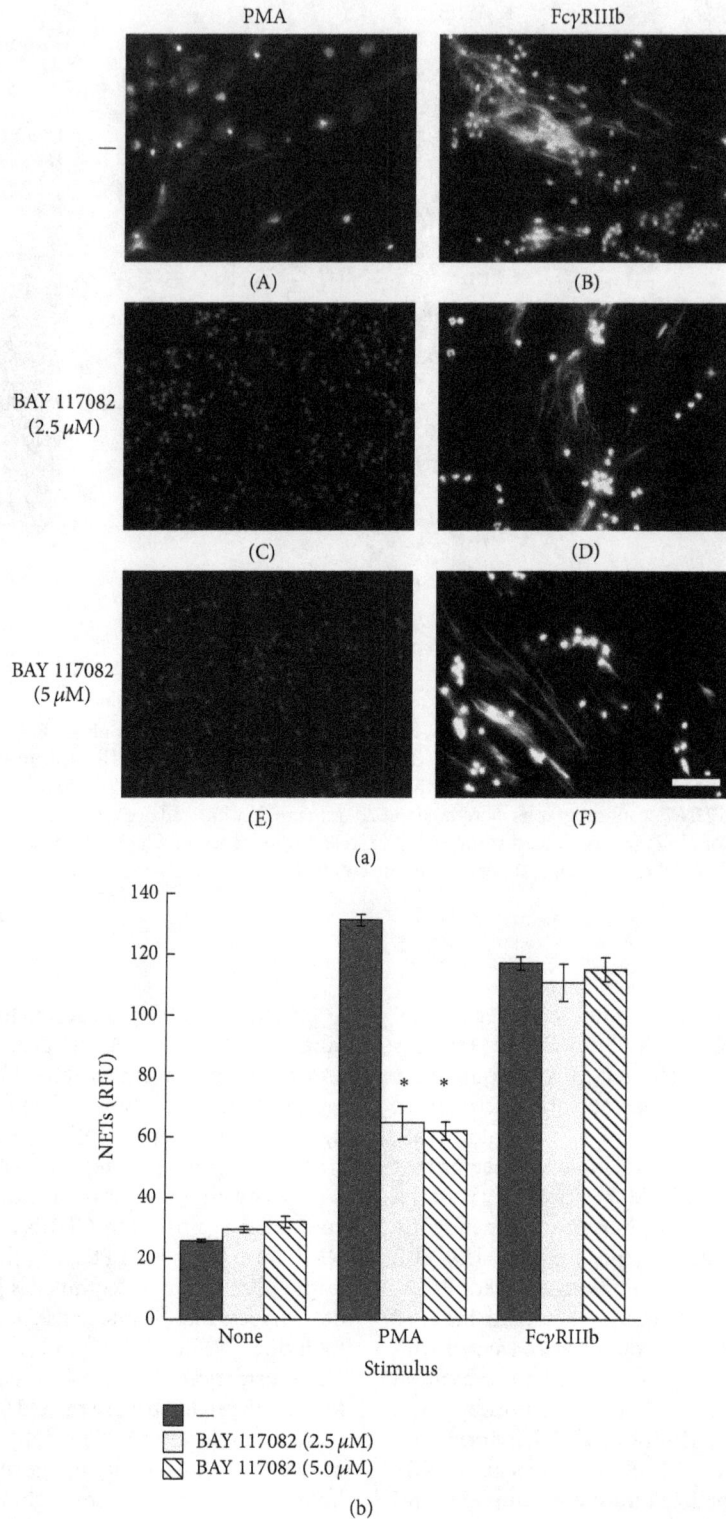

FIGURE 9: FcγRIIIb-induced NET formation is independent of NF-κB. (a) Human neutrophils (PMN) were not stimulated (None) or were stimulated with 20 nM phorbol 12-myristate 13-acetate (PMA) or by cross-linking FcγRIIIb with mAb 3G8. PMN were previously treated with solvent alone (—) or with the NF-κB inhibitor BAY 117082 at 2.5 μM and 5 μM. After four hours, PMN were fixed and stained for DNA (DAPI). Microphotographs were taken at 200x magnification and are representative of three experiments. Bar is 50 μm. (b) The relative amount of NETs was estimated from SYTOX Green fluorescence in relative fluorescent units (RFU) at 4 hours after stimulation. Data are mean ± SEM of 4 experiments. Asterisks denote conditions that are statistically different from control ($p < 0.05$).

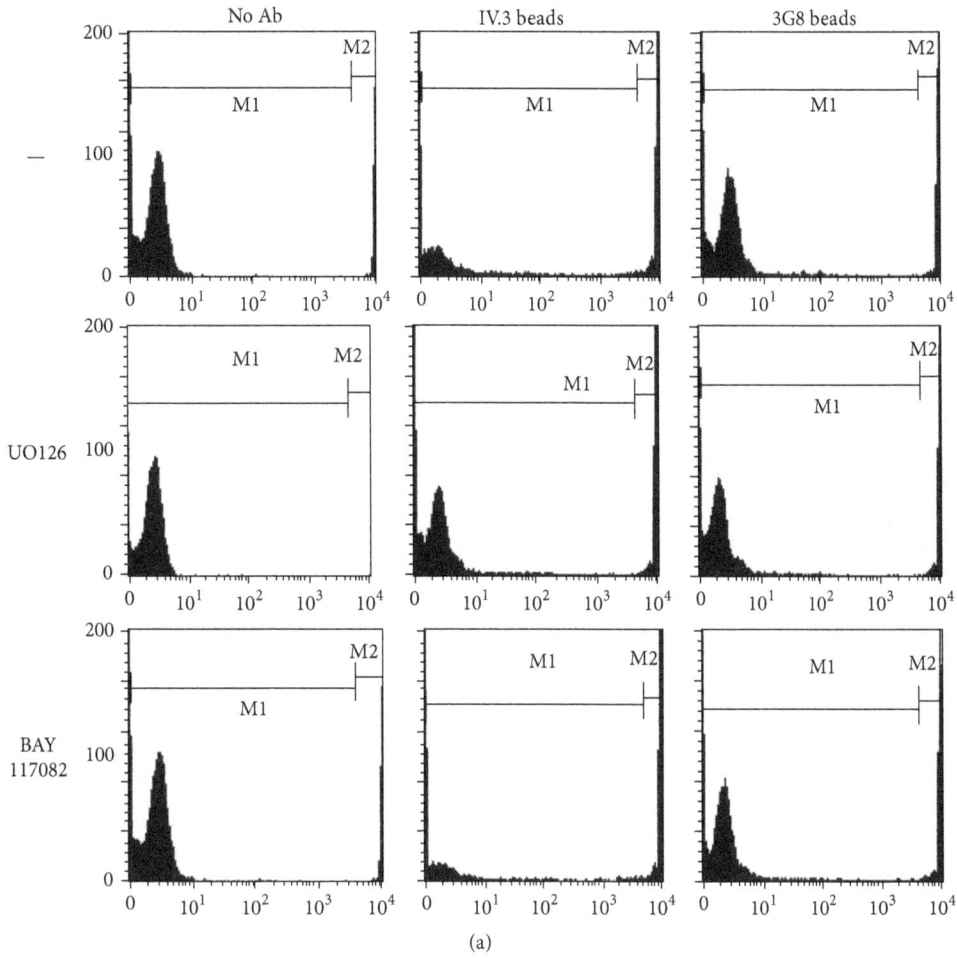

(a)

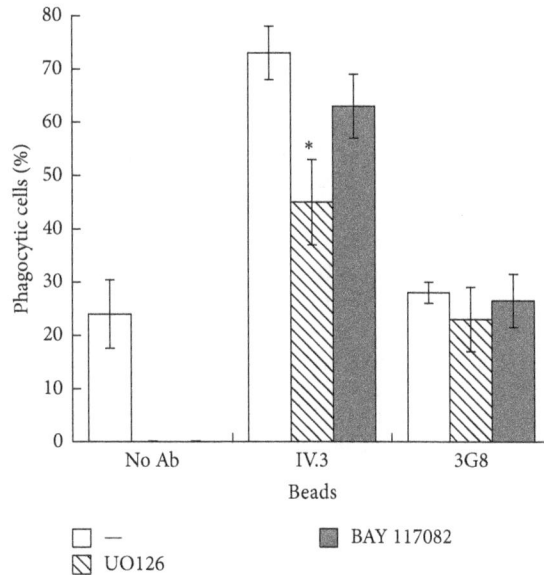

(b)

FIGURE 10: FcγRIIa induces efficient phagocytosis. (a) Human neutrophils were mixed with fluorescence latex particles. Particles were nonopsonized (no Ab) or opsonized with monoclonal antibody (mAb) IV.3 anti-FcγRIIa or with mAb 3G8 anti-FcγRIIIb. Cells were allowed to ingest the particles for 30 min. Phagocytosis of latex beads was also evaluated in the absence (None) or the presence of 50 μM UO126 (MEK inhibitor) or 2.5 μM BAY 117082 (NF-κB inhibitor). Phagocytosis was assessed by flow cytometry, detecting the reduced number of cells with low fluorescence (M1 marker), and the appearance of cells with high fluorescence in the far right side (M2 marker) of the histogram of gated PMN. (b) Phagocytosis was quantified by flow cytometry, as the percentage of high-fluorescence cells (marker M2) in the histogram of gated PMN. Data are representative of four separate experiments.

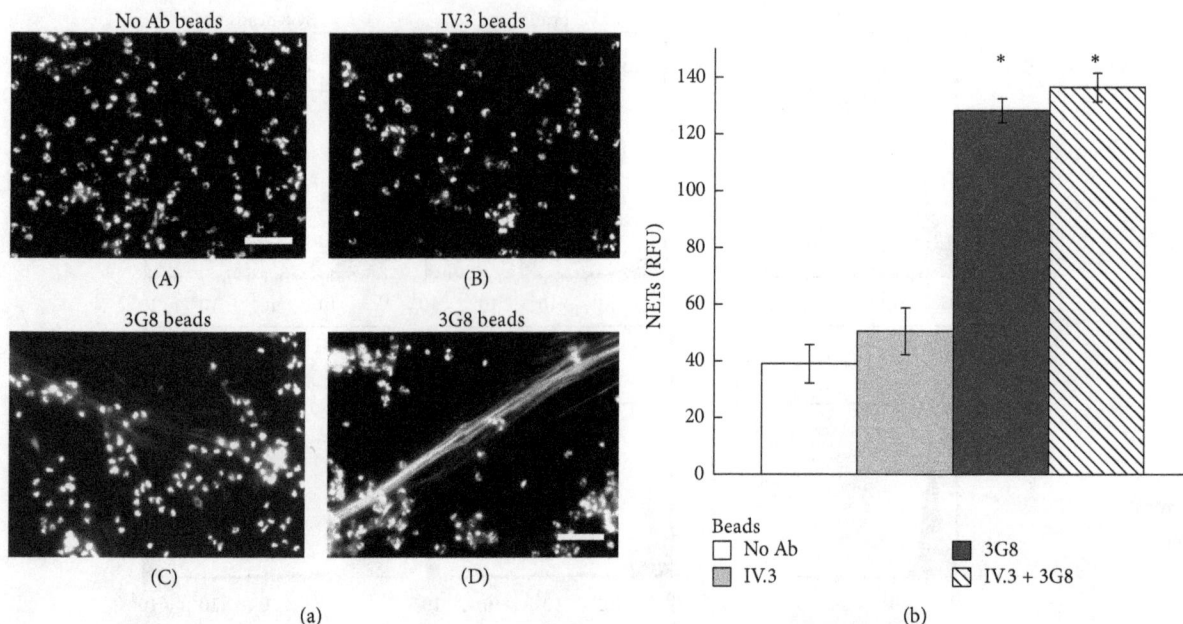

FIGURE 11: Anti-FcγRIIIb-opsonized particles induce NET formation. (a) Human neutrophils (PMN) mixed with latex particles nonopsonized (no Ab beads) or opsonized with monoclonal antibody IV.3, anti-FcγRIIa (IV.3 beads), or with monoclonal antibody 3G8, anti-FcγRIIIb (3G8 beads), were incubated for four hours and fixed and stained for DNA (DAPI). Microphotographs were taken at 200x magnification and are representative of three experiments. Bar is 50 μm. (b) The relative amount of NETs was estimated from SYTOX Green fluorescence in relative fluorescent units (RFU) at 4 hours after stimulation, as described in Materials and Methods. Data are mean ± SEM of four experiments. Asterisks denote conditions that are statistically different from control ($p < 0.02$).

ROS and NET formation [57]. However, invasin-mediated triggering of $\beta 1$ integrin was essential but not sufficient for NET production [57]. Additional, so far uncharacterized costimuli were required for NET formation. Clearly, integrins cooperate in different scenarios to activate NETosis after various stimuli including immune complexes, but the exact role they play in this process remains elusive.

Moreover, as mentioned above, selective cross-linking of FcγRIIa also did not promote NET formation. This was not due to a defect in FcγRIIa signaling because the same cross-linking procedure led to robust activation of ERK (Figure 6). In addition, latex beads opsonized with the specific anti-FcγRIIa mAb IV.3 were efficiently phagocytosed by neutrophils [30] (Figure 10). The same opsonized latex beads were not capable of inducing any NET formation. In contrast, latex beads opsonized with the specific anti-FcγRIIIb mAb 3G8 were poorly phagocytosed by neutrophils [30] (Figures 10 and 10S) but efficiently induced NET formation. Our results support the idea presented in a recent report showing that neutrophils sensed microbe size and selectively released NETs in response to large pathogens, such as Candida albicans hyphae and extracellular aggregates of Mycobacterium bovis, but not in response to small yeast or single bacteria [58]. In this study, phagocytosis via the receptor dectin-1 acted as a sensor of microbe size and prevented NET release by downregulating the translocation of neutrophil elastase to the nucleus [58]. Similarly, we present here that neutrophils responded via FcγRIIa with efficient phagocytosis; however NET formation was absent. In contrast, stimulation via FcγRIIIb led to poor phagocytosis but to significant NET

formation. Thus we conclude that NETs are not formed when an opsonized target can be efficiently phagocytosed via FcγRIIa. However, upon inefficient phagocytosis via FcγRIIIb engagement, NET formation is induced strongly. Together, these data support the idea that indeed each FcγR on the human neutrophil is capable of triggering specific responses. FcγRIIa promotes efficient phagocytosis, while FcγRIIIb induces NET formation instead. The inflammatory environment may be responsible for what receptor FcγRIIa or FcγRIIIb may predominate and initiate a particular cell response [11]. FcγRIIIb is expressed 4- to 5-fold more abundantly and has a higher affinity for IgG than FcγRIIa [59], thus probably becoming the preferred receptor to first engage immune complexes. At the same time, inflammatory stimuli can lead to FcγRIIIb shedding from the cell, favoring now immune complex interactions with FcγRIIa [60] to induce phagocytosis and cytotoxicity [13]. We believe that when a strong activating threshold is achieved by cross-linking FcγRIIIb an efficient induction of NET formation takes place.

In conclusion, our data show that FcγRIIIb governs Fc receptor-induced NET formation in human neutrophils. The signaling pathway used by FcγRIIIb to induce NETs involves PKC, PKC, and ERK 1. Our results also support the idea that different Fc receptors promote independent cell functions.

Conflict of Interests

The authors do not have any conflict of interests related to this paper.

Acknowledgments

The authors thank Dr. Martha Robles-Flores (Facultad de Medicina, UNAM) for her advice on PKC inhibitors, Dr. Leopoldo Santos Argumedo (CINVESTAV, IPN) and Dr. Yvonne Rosenstein (Instituto de Biotecnología, UNAM) for their help with the apoptosis assay, and Dr. Tzipe Govezensky (Instituto de Investigaciones Biomédicas, UNAM) for performing the statistical analysis of all data. Research in the authors' laboratory was supported by Grant 168098 from Consejo Nacional de Ciencia y Tecnología, Mexico (to Carlos Rosales), and by Grants PAPIIT IA202013-2 (to Eileen Uribe-Querol) and IN207514 (to Carlos Rosales) from Dirección General de Asuntos del Personal Académico, Universidad Nacional Autónoma de México, Mexico.

References

[1] A. Mócsai, "Diverse novel functions of neutrophils in immunity, inflammation, and beyond," *The Journal of Experimental Medicine*, vol. 210, no. 7, pp. 1283–1299, 2013.

[2] V. Brinkmann, U. Reichard, C. Goosmann et al., "Neutrophil extracellular traps kill bacteria," *Science*, vol. 303, no. 5663, pp. 1532–1535, 2004.

[3] B. G. Yipp, B. Petri, D. Salina et al., "Infection-induced NETosis is a dynamic process involving neutrophil multitasking in vivo," *Nature Medicine*, vol. 18, no. 9, pp. 1386–1393, 2012.

[4] T. A. Fuchs, U. Abed, C. Goosmann et al., "Novel cell death program leads to neutrophil extracellular traps," *Journal of Cell Biology*, vol. 176, no. 2, pp. 231–241, 2007.

[5] M. Bianchi, A. Hakkim, V. Brinkmann et al., "Restoration of NET formation by gene therapy in CGD controls aspergillosis," *Blood*, vol. 114, no. 13, pp. 2619–2622, 2009.

[6] Q. Remijsen, T. V. Berghe, E. Wirawan et al., "Neutrophil extracellular trap cell death requires both autophagy and superoxide generation," *Cell Research*, vol. 21, no. 2, pp. 290–304, 2011.

[7] I. Neeli and M. Radic, "Knotting the NETs: analyzing histone modifications in neutrophil extracellular traps," *Arthritis Research and Therapy*, vol. 14, article 115, 2012.

[8] H. Parker, M. Dragunow, M. B. Hampton, A. J. Kettle, and C. C. Winterbourn, "Requirements for NADPH oxidase and myeloperoxidase in neutrophil extracellular trap formation differ depending on the stimulus," *Journal of Leukocyte Biology*, vol. 92, no. 4, pp. 841–849, 2012.

[9] N. Branzk and V. Papayannopoulos, "Molecular mechanisms regulating NETosis in infection and disease," *Seminars in Immunopathology*, vol. 35, no. 4, pp. 513–530, 2013.

[10] V. Papayannopoulos and A. Zychlinsky, "NETs: a new strategy for using old weapons," *Trends in Immunology*, vol. 30, no. 11, pp. 513–521, 2009.

[11] C. Rosales and E. Uribe-Querol, "Antibody—Fc receptor interactions in antimicrobial functions," *Current Immunology Reviews*, vol. 9, no. 1, pp. 44–55, 2013.

[12] J. C. Unkeless, Z. Shen, C.-W. Lin, and E. DeBeus, "Function of human FcγRIIA and FcγRIIIB," *Seminars in Immunology*, vol. 7, no. 1, pp. 37–44, 1995.

[13] C. Rosales and E. Uribe-Querol, "Fc receptors: cell activators of antibody functions," *Advances in Bioscience and Biotechnology*, vol. 4, no. 4, pp. 21–33, 2013.

[14] P. Selvaraj, W. F. Rosse, R. Silber, and T. A. Springer, "The major Fc receptor in blood has a phosphatidylinositol anchor and is deficient in paroxysmal nocturnal haemoglobinuria," *Nature*, vol. 333, no. 6173, pp. 565–567, 1988.

[15] L. Marois, G. Paré, M. Vaillancourt, E. Rollet-Labelle, and P. H. Naccache, "FcγRIIIb triggers raft-dependent calcium influx in IgG-mediated responses in human neutrophils," *The Journal of Biological Chemistry*, vol. 286, no. 5, pp. 3509–3519, 2011.

[16] J. E. Salmon, N. L. Browle, J. C. Edberg, and R. P. Kimberly, "Fcγ receptor III induces actin polymerization in human neutrophils and primes phagocytosis mediated by Fcγ receptor II," *The Journal of Immunology*, vol. 146, no. 3, pp. 997–1004, 1991.

[17] A. Ortiz-Stern and C. Rosales, "FcγRIIIB stimulation promotes β1 integrin activation in human neutrophils," *Journal of Leukocyte Biology*, vol. 77, no. 5, pp. 787–799, 2005.

[18] E. García-García and C. Rosales, "Nuclear factor activation by FcγR in human peripheral blood neutrophils detected by a novel flow cytometry-based method," *Journal of Immunological Methods*, vol. 320, no. 1-2, pp. 104–118, 2007.

[19] I. Neeli, N. Dwivedi, S. Khan, and M. Radic, "Regulation of extracellular chromatin release from neutrophils," *Journal of Innate Immunity*, vol. 1, no. 3, pp. 194–201, 2009.

[20] I. Neeli, S. N. Khan, and M. Radic, "Histone deimination as a response to inflammatory stimuli in neutrophils," *The Journal of Immunology*, vol. 180, no. 3, pp. 1895–1902, 2008.

[21] A. K. Gupta, M. B. Joshi, M. Philippova et al., "Activated endothelial cells induce neutrophil extracellular traps and are susceptible to NETosis-mediated cell death," *FEBS Letters*, vol. 584, no. 14, pp. 3193–3197, 2010.

[22] K. Chen, H. Nishi, R. Travers et al., "Endocytosis of soluble immune complexes leads to their clearance by FcγRIIIB but induces neutrophil extracellular traps via FcγRIIA in vivo," *Blood*, vol. 120, no. 22, pp. 4421–4431, 2012.

[23] K. R. Short, M. von Köckritz-Blickwede, J. D. Langereis et al., "Antibodies mediate formation of neutrophil extracellular traps in the middle ear and facilitate secondary pneumococcal otitis media," *Infection and Immunity*, vol. 82, no. 1, pp. 364–370, 2014.

[24] M. Behnen, C. Leschczyk, S. Möller et al., "Immobilized immune complexes induce neutrophil extracellular trap release by human neutrophil granulocytes via FcγRIIIB and Mac-1," *Journal of Immunology*, vol. 193, no. 4, pp. 1954–1965, 2014.

[25] E. García-García, E. Uribe-Querol, and C. Rosales, "A simple and efficient method to detect nuclear factor activation in human neutrophils by flow cytometry," *Journal of Visualized Experiments*, no. 74, Article ID e50410, 2013.

[26] R. J. Looney, G. N. Abraham, and C. L. Anderson, "Human monocytes and U937 cells bear two distinct Fc receptors for IgG," *The Journal of Immunology*, vol. 136, no. 5, pp. 1641–1647, 1986.

[27] H. B. Fleit, S. D. Wright, and J. C. Unkeless, "Human neutrophil Fcγ receptor distribution and structure," *Proceedings of the National Academy of Sciences of the United States of America*, vol. 79, no. 10, pp. 3275–3279, 1982.

[28] V. Brinkmann, B. Laube, U. A. Abed, C. Goosmann, and A. Zychlinsky, "Neutrophil extracellular traps: how to generate and visualize them," *Journal of Visualized Experiments*, vol. 36, Article ID e1724, 2010.

[29] E. García-García, E. J. Brown, and C. Rosales, "Transmembrane mutations to FcγRIIA alter its association with lipid rafts: implications for receptor signaling," *The Journal of Immunology*, vol. 178, no. 5, pp. 3048–3058, 2007.

[30] S. Rivas-Fuentes, E. García-García, G. Nieto-Castañeda, and C. Rosales, "Fcγ receptors exhibit different phagocytosis potential

in human neutrophils," *Cellular Immunology*, vol. 263, no. 1, pp. 114–121, 2010.

[31] M. Reyes-Reyes, N. Mora, A. Zentella, and C. Rosales, "Phosphatidylinositol 3-kinase mediates integrin-dependent NF-κB and MAPK activation through separate signaling pathways," *Journal of Cell Science*, vol. 114, no. 8, pp. 1579–1589, 2001.

[32] J. F. Sweeney, P. K. Nguyen, G. M. Omann, and D. B. Hinshaw, "Ultraviolet irradiation accelerates apoptosis in human polymorphonuclear leukocytes: protection by LPS and GM-CSF," *Journal of Leukocyte Biology*, vol. 62, no. 4, pp. 517–523, 1997.

[33] J. T. McClave and T. T. Sincich, *Statistics*, Pearson, London, UK, 2012.

[34] C. H. Homburg, M. de Haas, A. E. von dem Borne, A. J. Verhoeven, C. P. Reutelingsperger, and D. Roos, "Human neutrophils lose their surface Fc gamma RIII and acquire Annexin V binding sites during apoptosis in vitro," *Blood*, vol. 85, no. 2, pp. 532–540, 1995.

[35] H. R. Luo and F. Loison, "Constitutive neutrophil apoptosis: mechanisms and regulation," *American Journal of Hematology*, vol. 83, no. 4, pp. 288–295, 2008.

[36] C. Akgul, D. A. Moulding, and S. W. Edwards, "Molecular control of neutrophil apoptosis," *FEBS Letters*, vol. 487, no. 3, pp. 318–322, 2001.

[37] A. Hakkim, T. A. Fuchs, N. E. Martinez et al., "Activation of the Raf-MEK-ERK pathway is required for neutrophil extracellular trap formation," *Nature Chemical Biology*, vol. 7, no. 2, pp. 75–77, 2011.

[38] E. García-García, G. Nieto-Castañeda, M. Ruiz-Saldaña, N. Mora, and C. Rosales, "FcγRIIA and FcγRIIIB mediate nuclear factor activation through separate signaling pathways in human neutrophils," *The Journal of Immunology*, vol. 182, no. 8, pp. 4547–4556, 2009.

[39] F. Y. S. Chuang, M. Sassaroli, and J. C. Unkeless, "Convergence of Fcγ receptor IIA and Fcγ receptor IIIB signaling pathways in human neutrophils," *Journal of Immunology*, vol. 164, no. 1, pp. 350–360, 2000.

[40] S. Patel, S. Kumar, A. Jyoti et al., "Nitric oxide donors release extracellular traps from human neutrophils by augmenting free radical generation," *Nitric Oxide*, vol. 22, no. 3, pp. 226–234, 2010.

[41] M. J. Lapponi, A. Carestia, V. I. Landoni et al., "Regulation of neutrophil extracellular trap formation by anti-inflammatory drugs," *Journal of Pharmacology and Experimental Therapeutics*, vol. 345, no. 3, pp. 430–437, 2013.

[42] E. Kolaczkowska and P. Kubes, "Neutrophil recruitment and function in health and inflammation," *Nature Reviews Immunology*, vol. 13, no. 3, pp. 159–175, 2013.

[43] K. Futosi, S. Fodor, and A. Mócsai, "Neutrophil cell surface receptors and their intracellular signal transduction pathways," *International Immunopharmacology*, vol. 17, no. 3, pp. 638–650, 2013.

[44] T. N. Mayadas, X. Cullere, and C. A. Lowell, "The multifaceted functions of neutrophils," *Annual Review of Pathology*, vol. 9, pp. 181–218, 2014.

[45] C. F. Urban, D. Ermert, M. Schmid et al., "Neutrophil extracellular traps contain calprotectin, a cytosolic protein complex involved in host defense against *Candida albicans*," *PLoS Pathogens*, vol. 5, no. 10, Article ID e1000639, 2009.

[46] E. Aleyd, M. W. M. van Hout, S. H. Ganzevles et al., "IgA enhances netosis and release of neutrophil extracellular traps by polymorphonuclear cells via FCα receptor I," *The Journal of Immunology*, vol. 192, no. 5, pp. 2374–2383, 2014.

[47] J. M. Kelley, P. A. Monach, C. Ji et al., "IgA and IgG antineutrophil cytoplasmic antibody engagement of Fc receptor genetic variants influences granulomatosis with polyangiitis," *Proceedings of the National Academy of Sciences of the United States of America*, vol. 108, no. 51, pp. 20736–20741, 2011.

[48] F. H. Pilsczek, D. Salina, K. K. H. Poon et al., "A novel mechanism of rapid nuclear neutrophil extracellular trap formation in response to *Staphylococcus aureus*," *The Journal of Immunology*, vol. 185, no. 12, pp. 7413–7425, 2010.

[49] I. Neeli and M. Radic, "Opposition between PKC isoforms regulates histone deimination and neutrophil extracellular chromatin release," *Frontiers in Immunology*, vol. 4, article 38, 2013.

[50] J. A. Van Ziffle and C. A. Lowell, "Neutrophil-specific deletion of Syk kinase results in reduced host defense to bacterial infection," *Blood*, vol. 114, no. 23, pp. 4871–4882, 2009.

[51] A. C. Newton, "Protein kinase C," *IUBMB life*, vol. 60, no. 11, pp. 765–768, 2008.

[52] O. Popa-Nita, S. Proulx, G. Paré, E. Rollet-Labelle, and P. H. Naccache, "Crystal-induced neutrophil activation. XI. Implication and novel roles of classical protein kinase C," *Journal of Immunology*, vol. 183, no. 3, pp. 2104–2114, 2009.

[53] V. Jancinova, T. Perecko, R. Nosal, K. Svitekova, and K. Drabikova, "The natural stilbenoid piceatannol decreases activity and accelerates apoptosis of human neutrophils: involvement of protein kinase C," *Oxidative Medicine and Cellular Longevity*, vol. 2013, Article ID 136539, 8 pages, 2013.

[54] R. S. Keshari, A. Verma, M. K. Barthwal, and M. Dikshit, "Reactive oxygen species-induced activation of ERK and p38 MAPK mediates PMA-induced NETs release from human neutrophils," *Journal of Cellular Biochemistry*, vol. 114, no. 3, pp. 532–540, 2013.

[55] M. J. Zhou and E. J. Brown, "CR3 (Mac-1, αMβ2, CD11b/CD18) and FcγRIII cooperate in generation of a neutrophil respiratory burst: requirement for FcγRIII and tyrosine phosphorylation," *The Journal of Cell Biology*, vol. 125, pp. 1407–1416, 1994.

[56] A. S. Byrd, X. M. O'Brien, C. M. Johnson, L. M. Lavigne, and J. S. Reichner, "An extracellular matrix-based mechanism of rapid neutrophil extracellular trap formation in response to *Candida albicans*," *The Journal of Immunology*, vol. 190, no. 8, pp. 4136–4148, 2013.

[57] E. Gillenius and C. F. Urban, "The adhesive protein invasin of *Yersinia pseudotuberculosis* induces neutrophil extracellular traps via β1 integrins," *Microbes and Infection*, vol. 17, no. 5, pp. 327–336, 2015.

[58] N. Branzk, A. Lubojemska, S. E. Hardison et al., "Neutrophils sense microbe size and selectively release neutrophil extracellular traps in response to large pathogens," *Nature Immunology*, vol. 15, no. 11, pp. 1017–1025, 2014.

[59] M. F. Tosi and M. Berger, "Functional differences between the 40 kDa and 50 to 70 kDa IgG Fc receptors on human neutrophils revealed by elastase treatment and antireceptor antibodies," *The Journal of Immunology*, vol. 141, no. 6, pp. 2097–2103, 1988.

[60] S. Nagarajan, K. Venkiteswaran, M. Anderson, U. Sayed, C. Zhu, and P. Selvaraj, "Cell-specific, activation-dependent regulation of neutrophil CD32A ligand-binding function," *Blood*, vol. 95, no. 3, pp. 1069–1077, 2000.

20

Heparin Interaction with the Primed Polymorphonuclear Leukocyte CD11b Induces Apoptosis and Prevents Cell Activation

Meital Cohen-Mazor,[1,2] **Rafi Mazor,**[1,2] **Batya Kristal,**[2,3] **Erik B. Kistler,**[4] **Inbal Ziv,**[1,2] **Judith Chezar,**[5] **and Shifra Sela**[1,2]

[1]*Eliachar Research Laboratory, Western Galilee Hospital, 22100 Nahariya, Israel*
[2]*Technion Faculty of Medicine, 3525433 Haifa, Israel*
[3]*Department of Nephrology and Hypertension, Western Galilee Hospital, 22100 Nahariya, Israel*
[4]*Department of Anesthesiology & Critical Care, VA San Diego Healthcare System, San Diego, CA 92161, USA*
[5]*Hematology Laboratory, Western Galilee Hospital, 22100 Nahariya, Israel*

Correspondence should be addressed to Rafi Mazor; mazrafi@gmail.com

Academic Editor: Eileen Uribe-Querol

Heparin is known to have anti-inflammatory effects, yet the mechanisms are not completely understood. In this study, we tested the hypothesis that heparin has a direct effect on activated polymorphonuclear leukocytes (PMNLs), changing their activation state, and can explain its anti-inflammatory effect. To test our hypothesis, we designed both *in vitro* and *ex vivo* studies to elucidate the mechanism by which heparin modulates PMNL functions and therefore the inflammatory response. We specifically tested the hypothesis that priming of PMNLs renders them more susceptible to heparin. Amplified levels of CD11b and increased rate of superoxide release manifested PMNL priming. Increase in cell priming resulted in a dose-dependent increase in heparin binding to PMNLs followed by augmented apoptosis. Blocking antibodies to CD11b inhibited heparin binding and abolished the apoptotic response. Moreover, heparin caused a significant dose-dependent decrease in the rate of superoxide release from PMNLs, which was blunted by blocking antibodies to CD11b. Altogether, this study shows that the interaction of heparin with the PMNL CD11b results in cell apoptosis and explains heparin's anti-inflammatory effects.

1. Introduction

In many inflammatory responses, polymorphonuclear leukocytes (PMNLs) are among the first cells to exit the blood stream and migrate to an inflammatory site, where they become fully activated. This activation is a two-stage process: PMNLs first encounter a stimulus that does not activate the cells directly but leaves them in a "primed" state. Then, upon encountering a second stimulus in the inflamed site, the transition into a fully activated state will occur [1, 2]. This process involves the production of free radicals and release of granule enzymes into the surrounding milieu. Therefore, tight regulation of PMNL activation is needed throughout the steps of infiltration from the blood stream to the inflamed

site in order to prevent damage to the vascular wall and the extracellular matrix (ECM).

One of the ECM components is heparin (in the form of heparan sulfate), a soluble molecule that plays a major role in defining the physical and chemical properties of the ECM [3]. Heparin, which is commonly used as a blood anticoagulant, is also known to have anti-inflammatory effects; however, the mechanism of these biological activities remains largely unknown [4, 5]. Some of heparin's anti-inflammatory effects are mediated through the modulation of cellular activation, particularly of PMNLs [6–9]. Heparin decreases phorbol myristate acetate (PMA), *N*-formyl-methionyl-leucyl-phenylalanine (fMLP), and opsonized zymosan-induced superoxide production [7], a decrease which is even greater when the PMNLs are primed by platelet activating factor (PAF) [9]. Heparin reduces fMLP-stimulated PMNL adhesion to endothelial cells and decreases the release of beta-glucuronidase and lysozyme from stimulated PMNLs [6]. In addition, heparin has been shown to inhibit leukocyte recruitment and chemotaxis in response to zymosan-activated serum [10].

Recently, it was shown that immobilized heparin can mediate cell adhesion via interaction with the PMNL integrin Mac-1 (CD11b/CD18, $\alpha_M\beta_2$) [11]. Mac-1 is one of the most versatile adhesion molecules, with ligands of various biological functions. One of these functions is the induction of a signal transduction cascade that substantially augments apoptosis of activated PMNLs [12].

The above data, especially the known apoptotic effect of heparin on PMNLs [13, 14], led us to hypothesize that priming of PMNLs renders them more susceptible to the apoptotic effects of heparin and that apoptosis induced by heparin is mediated in part by heparin interactions with CD11b, which is highly expressed on the surface of primed PMNLs [15]. In order to test our hypothesis, we used PMNLs isolated from hemodialysis (HD) patients as a model of *in vivo* primed cells [16] and PMNLs isolated from healthy controls (NC) primed *ex vivo* with PAF. Our results indicate that primed PMNLs, regardless of their priming origin (*ex vivo* or *in vivo*), are more susceptible to the apoptotic effect of heparin compared to nonprimed PMNLs. We also show that heparin binds to CD11b, leading to apoptosis that can be blocked with neutralizing antibodies against CD11b.

2. Methods

2.1. Patients and Blood Samples.
Blood was drawn from 17 patients on chronic hemodialysis and 24 age- and gender-matched healthy control subjects (NC). Blood for the determination of biochemical and hematological parameters and for the isolation of PMNLs was drawn after an overnight fast. Blood was collected into citrate tubes from the arterial line of all the HD patients immediately before a dialysis session. All patients underwent hemodialysis three times a week; each dialysis treatment lasted 4 hours and was carried out with low flux polysulfone membranes (F8, Fresenius Medical Care, Bad Homburg, Germany). The water for dialysis met the standards of the Association for the Advancement of Medical Instrumentation (AAMI). Patients with evidence of acute or chronic infection or malignancy or who had received blood transfusion within 3 months prior to blood sampling were excluded. All participants signed an informed consent for blood sampling, and the study was approved by the Institutional Committee in accordance with the Helsinki declaration.

2.2. PMNL Isolation and Analysis.
PMNLs were isolated as described previously [17]. Isolated PMNLs (>98% pure, approximately 10^7 cells per isolation) were resuspended and counted in phosphate buffered saline (PBS, Beit Haemek, Israel) containing 0.1% glucose. PMNL priming was assessed by the rate of superoxide release [17] and by the surface levels of CD11b, as described previously [15]. The rate of superoxide release was determined after cell stimulation with 0.32×10^{-7} M phorbol 12-myristate 13-acetate (PMA; Sigma, St. Louis, MO). The assay is based on superoxide dismutase (SOD) inhibitable reduction of 80 μM cytochrome C (Sigma, St. Louis, MO) to its ferrous form. The change in optical density was monitored at 549 nm, as described previously [17]. Expression of CD11b on PMNLs in whole blood was determined using the FC500 flow cytometer (Beckman-Coulter). 50 μL of blood was incubated for 10 min with anti-CD11b-PE conjugated monoclonal antibody (Immunotech, Marseille, France), followed by red blood cell lysis (Q-prep method; Coulter Corporation, Hialeah, FL, USA). To enable gating on the PMNL population, anti-CD16, conjugated to PC5 monoclonal antibody (IQ Products), was used. Surface levels of CD11b on PMNLs are expressed as mean fluorescence intensity (MFI), after subtracting the nonspecific background.

2.3. Priming of PMNLs by Platelet Activating Factor (PAF).
PAF (Sigma, USA), a known dose-dependent priming agent of PMNLs [18], was used for the *in vitro* priming of NC PMNLs in three concentrations: 1 pM, 1 nM, and 1 μM. Cells were incubated with PAF for 15 minutes at room temperature and then washed with PBS. In PAF-stimulated PMNLs where CD11b intensity was measured and in experiments where CD11b was blocked, 5 minutes after the initiation of incubation with PAF, mouse anti-human-CD11b-PE was added. CD11b expression was measured as described above for whole blood, but without the lysis step.

2.4. Effect of Heparin on PMNLs.
The effect of heparin was studied on three types of isolated PMNLs: normal control (NC) PMNLs, PAF-stimulated NC PMNLs, and HD PMNLs. All cells were incubated for 30 min at room temperature with 25, 50, and 100 U/mL sodium heparin (Kamada, Beit Kama, Israel) diluted in PBS. In order to measure time-dependent effects of heparin, NC and HD PMNLs were incubated with 100 U/mL sodium heparin for 300 min at room temperature.

2.5. Analysis of PMNL Apoptosis.
The percentage of apoptotic PMNLs was based on Annexin-V-FITC binding according to the manufacturer's recommendations (Annexin-V/FITC Kit, Bender MedSystems Diagnostics GmbH, Vienna, Austria). Annexin-V-FITC and propidium iodide (PI) were added to the cell suspension and incubated for 10 min in the dark at room temperature. PI staining is a dye-exclusion assay that discriminates between cells with intact membranes (PI negative) and permeabilized membranes (PI positive) [19]. The cell population showing Annexin-V−/PI− was considered viable; Annexin-V+/PI− was considered as an early apoptotic population. Late stage apoptotic or necrotic cells were represented by the Annexin-V+/PI+ population [19].

2.6. Analysis of PMNL Apoptosis after Preincubation with Anti-CD11b.
Separated PMNLs (5×10^5) were incubated with anti-CD11b-PE or its isotype control- (IC-) PE for 10 minutes, washed, and incubated for 30 minutes with 25 U/mL heparin. This dose of heparin was chosen since it is the minimal dose

that caused a statistically significant difference in apoptosis between primed and nonprimed PMNLs. Apoptosis in PMNLs was detected using the following: (A) Annexin-V-FITC binding was measured as mentioned above without the addition of PI. The percentage of apoptotic cells was compared with apoptosis detected using FITC-labeled Annexin-V, added after preincubation with IC-PE (Immunotech, Marseille, France). The positive cutoff point was determined by FITC-isotype controls (IQ Products, Netherlands), added after preincubation with IC-PE. (B) PMNLs (5×10^6) were cytospinned and apoptosis was detected with an Axioscop 2 upright fluorescence microscope, using the *In Situ* Cell Death detection kit (TUNEL staining, Roche Molecular Biochemicals). Nuclear staining was done with 5 μg/mL Hoechst (Calbiochem).

2.7. PMNL Viability. Cells (2×10^6) were incubated at room temperature for 0, 30, and 90 minutes in PBS with and without heparin (100 U/mL), stained with trypan blue solution (0.4% in HBSS), and counted.

2.8. Heparin Binding to PMNLs. Separated PMNLs (5×10^5) were incubated with anti-CD11b-PE or its isotype control for 10 minutes, washed, and assayed for heparin binding by two different methods: (A) the PMNLs were further incubated with 25 U/mL sodium heparin. The percentage of PMNLs that bound heparin and the intensity of heparin binding to PMNLs were determined by flow cytometry using mouse anti-human heparan sulfate-FITC (United States Biological, Massachusetts). The Ab was generated by immunization with liposome-intercalated membrane HS proteoglycans and recognizes an epitope present in many types of human heparan sulfate including heparin. The epitope includes N-sulfated glucosamine residues that are critical for the reactivity of the antibody. The Ab does not react with hyaluronan, chondroitin sulfate, dermatan sulfate, keratan sulfate, or DNA [20, 21]. The positive cutoff point was determined by FITC-isotype control (IQ Products, Netherlands), added after preincubation with anti-CD11b-PE. The percentage of heparin bound cells and the intensity of heparin binding to PMNLs detected in this experiment were compared with cells detected using FITC-labeled anti-heparan sulfate, added after preincubation with IC-PE (Immunotech, Marseille, France). The positive cutoff point was determined by FITC-isotype controls (IQ Products, Netherlands), added after preincubation with IC-PE. (B) The PMNLs were further incubated with 25 U/mL FITC-labeled heparin (Molecular Probes, Eugene, OR) in PBS for 30 minutes at room temperature. The intensity of heparin binding to PMNLs was determined by FC500 flow cytometer (Beckman-Coulter).

2.9. Statistical Analysis. Data are expressed as mean ± SD. In the box and whiskers presentations, the horizontal line in the middle shows the median (50th percentile), the top and bottom of the box indicate the 75th and 25th percentiles, respectively, and the whiskers show the maximum and the minimum values. The nonparametric Mann-Whitney test

was used for comparing two independent groups. The two-paired Wilcoxon Signed Ranks test was used for comparing two dependent groups. Statistical significance was considered at $P < 0.05$.

3. Results

3.1. PMNL Priming. PMNL priming was manifested by increased rates of superoxide release and amplified levels of membrane CD11b [16–18]. Preincubation of isolated normal control (NC) PMNLs with increasing concentrations of PAF caused a dose-dependent increase in the rate of superoxide release from PMA-stimulated PMNLs ([*]$P < 0.05$, Figure 1(a)). In addition, the expression of CD11b was higher in PAF-treated NC PMNLs compared to nontreated NC PMNLs ([*]$P < 0.05$, Figure 1(b)).

We reported previously that PMNLs from hemodialysis (HD) patients are primed [15]. To confirm these results, we isolated HD PMNLs and measured their priming. The rate of superoxide release following PMA stimulation was higher in PMNLs isolated from HD patients compared to PAF untreated NC cells (33.5 ± 4 versus 24.7 ± 5 nmoles/10^6 cells/10 min, resp., [*]$P < 0.05$, Figure 1(a)) and was similar to the rate achieved by stimulation with the highest concentration of PAF. The expression of CD11b was also higher in HD PMNLs than in NC PMNLs (61 ± 25 versus 29 ± 11 MFI, resp., [*]$P < 0.05$, Figure 1(b)) and comparable to the levels measured in NC cells stimulated with the highest concentration of PAF.

3.2. Dose-Dependent Effect of Heparin on PMNL Apoptosis and Priming. We have previously reported that heparin exerts an apoptotic effect on PMNLs [13]. To determine whether primed PMNLs are differently affected by heparin compared to nonprimed cells, we exposed 3 groups of PMNLs: NC, 1 μM PAF-stimulated NC, and HD PMNLs, to increasing concentrations of heparin for 30 min (Figure 2). We used 1 μM PAF-stimulated NC since the rate of superoxide release and the expression of CD11b on these *ex vivo* primed cells were similar to *in vivo* primed cells, isolated from HD patients (Figure 1). Incubation of PMNLs with increasing concentrations of heparin resulted in an increase in early apoptosis in all three groups, however to a much greater extent in HD PMNLs (Figure 2(b)). The increase in HD PMNL apoptosis was significant at all heparin concentrations versus without heparin ($P < 0.05$), while in NC PMNLs and PAF-stimulated NC PMNLs significance was achieved only at 100 U/mL of heparin ($P < 0.05$). Moreover, the maximal percentage of early apoptotic PMNLs was 8% in NC and 10% in PAF-stimulated NC whereas 17% apoptotic cells were detected in HD PMNLs.

Incubation of PMNLs with increasing concentrations of heparin caused a significant increase in apoptosis (early + late) in all three groups of PMNLs, however to a much greater extent in PAF-stimulated NC and HD PMNLs with both groups showing similar dose-dependent responses (Figure 2(c)). The increased degree of apoptosis in PAF-stimulated NC and HD PMNLs was significant at all heparin concentrations versus without heparin ($P < 0.05$), while in

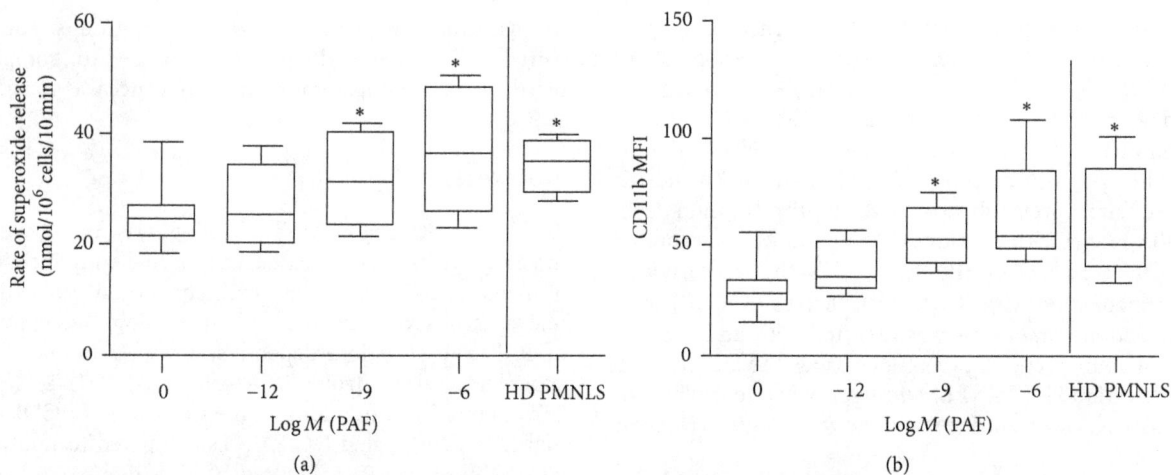

FIGURE 1: PMNL priming. (a) Rates of superoxide release from separated NC PMNLs after 15 min of stimulation by 1 pM, 1 nM, and 1 μM PAF and HD PMNLs activated with 0.32×10^{-7} M PMA. The changes in optical density were monitored at 549 nm continuously up to 10 min in the presence of 0.08 mM cytochrome C. Data are expressed as nmoles/10^6 cells/10 min; $^*P < 0.05$ for HD and PAF stimulated (10^{-9} M and 10^{-6} M) versus nonstimulated NC PMNLs (no PAF), $n = 10$. (b) Relative expression of surface CD11b on PMNLs measured by flow cytometry using specific PE-labeled antibody, as described in Section 2. Data are expressed as mean fluorescent intensity (MFI); $^*P < 0.05$ for HD and PAF stimulated (10^{-9} M and 10^{-6} M) versus nonstimulated NC PMNLs (no PAF), $n = 10$.

NC PMNLs significance was detected only at 100 U/mL of heparin ($P < 0.05$).

The effect of heparin on PAF-stimulated NC and HD PMNLs was much greater than its effect on NC PMNLs ($P < 0.05$ NC versus HD and PAF-stimulated NC at all heparin concentrations). The maximal percentage of apoptotic PMNLs in NC was only 14%, whereas 22% apoptotic cells were detected in PAF-stimulated NC and HD PMNLs.

Priming is also reflected by the rate of superoxide release from PMA-activated PMNLs. To determine whether apoptosis induced by heparin modulates activation of primed PMNLs, we investigated the dose-dependent effect of heparin on the rate of superoxide release. A significant reduction in the rate of superoxide release was observed in all groups of PMNLs ($P < 0.05$ for all heparin concentrations versus no heparin; Figure 2(d)). Moreover, PAF-stimulated NC and HD PMNLs showed lower rates of superoxide release versus NC PMNLs.

The decreased rate of superoxide release was maximized at heparin concentrations of 25 U/mL for NC PMNLs and 50 U/mL for 1 μM PAF-stimulated NC and HD PMNLs. This result suggests that the effect of heparin is greater with increased priming; the maximal inhibition in the rate of superoxide release from primed PMNLs was approximately three times higher than in unprimed cells.

3.3. Time-Dependent Effect of Heparin on PMNLs.

To determine whether heparin exerts a similar time-dependent apoptotic effect on primed versus quiescent cells, we incubated NC and HD PMNLs with 100 U/mL of heparin up to 300 min (Figure 3). We used 100 U/mL of heparin as it was the only heparin concentration that induced apoptosis in NC PMNLs (Figures 2(b) and 2(c)). Heparin induced early apoptosis in both HD and NC PMNLs at all time points during the incubation, while without heparin, these cells did not exhibit

enhanced early apoptosis at any time point (Figure 3(a)). Moreover, heparin caused an oscillatory apoptotic pattern of HD and NC PMNLs reaching apoptotic peaks at 30 and 210 min for HD PMNLs and 90 and 210 min for NC PMNLs. When detecting total apoptosis (early + late), the oscillatory apoptotic patterns of HD and NC PMNLs were similar regarding the apoptotic peaks, but with an augmented percentage of apoptotic cells at all points (Figure 3(b)). To test whether the oscillatory pattern could be explained by the loss of apoptotic cells in the *ex vivo* incubation, we counted the NC and HD PMNLs with and without heparin up to 90 min. This assay revealed that during the 30 min of incubation most of the cells (NC, HD) were still alive, while after 90 min a significant decrease in HD PMNL count was found (Figure 3(c)).

Based on these results, all incubation experiments were for 30 minutes to avoid significant cell disintegration *in vitro*.

3.4. The Effect of Priming on Heparin Binding to PMNLs.

PAF stimulation resulted in a dose-dependent increase in heparin binding to PMNLs (Figures 4(a)–4(c)). Pretreatment of PAF-stimulated PMNLs with anti-CD11b antibodies completely prevented heparin binding to PMNLs, indicating that heparin binds to PMNLs, at least partially, via CD11b (Figure 4(c)). These results were confirmed by additional studies using heparin that was conjugated to FITC. Heparin binding intensity to unstimulated NC PMNLs was 6.22 ± 0.19 MFI and increased to 13.15 ± 1.76 MFI after stimulation with 1 μM PAF, demonstrating increased heparin binding with increased priming. Pretreatment of PAF-stimulated PMNLs with anti-CD11b antibodies completely prevented heparin binding to PMNLs with heparin-FITC intensity reduced to 6.48 ± 0.57 MFI.

In a second set of experiments depicted in Figure 4(d), FITC-conjugated anti-heparin antibodies were used to detect

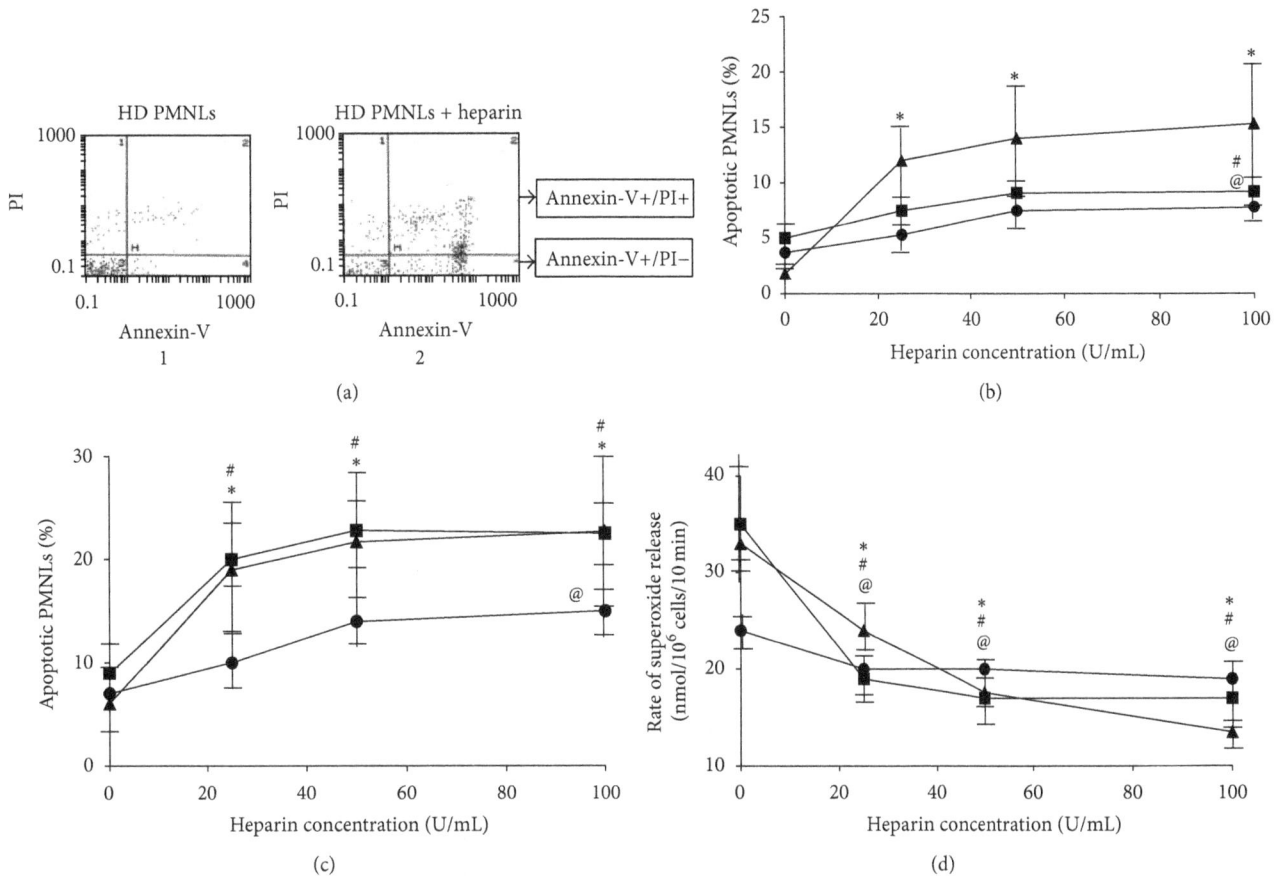

FIGURE 2: Dose-dependent effect of heparin on PMNL apoptosis and priming. (a) Representative histograms for apoptosis of HD PMNLs without heparin (1) and with 100 U/mL heparin (2) based on Annexin-V-FITC and PI binding. Cell populations: Annexin-V−/PI−, Annexin-V+/PI−, and Annexin-V+/PI+ were regarded as alive, early apoptotic, and late apoptotic or necrotic, respectively. (b) Early apoptosis (Annexin-V+/PI−) in NC PMNLs without stimulation (●) and after 15 min stimulation with 1 μM PAF (■) and HD PMNLs (▲). Cells were preincubated with PAF, washed, and incubated with increasing concentrations of heparin for 30 min. Apoptosis was determined by flow cytometer analysis, using a commercial kit for detection of Annexin-V as described in Section 2. Data are expressed as percentage of apoptotic PMNLs; $n = 10$. *$P < 0.05$ for HD at 25, 50, and 100 U/mL heparin versus no heparin. #$P < 0.05$ for NC pretreated with 1 μM PAF incubated with 100 U/mL heparin versus no heparin. @$P < 0.05$ for NC at 100 U/mL heparin versus no heparin. (c) Early and late (total) apoptosis (sum of Annexin-V+/PI− and Annexin-V+/PI+) in NC PMNLs without stimulation (●) and after 15 min stimulation with 1 μM PAF (■) and HD PMNLs (▲). *$P < 0.05$ for HD at 25, 50, and 100 U/mL heparin versus no heparin. #$P < 0.05$ for NC pretreated with 1 μM PAF incubated with 25, 50, and 100 U/mL heparin versus no heparin. @$P < 0.05$ for NC at 100 U/mL heparin versus no heparin. (d) Superoxide release from NC PMNLs without stimulation (●) and after 15 min stimulation with 1 μM PAF (■) and HD PMNLs (▲). Following preincubation with PAF, cells were washed and incubated with increasing concentrations of heparin for 30 min. The rate of superoxide release was determined after cells activation with 0.32×10^{-7} M PMA. The changes in optical density were monitored at 549 nm continuously in the presence of 0.08 mM cytochrome C. Data are represented by nmoles/10^6 cells/10 min; $n = 10$. *$P < 0.05$ for HD at 25, 50, and 100 U/mL heparin versus no heparin. #$P < 0.05$ for NC pretreated with 1 μM PAF incubated with 25, 50, and 100 U/mL heparin versus no heparin. @$P < 0.05$ for NC at 25, 50, and 100 U/mL heparin versus no heparin.

the percentage of PAF-stimulated PMNLs which bound heparin. The more primed the PMNLs, the higher the percentage of cells that bound heparin. This binding was also prevented by preincubation with anti-CD11b antibodies applied before the addition of heparin (Figure 4(d)). These results indicate that heparin binding is mediated by CD11b and that the higher the priming state is, the more the heparin binds to PMNLs.

3.5. The Effect of Priming on Apoptosis Induced by Heparin. PAF-stimulated NC PMNLs showed increased apoptosis dependent on the cell priming state when incubated with heparin (Figures 5(a) and 5(b)) and apoptosis was increased concomitantly with increases in cell priming. Anti-CD11b which prevents the binding of heparin to PMNLs abolished the apoptotic effect of heparin at all PAF concentrations (Figure 5(b)). In addition, anti-CD11b also prevented the binding of heparin to primed PMNLs isolated from HD patients and almost completely abolished the apoptosis induced by heparin (Figure 5(b)).

The effect of 25 U/mL heparin on apoptosis of NC PMNLs was also examined before and following the stimulation with 1 μM PAF, using the TUNEL assay. Representative results are shown in Figure 5(c). Very few apoptotic cells (with green

(a)

(b)

(c)

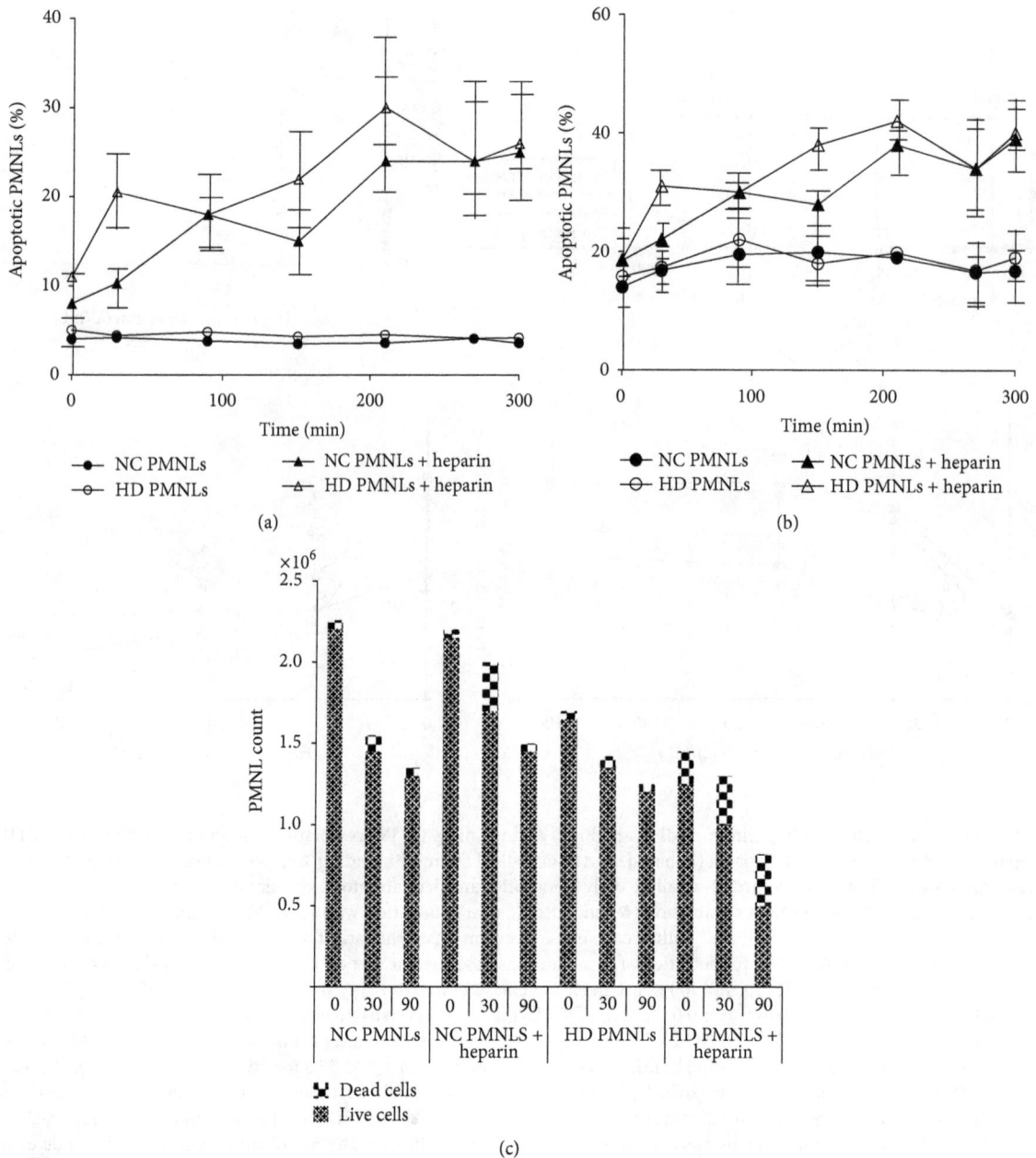

FIGURE 3: ((a), (b)) Early and total apoptosis (resp.) in PMNLs separated from NC (▲) and HD (△) after incubation with 100 U/mL of heparin for 300 min. The results of NC (●) and HD (○) represent the apoptotic levels throughout 300 min without heparin. Apoptosis was determined by flow cytometry using specific FITC-labeled Annexin-V, as described in Section 2. Data are expressed as percentage of apoptotic PMNLs; $n = 7$. (c) PMNL count using trypan blue exclusion assay: NC and HD PMNLs were incubated with 0 and 100 U/mL of heparin for 0, 30, and 90 minutes. Data is expressed as cells counts; $n = 3$.

nuclei, ~2%) were observed in NC PMNLs (Figure 5(c)(1)) and NC PMNLs stimulated by PAF (Figure 5(c)(2)) without exposure to heparin. When NC PMNLs were exposed to 25 U/mL heparin, the percentage of apoptotic cells increased to $6 \pm 2\%$, together with 25% cell loss (Figure 5(c)(3)). When PAF-stimulated NC PMNLs were exposed to 25 U/mL heparin, the percentage of apoptotic cells increased to approximately $22 \pm 5\%$ (Figure 5(c)(4)), concomitantly with 65% cell disappearance. Exposure of the cells to anti-CD11b-PE antibodies prior to the addition of heparin

completely abolished the apoptotic effects of heparin and cell disappearance (Figures 5(c)(5) and 5(c)(6)) on both NC PMNLs and NC PMNLs stimulated by PAF. Under the same conditions, exposure to isotype-controls- (IC-) PE (instead of to anti-CD11b-PE) did not prevent the apoptotic effects of heparin and cell disappearance (Figures 5(c)(7) and 5(c)(8)). These results clearly demonstrate that heparin-mediated apoptosis depends on PMNL priming.

In order to detect whether exposure of the cells to heparin causes loss of primed PMNLs, we further stained the

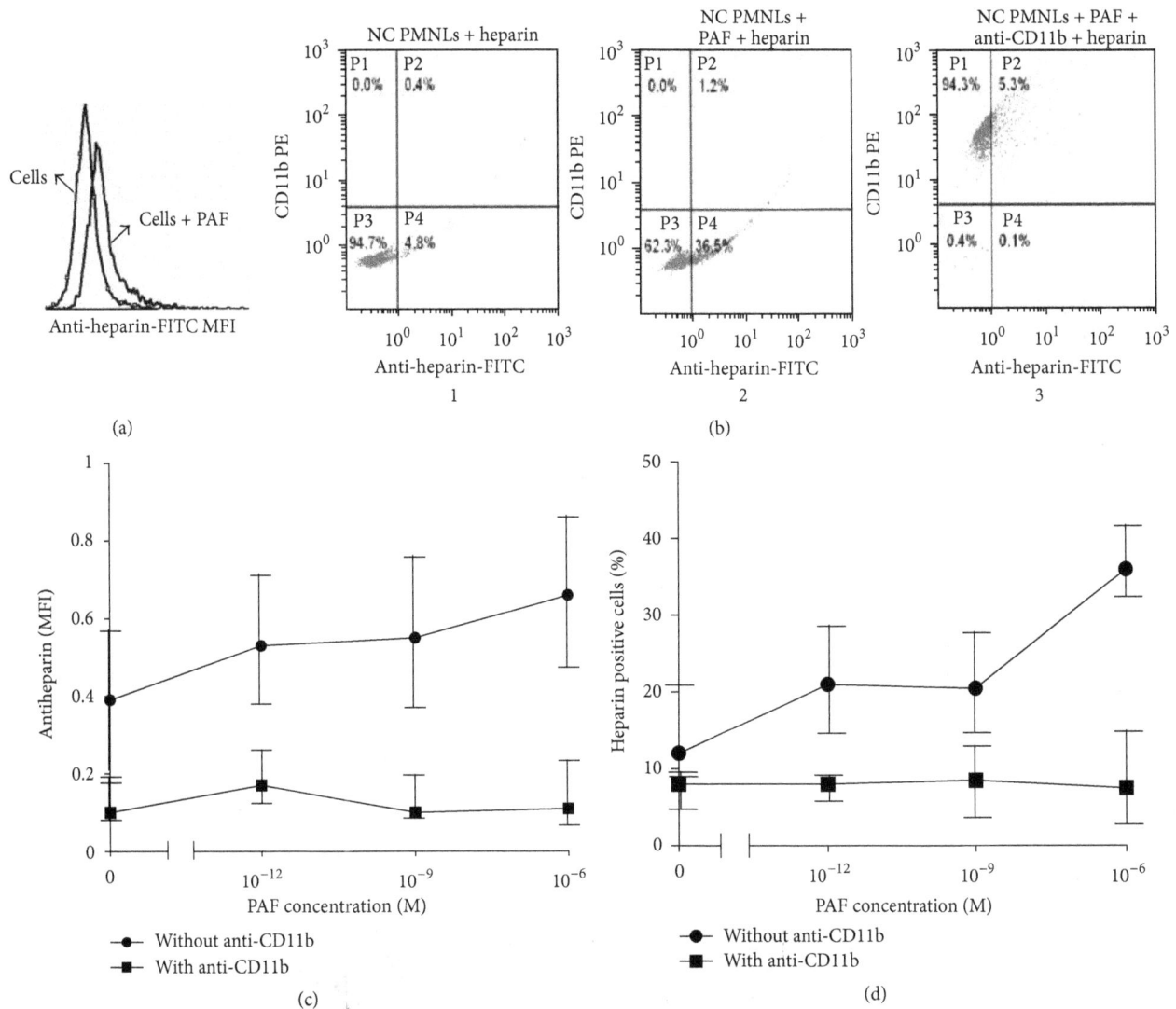

FIGURE 4: The effect of priming on heparin binding to PMNLs. (a) A representative histogram of flow cytometry, showing heparin binding intensity in NC PMNLs and NC PMNLs stimulated with 10^{-6} M PAF. (b) Representative histograms of flow cytometry showing percentage of heparin binding cells after incubation with 25 U/mL heparin for 30 min: NC PMNLs without PAF stimulation (1), NC PMNLs with 10^{-6} M PAF stimulation (2), and NC PMNLs with 10^{-6} M PAF stimulation and exposure to anti-CD11b-PE antibody (3). ((c), (d)) Levels of heparin bound to NC PMNLs (MFI) and percent of NC PMNLs that bind heparin, respectively, after preincubation with increasing concentration of PAF, determined by flow cytometry using specific FITC-labeled anti-heparin antibody, as described in Section 2 (●). Levels of heparin bound to PMNLs were also measured after preincubation of the cells with anti-CD11b antibodies (■) before the incubation with heparin ($n = 3$).

PAF-primed PMNLs with anti-CD11b-PE (Figure 6). Thirty percent of the PAF-treated cells that were not exposed to heparin showed elevated levels of CD11b, supporting their primed state. When these cells were exposed to heparin, no primed PMNLs or decreases in cell count could be seen.

3.6. The Effect of Anti-CD11b on Superoxide Release in the Presence of Heparin. Since heparin causes a decrease in superoxide release (Figure 2(d)) and at the same time it induces apoptosis via CD11b, it was interesting to find out whether blocking CD11b would have an effect on superoxide release. PAF-stimulated NC PMNLs incubated with IC showed increased

rates of superoxide release which were dependent on the extent of the cell priming: the greater the priming state, the greater the rate of superoxide release (PMNLs; Figure 7). Heparin (25 U/mL) prevented this increase in superoxide release (PMNLs + heparin; Figure 7). PAF-stimulated NC PMNLs, incubated with anti-CD11b but not with heparin, showed a similar increased rate of superoxide release as with IC, which was also dependent on the extent of the cell priming (PMNLs + anti-CD11b; Figure 7). When anti-CD11b was added to PMNLs prior to the incubation of the cells with heparin (PMNLs + anti-CD11b + heparin), the effect of heparin in terms of inhibition of superoxide release was abolished (Figure 7).

(a)

(b)

(c)

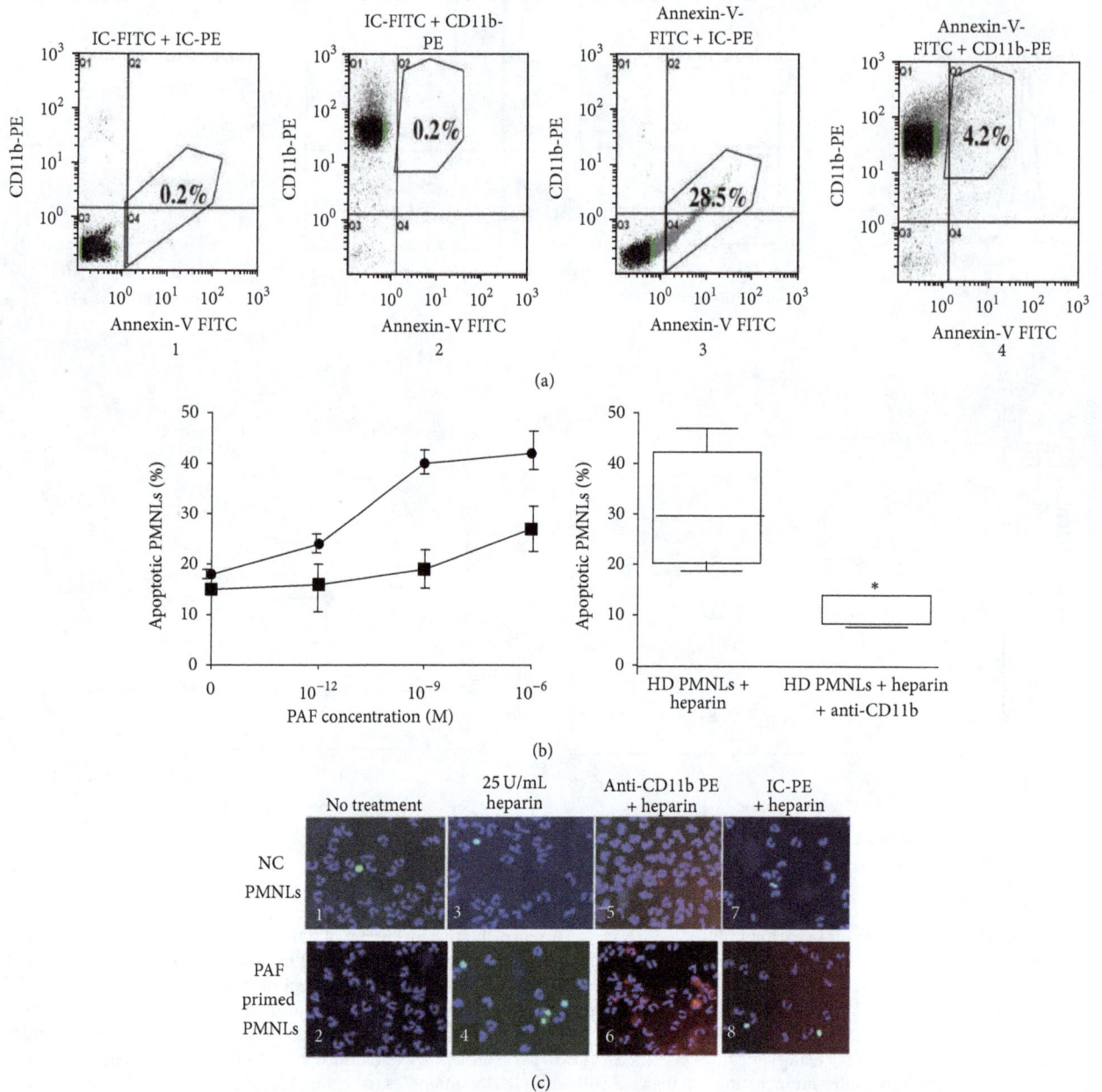

Figure 5: The effect of priming on apoptosis induced by heparin. (a) Representative histograms of flow cytometry showing the percentage of apoptotic cells after incubation with 25 U/mL heparin for 30 min: HD PMNLs with IC-FITC and IC-PE (1), HD PMNLs with IC-FITC and anti-CD11b-PE antibody (2), HD PMNLs with Annexin-V-FITC and IC-PE (3), and HD PMNLs with Annexin-V-FITC and anti-CD11b-PE antibody (4). (b) Apoptosis in NC PMNLs (●) after 15 min stimulation with increasing concentrations of PAF. Cells were preincubated with PAF, washed, and subjected to 30 min incubation with 25 U/mL heparin. Apoptosis was determined by flow cytometer analysis, using Annexin-V commercial kit as described in Section 2. Data are expressed as percentage of apoptotic PMNLs; $n = 3$. In addition, the percentage of apoptotic NC PMNLs that bind heparin was also measured after preincubation of NC separated PMNLs with PAF and anti-CD11b antibodies (■), before heparin incubation. The boxes and whiskers presentations represent apoptosis in HD PMNLs incubated with 25 U/mL heparin for 30 min, with and without incubation with anti-CD11b antibodies. (c) Apoptosis in NC PMNLs (upper left panel 1) and 15 min after stimulation with 10^{-6} M PAF (lower left panel 2). These cells were treated with 25 U/mL heparin for 30 min (panels 3 and 4). Apoptosis was evaluated by the TUNEL method (FITC green staining). Nuclei were stained with Hoechst reagent (blue staining). The percent of apoptotic NC PMNLs that bind heparin was measured after preincubation of the PMNLs with anti-CD11b antibodies (red staining) (panels 5 and 6) or IC-PE antibodies (red staining) (panels 7 and 8) before incubation with heparin. Quantification of apoptosis: over 300 cells were counted, from at least three independent experiments.

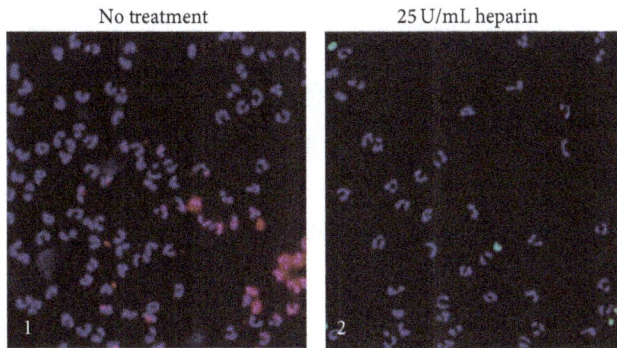

FIGURE 6: CD11b expression on primed PMNLs. CD11b expression on NC PMNLs after 15 min stimulation with 10^{-6} M PAF without an additional treatment (1) and with 30 min incubation with 25 U/mL heparin (2). Apoptosis was evaluated by the TUNEL method (FITC green staining). Nuclei were stained with Hoechst reagent (blue staining).

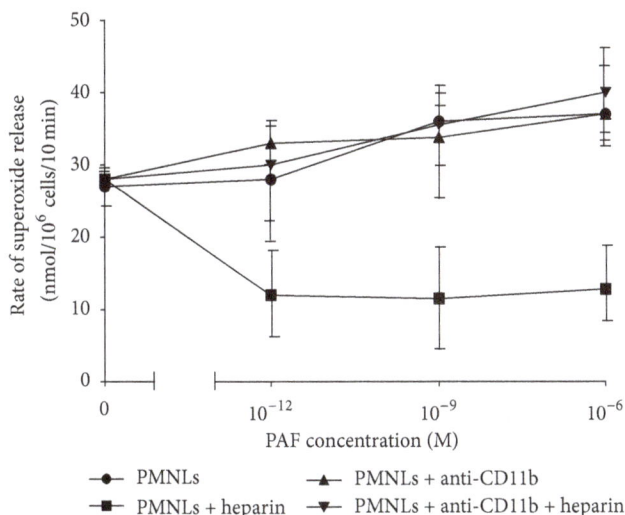

FIGURE 7: The effect of anti-CD11b on superoxide release in the presence of heparin. Superoxide release from NC PMNLs preincubated with increasing concentrations of PAF and IC-PE antibodies (●). In addition, superoxide release from NC PMNLs was also measured after 15 min preincubation with PAF and anti-CD11b-PE antibodies (▲). Furthermore, cells were washed and subjected to 30 min incubation with 25 U/mL of heparin (■). The rate of superoxide release from NC PMNLs was also measured after preincubation of NC PMNLs with PAF + anti-CD11b antibodies, before heparin incubation (▼). The rate of superoxide release was determined with 0.32×10^{-7} M PMA-stimulated PMNLs. The changes in optical density were monitored at 549 nm continuously in the presence of 0.08 mM cytochrome C. Data are represented as nmoles/10^6 cells/10 min; $n = 3$.

4. Discussion

In this study, we examined the effect of heparin on PMNLs. Our novel finding is that heparin exerts its apoptotic effect on primed PMNLs by binding to their CD11b. Moreover, heparin causes a significant dose-dependent decrease in the rate of superoxide release from PMNLs, blocking primed cells from further activation, partially explaining the anti-inflammatory effects of heparin.

It has been previously reported that heparin induces apoptosis in a dose-dependent manner in NC PMNLs [13]. In the present study, 30 min incubation with heparin enhanced apoptosis in separated human PMNLs in a dose-dependent fashion, however to a much greater extent in primed PAF-stimulated NC and HD PMNLs. In NC PMNLs, the increase in apoptosis was mild and became significant only at 100 U/mL of heparin. Interestingly, apoptosis time courses for NC or HD PMNLs incubated with heparin displayed an oscillatory pattern, with NC apoptosis lagging that of the HD PMNLs. This oscillatory behavior can be explained by the fact that 100 U/mL of heparin caused a time-dependent increase in apoptosis both in NC and in HD PMNLs (however faster and to a much greater extent in HD). The decline in apoptosis, for example, after 90 min for HD PMNLs and only after 150 min for NC PMNLs, can be explained by disappearance of the apoptotic cells as shown in our *ex vivo* survival studies: almost 40–50% of the HD PMNLs disappeared after 90 min, probably by disintegration. Why do we see another increase after the nadirs? We suggest that the next apoptotic peak is the result of an increase in CD11b expression *in vitro* during incubation in PBS (data not shown), which in the presence of heparin will result in apoptosis. Nevertheless, in the absence of heparin, such an increase in CD11b is not accompanied by enhanced apoptosis. Another possible explanation for increased apoptosis after 30 minutes can arise from a toxic effect. While we specifically measured priming and apoptosis, we do recognize that cell counts were decreasing over time (an effect we referred to as cell disintegration), which may suggest toxicity. Yet, when measuring cell activation, we made sure to count the same number of cells for each time point. Moreover, other markers of activation and priming were measured only on viable cells. Thus, even if cell toxicity is possible due to prolonged activation, the rate of superoxide release and levels of CD11b were measured on viable cells and support our conclusion that heparin can increase apoptosis through its actions mediated by CD11b.

Increases in PMNL priming as expressed by increased levels of CD11b and superoxide release resulted in dose-dependent increases of heparin binding to PMNLs. This increased binding is demonstrated both by the augmented intensity of heparin bound to the PMNLs and by the percentage of cells binding anti-heparin antibodies following incubation with heparin. In all experiments anti-CD11b antibodies competed with heparin for binding to CD11b, supporting the proposed mechanism of heparin-CD11b interactions as previously reported [11, 12]. Moreover, the percentage of PMNLs that bind heparin depends on the initial priming state of the cells; that is, a higher priming state results in a higher percentage of cells binding heparin. Finally, increases in cell priming resulted in augmented apoptosis by heparin in PMNLs, which was abolished by anti-CD11b antibodies added prior to the addition of heparin.

Heparin inhibited superoxide release from PMNLs and to a greater extent when cells were primed, such as HD and PAF-stimulated NC PMNLs. This indicates that heparin exerts its effect mainly on the subpopulation of cells that are primed and are more abundant in HD and PAF-stimulated PMNLs. Since the population of primed PMNLs is the major contributor to superoxide release, rendering them apoptotic by heparin results in a decreased rate of superoxide release. These important findings indicate that the rates of superoxide release are increased due to a primed subpopulation of cells. In addition, the inhibitory effect of heparin on superoxide release from PMNLs was also abolished by anti-CD11b antibodies added prior to the addition of heparin.

Altogether, this study suggests a novel role for the interaction of heparin and PMNL CD11b, resulting in cell apoptosis. Apoptosis induced by heparin occurs when CD11b levels are increased or, in other words, when a subpopulation of primed PMNLs exists. As a result, heparin plays an anti-inflammatory role by making the primed cells apoptotic and preventing leakage of PMNL contents into the surrounding milieu. Heparan sulfate, a less sulfated form of heparin, is also known to bind to the PMNL CD11b [11], and recently we found it can promote apoptosis in separated PMNLs (data not shown), a characteristic that is dose-dependently affecting superoxide release from stimulated PMNLs [22]. The higher the heparan sulfate concentration, the lower the rate of superoxide release. More interesting, however, is the *in vivo* presence of heparan sulfate in the ECM and on the endothelial cell surface of vascular walls. Our studies on heparin raise the intriguing possibility that heparan sulfate may limit and/or regulate, to a certain degree, tissue injury and vascular damage by uncontrolled degranulation and release of reactive oxygen species and toxic contents into the surrounding milieu by activated transmigrating PMNLs.

Conflict of Interests

The authors declare that there is no conflict of interests regarding the publication of this paper.

Authors' Contribution

Meital Cohen-Mazor and Rafi Mazor equally contributed to the preparation of this paper.

References

[1] S. D. Swain, T. T. Rohn, and M. T. Quinn, "Neutrophil priming in host defense: role of oxidants as priming agents," *Antioxidants and Redox Signaling*, vol. 4, no. 1, pp. 69–83, 2002.

[2] M. B. Hallett and D. Lloyds, "Neutrophil priming: the cellular signals that say 'amber' but not 'green'," *Immunology Today*, vol. 16, no. 6, pp. 264–268, 1995.

[3] A. Sharma, J. A. Askari, M. J. Humphries, E. Y. Jones, and D. I. Stuart, "Crystal structure of a heparin- and integrin-binding segment of human fibronectin," *The EMBO Journal*, vol. 18, no. 6, pp. 1468–1479, 1999.

[4] A. K. Mandal, T. W. Lyden, and M. G. Saklayen, "Heparin lowers blood pressure: biological and clinical perspectives," *Kidney International*, vol. 47, no. 4, pp. 1017–1022, 1995.

[5] R. M. Nelson, O. Cecconi, W. G. Roberts, A. Aruffo, R. J. Linhardt, and M. P. Bevilacqua, "Heparin oligosaccharides bind L- and P-selectin and inhibit acute inflammation," *Blood*, vol. 82, no. 11, pp. 3253–3258, 1993.

[6] G. Bazzoni, A. Beltran Nunez, G. Mascellani, P. Bianchini, E. Dejana, and A. Del Maschio, "Effect of heparin, dermatan sulfate, and related oligo-derivatives on human polymorphonuclear leukocyte functions," *The Journal of Laboratory and Clinical Medicine*, vol. 121, no. 2, pp. 268–275, 1993.

[7] K. Itoh, A. Nakao, W. Kishimoto, and H. Takagi, "Heparin effects on superoxide production by neutrophils," *European Surgical Research*, vol. 27, no. 3, pp. 184–188, 1995.

[8] C. Léculier, N. Couprie, P. Adeleine, P. Leitienne, A. Francina, and M. Richard, "The effects of high molecular weight- and low molecular weight-heparins on superoxide ion production and degranulation by human polymorphonuclear leukocytes," *Thrombosis Research*, vol. 69, no. 6, pp. 519–531, 1993.

[9] K. T. Kruse-Elliott, K. Chaban, J. E. Grossman, S. Tomasko, C. Kamke, and B. Darien, "Low molecular weight heparin alters porcine neutrophil responses to platelet-activating factor," *Shock*, vol. 10, no. 3, pp. 198–202, 1998.

[10] Y. Matzner, G. Marx, R. Drexler, and A. Eldor, "The inhibitory effect of heparin and related glycosaminoglycans on neutrophil chemotaxis," *Thrombosis and Haemostasis*, vol. 52, no. 2, pp. 134–137, 1984.

[11] M. S. Diamond, R. Alon, C. A. Parkos, M. T. Quinn, and T. A. Springer, "Heparin is an adhesive ligand for the leukocyte integrin Mac-1 (CD11b/CD18)," *The Journal of Cell Biology*, vol. 130, no. 6, pp. 1473–1482, 1995.

[12] B. Walzog, F. Jeblonski, A. Zakrzewicz, and P. Gaehtgens, "β2 Integrins (CD11/CD18) promote apoptosis of human neutrophils," *The FASEB Journal*, vol. 11, no. 13, pp. 1177–1186, 1997.

[13] J. Manaster, J. Chezar, R. Shertz-Swirski et al., "Heparin induces apoptosis in human peripheral blood neutrophils," *British Journal of Haematology*, vol. 94, no. 1, pp. 48–52, 1996.

[14] S. Sela, R. Shurtz-Swirski, G. Shapiro et al., "Oxidative stress during hemodialysis: effect of heparin," *Kidney International Supplements*, vol. 78, pp. S159–S163, 2001.

[15] J. W. Yoon, M. V. Pahl, and N. D. Vaziri, "Spontaneous leukocyte activation and oxygen-free radical generation in end-stage renal disease," *Kidney International*, vol. 71, no. 2, pp. 167–172, 2007.

[16] S. Sela, R. Shurtz-Swirski, M. Cohen-Mazor et al., "Primed peripheral polymorphonuclear leukocyte: a culprit underlying chronic low-grade inflammation and systemic oxidative stress in chronic kidney disease," *Journal of the American Society of Nephrology*, vol. 16, no. 8, pp. 2431–2438, 2005.

[17] B. Kristal, R. Shurtz-Swirski, J. Chezar et al., "Participation of peripheral polymorphonuclear leukocytes in the oxidative stress and inflammation in patients with essential hypertension," *American Journal of Hypertension*, vol. 11, no. 8, pp. 921–928, 1998.

[18] J. C. Gray, "Priming of neutrophil oxidative responses by platelet-activating factor," *Journal of Lipid Mediators*, vol. 2, supplement, pp. S161–S175, 1990.

[19] E. Majewska, Z. Sulowska, and Z. Baj, "Spontaneous apoptosis of neutrophils in whole blood and its relation to apoptosis gene proteins," *Scandinavian Journal of Immunology*, vol. 52, no. 5, pp. 496–501, 2000.

[20] M. A. B. A. Dennissen, G. J. Jenniskens, M. Pieffers et al., "Large, tissue-regulated domain diversity of heparan sulfates demonstrated by phage display antibodies," *The Journal of Biological Chemistry*, vol. 277, no. 13, pp. 10982–10986, 2002.

[21] J. van den Born, K. Salmivirta, T. Henttinen et al., "Novel heparan sulfate structures revealed by monoclonal antibodies," *Journal of Biological Chemistry*, vol. 280, no. 21, pp. 20516–20523, 2005.

[22] P. L. Capecchi, L. Ceccatelli, F. Laghi Pasini, and T. Di Perri, "Inhibition of neutrophil function in vitro by heparan sulfate," *International Journal of Tissue Reactions*, vol. 15, no. 2, pp. 71–76, 1993.

21

Sirtuins Link Inflammation and Metabolism

Vidula T. Vachharajani,[1,2] Tiefu Liu,[2,3] Xianfeng Wang,[1] Jason J. Hoth,[4] Barbara K. Yoza,[4] and Charles E. McCall[1]

[1]Department of Anesthesiology, Wake Forest School of Medicine, Winston-Salem, NC 27157, USA
[2]Department of Internal Medicine, Wake Forest School of Medicine, Winston-Salem, NC 27157, USA
[3]Fudan University, Shanghai Public Health Clinical Center, Shanghai 201508, China
[4]Department of Surgery, Wake Forest School of Medicine, Winston-Salem, NC 27157, USA

Correspondence should be addressed to Vidula T. Vachharajani; vvachhar@wakehealth.edu

Academic Editor: Ethan M. Shevach

Sirtuins (SIRT), first discovered in yeast as NAD+ dependent epigenetic and metabolic regulators, have comparable activities in human physiology and disease. Mounting evidence supports that the seven-member mammalian sirtuin family (SIRT1-7) guard homeostasis by sensing bioenergy needs and responding by making alterations in the cell nutrients. Sirtuins play a critical role in restoring homeostasis during stress responses. Inflammation is designed to "defend and mend" against the invading organisms. Emerging evidence supports that metabolism and bioenergy reprogramming direct the sequential course of inflammation; failure of homeostasis retrieval results in many chronic and acute inflammatory diseases. Anabolic glycolysis quickly induced (compared to oxidative phosphorylation) for ROS and ATP generation is needed for immune activation to "defend" against invading microorganisms. Lipolysis/fatty acid oxidation, essential for cellular protection/hibernation and cell survival in order to "mend," leads to immune repression. Acute/chronic inflammations are linked to altered glycolysis and fatty acid oxidation, at least in part, by NAD+ dependent function of sirtuins. Therapeutically targeting sirtuins may provide a new class of inflammation and immune regulators. This review discusses how sirtuins integrate metabolism, bioenergetics, and immunity during inflammation and how sirtuin-directed treatment improves outcome in chronic inflammatory diseases and in the extreme stress response of sepsis.

1. Introduction

Sirtuins are a highly conserved family of proteins [1]. The silent information regulator 2 (SIR2) gene was first described in budding yeast as a regulator of chromatin structure and named MAR1 (mating-type regulator 1) [2]. A set of four genes, SIR1-4 described later, replaced the name "MAR" with "SIR" [3]. Subsequently, SIR2 homologues were identified in bacteria, plants, and mammals, representing a large family of highly conserved proteins called "sirtuins" [4]. Sirtuins belong to class III histone deacetylase family of enzymes. There are 7 mammalian sirtuins with distinct protein structure, varied subcellular location, and unique functional properties. The requirement for NAD+ as a cosubstrate for SIR2 deacetylase activity suggests that sirtuins may have developed as energy sensors and the redox state of cells [4].

Metabolism is known to influence aging in rodents and a number of other species of organisms [5-9]. Several lines of evidence suggest that benefits of calorie restriction are mediated through sirtuins [10-12]. The most convincing link between aging and sirtuins was established after the effects of aging on NAD+ were studied [13]. In addition to its role as a cofactor in many enzymatic processes, NAD+ regulates key metabolic processes. Sirtuins are NAD+ sensors. SIRT1 and SIRT6 are known aging related sirtuins. Evidence suggests that NAD+ levels are decreased in aging; NAD+ replenishment in aged mice restores mitochondrial homeostasis in a SIRT1 dependent manner [14]. SIRT6 deficient mice show signs of accelerated aging and early death from hypoglycemia [15, 16].

Inflammation defends against severe stress responses and if successful must resolve. SIRT1, known as a major metabolic regulator, epigenetically reprograms inflammation by altering histones and transcription factors such as NFκB and AP1 [17]. Mounting evidence supports that inflammation sequentially links immune, metabolic, and mitochondrial bioenergy networks; sirtuins are essential regulators of these networks. This review focuses on how sirtuins contribute to dynamic shifts in immunity, metabolism, and bioenergy during inflammation and selective chronic and acute inflammatory diseases and may provide novel therapeutic targets.

Several general concepts are relevant to the role of sirtuins in inflammation:

(1) The requirement for NAD+ as cofactor supports sirtuin function in redox and bioenergy sensing.

(2) While sirtuin-dependent deacetylation activities dominateour present understanding of the functional roles of sirtuins in inflammation, other attributes such as ADP ribosylation (SIRT4) and removal of succinyl, malonyl, and glutamyl groups from lysine residues (SIRT5) may be important in inflammation [18, 19].

(3) Acetyl CoA levels and its support of histone-acetylation and other proteins are linked to nutritional status of cell. Fasted or survival state of cell utilizes protein deacetylation with SIRT [20].

(4) SIRT effects on inflammation can be a double edged sword, since low levels accentuate early acute inflammation-related autotoxicity by increasing NFκB RelA/p65 activity, and prolonged increases in SIRT1 during late inflammation are associated with immunosuppression and increased mortality [21].

2. Inflammation and Metabolism

Evidence suggests that the sequential course of inflammation is linked with metabolism. Several recent studies have connected inflammation with glycolysis and fatty acids to provide nutritional needs of immune cells for fueling phase shifts after stress sensing [21].

Glycolysis was considered as strictly an anaerobic process until Warburg described aerobic glycolysis in cancer cells for the first time in 1927. Warburg showed that cancer cells, under normoxic conditions, undergo glycolysis and produce lactate. It was deemed, however, that leukocytes/macrophages do not simulate "cancer metabolism" [22, 23]. Although glycolysis is metabolically less efficient per molecule of glucose (a net gain of 2 ATP) compared to oxidative phosphorylation (net gain of 36 ATP), marked increases in glycolysis rapidly respond to high metabolic demands of effector immunity [24]. Glycolysis activates pentose phosphate pathway to aid bacterial killing via NADPH oxidase and also provides fatty acids and amino acids for anabolic processes of cell. Glycolysis and glucose fueling are regulated via increased expression of and genes regulating glycolysis [21]. Additionally, there is disruption of mitochondrial glucose oxidation by PDHK which deactivates mitochondrial PDH. Thus, there is decreased mitochondrial glucose oxidation resulting in increased lactate and pyruvate accumulation. This glycolysis

surge and decrease in mitochondrial glucose oxidation are dependent upon HIF-1α [25, 26]. HIF-1α in turn is regulated by PKM2 and NF kappa B [27, 28]. Thus, HIF1-α provides a bridge between glucose metabolism and inflammation [29]. Sirtuins, especially SIRT6, are known to be a master regulator of glycolysis. Evidence suggests that SIRT6 is a corepressor of glycolysis [30, 31]. Thus, glucose use for glycolysis generates effector responses needed for microbial defense including (1) ROS generation from NOX proteins and release of antimicrobial proteins such as porins, (2) anabolic pathways coupled to nucleus acid, fatty acid, and protein synthetic pathways, and (3) aerobic and anaerobic glycolysis which also supply rapidly needed ATP from high glucose flux as well as very early pyruvate oxidation to feed electron transport chain. Later this fuel is shifted to fatty acids because of closure of the pyruvate portal.

The switch away from high levels of reducing agents (e.g., NADH and NADPH) to NAD+ dominance supports the cellular "mending" pathway, which is a low ATP generating catabolic state. The anti-inflammatory response of macrophages (so-called M2) requires fatty acid oxidation [22]. We now know that a metabolism shifts from glycolysis to fatty acid oxidation in macrophages after LPS stimulation [22, 32, 33]. This increase in fatty acid oxidation occurs via expression of PGC-1α and PGC-1β [34]. SIRT1 and SIRT6 regulate the metabolic switch in monocytes from glycolysis to fatty acid oxidation during adaptation to acute inflammation [30]. This catabolic state supports repressor not only M2 like monocytes and macrophages, but also T repressor cells.

The immunosuppression that accompanies severe systemic inflammation is generated by an inflexible persistence of the repressor homeostasis axis, which limits a secondary response to new stress—for example, like bacterial and viral original or secondary opportunistic infections (discussed subsequently).

3. Sirtuins and Chronic Inflammation

Normal physiologic processes are accompanied by changes in levels and activity of sirtuins [35]. For example, circadian rhythm is controlled by NAD+ generation and cyclical activation and deactivation of SIRT1 and SIRT6. The circadian clock can influence chronic or acute inflammation [36].

How do the functions of sirtuins contribute to chronic inflammation? Nuclear sirtuins SIRT1, SIRT6, and mitochondrial SIRT3—and likely other less well studied members of the sirtuin family—sense nutrient availability and changes in NAD+ production or ratios of NAD/NADH in macrophages or tissue cells. They then respond by reprogramming immune, metabolic, and bioenergy pathways [21, 37]. For example, SIRT1 supports insulin secretion in pancreatic β cells [38], gluconeogenesis in hepatocytes [39], and lipolysis/fatty acid oxidation in macrophages [40].

While research on the role of SIRT in chronic inflammation is in a very early stage, mounting evidence shows that NAD+ levels and SIRT transcription and/or protein levels are persistently reduced in specific tissue during chronic inflammation. Examples include fat deposits in obesity with

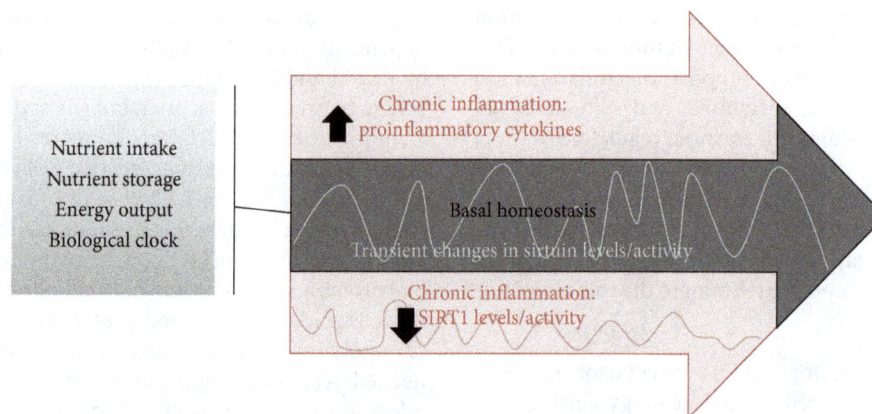

FIGURE 1: Sirtuins and chronic inflammation: during homeostasis (grey arrow), there are small perturbations in sirtuin levels without inflammation. During chronic inflammatory states (denoted by pink), persistent decreases in SIRT1 levels/activity sustain glycolysis-dependent proinflammatory pathways. This immunometabolic inflexibility alters the bioenergy homeostasis set point, which is rebalanced by increasing SIRT1 activity.

inflammation [41], brain in Alzheimer's disease [42], and arterial inflammation in atherosclerosis, using several types of chronic inflammation. Not unexpectedly, chronic inflammation also is accompanied by increased levels of activated proinflammatory transcription factor NFκB RelA/p65 [43]. Since nuclear SIRT1 and SIRT6 deacetylate RelA/p65 and support its proteasome degradation, decreased nuclear SIRT1 or SIRT6 levels/activity increase NFκB RelA/p65 activity and amplify proinflammatory gene expression during chronic inflammation. Further supporting of a role of SIRT1 in chronic inflammation is that increasing NAD+ levels [1] or activating SIRT1 by the polyphenol resveratrol reduces chronic inflammation and rebalances metabolism and bioenergetics toward homeostasis [44].

A schematic representation of relationship between chronic inflammation and sirtuin expression/activity is depicted in Figure 1.

3.1. Examples of Sirtuin Links to Chronic Inflammatory Diseases

3.1.1. Obesity, Diabetes, and Metabolic Syndrome. In mature adipocytes, PPAR-γ regulates genes involved in fatty acid uptake and triglyceride synthesis to increase white adipose tissue (WAT) capacity to store fat [39]. SIRT1 suppresses PPAR-γ and decreases accumulation of fat. In obesity, with increased number and size of adipocytes, there is a decrease in SIRT1 levels and activity. Increased adiposity leads to increased adipose tissue macrophages prone to secreting TNF-α, IL-6, and iNOS, with heightened inflammation [45]. Thus, obesity is associated with low SIRT1 activity, increased inflammatory response, and expansion of WAT [39, 46].

Literature suggests that SIRT1 counters insulin resistance [47]. Increased SIRT1 expression and activation elevate insulin secretion [38], while SIRT1 deficient mice show blunted insulin response to glucose stimulation. Mechanistically, SIRT1 promotes insulin secretion in pancreatic beta cells by repressing uncoupling protein UCP 2 expression

[48]. In animal models of diabetes, SIRT1 activation increases energy expenditure and improves insulin sensitivity [49, 50]. Taken together, substantial data support that increased SIRT1 activity counters obesity, metabolic syndrome, and diabetes with or without obesity.

3.1.2. Atherosclerosis and Cardiovascular Diseases. Evidence supports an anti-inflammatory role for sirtuins in atherosclerosis. SIRT1 downregulates expression of the NFκB signaling pathway during atherosclerosis by deacetylating RelA/p65-NFκB in macrophages and decreasing foam cell formation [51]. The role of SIRT1 as a positive regulator of nuclear receptor and liver X receptor (LXR) that function as cholesterol sensors to regulate whole-body cholesterol and lipid homeostasis is evident from studies by Li et al. [52].

Caloric restriction is shown to be associated with not only increased longevity, but also improved cardiovascular health [53]. Cardiovascular protective benefits of caloric restriction support SIRT1's ability to promote lipolysis, improve insulin sensitivity, and limit proinflammatory macrophage activity [52, 54]. SIRT1 and SIRT3 activation reduces ischemia reperfusion injury in rodents [54–56]; nuclear-cytoplasmic shuttling of SIRT1 plays an important role in this protection [57]. Thus, accumulating data supports an overall protective effect of SIRT1 activation on the chronic inflammation associated with atherosclerosis [58–60].

3.1.3. Alzheimer's Disease. Sirtuins contribute to chronic inflammation associated with Alzheimer's disease and neurodegenerative diseases. The protective effect of caloric restriction with increased SIRT1 expression on Alzheimer's disease was first reported in 2006 [42]. Consistent with a role for SIRT1 in brain dysfunction, animal models of ALS and Alzheimer's disease respond to resveratrol induced SIRT1 activation by both promoting α-secretase nonamyloidogenic activity and attenuating Aβ generation, a hallmark for Alzheimer's disease [61]. Resveratrol delays the onset of

Alzheimer's disease and neurodegeneration [62] by decreasing plaque accumulation in rodents [63].

3.1.4. Chronic Kidney Disease. Sirtuins regulate chronic renal inflammation. In cisplatin-induced chronic inflammatory kidney injury in animals, SIRT1 deacetylated NFκB RelA/p65 [64] and p53 [65] leading to reduced inflammation and apoptosis in an ischemia/reperfusion injury model [66]. Evidence also suggests administration of antioxidant agent acetyl-l-carnitine (AICAR) improves mitochondrial dynamics and protects mice from cisplatin-induced kidney injury in a SIRT3-dependent manner [67].

3.1.5. Tobacco Smoke-Induced Inflammation. Detailed studies of chronic inflammation associated with smoking implicate sirtuins in the process and support their potential role in prevention/intervention [68] and also implicated generation of reactive oxygen species in modifying the sirtuin axis [69]. SIRT1 deficient mice markedly amplify protein oxidation and lipid peroxidation induced by cigarette smoke. Genetic alterations of FOXO3 recapitulate these effects, and SIRT1 activation protects against smoke-induced lung injury. Improvement correlates with increased antioxidant activities of mitochondrial manganese superoxide dismutase (SOD2) and heme oxygenase 1 (HO1). SIRT1 and FOXO1 epigenetically control this balance in oxidation/reduction and ROS-dependent damage.

3.1.6. Sirtuins and Other Mediators of Chronic Inflammatory Diseases. It is important to emphasize that changes in SIRT1 or other sirtuins do not exist in isolation as a family of immunometabolic and bioenergy sensors and controllers of chronic inflammation. Most clearly documented are the connections between decreases in ATP with reciprocal increases in AMP with AMPK activation. SIRT1 and AMPK activation are commonly coupled and support reprogramming of shared pathways of metabolism and bioenergetics [70]; in some cases AMPK activation precedes that of SIRT1 and in others it follows. AMPK reduces anabolism by blocking protein synthesis via mTOR signaling. These interactions between SIRT redox sensing (NAD/NADH) and AMPK energy (ATP/ADP/AMP) sensing are at a crossroad for reducing glucose and protein synthesis proinflammatory anabolic processes and increasing fatty acid oxidation anti-inflammatory catabolic pathways. Dysregulation of this balance is a common feature of chronic inflammation.

4. Sirtuins in Acute Inflammation

Energy homeostasis maintains an intricate balance between cell nutrient sources and their storage (glycogen or triglyceride) or consumption (glycolysis or lipolysis) to meet cellular energy demands. For example, boundaries of basal homeostasis are temporarily exceeded and then restored during transient exercise, increased food intake, or fasting. Inflammatory reactions deviate from physiologic homeostasis boundaries and ultimately restore balance when successful [71]. Acute proinflammatory and immune effector pathways require increased glucose uptake, pentose phosphate pathway activation, and glycolysis leading to lactic acid accumulation. In a major stress response with acute systemic inflammation, this initial immune defensive pathway rapidly becomes autotoxic to cells and tissues by generating excessive ROS and prompting cell death pathways. These processes are described in detail below.

Unlike chronic inflammation, a major stress response with acute inflammation shifts from an anabolic glucose fueling aerobic glycolysis (Warburg response) to a fatty acid fueling catabolic/adaptation response. This fuel source enters mitochondria and generates acetyl CoA, which undergoes the tricarboxylic acid (TCA) cycle. The TCA cycle ultimately provides NADH and FADH as reducing agents for oxygen support of ATP generation. Importantly, the effector immune cell requires glycolysis as primary energy, whereas the repressor cell needs fatty acid. This concept emerges as a critical determinant of acute inflammatory injury and restoration of homeostasis and is a bedrock of the emerging concept of how metabolism and immunity are integrated based on bioenergy requirements.

Emerging data indicate that this "switch" from aerobic glycolysis to fatty acid fueling/adaptation response is modulated by sirtuins. We describe the role of SIRT1, SIRT3, and SIRT6 in subsequent sections in various conditions associated with acute inflammation.

4.1. Examples of Sirtuin Links to Acute Inflammatory Diseases

4.1.1. Sirtuins in Acute Systemic Inflammation of Sepsis. Sepsis is an example in which an extreme and highly lethal stress response induces marked deviations in homeostasis caused by an acute systemic inflammatory response. At an organism level, cardiovascular and microvascular functions are impaired leading to multiple organ failure. Within a few hours of sepsis and septic shock, the early initiating hyperinflammatory phase shifts to anti-inflammatory adaptation phase, which can persist for days to weeks in humans [72, 73]. Historically, the first recognition that extreme stress from bacterial products generates resistance to the products was endotoxin tolerance [74]. It is now known that endotoxin tolerance in neutrophils and monocyte/macrophages and dendritic cells frequently accompanies sepsis in humans and animals [75, 76]. Endotoxin tolerance, which is similar to the sepsis adaptation phase, requires changes in TLR-dependent signaling pathways, which culminate in epigenetic reprogramming of NFκB and other proinflammatory pathways [76–78]. It is important to emphasize that endotoxin tolerance or adaptation develops very quickly [79]. Septic patients are likely to spend less than a day, if not only a few hours, in the cytokine storm of hyperinflammation. This quick switch makes it appear as if there is only one phase of human sepsis [80], which obscures sepsis molecular reprogramming and complicated treatment design and interpretations. Moreover, the acute systemic inflammation with sepsis prolongs the adaptation or immunometabolic phase, thereby generating clinically important immunosuppression [81, 82]. This has major implications for understanding the molecular basis of sepsis and its treatment.

The shift in NAD+ availability and decreased ATP availability during the transition from hyperinflammation to adaptation is the key to understanding the role of sirtuins in sepsis [83]. Increase in nuclear NAD+ activates SIRT1, which promotes gene silencing facultative heterochromatin formation at the promotors of proinflammatory genes such as TNF-α and IL-1β [30, 84]. Mechanistically, activated SIRT1 first directly binds and deactivates NF-κB RelA/p65 through deacetylation and proteasome degradation [85]. SIRT1 also induces RelB transcription and promotes its binding to NF-κB RelA/p65 sites, perhaps replacing RelA/p65. The SIRT1 and RelB partnership also deacetylates histone (H1) and recruits a multiunit repressor complex to form heterochromatin [21, 86].

Acute inflammation-dependent immunometabolic reprogramming also requires communication between nuclear SIRT1 and SIRT6 [30]. Mechanistically, SIRT1 activation increases fatty acid flux, lipolysis, and fatty acid β oxidation in mitochondria by deacetylating and deactivating fork head box subgroup O (FOXO) family of transcription factors and other pathway regulators. This couples with activating nuclear receptors peroxisome proliferator-activated receptor gamma (PPAR-γ) by deacetylating PPAR-γ coactivator 1 alpha (PGC-1α). In a reciprocal process, SIRT6 directs deacetylation of histone H3K9 and hypoxia inducing factor alpha (HIF1-α), represses glucose flux and glycolysis, and limits pentose phosphate pathway-related oxidative (NADPH oxidase) and nonoxidative signaling (anabolism of nucleic acids). Thus, nuclear SIRT1 and SIRT6 acting through epigenetic chromatin are essential for switching glucose anabolic pathways to fatty acid oxidation catabolic pathways. This flexibility/polarity is required for inflammation to progress through its initiating effector phase to adaptation [21, 87]. This switch is essential for directing acute inflammation beyond the proinflammatory state typical of chronic inflammation, which appears to interfere with adaptation. Concomitant with this immune and metabolic switch, SIRT1 interactions with RelB induce transcription of mitochondrial SIRT3, which is needed in mitochondria to support SIRT1 dependent increases in fatty acid oxidation; SIRT3 is a master regulator of the majority of mitochondrial structural and functional proteins [88].

We have studied the role of SIRT1 in rodent sepsis with the focus on microvasculature. We also have shown that similar to the cell models of sepsis there are three distinct phases in the microvasculature of rodent sepsis: the hyperinflammatory/endotoxin responsive phase in early sepsis, a hypoinflammatory/endotoxin tolerant phase in late sepsis [79], and with return of endotoxin responsiveness in resolution phase in survivors.

We show that the SIRT1 levels are increased during the hypoinflammatory (endotoxin tolerant: adaptation) phase of sepsis adaptation in mice. Importantly, SIRT1 inhibition with a specific inhibitor during the adaptation state significantly improves survival, concomitant with early reversal

of microvascular endotoxin tolerance and decreased bacterial load [79]. Along with reversal of endotoxin tolerance, SIRT1 inhibition reshifts fatty acid oxidation to glycolysis in septic mouse splenocytes and human blood monocytes [37]. Together, these data emphasize the crucial role that sirtuins play in generating and prolonging adaptation and immunosuppression during the severe stress response of acute systemic inflammation from sepsis.

As an axis of immunometabolic regulation of acute inflammation, low levels of SIRT1 amplify the initial stage of acute inflammation, at least in part by increasing NFκB RelA/p65 activity. Accordingly, SIRT1 activation before sepsis onset or preceding administration of bacterial endotoxin protects against the initial "hyperinflammation" of sepsis. In the endotoxin shock model, resveratrol, a putative SIRT1 activator, decreases the initial inflammatory response [83]. Calorie restriction with increased SIRT1 improves outcome in polymicrobial sepsis in mice via activation of SIRT1 [89]. A schematic representation of relationship between acute inflammation and sirtuin expression/activity is depicted in Figure 2.

4.1.2. Obesity and Acute Inflammation from Sepsis. As discussed, obesity with chronic inflammation and the metabolic syndrome are associated with reduced levels of SIRT1 [90]. We have found that SIRT1 deficient *ob/ob* mice show exaggerated microvascular inflammation during sepsis, which markedly increases mortality in comparison with lean mice [91]. As shown in Figure 3, sirtuin deficient obese mice show exaggerated hyperinflammatory phase of sepsis. We speculate that this exaggeration in hyperinflammation dictates prolongation of hypoinflammation/adaptation in sepsis. Moreover, pretreatment of *ob/ob* mice with resveratrol before sepsis reduces the accentuated microvascular inflammation and improves survival. The beneficial effect of resveratrol can be reversed by inhibiting SIRT1, supporting the amplified inflammatory response and perhaps high mortality in SIRT1 dependent manner [92].

4.1.3. Traumatic Lung Injury with Acute Inflammation. Traumatic injury induces an acute inflammatory response similar to that seen after acute infection and depends on TLR and NFκB-dependent transcriptional activation of IL-1β, TNF-α, and IL-6. In our model of traumatic lung injury, SIRT1 mRNA, protein, and activity are reduced for up to 24 hrs after injury [93]. In distinct contrast to immunosuppression observed after sepsis, trauma in this model sensitizes or "primes" the lung for a hyperinflammatory response to subsequent TLR stimulation, reflecting the clinically important "2nd hit response." Resveratrol treatment prevents the trauma induced, neutrophil-dependent inflammatory response. Moreover, treating animals with resveratrol before the second hit rescues injured mice subjected to a TLR stimulus 24 hours after lung injury. Together, these data support that, like obesity with low SIRT1, acute trauma generates an inflammatory reaction in which insufficiently available SIRT1 leads to excessive inflammatory injury if an acute infection occurs.

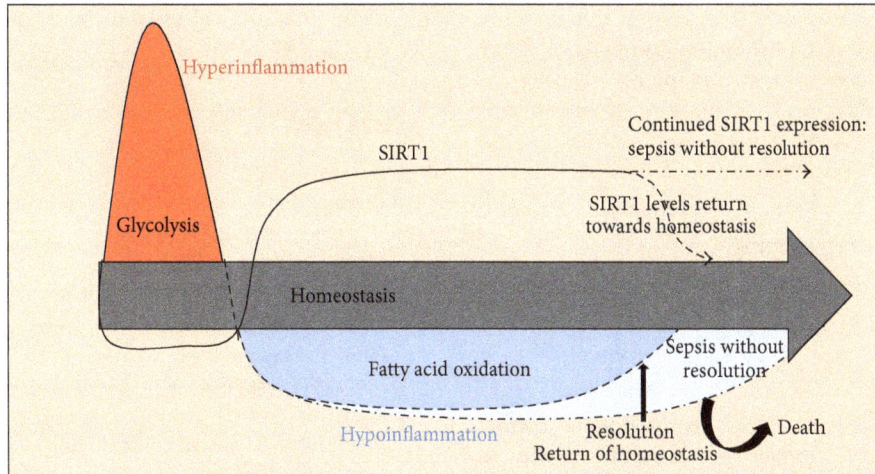

FIGURE 2: Sirtuins and acute inflammation of sepsis: the extreme stress response of sepsis rapidly induces a systemic and potentially lethal hyperinflammatory state (red), which shifts within hours to a counterreactive hypoinflammation/adaptation phase (blue). NAD+ activation of sirtuins directs this switch. Mechanistically, nuclear SIRT1 levels briefly drop when homeostasis deviation initiates the glycolysis-dependent hyperinflammation, but within hours nuclear and mitochondrial sirtuin activation shifts glycolysis to fatty acid oxidation. This metabolic reprogramming globally represses immunity, affecting neutrophils, monocytes, dendritic cells, NK cells, and T lymphocytes. Resolution of acute inflammation and sepsis rebalances sirtuins and inflammation to restore homeostasis. Persistent elevation of sirtuins and hypoinflammation as a result lead to death (denoted by light blue area).

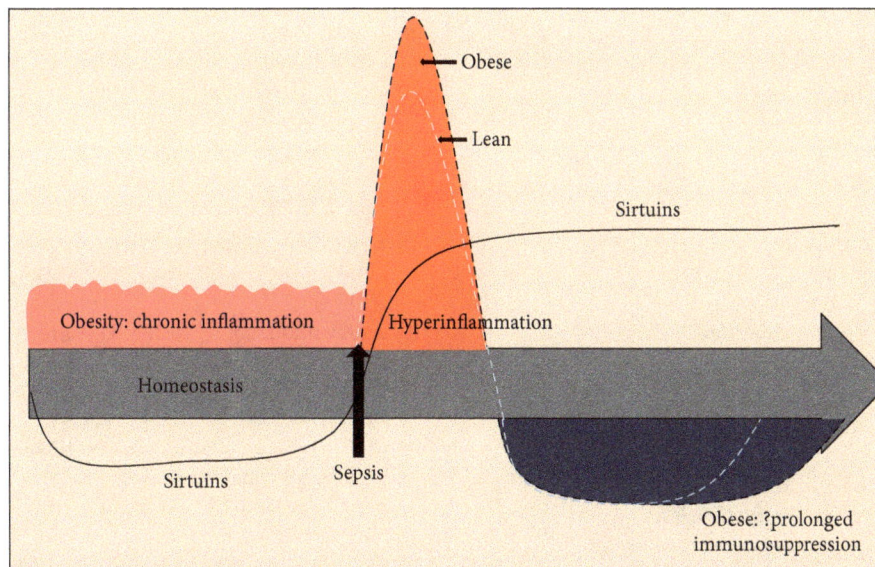

FIGURE 3: Sirtuins and obesity with sepsis: obesity is associated with low-sirtuin levels/activity, but mechanisms responsible for this imbalance are unknown. If sepsis occurs in obese individuals with low SIRT1, the early hyperinflammatory phase is accentuated and counteractive adaptation stage may be prolonged. Activating SIRT1 before obesity-associated sepsis prevents the accentuated acute inflammatory reaction.

5. Summary

Substantial evidence supports that NAD+ dependent sirtuins play essential, but distinct, roles, in chronic and acute inflammation. Chronic inflammatory diseases often persist in a "low-sirtuin" state, and increasing SIRT1 levels or activity is beneficial. In acute inflammation, nuclear SIRT1 activation induces SIRT6 and SIRT3 and the combined functions of this nuclear-mitochondrial triad switch glycolysis to fatty acid oxidation and immunity from activation to repression.

In the severe stress of sepsis, SIRT1 dependent control over immunometabolic reprogramming during adaptation, which counters the initial hyperinflammatory response, is prolonged. Sustaining the adaptation phenotype is supported by continued NAD+ generation coupled with increased SIRT1 expression and activation. This apparent inflexibility of adaptation during sepsis overrides inflammation resolution and homeostasis retrieval. SIRT1 dependent control over adaptation can be reversed in vitro by blocking SIRT1, which results in rebalanced mitochondrial fueling and restored immune competence. Moreover, blocking SIRT1 in septic mice during adaptation restores immune competence, rebalances mitochondrial bioenergetics, and improves survival.

Better understanding of SIRT biology and its role in regulation of inflammation is in its infancy. Among the important unanswered questions are the following:

(i) Do all sirtuin family members participate in immunometabolic reprogramming?

(ii) What markers identify when to start anti-SIRT1 treatment for sepsis?

(iii) What blocks "low SIRT1 states" from shifting to adaptation?

(iv) What are the effects of SIRT1 modulators on various acute/chronic inflammatory conditions in patients with obesity/metabolic syndrome/aging/sepsis, and so forth?

(v) What epigenetic/metabolic signatures occur during anti-SIRT1 sepsis rescue?

(vi) What pathways link redox and ATP/AMP sensing?

(vii) What informs the SIRT axis to shift from glycolysis to fatty acid oxidation?

(viii) How is acute inflammation adaptation shift to resolution?

(ix) What prevents "low SIRT1" proinflammatory states from entering adaptation?

Abbreviations

SIRT:	Sirtuin
NAD+:	Nicotinamide dinucleotide
SIR 2:	Silent information regulator 2
ATP:	Adenosine triphosphate
ADP:	Adenosine dinucleotide
AMP:	Adenosine monophosphate
Acetyl CoA:	Acetyl coenzyme A
PPAR-γ:	Peroxisome proliferator-activated receptor gamma
PGC-1α:	PPAR-γ coactivator 1 alpha
HIF-1α:	Hypoxia inducing factor alpha
NADPH:	Nicotinamide adenine dinucleotide phosphate
UCP:	Uncoupling protein
NFκB:	Nuclear factor κ B
ROS:	Reactive oxygen species
AMPK:	Adenosine monophosphate-activated protein kinase
mTOR:	Mammalian target of rapamycin.

Conflict of Interests

The authors have no significant conflict of interests.

Acknowledgments

This work was supported by the following NIH grants: Vidula T. Vachharajani: (1) K08GM086470 and (2) R01GM099807; Charles E. McCall: (1) R01AI065791, (2) R01AI079144, and (3) R01 GM102497.

References

[1] S.-I. Imai and L. Guarente, "NAD$^+$ and sirtuins in aging and disease," *Trends in Cell Biology*, vol. 24, no. 8, pp. 464–471, 2014.

[2] A. J. S. Klar, S. Fogel, and K. Macleod, "Mar1—a regulator of the HMa and HMα loci in *Saccharomyces cerevisiae*," *Genetics*, vol. 93, no. 1, pp. 37–50, 1979.

[3] J. Rine and I. Herskowitz, "Four genes responsible for a position effect on expression from HML and HMR in *Saccharomyces cerevisiae*," *Genetics*, vol. 116, no. 1, pp. 9–22, 1987.

[4] S. Michan and D. Sinclair, "Sirtuins in mammals: insights into their biological function," *The Biochemical Journal*, vol. 404, no. 1, pp. 1–13, 2007.

[5] R. Weindruch, R. L. Walford, S. Fligiel, and D. Guthrie, "The retardation of aging in mice by dietary restriction: longevity, cancer, immunity and lifetime energy intake," *The Journal of Nutrition*, vol. 116, no. 4, pp. 641–654, 1986.

[6] L. Guarente, "Sir2 links chromatin silencing, metabolism, and aging," *Genes & Development*, vol. 14, no. 9, pp. 1021–1026, 2000.

[7] B. Lakowski and S. Hekimi, "Determination of life-span in *Caenorhabditis elegans* by four clock genes," *Science*, vol. 272, no. 5264, pp. 1010–1013, 1996.

[8] I. Müller, M. Zimmermann, D. Becker, and M. Flömer, "Calendar life span versus budding lifespan of *Saccharomyces cerevisiae*," *Mechanisms of Ageing and Development*, vol. 12, no. 1, pp. 47–52, 1980.

[9] G. S. Roth, D. K. Ingram, and M. A. Lane, "Calorie restriction in primates: will it work and how will we know?" *Journal of the American Geriatrics Society*, vol. 47, no. 7, pp. 896–903, 1999.

[10] L. Guarente, "Sirtuins, aging, and metabolism," *Cold Spring Harbor Symposia on Quantitative Biology*, vol. 76, pp. 81–90, 2011.

[11] A. Purushotham, T. T. Schug, Q. Xu, S. Surapureddi, X. Guo, and X. Li, "Hepatocyte-specific deletion of SIRT1 alters fatty acid metabolism and results in hepatic steatosis and inflammation," *Cell Metabolism*, vol. 9, no. 4, pp. 327–338, 2009.

[12] M. C. Haigis, R. Mostoslavsky, K. M. Haigis et al., "SIRT4 inhibits glutamate dehydrogenase and opposes the effects of calorie restriction in pancreatic β cells," *Cell*, vol. 126, no. 5, pp. 941–954, 2006.

[13] S.-I. Imai, "The NAD world: a new systemic regulatory network for metabolism and aaging—Sirt1, systemic NAD biosynthesis, and their importance," *Cell Biochemistry and Biophysics*, vol. 53, no. 2, pp. 65–74, 2009.

[14] A. P. Gomes, N. L. Price, A. J. Y. Ling et al., "Declining NAD$^+$ induces a pseudohypoxic state disrupting nuclear-mitochondrial communication during aging," *Cell*, vol. 155, no. 7, pp. 1624–1638, 2013.

[15] S. Kugel and R. Mostoslavsky, "Chromatin and beyond: the multitasking roles for SIRT6," *Trends in Biochemical Sciences*, vol. 39, no. 2, pp. 72–81, 2014.

[16] R. Mostoslavsky, K. F. Chua, D. B. Lombard et al., "Genomic instability and aging-like phenotype in the absence of mammalian SIRT6," *Cell*, vol. 124, no. 2, pp. 315–329, 2006.

[17] J. Xie, X. Zhang, and L. Zhang, "Negative regulation of inflammation by SIRT1," *Pharmacological Research*, vol. 67, no. 1, pp. 60–67, 2013.

[18] Y. Tao, C. Huang, Y. Huang et al., "SIRT4 suppresses inflammatory responses in human umbilical vein endothelial cells," *Cardiovascular Toxicology*, vol. 15, no. 3, pp. 217–223, 2015.

[19] J. Du, Y. Zhou, X. Su et al., "Sirt5 is a NAD-dependent protein lysine demalonylase and desuccinylase," *Science*, vol. 334, no. 6057, pp. 806–809, 2011.

[20] L. Shi and B. P. Tu, "Acetyl-CoA and the regulation of metabolism: mechanisms and consequences," *Current Opinion in Cell Biology*, vol. 33, pp. 125–131, 2015.

[21] T. F. Liu, C. M. Brown, M. E. Gazzar et al., "Fueling the flame: bioenergy couples metabolism and inflammation," *Journal of Leukocyte Biology*, vol. 92, no. 3, pp. 499–507, 2012.

[22] A. F. McGettrick and L. A. J. O'Neill, "How metabolism generates signals during innate immunity and inflammation," *The Journal of Biological Chemistry*, vol. 288, no. 32, pp. 22893–22898, 2013.

[23] O. Warburg, K. Gawehn, and A. W. Geissler AW, "Metabolism of leukocytes," *Zeitschrift für Naturforschung—Teil B: Chemie, Biochemie, Biophysik, Biologie*, vol. 13, no. 8, pp. 515–516, 1958.

[24] A. Vazquez, J. Liu, Y. Zhou, and Z. N. Oltvai, "Catabolic efficiency of aerobic glycolysis: the Warburg effect revisited," *BMC Systems Biology*, vol. 4, article 58, 2010.

[25] J.-W. Kim, I. Tchernyshyov, G. L. Semenza, and C. V. Dang, "HIF-1-mediated expression of pyruvate dehydrogenase kinase: a metabolic switch required for cellular adaptation to hypoxia," *Cell Metabolism*, vol. 3, no. 3, pp. 177–185, 2006.

[26] G. L. Semenza, "Oxygen-dependent regulation of mitochondrial respiration by hypoxia-inducible factor 1," *The Biochemical Journal*, vol. 405, no. 1, pp. 1–9, 2007.

[27] G. L. Semenza, "Regulation of metabolism by hypoxia-inducible factor 1," *Cold Spring Harbor Symposia on Quantitative Biology*, vol. 76, pp. 347–353, 2011.

[28] K. Nishi, T. Oda, S. Takabuchi et al., "LPS induces hypoxia-inducible factor 1 activation in macrophage-differentiated cells in a reactive oxygen species-dependent manner," *Antioxidants & Redox Signaling*, vol. 10, no. 5, pp. 983–995, 2008.

[29] S. R. Walmsley, C. Print, N. Farahi et al., "Hypoxia-induced neutrophil survival is mediated by HIF-1alpha-dependent NF-kappaB activity," *Journal of Experimental Medicine*, vol. 201, no. 1, pp. 105–115, 2005.

[30] T. F. Liu, V. T. Vachharajani, B. K. Yoza, and C. E. McCall, "NAD$^+$-dependent sirtuin 1 and 6 proteins coordinate a switch from glucose to fatty acid oxidation during the acute inflammatory response," *The Journal of Biological Chemistry*, vol. 287, no. 31, pp. 25758–25769, 2012.

[31] L. Zhong, A. D'Urso, D. Toiber et al., "The histone deacetylase Sirt6 regulates glucose homeostasis via Hif1α," *Cell*, vol. 140, no. 2, pp. 280–293, 2010.

[32] G. M. Tannahill, A. M. Curtis, J. Adamik et al., "Succinate is an inflammatory signal that induces IL-1β through HIF-1α," *Nature*, vol. 496, no. 7444, pp. 238–242, 2013.

[33] C. M. Krawczyk, T. Holowka, J. Sun et al., "Toll-like receptor-induced changes in glycolytic metabolism regulate dendritic cell activation," *Blood*, vol. 115, no. 23, pp. 4742–4749, 2010.

[34] P. J. Fernandez-Marcos and J. Auwerx, "Regulation of PGC-1alpha, a nodal regulator of mitochondrial biogenesis," *The American Journal of Clinical Nutrition*, vol. 93, no. 4, pp. 884S–890S, 2011.

[35] R. Nogueiras, K. M. Habegger, N. Chaudhary et al., "Sirtuin 1 and sirtuin 3: physiological modulators of metabolism," *Physiological Reviews*, vol. 92, no. 3, pp. 1479–1514, 2012.

[36] X. Li, "SIRT1 and energy metabolism," *Acta Biochimica et Biophysica Sinica*, vol. 45, no. 1, pp. 51–60, 2013.

[37] T. F. Liu, V. Vachharajani, P. Millet, M. S. Bharadwaj, A. J. Molina, and C. E. McCall, "Sequential actions of SIRT1-RELB-SIRT3 coordinate nuclear-mitochondrial communication during immunometabolic adaptation to acute inflammation and sepsis," *The Journal of Biological Chemistry*, vol. 290, no. 1, pp. 396–408, 2015.

[38] K. A. Moynihan, A. A. Grimm, M. M. Plueger et al., "Increased dosage of mammalian Sir2 in pancreatic β cells enhances glucose-stimulated insulin secretion in mice," *Cell Metabolism*, vol. 2, no. 2, pp. 105–117, 2005.

[39] T. T. Schug and X. Li, "Sirtuin 1 in lipid metabolism and obesity," *Annals of Medicine*, vol. 43, no. 3, pp. 198–211, 2011.

[40] J. I. Odegaard, R. R. Ricardo-Gonzalez, A. Red Eagle et al., "Alternative M2 activation of Kupffer cells by PPARdelta ameliorates obesity-induced insulin resistance," *Cell Metabolism*, vol. 7, no. 6, pp. 496–507, 2008.

[41] T. T. Schug and X. Li, "Surprising sirtuin crosstalk in the heart," *Aging*, vol. 2, no. 3, pp. 129–132, 2010.

[42] W. Qin, T. Yang, L. Ho et al., "Neuronal SIRT1 activation as a novel mechanism underlying the prevention of alzheimer disease amyloid neuropathology by calorie restriction," *The Journal of Biological Chemistry*, vol. 281, no. 31, pp. 21745–21754, 2006.

[43] L. Serrano-Marco, M. R. Chacón, E. Maymó-Masip et al., "TNF-α inhibits PPARβ/δ activity and SIRT1 expression through NF-κB in human adipocytes," *Biochimica et Biophysica Acta*, vol. 1821, no. 9, pp. 1177–1185, 2012.

[44] M. C. Haigis and D. A. Sinclair, "Mammalian sirtuins: biological insights and disease relevance," *Annual Review of Pathology: Mechanisms of Disease*, vol. 5, pp. 253–295, 2010.

[45] J. I. Odegaard and A. Chawla, "Mechanisms of macrophage activation in obesity-induced insulin resistance," *Nature Clinical Practice Endocrinology and Metabolism*, vol. 4, no. 11, pp. 619–626, 2008.

[46] F. Picard, M. Kurtev, N. Chung et al., "Sirt1 promotes fat mobilization in white adipocytes by repressing PPAR-α," *Nature*, vol. 429, no. 6993, pp. 771–776, 2004.

[47] S.-I. Imai and W. Kiess, "Therapeutic potential of SIRT1 and NAMPT-mediated NAD biosynthesis in type 2 diabetes," *Frontiers in Bioscience*, vol. 14, no. 8, pp. 2983–2995, 2009.

[48] L. Bordone, M. C. Motta, F. Picard et al., "Sirt1 regulates insulin secretion by repressing UCP2 in pancreatic beta cells," *PLoS Biology*, vol. 4, no. 2, article e31, 2006.

[49] S. Sharma, C. S. Misra, S. Arumugam et al., "Antidiabetic activity of resveratrol, a known SIRT1 activator in a genetic model for type-2 diabetes," *Phytotherapy Research*, vol. 25, no. 1, pp. 67–73, 2011.

[50] K. P. Goh, H. Y. Lee, D. P. Lau, W. Supaat, Y. H. Chan, and A. F. Y. Koh, "Effects of resveratrol in patients with type 2 diabetes mellitus on skeletal muscle SIRT1 expression and energy expenditure," *International Journal of Sport Nutrition and Exercise Metabolism*, vol. 24, no. 1, pp. 2–13, 2014.

[51] S. Stein, C. Lohmann, N. Schäfer et al., "SIRT1 decreases Lox-1-mediated foam cell formation in atherogenesis," *European Heart Journal*, vol. 31, no. 18, pp. 2301–2309, 2010.

[52] X. Li, S. Zhang, G. Blander, J. G. Tse, M. Krieger, and L. Guarente, "SIRT1 deacetylates and positively regulates the nuclear receptor LXR," *Molecular Cell*, vol. 28, no. 1, pp. 91–106, 2007.

[53] C. W. Bales and W. E. Kraus, "Caloric restriction: implications for human cardiometabolic health," *Journal of Cardiopulmonary Rehabilitation and Prevention*, vol. 33, no. 4, pp. 201–208, 2013.

[54] T. Yamamoto, J. Byun, P. Zhai, Y. Ikeda, S. Oka, and J. Sadoshima, "Nicotinamide mononucleotide, an intermediate of NAD$^+$ synthesis, protects the heart from ischemia and reperfusion," *PLoS ONE*, vol. 9, no. 6, Article ID e98972, 2014.

[55] G. A. Porter, W. R. Urciuoli, P. S. Brookes, and S. M. Nadtochiy, "SIRT3 deficiency exacerbates ischemia-reperfusion injury: implication for aged hearts," *American Journal of Physiology—Heart and Circulatory Physiology*, vol. 306, no. 12, pp. H1602–H1609, 2014.

[56] M. Shalwala, S.-G. Zhu, A. Das, F. N. Salloum, L. Xi, and R. C. Kukreja, "Sirtuin 1 (SIRT1) activation mediates sildenafil induced delayed cardioprotection against ischemia-reperfusion injury in mice," *PLoS ONE*, vol. 9, no. 1, Article ID e86977, 2014.

[57] C. Tong, A. Morrison, S. Mattison et al., "Impaired SIRT1 nucleocytoplasmic shuttling in the senescent heart during ischemic stress," *The FASEB Journal*, vol. 27, no. 11, pp. 4332–4342, 2013.

[58] H.-T. Zeng, Y.-C. Fu, W. Yu et al., "SIRT1 prevents atherosclerosis via liver-X-receptor and NF-κB signaling in a U937 cell model," *Molecular Medicine Reports*, vol. 8, no. 1, pp. 23–28, 2013.

[59] B. Bai, P. M. Vanhoutte, and Y. Wang, "Loss-of-SIRT1 function during vascular ageing: hyperphosphorylation mediated by cyclin-dependent kinase 5," *Trends in Cardiovascular Medicine*, vol. 24, no. 2, pp. 81–84, 2014.

[60] A. Toniolo, E. A. Warden, A. Nassi, A. Cignarella, and C. Bolego, "Regulation of SIRT1 in vascular smooth muscle cells from streptozotocin-diabetic rats," *PLoS ONE*, vol. 8, no. 5, Article ID e65666, 2013.

[61] D. Kim, M. D. Nguyen, M. M. Dobbin et al., "SIRT1 deacetylase protects against neurodegeneration in models for Alzheimer's disease and amyotrophic lateral sclerosis," *The EMBO Journal*, vol. 26, no. 13, pp. 3169–3179, 2007.

[62] S. S. Karuppagounder, J. T. Pinto, H. Xu, H.-L. Chen, M. F. Beal, and G. E. Gibson, "Dietary supplementation with resveratrol reduces plaque pathology in a transgenic model of Alzheimer's disease," *Neurochemistry International*, vol. 54, no. 2, pp. 111–118, 2009.

[63] G. Donmez, D. Wang, D. E. Cohen, and L. Guarente, "SIRT1 suppresses β-amyloid production by activating the α-secretase gene ADAM10," *Cell*, vol. 142, no. 2, pp. 320–332, 2010.

[64] Y. J. Jung, J. E. Lee, A. S. Lee et al., "SIRT1 overexpression decreases cisplatin-induced acetylation of NF-κB p65 subunit and cytotoxicity in renal proximal tubule cells," *Biochemical and Biophysical Research Communications*, vol. 419, no. 2, pp. 206–210, 2012.

[65] D. H. Kim, Y. J. Jung, J. E. Lee et al., "Sirt1 activation by resveratrol ameliorates cisplatin-induced renal injury through deacetylation of p53," *American Journal of Physiology—Renal Physiology*, vol. 301, no. 2, pp. F427–F435, 2011.

[66] H. Fan, H.-C. Yang, L. You, Y.-Y. Wang, W.-J. He, and C.-M. Hao, "The histone deacetylase, SIRT1, contributes to the resistance of young mice to ischemia/reperfusion-induced acute kidney injury," *Kidney International*, vol. 83, no. 3, pp. 404–413, 2013.

[67] M. Morigi, L. Perico, C. Rota et al., "Sirtuin 3-dependent mitochondrial dynamic improvements protect against acute kidney injury," *The Journal of Clinical Investigation*, vol. 125, no. 2, pp. 715–726, 2015.

[68] H. Yao, I. K. Sundar, T. Ahmad et al., "SIRT1 protects against cigarette smoke-induced lung oxidative stress via a FOXO$_3$-dependent mechanism," *The American Journal of Physiology—Lung Cellular and Molecular Physiology*, vol. 306, no. 9, pp. L816–L828, 2014.

[69] J.-W. Hwang, H. Yao, S. Caito, I. K. Sundar, and I. Rahman, "Redox regulation of SIRT1 in inflammation and cellular senescence," *Free Radical Biology & Medicine*, vol. 61, pp. 95–110, 2013.

[70] C. Cantó and J. Auwerx, "PGC-1α, SIRT1 and AMPK, an energy sensing network that controls energy expenditure," *Current Opinion in Lipidology*, vol. 20, no. 2, pp. 98–105, 2009.

[71] R. Medzhitov, "Inflammation 2010: new Adventures of an Old Flame," *Cell*, vol. 140, no. 6, pp. 771–776, 2010.

[72] J. Chang, S. L. Kunkel, and C.-H. Chang, "Negative regulation of MyD88-dependent signaling by IL-10 in dendritic cells," *Proceedings of the National Academy of Sciences of the United States of America*, vol. 106, no. 43, pp. 18327–18332, 2009.

[73] L. Li, S. Cousart, J. Hu, and C. E. McCall, "Characterization of interleukin-1 receptor-associated kinase in normal and endotoxin-tolerant cells," *The Journal of Biological Chemistry*, vol. 275, no. 30, pp. 23340–23345, 2000.

[74] P. B. Beeson, "Tolerance to bacterial pyrogens," *The Journal of Experimental Medicine*, vol. 86, pp. 29–41, 1947.

[75] J. A. Cook, "Molecular basis of endotoxin tolerance," *Annals of the New York Academy of Sciences*, vol. 851, pp. 426–428, 1998.

[76] C. E. McCall, B. Yoza, T. Liu, and M. El Gazzar, "Gene-specific epigenetic regulation in serious infections with systemic inflammation," *Journal of Innate Immunity*, vol. 2, no. 5, pp. 395–405, 2010.

[77] R. Medzhitov, "Origin and physiological roles of inflammation," *Nature*, vol. 454, no. 7203, pp. 428–435, 2008.

[78] C. Chan, L. Li, C. E. McCall, and B. K. Yoza, "Endotoxin tolerance disrupts chromatin remodeling and NF-κB transactivation at the IL-1β promoter," *Journal of Immunology*, vol. 175, no. 1, pp. 461–468, 2005.

[79] V. T. Vachharajani, T. Liu, C. M. Brown et al., "SIRT1 inhibition during the hypoinflammatory phenotype of sepsis enhances immunity and improves outcome," *Journal of Leukocyte Biology*, vol. 96, no. 5, pp. 785–796, 2014.

[80] W. Xiao, M. N. Mindrinos, J. Seok et al., "A genomic storm in critically injured humans," *Journal of Experimental Medicine*, vol. 208, no. 13, pp. 2581–2590, 2011.

[81] R. S. Hotchkiss, C. M. Coopersmith, J. E. McDunn, and T. A. Ferguson, "The sepsis seesaw: tilting toward immunosuppression," *Nature Medicine*, vol. 15, no. 5, pp. 496–497, 2009.

[82] J. S. Boomer, K. To, K. C. Chang et al., "Immunosuppression in patients who die of sepsis and multiple organ failure," *The Journal of the American Medical Association*, vol. 306, no. 23, pp. 2594–2605, 2011.

[83] Z. Zhang, S. F. Lowry, L. Guarente, and B. Haimovich, "Roles of SIRT1 in the acute and restorative phases following induction of inflammation," *The Journal of Biological Chemistry*, vol. 285, no. 53, pp. 41391–41401, 2010.

[84] T. F. Liu, B. K. Yoza, M. El Gazzar, V. T. Vachharajani, and C. E. McCall, "NAD$^+$-dependent SIRT1 deacetylase participates in epigenetic reprogramming during endotoxin tolerance," *The Journal of Biological Chemistry*, vol. 286, no. 11, pp. 9856–9864, 2011.

[85] M. Lei, J.-G. Wang, D.-M. Xiao et al., "Resveratrol inhibits interleukin 1β-mediated inducible nitric oxide synthase expression in articular chondrocytes by activating SIRT1 and thereby

suppressing nuclear factor-κB activity," *European Journal of Pharmacology*, vol. 674, no. 2-3, pp. 73–79, 2012.

[86] M. El Gazzar, B. K. Yoza, X. Chen, J. Hu, G. A. Hawkins, and C. E. McCall, "G9a and HP1 couple histone and DNA methylation to TNFα transcription silencing during endotoxin tolerance," *The Journal of Biological Chemistry*, vol. 283, no. 47, pp. 32198–32208, 2008.

[87] V. Vachharajani, T. Liu, and C. E. McCall, "Epigenetic coordination of acute systemic inflammation: potential therapeutic targets," *Expert Review of Clinical Immunology*, vol. 10, no. 9, pp. 1141–1150, 2014.

[88] J. C. Newman, W. He, and E. Verdin, "Mitochondrial protein acylation and intermediary metabolism: regulation by sirtuins and implications for metabolic disease," *The Journal of Biological Chemistry*, vol. 287, no. 51, pp. 42436–42443, 2012.

[89] A. Hasegawa, H. Iwasaka, S. Hagiwara, N. Asai, T. Nishida, and T. Noguchi, "Alternate day calorie restriction improves systemic inflammation in a mouse model of sepsis induced by cecal ligation and puncture," *The Journal of Surgical Research*, vol. 174, no. 1, pp. 136–141, 2012.

[90] M. M. Poulsen, J. O. L. Jørgensen, N. Jessen, B. Richelsen, and S. B. Pedersen, "Resveratrol in metabolic health: an overview of the current evidence and perspectives," *Annals of the New York Academy of Sciences*, vol. 1290, no. 1, pp. 74–82, 2013.

[91] V. Vachharajani, J. M. Russell, K. L. Scott et al., "Obesity exacerbates sepsis-induced inflammation and microvascular dysfunction in mouse brain," *Microcirculation*, vol. 12, no. 2, pp. 183–194, 2005.

[92] X. Wang, N. L. Buechler, B. K. Yoza, C. E. McCall, and V. T. Vachharajani, "Resveratrol attenuates microvascular inflammation in sepsis via SIRT-1-Induced modulation of adhesion molecules in ob/ob mice," *Obesity*, vol. 23, no. 6, pp. 1209–1217, 2015.

[93] L. M. Smith, J. D. Wells, V. T. Vachharajani, B. K. Yoza, C. E. McCall, and J. J. Hoth, "SIRT1 mediates a primed response to immune challenge after traumatic lung injury," *The Journal of Trauma and Acute Care Surgery*, vol. 78, no. 5, pp. 1034–1038, 2015.

22

Hib Vaccines: Past, Present, and Future Perspectives

Adi Essam Zarei,[1,2] **Hussein A. Almehdar,**[1] **and Elrashdy M. Redwan**[1,3]

[1]*Biological Sciences Department, Faculty of Science, King Abdulaziz University, P.O. Box 80203, Jeddah 21589, Saudi Arabia*
[2]*Main Medical Laboratory, Medical Services, Saudi Airlines, P.O. Box 167, Cost Center 507, Jeddah 21231, Saudi Arabia*
[3]*Therapeutic and Protective Proteins Laboratory, Protein Research Department, Genetic Engineering and Biotechnology
Research Institute, City for Scientific Research and Technology Applications, New Borg EL-Arab, Alexandria 21934, Egypt*

Correspondence should be addressed to Elrashdy M. Redwan; redwan1961@yahoo.com

Academic Editor: Clelia M. Riera

Haemophilus influenzae type b (Hib) causes many severe diseases, including epiglottitis, pneumonia, sepsis, and meningitis. In developed countries, the annual incidence of meningitis caused by bacteria is approximately 5–10 cases per population of 100,000. The Hib conjugate vaccine is considered protective and safe. Adjuvants, molecules that can enhance and/or regulate the fundamental immunogenicity of an antigen, comprise a wide range of diverse compounds. While earlier developments of adjuvants created effective products, there is still a need to create new generations, rationally designed based on recent discoveries in immunology, mainly in innate immunity. Many factors may play a role in the immunogenicity of Hib conjugate vaccines, such as the polysaccharides and proteins carrier used in vaccine construction, as well as the method of conjugation. A Hib conjugate vaccine has been constructed via chemical synthesis of a Hib saccharide antigen. Two models of carbohydrate-protein conjugate have been established, the single ended model (terminal amination-single method) and cross-linked lattice matrix (dual amination method). Increased knowledge in the fields of immunology, molecular biology, glycobiology, glycoimmunology, and the biology of infectious microorganisms has led to a dramatic increase in vaccine efficacy.

1. Introduction

Encapsulated *H. influenzae* type b (Hib) causes many severe infections, including sepsis, epiglottitis, pneumonia, and meningitis. Occasionally, encapsulated nontype b strains of *H. influenzae*, mostly type a, are able to produce invasive infections similar to Hib infections. In contrast, nontypeable (unencapsulated) strains are rarely a source of severe infections but most frequently generate infections of mucus membrane, such as conjunctivitis, sinusitis, and otitis media [1, 2]. Hib meningitis has been common in developed countries and hence must be presented along with the other Hib systemic diseases. In 1972, it was approximated that one in 280 newborns are infected with Hib in the first 5 years of life [3]. In a number of populations, including Australian aboriginal and Alaskan Eskimo children, incidence of meningitis caused by Hib has reached 1/50 to 1/30 newborns per year [4, 5]. The Hib meningitis mortality rate is about 5 to 10%, and around 30%

of cured infected children have deficits of the central nervous system (CNS) varying from seizures, to deafness, to mental retardation [6]. Furthermore, Hib antibiotics resistance is increasing; around 30% of isolated Hib is ampicillin-resistant, and Hib meningitis in children is tenfold more transmissible than *Neisseria meningitidis* meningitis [7, 8]. In the prevaccination era, Hib epiglottitis caused much more morbidity and mortality than Hib meningitis and was second to Hib meningitis as the most common systemic Hib infection in Sweden [9].

According to the Global Alliance for Vaccines and Immunization (GAVI), more than 1.5 million children (around three per minute) die each year from diseases that could be prevented by vaccines. Enhancements in related fields such as biotechnology, virology, synthetic biology, and genetics offer a novel array of tools to advance vaccinology [10].

Capsular polysaccharide (CPS) covers the surface of some pathogenic bacteria, such as Hib, and is accessible for detection by cells of the immune system including macrophages, B cells, and dendritic cells. Moreover, most CPSs have unique structures that differ from those of mammalian glycans; and their accessibility by the immune cells and induction of immune responses specific for CPS make them excellent vaccine candidates [11]. The structure of the replicating disaccharide units of CPS of Hib is presented in Figure 1 [12]. These units are linked through phosphor-diester bonds, which generate the acidity of the polysaccharide Hib molecule [13].

The immunogenicity of CPS antigens leads to their categorization as T cell independent type 2 (TI-2) immune response, which stimulate protective antibodies without help from MHC-II classified T cells. CPSs trigger activation of the complement factor C3d by the complement alternative pathway; subsequently, primed marginal-zone B cells in the spleen travel to the germinal center and connect to polysaccharide-C3d via their CD21 complement receptor [14]. However, isotype switching follows, and responses against CPSs antigens occurred not only by IgM, but also by IgG and IgA [15, 16]. A specific signaling system might manage the vital responses of these antibodies [17], which differ in character and size among individuals [18] according to their age and earlier infections [19].

The naivety of the immune systems of young children and their relative incompetence compared to those of adults render children more vulnerable to Hib infections. Moreover, the integument and mucosa delicacy, as a kind of structural naivety, may play a role in susceptibility. Many studies have compared the immune systems of infants and adults, considering the role and potency of nearly every constituent of the immune system, humoral and cellular, innate and adaptive, that may make the infant immune system vulnerable [20]. The marginal zone of the human spleen is not completely formed until one to two years of age, numbers of CD21-expressing B cells in the marginal zone and complement are small at childbirth, and CPS-specific antibodies productions are limited or absent in newborns [21, 22]. At delivery, very little IL12 is produced from antigen presenting cells (APCs), and with the exception of live attenuated vaccines, which have a maturation effect on neonatal APC, most vaccines have little capability to prime protective T-helper 1 responses in newborns [23–28]. The suppression of antibody responses (mainly against protein antigens) in early life may be caused partly by transplacentally acquired IgG, which fades after birth according to a half-life of about 28 days; this transplacental IgG does not cause downregulation of T cell function [29].

When used as vaccines, CPS antigens of several infectious bacteria stimulate considerable protection by inducing antibody production [30]. Without considering herd immunity, the effectiveness of the conjugate Hib vaccine may range between a 46% and 93% reduction in invasive disease caused by Hib. The success and safety of the Hib conjugate vaccine have been confirmed in pharmacovigilance screening. Adverse reactions to the conjugate Hib vaccine are rare; only individuals with hypersensitivity to the vaccine's constituents are subject to contraindications [31]. However, children who contract Hib disease regardless of proper immunization must

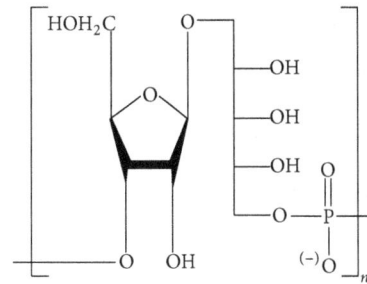

FIGURE 1: *H. influenzae* type b capsular polysaccharides repeating unit.

be examined for suspected malfunctions in their immune system that make them sensitive to the infection [32].

Several factors may explain the low introduction level of Hib conjugate vaccines in the majority of developing countries, such as the absence of statistics that reflect the burden of disease and the troubles facing its estimation and calculation, political failure to consider Hib infection a health crisis, and the absence of practices related to vaccinology [33, 34]. The use of smaller doses of antigen and smaller quantities for vaccine injection in developing countries could support the introduction of vaccines by immunization schedules such as those routinely planned for children [35].

The use of the Hib vaccine in Saudi Arabia began in April 1998 at King Fahad National Guard Hospital, where it was used routinely for all infants in the hospital [36]. Subsequently, vaccine became obligatory in the national immunization program in 2000 and since then cases of Hib have declined considerably. During three years (2001–2003) there were 30 cases of *H. Influenzae* invasive disease, compared to only 6 cases in the following three years (2004–2007) [37]. According to the Saudi Ministry of Health 2013 Statistics Book, coverage of the pentavalent vaccine (which includes diphtheria, pertussis, tetanus, Hib, and hepatitis B) is 97.7% [38]. This review on the vaccinology of Hib will serve as a valuable source of information for public health officials and decision-makers.

2. Hib Vaccines

2.1. CPS Vaccines and Adjuvants. The idea of using the bacterial CPS in vaccines dates back to 1930s and involves inducing polysaccharide-specific antibodies to protect against pathogenic bacteria [39–41]. The CPS of Hib, polyribosylribitol phosphate (PRP, Figure 1), has several significant characters, such as immunogenicity in humans, the same antigenic properties in all strains of type b, and stimulation of anti-Hib antibodies. In 1985 purified PRP was certified for use in a vaccine in the United States. However, rapid reduction of antibodies stimulated by purified PRP was the main drawback, as it offered no immunological memory [42]. The solution was to give more injections as boosters that took dropping levels of antibodies back up to postvaccination levels, but this failed to generate either strong response nor immunological memory, as injection of the booster did not stimulate IgM class switching to IgG [43]. In Finland, the vaccine was very successful in experiments in children 18 months and older, while in the United States postmarketing surveillance showed fluctuating efficiency (from 69% to 88%) [44]. However, the level of $\geq 0.15\,\mu g/mL$ of anti-PRP in unvaccinated children and level of $\geq 1.0\,\mu g/mL$ in vaccinated children were considered protective against Hib infections, as suggested by many studies [45].

CPS-specific receptors on the surfaces of native B cells (BCRs) recognize the multivalency and large size of CPSs. Upon immunization with pure CPS, these BCRs bind to the CPSs and the BCR-CPS complex stimulates the B cell to induce and secrete IgM antibodies against CPS. In the event of bacterial infection following CPS immunization, IgM antibodies bind to the CPS expressed on the surface of the particular pathogenic bacteria and help eradicate that pathogen [11, 46].

The compounds that are able to enhance and/or regulate the antigen's immunogenicity are called adjuvants and represent a varied collection of compounds. Put simply, an adjuvant is a vaccine assistant (*adjuvare* is a Latin word meaning "to help") and is a synonym of immunostimulant. It can be a combination of one or more compounds that act and function differently: that is, a molecule, carrier or depot, immunomodulator, and/or immunostimulant. The adjuvant industry has grown to meet demand for enhancing the immunogenicity of insufficient vaccines. The two main basic mechanisms by which adjuvants act are enhancing antigen presentation to the immune elements and stimulating immunity so that a stronger or wider response is reached. By these means, immunogenicity can be improved and/or doses of the vaccines can be decreased to a level that has no negative effect on immunogenicity [47, 48].

Animals, plants, and bacteria are sources of widespread immunostimulatory constituents of several adjuvants that function as stimulators of immunological components. One highly effective method of adjuvanticity is the conjugation of inactivated toxoids to purified PRP. This method has been used successfully in anti-Hib, anti-*N. meningitidis*, and anti-*Streptococcus pneumoniae* conjugate vaccines. Compounds such as alum and calcium phosphate are the only mineral salts authorized for use as adjuvants with vaccines in the United States since the 1920s. The primary mineral salt adjuvant for use in humans is alum, either as aluminum hydroxide or as aluminum phosphate. It acts by creating a depot spot, such that mild and constant release of the antigen improves presentation to immunological components [47, 48].

Studies have investigated the role of innate cells in adjusting adaptive immunity. Numerous antigen presenting cell (APC) signals are needed to start T-helper responses. First, a signal is activated by presentation of a certain peptide by class II molecules to the T cell receptor (TCR). Without the contribution of an additional signal, abortive and anergy responses are stimulated; a costimulatory second signal is required, via receptor-ligand contacts among APC/T antigens. It appears that another (preceding) signal, the zero signal, is required to stimulate APCs and orient subsequent Th responses, for example, throughout IL12 for Th1 responses. Zero signals are typically stimulated by detection of pathogen-associated molecular patterns (PAMPs) through pathogen recognition

receptors (PRR), involving toll-like receptors (TLRs). APCs class I presentation for CD8 stimulation may be controlled by these signals. Promotion of CD4 cells that secrete interferon gamma (IFNg) by Th1 adjuvants is not enough to activate CD8 cytotoxic T cells, which also need class I antigen presentation [48]. These outcomes closely connect native immunity and the following adaptive immunity. The essential signals and steps needed to stimulate T and B cell responses suggest that signals of innate immunity also control the quality (not only the degree) of adaptive immunity. For example, innate cells permit adaptive T and B cells to differentiate and grow, and Th1 polarization is observed throughout IL12 secretion [48]. Adjuvants may be able to perform on any of these signals. Affecting exactly costimulatory molecules (second signal) throughout antibodies, chemokines, or cytokines is an attractive option [49], but it may lead to unfocused overreaction status [48].

While earlier development of adjuvants generated effective products, there is still a need to create new generations, rationally designed based on recent discoveries in immunology, especially innate immunity. The safe and optimal preparation of adjuvants is the most challenging task in the field. Little work has been dedicated to adjuvants with free PRP or with glycoconjugate vaccines, compared to protein vaccines. However, a number of researchers have examined the capacity of several molecules, especially TLR agonists, to increase the immunogenicity of conjugated or free carbohydrate antigens [48]. Free PRP vaccines against Hib are no longer used in the United States [50].

2.2. Conjugate Vaccines and Adjuvants. Most proteins need participation of T cells to stimulate antibody synthesis and consequently are considered T cell dependent (TD) antigens [51]. These proteins promote increased response of antibodies in the booster vaccine and encourage class switching from IgM to IgG via the involvement of T-helper cells in the immune process. Moreover, subsets of B-memory cells are generated from B cells in TD immunity, resulting in the establishment of memory against a specific antigen. This is accomplished by covalently connecting PRP to protein carriers, which results in production of Hib glycoconjugate vaccines [52]. By this kind of conjugation, the humoral immune response is induced with features of TD immunity reactions, such as affinity maturation, memory, and, crucially, the presence of immunogenicity in children aged more than 2 months [30]. Development of protein-conjugated polysaccharide vaccines has been accelerated by increasing antibiotic resistance and the need to stop Hib infections in high-risk populations [12].

In 1931, Avery and Goebel invented the improvement of polysaccharide immunogenicity by the tool of conjugation to proteins. Nevertheless, this was not widely practiced until the invention of polysaccharide conjugate vaccines. In the 1970s through 1980s, the application of bacterial polysaccharides and proteins for stimulating immunity increased. Conjugate Hib vaccines are created by Hib CPS (polyribosylribitol phosphate; 5-D-ribitol-$(1 \rightarrow 1)$-β-D-ribose-3-phosphate; PRP) attached to proteins, with excellent safety and distinctly different structures and conformations [53–55]. The first invented and approved conjugate vaccine in the United States was created from PRP conjugated to diphtheria toxoid (PRP-D), which was withdrawn from the market soon after introduction of more effective vaccines using meningococcal outer membrane protein (PRP-OMP), CRM_{197} (PRP-CRM) protein carriers, or tetanus toxoid (PRP-T) [56].

The structure of polysaccharides and carrier proteins properties largely determine the immunogenicity of the conjugates, and the techniques used in the conjugation process can play a central effect. The conjugation process should be uncomplicated and mild and cause little alteration to the constituents, such that it does not damage important epitopes on either the protein or the PS, cause undesired depolymerization of the PS, or introduce any harmful epitopes. While a number of conjugation chemistries are available for the synthesis of PS-protein conjugates [57], only a few have been used in licensed vaccines. For proteins, surface-exposed amines (e.g., ε amines of lysine residues) and carboxyls (e.g., the side chains of carboxyl of aspartic and glutamic acid residues) are the major groups used for conjugation [58, 59]. Prior to the conjugation process, fermentation/isolation techniques of Hib CPS are used to produce Hib conjugate vaccines on a large scale [60].

Chemical synthesis of the Hib saccharide antigen was a breakthrough in conjugated vaccines, which led to development of a novel type of Hib conjugate vaccine. This generally includes the formulation of the oligosaccharide moiety by chemical or enzymatic methods, which represents the immunological specificity for the vaccine and then attachment of this to an immunogenic protein by a linker. Chemical synthesis of these complex oligosaccharides is difficult and requires a suitable mixture of techniques that allow appropriate treatments by applicable glycosyl donors, acceptors, protecting groups, and coupling reactions settings. This option has come to be accessible due to notable growth of enzymatic and chemical oligosaccharides preparation [61–64]. Currently, the synthetic Quimi-Hib vaccine is approved for use in the National Immunization Program in Cuba [64]. Figure 2 summarizes the types of currently used Hib vaccines according to the type of PRP.

Glycoconjugate syntheses include the usage of well-defined or random activation sites in the polysaccharide as possible attachment sites for proteins. The choice of method for activation is mainly governed by the molecular size of the polysaccharide. Large polysaccharides are frequently arbitrarily activated, while selective activation at the reducing end is typical for oligosaccharides [12]. Molecular differences between conjugation methods do not affect their clinical performance but do influence strategies for quality control [57].

The conjugation process can be divided into the following steps (Figure 3): (I) preparing the carbohydrate, (II) preparing the protein carrier, (III) performing the conjugation, and (IV) finishing. Some conjugation schemes combine several steps, whereas in others a particular step may be unnecessary [58].

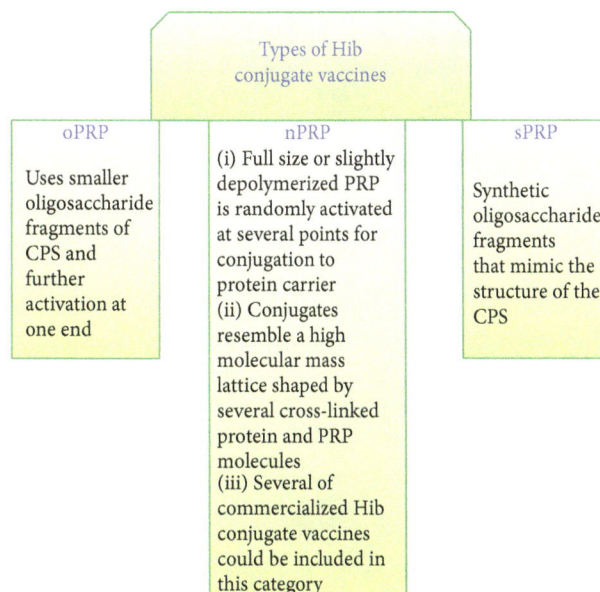

FIGURE 2: Schematic diagram summarizing the types of currently used Hib vaccines according to the type of PRP (nPRP-native PRP, oPRP-oligosaccharide PRP, and sPRP-synthetic PRP).

Preparation of the Carbohydrate

(1) *Sizing.* Native CPSs have molecular sizes in the millions of Daltons, and solutions tend to be viscous. Reducing the molecular size of the PSs decreases their viscosity and makes the solutions easier to handle.

(2) *Activation.* Carbohydrates have hydroxyl groups, which are relatively inactive and must be translated into a more reactive form (functional group). The activated PS can be either immediately conjugated to the protein or further functionalized. The positions of the activated groups determine the positions of the linkages on the PS.

(3) *Functionalization.* This procedure adds reactive chemical groups to the carbohydrate or converts the activated PS into a more stable form while maintaining its reactivity. Functionalization can include the addition of a spacer molecule between the carbohydrate and the reactive group and in some cases is a multistep process [58].

Protein Carrier Preparation. Amines (the ε amines of lysines) and carboxyls (glutamic and aspartic acids) can be applied to link directly to the activated or functionalized carbohydrate. However, some protocols rely on the addition of chemical groups that are more reactive and/or more specific in their reaction with the activated or functionalized carbohydrate than carboxyls or amines. Functionalization of the protein can also provide a spacer molecule such that the reactive groups on the protein are more accessible to the carbohydrate [58].

Conjugation. Conditions that promote conjugation-high concentrations of protein and PS and high numbers of reactive

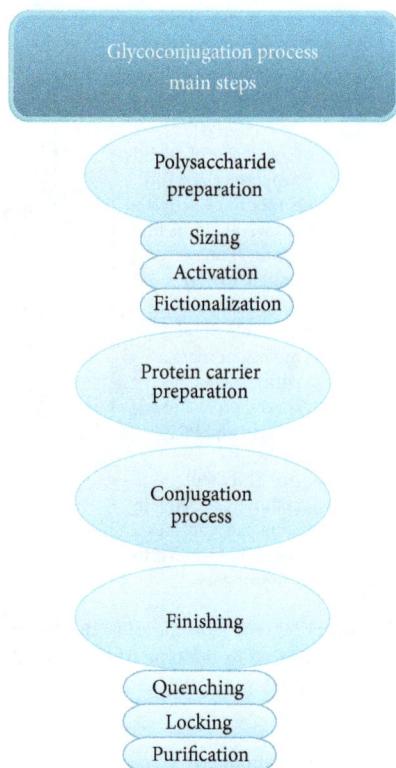

FIGURE 3: Main steps in the glycoconjugate process.

groups bring the risk of excessive cross-linking when both the protein and the PS have multiple reactive groups. Also of concern is the need to confirm uniform mixing and reaction, which can be challenging on a production scale due to the high viscosity of the PSs. Careful control over factors relevant to the particular chemistry is crucial for successful conjugation. These factors include pH, temperature, the ratio of protein to PS, and the concentration of each. The type of linkage achieved depends on the chemistry and may be reversible or irreversible [58].

Finishing

(1) *Quenching.* Quenching inactivates any residual groups to prevent further cross-linking. This step is commonly completed with monovalent blocking reagents, such as ethanolamine or glycine.

(2) *Locking.* A locking (or blocking) step makes the conjugation linkage fundamentally irreversible.

(3) *Purification.* The conjugate must be purified to elim-inate the conjugation reagents and to guarantee low levels of unconjugated carbohydrate and protein. Unconjugated PS has been shown to decrease the immune response to the conjugate [65, 66].

Two models for carbohydrate-protein conjugation have been established: the single ended model (terminal amina-tion-single method) and cross-linked lattice matrix (dual amination method) [12, 57].

2.2.1. Terminal Amination-Single Method. This method imi-tates the structural features of glycoproteins by which protein is connected to the oligosaccharides across its reducing end, resulting in the single ended model (Figure 4) [57]. The model differs from native glycoproteins in terms of polymeric carbohydrate chain length, connection sites, and structure. The antigenic carbohydrate positions of this model of neoglycoprotein are instantly available to antibodies. The carbohydrate hapten density is the main factor that influences the antigenicity of these neoglycoproteins [12].

2.2.2. Dual Amination Method. A cross-linked lattice matrix is molded by several connection points formed by con-jugation of an antigenic carbohydrate and a protein car-rier (Figure 5) [57]. Vaccine solubility can be enhanced by decreasing the quantity of cross-linked points on the polysac-charide chain, which shrinks the conjugate matrix and cross-linking. The large number of reachable antigenic spots on the superficial cross-linked lattice matrix guarantees the molecule's extraordinary immunogenicity, despite the quan-tity of cross-linking [12].

The tendency of the carrier protein to denature is a lim-iting factor for conjugation. However, immunogenicity can be maintained if an alteration in the tertiary geometric shape is able to influence the antibody specificity. The modification of hydroxyl, carboxyl, hemiacetal, phenoxyl, amino/imino, or mercapto/disulfide functional group is thus an important step in the conjugation process. Sodium cyanoborohydrate is used in conjugation chemistry involving reductive amination to selectively reduce intermediate imine adducts known as Schiff bases [67, 68]. This reduction pushes the system to equilibrium, affording stable adducts, despite the formation of Schiff bases being a disfavored equilibrium technique in water. Glycosylamine formation is straightforward reaction whereby carbohydrates are treated with saturated solution of ammonium bicarbonate for 5–7 days at room temperature. Catching the glycosyl amine by creation of the peptide with iodoacetic acid and reaction of the cysteine residue of the protein to the thiol reactive iodoacyl group produces neoglycoconjugates [69–71]. The spacer arm, an allyl group presented at the reducing end, may be employed to make aldehyde by ozonolysis and can be joined to the protein amine groups by reductive amination.

A thiol reactive maleimide group can be connected to a carbohydrate over a spacer arm to increase the availability of functional groups and reactive centers [72]. Methods using N,N′-dicyclohexylcarbodiimide (DCC), water soluble 1-ethyl-3-(3-dimethylaminopropyl) carbodiimide (EDC), or activation of carboxylic groups by sulfo-NHS for combined amino functionality in a carbohydrate or protein have been broadly applied to the production of neoglycoproteins [73, 74]. *p*-Nitrophenyl glycosides may be converted to highly reactive diazonium salts to create electron-rich adducts, aromatic tyrosine, or tryptophan residues [75]. Although regarded as limited by recent measures, diazo coupling grants strong conjugates immunogenicity and has been broadly utilized for preparation of conjugate vaccines such as the type 3 *S. pneumoniae* CPS vaccine. By nonspecific activation of hydroxyl groups and creation of reactive cyanate esters,

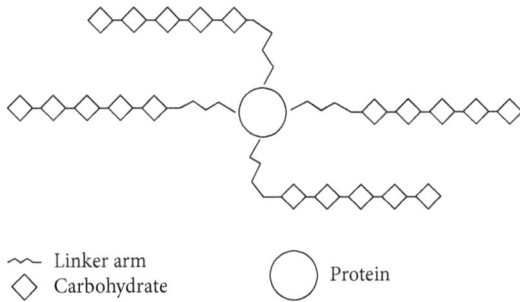

~~ Linker arm
◇ Carbohydrate
◯ Protein

FIGURE 4: Single ended model (neoglycoprotein).

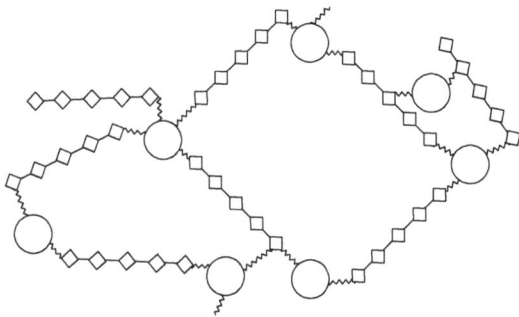

FIGURE 5: Cross-linked lattice model.

cyanogen bromide has been employed to conjugate carbohydrates and protein amino groups in aqueous alkaline solution via a stable O-alkyl isourea linkage [76]. When a phosphate presents at the terminal end, it frequently appears in an internal ester, because of the closeness of the adjoining hydroxyl group on the ribitol moiety to the phosphate hydroxyl; this internal esterification triggers Hib PS hydrolytic lability at both alkaline and acid pH and at elevated temperature [77].

Adjuvants for conjugate vaccines include salts of aluminum. Depending on the conjugate, the adjuvant may be unimportant or crucial [78]; or it may have a harmful influence on the stability of the conjugate, as with Hib conjugates vaccines [79]. Toll-like receptor 9 (TLR9) agonists have also been employed as adjuvants, helping to compensate for immunodeficiency such as that faced in late or early life [80–82]. Immune interference arising in polyvalent conjugate vaccines could be lessened by adjuvants via suppression of the B or T cell dependent carrier, among other methods [83–85].

Quality control of Hib conjugate vaccines by laboratories, manufacturers, and the government depends on physicochemical procedures for screening of production consistency and recognition of any defects in batches over time. Biological tests are performed by manufacturers only during vaccine production to confirm stimulation of TD immunity by conjugate vaccines and to guarantee their safety [86].

Since 1997, the World Health Organization (WHO) has recommended the Hib conjugate vaccine for national immunization programs anywhere resources exist and disease burden data support its priority [39, 87–89]. Before 1997, however, only a minority of children in developing countries had access to the Hib conjugate vaccine, due to shortages

arising from sparse statistics on disease burden [90], lack of belief in the vaccination value, lack of awareness, and greater priority of other concerns [91]. The vaccine was supplied by only one manufacturer to the United Nations International Children's Emergency Fund (UNICEF) [92], and its three-dose course was much more expensive than the combined price of all other vaccines in the standard immunization for infants specified by the WHO Expanded Program on Immunization (EPI). The estimated price of the Hib conjugate vaccine was twofold higher than the measles, mumps, and rubella multivalent vaccine, and it was more costly than conventional vaccines in EPI (3.15 versus US$1.4/dose) [93]. Because of a lack of competition, the vaccine price remained high for several years [92]. The vaccine formulation choice (monovalent or multivalent) (Table 1) and final product vialing (1- or 10-dose vial) were crucial factors in the introduction of the Hib vaccine in North and South America. These two factors affect the vaccine wastage level, cost, reconstitution necessity, space of cold chain, and education events for medical employees [94, 95].

The regimen of three doses in the first year of life, with a fourth dose given in the second year, is followed in majority of the world. A three-dose regimen without the fourth dose is typical in low-income countries. Generally the Hib conjugate vaccine is given as a one-injection polyvalent together with tetanus toxoid, diphtheria toxoid, and whole-cell or acellular pertussis (DTwP or DTaP), and sometimes additionally with hepatitis B antigen (Table 1) and/or inactivated poliovirus [47].

In the 1990s patent law prevented vaccine manufacturers in developing countries from acquiring the techniques for making Hib conjugates [96, 97]; and markets were cautious due to a lack of dependable estimation. Additionally, manufacturers in developed countries began cancelling conventional manufacture of DTwP vaccines, which were less costly and hence obtainable to UNICEF for developing countries [98]. To deal with these obstacles, the National Institute for Public Health and the Environment/Netherlands Vaccine Institute (RIVM/NVI, Bilthoven, Netherlands) initiated a plan in 1998 to develop commercially viable and scalable Hib conjugate vaccine production, without patent violation, by employing technology transmissible to manufacturers in developing countries. Further assistance for the growth of combined vaccines containing the Hib conjugate indicated that manufacturers, by acquisition of entrance to technology for the Hib conjugate vaccine, could subsequently confirm a sustainable supply of inexpensive and valuable vaccines [98].

Founded in 2000, the Developing Countries Vaccine Manufactures Network (DCVMN) was formed to distribute surveillance against identified and emergent contagious infections, with the goal of raising the obtainability and quality of vaccines inexpensive to everyone. DCVMN is an international alliance of manufacturers that provides data and professional education plans, development of technology, inspiring transfer of technologies, advanced research and development, and community teaching regarding the accessibility of secure, cheap, and effective vaccines. The network grew to involve 44 manufacturers in 16 territories and countries, creating and distributing >40 several vaccine

TABLE 1: Summary of the most important Hib vaccines in U.S. Food and Drug Administration (FDA) and The European Medicines Agency (EMA) up to 20 December 2015.

Vaccine name	Approval date	Valency	Description	Manufacture and marketing
b-CAPSA 1 Hib-VAX Hib-IMUNE	1985 US	Monovalent	Pure polysaccharide CPS vaccine (unconjugated). The vaccine was recommended routinely for children at 24 months of age and for children at 15 months of age enrolled in child care facilities. The vaccine was not consistently immunogenic in children <18 months of age and was withdrawn from the market in 1988.	b-CAPSA 1 by Praxis, Biologics, Hib-VAX by Connaught, and Hib-IMUNE by Lederle
ProHIBIT	1987 US	Monovalent	First conjugate *Haemophilusinfluenzae* b vaccine to be approved by FDA. ProHIBIT is no longer available in the United States.	Connaught Laboratories, Inc.
HibTITER	1990 US	Monovalent	Hib conjugate vaccine (diphtheria CRM197 protein conjugate). Discontinued 2007.	Wyeth Pharmaceuticals Inc.
PedvaxHIB	1989 US	Monovalent	Hib conjugate vaccine (meningococcal protein conjugate).	Merck & Co., Inc. http://www.merck.com/product/vaccines/home.html
ActHIB	1993 US	Monovalent	Approved for use as a four-dose series in infants and children 2 months through 5 years of age.	Sanofi Pasteur http://www.sanofipasteur.com/en/
OmniHib	1993 US	Monovalent	Hib conjugate vaccine. No longer available in the United States.	SmithKline Beecham
TriHIBit	1996 US	Polyvalent	Combination of DTaP and Hib vaccine, licensed for the fourth dose in the DTaP and Hib series. Discontinued on 2011 according to CDC.	Sanofi Pasteur http://www.sanofipasteur.com/en/
Comvax	1996 US	Polyvalent	Mixed vaccines of recombinant hepatitis B antigen and *Haemophilusinfluenzae* type b conjugated vaccine. Discontinued on 2014 according to Merck.	Merck & Co., Inc. http://www.merck.com/product/vaccines/home.html
Tetramune	1996 US	Polyvalent	DTP and Hib conjugate vaccine. Discontinued according to CDC.	Wyeth Pharmaceuticals Inc.
PROCOMVAX	1999 EU	Polyvalent	Hib conjugate and hepatitis B (recombinant) vaccine. Withdrawn on 2009 according to EMA.	Sanofi Pasteur MSD http://www.spmsd.com/
Hexavac	2000 EU	Polyvalent	Diphtheria, tetanus, acellular pertussis, inactivated poliomyelitis, hepatitis B (recombinant), and Hib conjugate vaccine, adjuvant. Suspended 2005, withdrawn on 2012 according to EMA.	Sanofi Pasteur http://www.sanofipasteur.com/en/
Infanrix-Hib	2000 EU 2002 US	Polyvalent	DTaP and adsorbed conjugated Hib vaccine.	GlaxoSmithKline Biologicals https://www.gsk.com/
Infanrix Hexa	2000 EU	Polyvalent	DTaP, hepatitis B (recombinant), inactivated poliomyelitis, and adsorbed conjugated Hib vaccine.	GlaxoSmithKline Biologicals https://www.gsk.com/
Quintanrix	2005 EU	Polyvalent	DTP, hepatitis B (rDNA), and adsorbed Hib conjugate vaccine. Withdrawn on 2008 according to EMA.	GlaxoSmithKline Biologicals https://www.gsk.com/
Pentacel	2008 US	Polyvalent	DTaP adsorbed, inactivated poliovirus, and Hib conjugate.	Sanofi Pasteur http://www.sanofipasteur.com/en/

TABLE 1: Continued.

Vaccine name	Approval date	Valency	Description	Manufacture and marketing
Hiberix	2009 US	Monovalent	Hib conjugate vaccine (tetanus toxoid conjugate). Approved only as a booster dose of the Hib schedule among children 12 months and older.	GlaxoSmithKline Biologicals https://www.gsk.com/
MenHibrix	2012 US	Polyvalent	Meningococcal groups C and Y and Hib tetanus toxoid conjugate vaccine for infants at increased risk of meningococcal disease.	GlaxoSmithKline Biologicals https://www.gsk.com/
Hexacima	2013 EU	Polyvalent	DTaP, hepatitis B (rDNA), poliomyelitis (inactivated), and adsorbed Hib conjugate vaccine.	Sanofi Pasteur http://www.sanofipasteur.com/en/
Hexyon	2013 EU	Polyvalent	DTaP, hepatitis B (rDNA), inactivated poliomyelitis, and Hib conjugate vaccine (adsorbed).	Sanofi Pasteur http://www.sanofipasteur.com/en/
INFANRIX-IPV/Hib	2015 US	Polyvalent	DTaP, inactivated poliomyelitis, and Hib vaccine.	GlaxoSmithKline Biologicals https://www.gsk.com/

CRM197: enzymatically inactive and nontoxic form of diphtheria toxin that contains a single amino acid substitution.

DTaP: diphtheria, tetanus, and acellular pertussis.

DTP: Diphtheria and tetanus toxoids and whole-cell pertussis.

CDC discontinued vaccines:

http://www.cdc.gov/vaccines/pubs/pinkbook/downloads/appendices/B/discontinued_vaccines.pdf.

CDC, Morbidity and Mortality Weekly Report (MMWR):

http://www.cdc.gov/mmwr/preview/mmwrhtml/00000696.htm.

EMA, European public assessment reports:

http://www.ema.europa.eu/ema/index.jsp?curl=pages/medicines/landing/epar_search.jsp&mid=WC0b01ac05800ld124.

MERCK, COMVAX vaccines discontinue report:

https://www.merckvaccines.com/is-bin/intershop.static/WFS/Merck-MerckVaccines-Site/Merck-MerckVaccines/en_US/Professional-Resources/Documents/announcements/VACC-1114028-0000,pdf.

types [99]. Arabio, founded in 2005, was the first biopharmaceutical company in the Gulf Cooperation Council (GCC), located in Jeddah BioCity with Vacsera as a limited liability company, and is a member of DCVMN. Arabio focuses on plasma, biopharmaceutical, and vaccine products. The range of developments planned by Arabio could establish it as the leading biological company of its category in the Middle East [100].

3. Future Perspectives

The immune and central nervous systems are characterized by their ability to retain memory. This exceptional quality creates many opportunities for health interventions, such as prophylactic immunization. Advances in molecular chemistry and biology, glycobiology, glycoimmunology, pathogen biology, and immunology have led to substantial increases in vaccine efficacy. Current vaccines are commonly made from highly purified antigens or hapten obtained from or designed on the most immunogenic parts of pathogens. The latest molecular biology advances also promote techniques helping in immune system stimulation [12]. Figure 6 summarizes the most important fields in the future of vaccinology as whole and Hib vaccines in particular. In addition, new vaccinology concentrates on tools that offer sustained immunogenicity with better safety. These technologies consist of employing engineered antigens, subunits from pathogens (polysaccharides or proteins), or vectored antigens. The vector is a harmless virus or bacterium in which a gene can be enclosed and expressed. This technique has come to dominate the field due to its usefulness for hard-to-reach pathogens, such as intracellular pathogens [101].

Vaccinology is further improving via development of more adjuvants, combination vaccines, and new methods of administration. New administration methods include transcutaneous (intradermal) immunization (TCI), which has potential for use in humans, whereby antigens are transported by Langerhans antigen presenting cells to nearby lymph nodes, directly stimulating systemic immunity. A major model for this method is the intradermal influenza vaccine, which penetrates the epidermis with a microneedle and creates the same immune responses as intramuscular vaccines [101, 102]. Moreover, via an ADP-ribosylating exotoxin in mouse, such as the heat-labile enterotoxin of *Escherichia coli* or its mutants (LTK63 and LTR72) or cholera toxin, TCI activates antitoxin protecting responses and the coadministered antigen [103–108].

Combination vaccines are increasingly significant for efforts to improve vaccination acceptance by the public, as they reduce the number of injections essential for complete immunization (Table 1). Combined vaccines help to achieve high vaccination coverage and well-timed vaccination by minimizing occurrences of delay. Including novel antigens on current high-coverage vaccines is an effective method for presenting novel antigens to schedules of vaccination [109]. Studies conducted in Germany [110] and the United States [39, 111] confirm that combined vaccines can lead to improved coverage of specific antigens, and with further well-timed

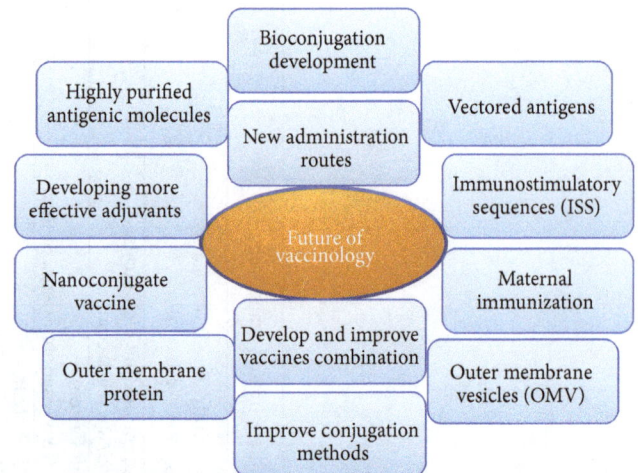

FIGURE 6: The most important fields in the future of vaccinology as a whole and Hib vaccines in particular.

vaccination, a greater proportion of children can obtain all recommended vaccines at the appropriate age [112].

In Germany, 5-year surveillance was conducted to inspect the efficiency of hexavalent vaccines and found that DTPa-HBV-IPV/Hib was 90.4% effective for a complete three-dose primary series and 100% for a complete primary series with a booster (regardless of the priming Hib vaccine) [113]. Long-standing effectiveness of a combined Hib-DTPa-based vaccine on a 3-, 5-, and 11-month schedule has also been confirmed in Sweden, as incidence in children younger than 4 years was approximately 0.4/100,000 in between 2005 and 2008 [114].

Maternal immunization to protect from pathogenic organisms has been suggested as a technique to protect newborns, as maternofetal immunoglobulin transfer occurs through the placenta and maternal immunoglobulins appear in the fetus blood. Maternal immunization with Hib polysaccharide and conjugate vaccines appears to be a successful approach for delivering antibodies protective levels to infants. Maternal immunization studies [115, 116] have recognized several factors affecting the placental passage of immunoglobulins. Compared to IgM and IgA antibodies, IgG antibodies more effectively cross the placenta, and antibodies in the IgGl subclass are better for transport than those in the IgG2 subclass [117]. Antibody placental crossing is moreover subject to the vaccination time through pregnancy [116]. The detection of factors affecting antibody placental crossing may be fundamental to choosing plans for future maternal immunization [118].

Synthetic oligodeoxynucleotides enclosing cytosine triphosphate deoxynucleotide-phospho-diester-guanine triphosphate deoxynucleotide (CpG) immunostimulatory sequences (ISS) may function as danger signals of bacterial attacks and trigger immune warfare [119, 120]. While the exact mechanism of action is not fully understood, it is thought that ISS act as PAMPs able to connect PRR, mainly expressed on the surface of antigen nonspecific innate immune cells [121]. The presence of APC-expressed PRR by PAMPs activates innate cells that gain the power to stimulate adaptive immunity cells, which in turn support the launch of an antigen-specific immune action. ISS are made in accordance with DNA sequences of bacteria that may stimulate innate immunity cells [122]. ISS stimulate innate immunity in the same way as bacterial infections, therefore supporting the specific immunity to the antigen, in contrast to other adjuvants, such as mineral oils or alum, whose immunostimulatory action extends delivery of antigens [120]. The danger signals produced by ISS provide a powerful adjuvant to stimulate the anti-conjugated PS type one immunity response.

The adjuvant effect of ISS effectively improves the anti-carrier immunity response. Anti-diphtheria toxoid (anti-DT) and anti-tetanus toxoid (anti-TT) antibody titers were greatly improved by ISS in the Hib-CRM and Hib-TT vaccines. Moreover, the pattern of the anti-carrier IgG subclass was affected by ISS, as IgG2a and IgG2b increased in the presence of ISS. A considerable rise in IgG3 was distinguished only in the anti-TT immune response. IgG3 is the major IgG subclass in several humoral immunity responses in the mouse that are stimulated by polysaccharide antigens but is a minor constituent of the anti-protein immune response [123]. Therefore, TT but not CRM stimulates IgG3 production in the similar cytokine milieu resulting from ISS, supporting the suggestion that the antigen structure is included in the immunoglobulin isotype switch of B-lymphocyte differentiation [124].

H. influenzae outer membrane proteins have received attention due to their antigenic excellence as potential vaccine candidates [125]. However, one significant criterion that must be met for a Hib outer membrane protein to be an effective vaccine is that the protein must have surface-exposed and antibody-accessible antigenic determinants that are common to most strains of the pathogen. At least three Hib outer membrane proteins appear to fulfill this requirement. Data on the P6 protein show that this protein has at least one surface epitope that is common to all strains [126]. To date, P2 and P6 are the best candidates for anti-nontypeable *H. influenza* vaccines [127]. Another method in vaccine development inserts surface-exposed proteins in outer membrane vesicles (OMV), which, in clinical trials, stimulates responses of serum bactericidal antibodies and gives rise to antimeningococcal activity [128].

3.1. Conjugation Development. The classic antigen presentation hypothesis for glycoconjugate vaccines suggests that helper CD4$^+$ T cells identify a peptide originated from the carrier protein [129]. According to the traditional pattern, the glycoconjugate binds to the surface of a B cell whose specific job is to make antibodies to the polysaccharide component. The B cell deals with the protein portion of the glycoconjugate and exhibits a peptide from the covalently linked carrier protein in the setting of the major histocompatibility complex class II (MHC II) to the $\alpha\beta$-TCR of CD4$^+$ T-helper cells. Stimulation of T cells by peptide-MHC II complexes and other costimulatory molecules leads to production of the cytokine interleukin 4 (IL-4) by the T cell, which in sequence encourages cognate B cell maturation and subsequent creation of carbohydrate-specific antibodies, with associated class

switching of immunoglobulin to IgG and memory responses. This hypothesis was originally based on the theory that only protein antigens can be presented to and identified by T cells. Initial research on hapten-carrier conjugates (i.e., small molecular weight noncarbohydrate molecules connected to carrier proteins) suggested that peptide presentation is the triggering tool for glycoconjugate induced T cell activation [130].

A new study [129] strongly suggests that carbohydrate-recognizing T cells, not peptide-recognizing T cells, are the principal T cell population driving the T cell-mediated adaptive immune response. It shows that carbohydrates, which were previously thought to be "T cell-independent" antigens, can be precisely distinguished by T cells, as they are conjugated with carrier peptides that permit their presentation by MHC II molecules on the surface of APCs. These conclusions are different from the classical understanding that T cells can only recognize peptides [129]. A model new-generation glycoconjugate vaccine [129] has enriched carbohydrate T cell epitopes compared to a glycoconjugate vaccine made by traditional conjugation methods. This model vaccine is 50–100 times more immunogenic than classical vaccines. This type of carbohydrate-recognition T cell may lead to significantly better vaccines against infectious diseases. Elucidation of the T cell epitopes of glycoconjugate vaccines would allow us to imitate those epitopes and enhance vaccines by joining carbohydrate epitopes at a frequency and density that enhances immunogenicity and protection through APCs proficient processing and presentation and highly specific T cell recognition [131]. The zwitterionic polysaccharides are a class of complex carbohydrates that activate T cells [131, 132]. Figure 7 summarizes the most important approaches to the improvement of glycoconjugate vaccines.

The conjugation of biomolecules to metal nanoclusters and nanoemulsions has opened new opportunities in the design and synthesis of multifunctional and multimodal built systems for biomedical uses. Gold nanoparticles have been widely studied for their low toxicity, relative inertness, easy handling, and easy chemistry of surface control. The surface of gold can be shaped in a controlled way with various ligands through thiol chemistry, producing multifunctional and multivalent nanoparticles [101, 133].

Carrier proteins are fundamental components of classical conjugate vaccines. Peptides offer covalently bound carbohydrate epitopes to the TCR of CD4$^+$ T cells [134]. Thus, optimization of the MHC II-binding peptide concentration in a conjugate vaccine would theoretically enhance the immunogenicity of the conjugate vaccine by increasing the number of carbohydrates that can be presented on MHC II proteins. The best approach to accomplish this is to connect polysaccharides to MHC II-binding peptides in place of the intact proteins. This would allow the presentation of significantly greater amounts of peptide-bound carbohydrate epitopes to T cells, compared to when intact proteins are. In fact, many studies have shown that conjugating peptides to polysaccharides creates highly effective conjugate vaccines [134–137]. In one study, three polypeptides consisting of strings of 6, 10, or 19 human MHC II-binding peptides from several antigenic proteins were created [138]. In each

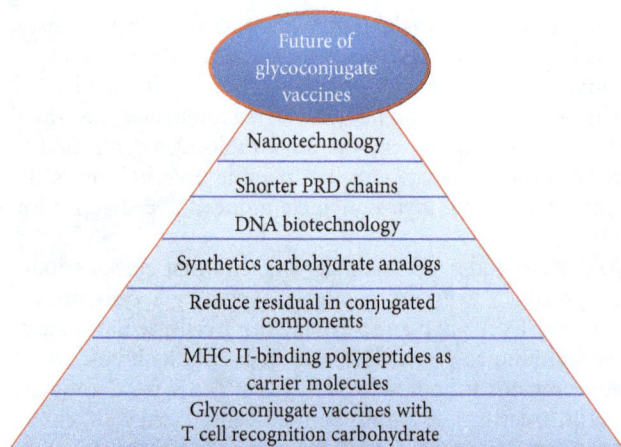

FIGURE 7: The most important approaches to improve glycoconjugate vaccines.

construct, the MHC II-binding peptides were separated by the lysine-glycine spacer to give flexibility to the polypeptide and to permit the conjugation of the glycan to the amino side chains of the lysine spacer. The 19-valent polypeptide was then conjugated with CPSs of *N. meningitides* serogroups A, C, W-135, and Y [139]. In immunization tests, the polypeptide-containing glycoconjugate vaccines had greater immunogenicity than glycoconjugates that contained CRM_{197} as carrier protein. Compared to CRM_{197}-based conjugates, smaller quantities of polypeptide-based conjugates stimulated a higher bactericidal antibody titer against all four meningococcal polysaccharides. This strategy illustrates the use of MHC II-binding polypeptides as carrier molecules to create greatly effective glycoconjugate vaccines. The main improvement enabled by this strategy is that these synthetic polypeptide carriers can be identified by most of the human MHCII haplotypes. Furthermore, peptide carriers can be expressed in *E. coli*, which makes them easy to produce for production of glycoconjugate vaccines [11].

An important step in conjugation chemistry is to improve conjugation efficiencies to levels at which residual unconjugated components, particularly free PSs, do not affect the stimulation of protective immune responses. The use of an effective, mild conjugation chemistry would allow for higher yields of vaccine. For example, reaching more than 90% efficiency of coupling of the PS may allow for a simplified purification process. It would also be needed for development of conjugate vaccines that do not require refrigeration [58].

Current improvements in carbohydrate synthesis must simplify the enzymatic and chemical preparation of well-characterized and well-defined homogenous carbohydrate antigens for further development of glycoconjugate vaccines. Several carbohydrate antigens analogs that are stable metabolically, such as S-glycosides and C-glycosides, may enhance the immunogenicity and antigenicity of the glycoconjugate vaccines. Moreover, such analogs should expand our knowledge of antibody carbohydrate identification, processing and presentation of antigens, and immune system stimulation. Such improved knowledge of glycoimmunology

would facilitate the creation of the ideal glycoconjugate vaccine for a particular disease or infection. Synthetic C-glycoside analogs of tumor-combined antigens, which are metabolically stable, nonhydrolysable carbohydrates, would similarly enhance batch-to-batch consistency in vaccine manufacturing and bypass the cold storage that is generally needed to preserve and guarantee effectiveness of existing carbohydrate-based vaccines [12].

Recently, a study reported highly immunogenic PRP-TT conjugates generated from shorter chain PRP, compared to both their high-molecular-weight counterparts from the same laboratory and licensed vaccines. The authors have optimized methods to prepare more immunogenic low-molecular-weight PRP-TT conjugates in a reproducible manner. The higher reactivity of hydrazide groups compared to the lysine ε-amino group resulted in a shorter conjugation time and an optimal yield. The conjugates thus created are immunogenic in rats. A hallmark of this study is the development of highly immunogenic PRP-TT conjugates using short-chain PRP, which forms the basis for further development of oligosaccharide conjugates as successful vaccine candidates alone or in combination [140].

3.2. Conjugation through DNA Biotechnology. Generally, chemical approaches that allow for well-controlled conjugation reactions between distinct-length glycans and proteins [141–143] are vital for designing highly immunogenic vaccines. To date, the most effective vaccines used for protection from invasive pathogenic bacterial infection are the glycoconjugate vaccines, mainly consisting of bacterial capsular polysaccharides coupling to a desired protein carrier. Within the pathogenic bacterial strains there is effective single CPS component and/or multiple CPS from different strains. The later condition makes glycoconjugate vaccine production a very hard process, since each strain requires extraction, hydrolysis, chemical activation, and conjugation to a carrier protein. To avoid this hard situation for conserved and/or nonconserved CPS of different bacterial pathogen, the use of bioglycoconjugates machinery of innovative *E. coli* will substantially simplify the production of glycoconjugate vaccines.

DNA biotechnology has revolutionized vaccinology and generated new methods for vaccine discovery, such as antigenome technology, reverse vaccinology, surfome analysis, genetics vaccinology, and immunoproteomics to uncover innovative immunogenic antigens [144]. Genetically engineered vaccines are expected to be a major type of future vaccines due to their high safety level, improved immunogenicity, and decreased reactogenicity. However, absence of posttranslational modifications (PTMs) machinery in *E. coli* limits its use for the production of recombinant biopharmaceuticals and/or biosimilars [145–152]. Various posttranslational modifications including glycosylation and phosphorylation, which are critical for functional activity, do not take place in *E. coli* [149–153]. Protein glycan coupling technology (PGCT) is a strategy that has been used to move toward the target of making structurally defined, homogenous glycoconjugate vaccines with a well-controlled conjugation reaction [154–156]. N-linked glycosylation of proteins is one of the most important posttranslational modifications in eukaryotes. Kowarik et al. identified a novel N-linked glycosylation pathway in the bacterium *Campylobacter jejuni* and also showed the successful transfer of functionally active N-glycosylation pathway into *E. coli* [157]. PGCT uses the bacterial glycosyltransferase enzyme PglB, an oligotransferase expressed in *Campylobacter jejuni*, to enzymatically link a bacterial polysaccharide with a carrier protein. PglB specifically recognizes a 2-acetamido-containing a reducing end sugar and glycosidically links it to a carrier protein that has a specific sequence identified by the PglB enzyme for N-linked glycosidation. The enzymatic conjugation, and glycan and protein biosynthesis, occurs in an *E. coli* host strain. The target glycan, protein, and PglB are cloned and expressed in *E. coli*. This technology removes the necessity for multistep production and purification of the glycan and protein and several steps of chemical conjugation. Consequently, the process of creating glycoconjugate vaccines is shortened and vaccine production is enhanced. Furthermore, current chemical conjugation strategies require alteration of the polysaccharides or proteins (e.g., random oxidation of the sugar chain), which may change the natural epitopes and lead to generation of less-effective conjugates. Additionally, enzymatic conjugation uses highly specific substrates with distinct binding domains, and as a result, the conjugation outcomes are homogenous and structurally defined. Finally, PGCT avoids the need for pathogenic bacteria from which polysaccharides and/or proteins are isolated, as both glycan and protein synthesis and glycoconjugate assembly take place completely in an *E. coli* system [156].

Although the bacterial N-glycan structure is not similar to that seen in eukaryotes, engineering of glycosylation pathway of *C. jejuni* into *E. coli* has not paved the way for expressing and production of glycosylated protein *E. coli* [158, 159], but the glycoconjugate vaccines too [154, 156, 160–164], which will avoid the chemical conjugation vaccines producers for the harsh capsular polysaccharide-protein conjugation chemical reactions. The coming challenge for synthesis of glycosylated proteins in the engineering *E. coli* is the robotic machinery for secretory and extracellular N-linked glycoproteins production [165].

4. Conclusion

Heterogeneity in antibody responses between individuals and racial groups is controlled by genetic allotypes, which are still only partly understood and may be well-defined for governing T-independent and T-dependent antibody responses in certain circumstances. Moreover, as immunity weakens with age and fluctuates due to previous pathogen contact, life-cycle controlling vaccines implemented for several periods of life can make the most of defense at all ages. The recent concept of "one vaccine suits everyone" to immunize individuals is the only practical concept at the current time, but it is possible that future vaccines will be developed according to national boundaries and personalized to each individual beneficiary; this is termed "vaccinomics." Sustainment of surveillance of colonization and isolates from diseases will be a vital part of a planned strategy for immunization in coming years.

Several populations remain vulnerable to Hib disease even with vaccination. Native American populations are up to six times more susceptible to Hib infection, and Alaskan natives and Navajo Indians still get Hib disease. Studies in Europe and the United States raise the question of whether three primary injections and one boost at around 15 months of age are sufficient, or if something more is needed to protect these populations, especially if the number or people around them who carry *H. influenzae* or other bacteria will not give them a boost in immunity. It has long been established that vaccine manufacturers in developing countries are able to manufacture high quality new vaccines that can satisfy WHO requisites. The Hib conjugate vaccine RIVM/NVI can offer an effective prototype for the efficacious resettlement of technology of up-to-date vaccine to the Arab Gulf and developing nations, including Saudi Arabia.

Conflict of Interests

The authors confirm that this paper content has no conflict of interests.

Acknowledgments

The current work is a part of the Ph.D. thesis of Mr. Adi Essam Zarei (Department of Biology, Faculty of Science, King Abdulaziz University). This work was supported in part by King Abdulaziz City for Scientific Research and Technology (KACST, PGP-37-56), Saudi Arabia.

References

[1] E. E. Adderson, C. L. Byington, L. Spencer et al., "Invasive serotype a *Haemophilus influenzae* infections with a virulence genotype resembling *Haemophilus influenzae* type b: emerging pathogen in the vaccine era?" *Pediatrics*, vol. 108, no. 1, article E18, 2001.

[2] M. G. Bruce, S. L. Deeks, T. Zulz et al., "Epidemiology of *Haemophilus influenzae* serotype a, North American Arctic, 2000–2005," *Emerging Infectious Diseases*, vol. 14, no. 1, pp. 48–55, 2008.

[3] J. C. Parke Jr., R. Schneerson, and J. B. Robbins, "The attack rate, age incidence, racial distribution, and case fatality rate of *Hemophilus influenzae* type b meningitis in Mecklenburg County, North Carolina," *The Journal of Pediatrics*, vol. 81, no. 4, pp. 765–769, 1972.

[4] J. N. Hanna, "The epidemiology of invasive *Haemophilus influenzae* infections in children under five years of age in the Northern Territory: a three-year study," *Medical Journal of Australia*, vol. 152, no. 5, pp. 234–240, 1990.

[5] J. I. Ward, H. S. Margolis, M. K. Lum, D. W. Fraser, T. R. Bender, and P. Anderson, "*Haemophilus influenzae* disease in Alaskan Eskimos: characteristics of a population with an unusual incidence of invasive disease," *The Lancet*, vol. 1, no. 8233, pp. 1281–1285, 1981.

[6] S. H. Sell, R. E. Merrill, E. O. Doyne, and E. P. Zimsky Jr., "Long-term sequelae of *Hemophilus influenzae* meningitis," *Pediatrics*, vol. 49, no. 2, pp. 206–211, 1972.

[7] M. Glode, R. S. Daum, D. A. Goldmann, J. Leclair, and A. Smith, "*Haemophilus influenzae* type B meningitis: a contagious

disease of children," *The British Medical Journal*, vol. 280, no. 6218, pp. 899–901, 1980.

[8] M. P. Glode, M. S. Schiffer, J. B. Robbins, W. Khan, U. Battle, and E. Armenta, "An outbreak of *Hemophilus influenzae* type b meningitis in an enclosed hospital population," *The Journal of Pediatrics*, vol. 88, no. 1, pp. 36–40, 1976.

[9] B. Claesson, B. Trollfors, B. Ekstrom-Jodal et al., "Incidence and prognosis of acute epiglottitis in children in a Swedish region," *Pediatric Infectious Disease*, vol. 3, no. 6, pp. 534–538, 1984.

[10] G. J. Nabel, "Designing tomorrow's vaccines," *The New England Journal of Medicine*, vol. 368, no. 6, pp. 551–560, 2013.

[11] F. Y. Avci, "Novel strategies for development of next-generation glycoconjugate vaccines," *Current Topics in Medicinal Chemistry*, vol. 13, no. 20, pp. 2535–2540, 2013.

[12] B. Kuberan and R. J. Linhardt, "Carbohydrate based vaccines," *Current Organic Chemistry*, vol. 4, no. 6, pp. 653–677, 2000.

[13] P. T. Heath, "*Haemophilus influenzae* type b conjugate vaccines: a review of efficacy data," *Pediatric Infectious Disease Journal*, vol. 17, no. 9, pp. S117–S122, 1998.

[14] A. Zandvoort and W. Timens, "The dual function of the splenic marginal zone: essential for initiation of anti-TI-2 responses but also vital in the general first-line defense against blood-borne antigens," *Clinical and Experimental Immunology*, vol. 130, no. 1, pp. 4–11, 2002.

[15] T. Nieminen, H. Käyhty, A. Virolainen, and J. Eskola, "Circulating antibody secreting cell response to parenteral pneumococcal vaccines as an indicator of a salivary IgA antibody response," *Vaccine*, vol. 16, no. 2-3, pp. 313–319, 1998.

[16] Q. Zhang, S. Choo, J. Everard, R. Jennings, and A. Finn, "Mucosal immune responses to meningococcal group C conjugate and group A and C polysaccharide vaccines in adolescents," *Infection and Immunity*, vol. 68, no. 5, pp. 2692–2697, 2000.

[17] Q. Vos, A. Lees, Z.-Q. Wu, C. M. Snapper, and J. J. Mond, "B-cell activation by T-cell-independent type 2 antigens as an integral part of the humoral immune response to pathogenic microorganisms," *Immunological Reviews*, vol. 176, pp. 154–170, 2000.

[18] D. M. Musher, J. E. Groover, D. A. Watson et al., "Genetic regulation of the capacity to make immunoglobulin G to pneumococcal capsular polysaccharides," *Journal of Investigative Medicine*, vol. 45, no. 2, pp. 57–68, 1997.

[19] D. M. Granoff, R. K. Gupta, R. B. Belshe, and E. L. Andersen, "Induction of immunologic refractoriness in adults by meningococcal C polysaccharide vaccination," *Journal of Infectious Diseases*, vol. 178, no. 3, pp. 870–874, 1998.

[20] C. B. Wilson, D. B. Lewis, and L. A. Penix, "The physiologic immunodeficiency of immaturity," in *Immunologic Disorders in Infants and Children*, E. R. Stiehm, Ed., pp. 253–295, W.B. Saunders, Philadelphia, Pa, USA, 4th edition, 1996.

[21] C. Laferriere, "The immunogenicity of pneumococcal polysaccharides in infants and children: a meta-regression," *Vaccine*, vol. 29, no. 40, pp. 6838–6847, 2011.

[22] W. S. Pomat, D. Lehmann, R. C. Sanders et al., "Immunoglobulin G antibody responses to polyvalent pneumococcal vaccine in children in the highlands of Papua New Guinea," *Infection and Immunity*, vol. 62, no. 5, pp. 1848–1853, 1994.

[23] B. P. Arulanandam, J. N. Mittler, W. T. Lee, M. O'Toole, and D. W. Metzger, "Neonatal administration of IL-12 enhances the protective efficacy of antiviral vaccines," *The Journal of Immunology*, vol. 164, no. 7, pp. 3698–3704, 2000.

[24] M. O. C. Ota, J. Vekemans, S. E. Schlegel-Haueter et al., "Hepatitis B immunisation induces higher antibody and memory Th2 responses in new-borns than in adults," *Vaccine*, vol. 22, no. 3-4, pp. 511–519, 2004.

[25] J. Rowe, C. Macaubas, T. Monger et al., "Heterogeneity in diphtheria-tetanus-acellular pertussis vaccine-specific cellular immunity during infancy: relationship to variations in the kinetics of postnatal maturation of systemic Th1 function," *Journal of Infectious Diseases*, vol. 184, no. 1, pp. 80–88, 2001.

[26] J. Vekemans, M. O. C. Ota, E. C. Y. Wang et al., "T cell responses to vaccines in infants: defective IFNγ production after oral polio vaccination," *Clinical and Experimental Immunology*, vol. 127, no. 3, pp. 495–498, 2002.

[27] O. J. White, K. L. McKenna, A. Bosco, A. H. J. van den Biggelaar, P. Richmond, and P. G. Holt, "A genomics-based approach to assessment of vaccine safety and immunogenicity in children," *Vaccine*, vol. 30, no. 10, pp. 1865–1874, 2012.

[28] O. J. White, J. Rowe, P. Richmond et al., "Th2-polarisation of cellular immune memory to neonatal pertussis vaccination," *Vaccine*, vol. 28, no. 14, pp. 2648–2652, 2010.

[29] C.-A. Siegrist, "Neonatal and early life vaccinology," *Vaccine*, vol. 19, no. 25-26, pp. 3331–3346, 2001.

[30] A. Finn, "Bacterial polysaccharide-protein conjugate vaccines," *British Medical Bulletin*, vol. 70, pp. 1–14, 2004.

[31] G. Swingler, D. Fransman, and G. Hussey, "Conjugate vaccines for preventing *Haemophilus influenzae* type b infections," *Cochrane Database of Systematic Reviews*, vol. 4, Article ID CD001729, 2003.

[32] P. T. Heath, R. Booy, H. Griffiths et al., "Clinical and immunological risk factors associated with haemophilus influenzae type b conjugate vaccine failure in childhood," *Clinical Infectious Diseases*, vol. 31, no. 4, pp. 973–980, 2000.

[33] S. R. Dominguez and R. S. Daum, "Toward global *Haemophilus influenzae* type b immunization," *Clinical Infectious Diseases*, vol. 37, no. 12, pp. 1600–1602, 2003.

[34] R. T. Mahoney and J. E. Maynard, "The introduction of new vaccines into developing countries," *Vaccine*, vol. 17, no. 7-8, pp. 646–652, 1999.

[35] A. Arvas, E. Gur, H. Bahar et al., "*Haemophilus influenzae* type b antibodies in vaccinated and non-vaccinated children," *Pediatrics International*, vol. 50, no. 4, pp. 469–473, 2008.

[36] M. Almuneef, M. Alshaalan, Z. Memish, and S. Alalola, "Bacterial meningitis in Saudi Arabia: the impact of *Haemophilus influenzae* type b vaccination," *Journal of Chemotherapy*, vol. 13, supplement 1, pp. 34–39, 2001.

[37] F. A. Al-Zamil, "Conjugated pneumococcal vaccine for children in Saudi Arabia: following the footsteps of hib vaccine," *The Journal of the Egyptian Public Health Association*, vol. 83, no. 1-2, pp. 35–47, 2008.

[38] Health Statistic Annual Book: Kingdom of Saudi Arabia Ministry of Health, 2013, http://www.moh.gov.sa/en/Ministry/Statistics/book/Documents/Statistics-Book-1434.pdf.

[39] Global Programme for Vaccines and Immunization (GPV), "The WHO position paper on Haemophilus influenzae type b conjugate vaccines," *The Weekly Epidemiological Record*, vol. 73, no. 10, pp. 64–68, 1998.

[40] M. Finland and W. D. Sutliff, "Specific antibody response of human subjects to intracutaneous injection of pneumococcus products," *The Journal of Experimental Medicine*, vol. 55, no. 6, pp. 853–865, 1932.

[41] C. L. Hoagland, P. B. Beeson, and W. F. Goebel, "The capsular polysaccharide of the type XIV pneumococcus and its relationship to the specific substances of human blood," *Science*, vol. 88, no. 2281, pp. 261–263, 1938.

[42] H. Kayhty, V. Karanko, H. Peltola, and P. H. Makela, "Serum antibodies after vaccination with *Haemophilus influenzae* type b capsular polysaccharide and responses to reimmunization: no evidence of immunologic tolerance or memory," *Pediatrics*, vol. 74, no. 5, pp. 857–865, 1984.

[43] J. B. Robbins and R. Schneerson, "Polysaccharide-protein conjugates: a new generation of vaccines," *The Journal of Infectious Diseases*, vol. 161, no. 5, pp. 821–832, 1990.

[44] J. I. Ward, C. V. Broome, L. H. Harrison, H. Shinefield, and S. Black, "*Haemophilus influenzae* type b vaccines: lessons for the future," *Pediatrics*, vol. 81, no. 6, pp. 886–893, 1988.

[45] H. Kayhty, H. Peltola, V. Karanko, and P. H. Makela, "The protective level of serum antibodies to the capsular polysaccharide of *Haemophilus influenzae* type b," *Journal of Infectious Diseases*, vol. 147, no. 6, p. 1100, 1983.

[46] R. Z. Dintzis, M. Okajima, M. H. Middleton, G. Greene, and H. M. Dintzis, "The immunogenicity of soluble haptenated polymers is determined by molecular mass and hapten valence," *The Journal of Immunology*, vol. 143, no. 4, pp. 1239–1244, 1989.

[47] J. C. Aguilar and E. G. Rodríguez, "Vaccine adjuvants revisited," *Vaccine*, vol. 25, no. 19, pp. 3752–3762, 2007.

[48] B. Guy, "Adjuvants for protein- and carbohydrate-based vaccines," in *Carbohydrate-Based Vaccines and Immunotherapies*, pp. 89–115, John Wiley & Sons, New York, NY, USA, 2008.

[49] T. A. Barr, J. Carlring, and A. W. Heath, "Co-stimulatory agonists as immunological adjuvants," *Vaccine*, vol. 24, no. 17, pp. 3399–3407, 2006.

[50] E. C. Briere, L. Rubin, P. L. Moro, A. Cohn, T. Clark, and N. Messonnier, "Prevention and control of haemophilus influenzae type b disease: recommendations of the advisory committee on immunization practices (ACIP)," *Morbidity and Mortality Weekly Report*, vol. 63, no. 1, pp. 1–14, 2014.

[51] R. Z. Dintzis, "Rational design of conjugate vaccines," *Pediatric Research*, vol. 32, no. 4, pp. 376–385, 1992.

[52] K. E. Stein, "Glycoconjugate vaccines. What next?" *International Journal of Technology Assessment in Health Care*, vol. 10, no. 1, pp. 167–176, 1994.

[53] A. A. Lindberg, "Glycoprotein conjugate vaccines," *Vaccine*, vol. 17, supplement 2, pp. S28–S36, 1999.

[54] J. L. Hsu, "A brief history of vaccines: smallpox to the present," *South Dakota Medicine*, Special no. 33–37, 2013.

[55] S. A. Plotkin and S. L. Plotkin, "The development of vaccines: how the past led to the future," *Nature Reviews Microbiology*, vol. 9, no. 12, pp. 889–893, 2011.

[56] A. H. J. van den Biggelaar and W. S. Pomat, "Immunization of newborns with bacterial conjugate vaccines," *Vaccine*, vol. 31, no. 21, pp. 2525–2530, 2013.

[57] W. E. Dick Jr. and M. Beurret, "Glycoconjugates of bacterial carbohydrate antigens. A survey and consideration of design and preparation factors," *Contributions to Microbiology and Immunology*, vol. 10, pp. 48–114, 1989.

[58] A. Lees, V. Puvanesarajah, and C. E. Frasch, "Conjugation chemistry," in *Pneumococcal Vaccines*, pp. 163–174, American Society of Microbiology, 2008.

[59] W. Zou and H. J. Jennings, "Preparation of glycoconjugate vaccines," in *Carbohydrate-Based Vaccines and Immunotherapies*, Z. Guo and G.-J. Boons, Eds., John Wiley & Sons, New York, NY, USA, 2009.

[60] G. Toraño, M. E. Toledo, A. Baly et al., "Phase I clinical evaluation of a synthetic oligosaccharide-protein conjugate vaccine against *Haemophilus influenzae* type b in human adult volunteers," *Clinical and Vaccine Immunology*, vol. 13, no. 9, pp. 1052–1056, 2006.

[61] S. Bay, V. Huteau, M.-L. Zarantonelli et al., "Phosphorylcholine-carbohydrate-protein conjugates efficiently induce hapten-specific antibodies which recognize both *Streptococcus pneumoniae* and *Neisseria meningitidis*: a potential multitarget vaccine against respiratory infections," *Journal of Medicinal Chemistry*, vol. 47, no. 16, pp. 3916–3919, 2004.

[62] T. Buskas, Y. Li, and G. J. Boons, "The immunogenicity of the tumor-associated antigen Lewis(y) may be suppressed by a bifunctional cross-linker required for coupling to a carrier protein," *Chemistry*, vol. 10, no. 14, pp. 3517–3524, 2004.

[63] P. H. Seeberger, R. L. Soucy, Y.-U. Kwon, D. A. Snyder, and T. Kanemitsu, "A convergent, versatile route to two synthetic conjugate anti-toxin malaria vaccines," *Chemical Communications*, vol. 10, no. 15, pp. 1706–1707, 2004.

[64] V. Verez-Bencomo, V. Fernández-Santana, E. Hardy et al., "A synthetic conjugate polysaccharide vaccine against *Haemophilus influenzae* type b," *Science*, vol. 305, no. 5683, pp. 522–525, 2004.

[65] C. C. A. M. Peeters, A.-M. J. Tenbergen-Meekes, J. T. Poolman, B. J. M. Zegers, and G. T. Rijkers, "Immunogenicity of a *Streptococcus pneumoniae* type 4 polysaccharide-protein conjugate vaccine is decreased by admixture of high doses of free saccharide," *Vaccine*, vol. 10, no. 12, pp. 833–840, 1992.

[66] M. E. Rodriguez, G. P. J. M. van den Dobbelsteen, L. A. Oomen et al., "Immunogenicity of *Streptococcus pneumoniae* type 6B and 14 polysaccharide-tetanus toxoid conjugates and the effect of uncoupled polysaccharide on the antigen-specific immune response," *Vaccine*, vol. 16, no. 20, pp. 1941–1949, 1998.

[67] G. R. Gray, "Antibodies to carbohydrates: preparation of antigens by coupling carbohydrates to proteins by reductive amination with cyanoborohydride," *Methods in Enzymology*, vol. 50, pp. 155–160, 1978.

[68] B. A. Schwartz and G. R. Gray, "Proteins containing reductively aminated disaccharides. Synthesis and chemical characterization," *Archives of Biochemistry and Biophysics*, vol. 181, no. 2, pp. 542–549, 1977.

[69] M. L. C. Da Silva, T. Tamura, T. McBroom, and K. G. Rice, "Tyrosine derivatization and preparative purification of the sialyl and asialyl N-linked oligosaccharides from porcine fibrinogen," *Archives of Biochemistry and Biophysics*, vol. 312, no. 1, pp. 151–157, 1994.

[70] S. Y. C. Wong, G. R. Guile, R. A. Dwek, and G. Arsequell, "Synthetic glycosylation of proteins using *N*-(β-saccharide) iodoacetamides: applications in site-specific glycosylation and solid-phase enzymic oligosaccharide synthesis," *Biochemical Journal*, vol. 300, no. 3, pp. 843–850, 1994.

[71] S. Y. C. Wong, G. R. Guile, T. W. Rademacher, and R. A. Dwek, "Synthetic glycosylation of peptides using unprotected saccharide beta-glycosylamines," *Glycoconjugate Journal*, vol. 10, no. 3, pp. 227–234, 1993.

[72] G. Ragupathi, R. R. Koganty, D. Qiu, K. O. Lloyd, and P. O. Livingston, "A novel and efficient method for synthetic carbohydrate conjugate vaccine preparation: synthesis of sialyl Tn-KLH conjugate using a 4-(4-N-maleimidomethyl) cyclohexane-1-carboxyl hydrazide (MMCCH) linker arm," *Glycoconjugate Journal*, vol. 15, no. 3, pp. 217–221, 1998.

[73] E. C. Beuvery, G. J. Speijers, B. I. Lutz et al., "Analytical, toxicological and immunological consequences of the use of N-ethyl-N'-(3-dimethylaminopropyl) carbodiimide as coupling reagent for the preparation of meningococcal group C polysaccharide-tetanus toxoid conjugate as vaccine for human use," *Developments in Biological Standardization*, vol. 63, pp. 117–128, 1986.

[74] J. V. Staros, R. W. Wright, and D. M. Swingle, "Enhancement by N-hydroxysulfosuccinimide of water-soluble carbodiimide-mediated coupling reactions," *Analytical Biochemistry*, vol. 156, no. 1, pp. 220–222, 1986.

[75] O. T. Avery and W. F. Goebel, "Chemo-immunological studies on conjugated carbohydrate-proteins: V. The immunological specifity of an antigen prepared by combining the capsular polysaccharide of type III pneumococcus with foreign protein," *The Journal of Experimental Medicine*, vol. 54, no. 3, pp. 437–447, 1931.

[76] R. Axén, J. Porath, and S. Ernback, "Chemical coupling of peptides and proteins to polysaccharides by means of cyanogen halides," *Nature*, vol. 214, no. 5095, pp. 1302–1304, 1967.

[77] L. Chi-Jen, "Bacterial capsular polysaccharides—biochemistry, immunity and vaccine," *Molecular Immunology*, vol. 24, no. 10, pp. 1005–1019, 1987.

[78] L. C. Paoletti, M. A. Rench, D. L. Kasper, D. Molrine, D. Ambrosino, and C. J. Baker, "Effects of alum adjuvant or a booster dose on immunogenicity during clinical trials of group B streptococcal type III conjugate vaccines," *Infection and Immunity*, vol. 69, no. 11, pp. 6696–6701, 2001.

[79] A. W. Sturgess, K. Rush, R. J. Charbonneau et al., "*Haemophilus influenzae* type b conjugate vaccine stability: catalytic depolymerization of PRP in the presence of aluminum hydroxide," *Vaccine*, vol. 17, no. 9-10, pp. 1169–1178, 1999.

[80] R. S. Chu, T. McCool, N. S. Greenspan, J. R. Schreiber, and C. V. Harding, "CpG oligodeoxynucleotides act as adjuvants for pneumococcal polysaccharide-protein conjugate vaccines and enhance antipolysaccharide immunoglobulin G2a (IgG2a) and IgG3 antibodies," *Infection and Immunity*, vol. 68, no. 3, pp. 1450–1456, 2000.

[81] T. A. Olafsdottir, S. G. Hannesdottir, G. D. Giudice, E. Trannoy, and I. Jonsdottir, "Effects of LT-K63 and CpG2006 on phenotype and function of murine neonatal lymphoid cells," *Scandinavian Journal of Immunology*, vol. 66, no. 4, pp. 426–434, 2007.

[82] G. Sen, Q. Chen, and C. M. Snapper, "Immunization of aged mice with a pneumococcal conjugate vaccine combined with an unmethylated CpG-containing oligodeoxynucleotide restores defective immunoglobulin G antipolysaccharide responses and specific CD4$^+$-T-cell priming to young adult levels," *Infection and Immunity*, vol. 74, no. 4, pp. 2177–2186, 2006.

[83] T. Barington, M. Skettrup, L. Juul, and C. Heilmann, "Non-epitope-specific suppression of the antibody response to *Haemophilus influenzae* type b conjugate vaccines by preimmunization with vaccine components," *Infection and Immunity*, vol. 61, no. 2, pp. 432–438, 1993.

[84] A. Fattom, Y. H. Cho, C. Chu, S. Fuller, L. Fries, and R. Naso, "Epitopic overload at the site of injection may result in suppression of the immune response to combined capsular polysaccharide conjugate vaccines," *Vaccine*, vol. 17, no. 2, pp. 126–133, 1999.

[85] M.-P. Schutze, E. Deriaud, G. Przewlocki, and C. LeClerc, "Carrier-induced epitopic suppression is initiated through clonal dominance," *The Journal of Immunology*, vol. 142, no. 8, pp. 2635–2640, 1989.

[86] Organization WHO, "Recommendations for the production and control of *Haemophilus influenzae* type b conjugate vaccines," *WHO Technical Report Series*, no. 897, pp. 27–60, 2000.

[87] World Health Organization, "WHO position paper on *Haemophilus influenzae* type b conjugate vaccines. (Replaces WHO position paper on Hib vaccines previously published in the Weekly Epidemiological Record," *The Weekly Epidemiological Record*, vol. 81, no. 47, pp. 445–452, 2006.

[88] "Progress introducing *Haemophilus influenzae* type b vaccine in low-income countries, 2004–2008," *Weekly Epidemiological Record*, vol. 83, no. 7, pp. 61–67, 2008.

[89] B. D. Gessner, A. Sutanto, M. Linehan et al., "Incidences of vaccine-preventable *Haemophilus influenzae* type b pneumonia and meningitis in Indonesian children: hamlet-randomised vaccine-probe trial," *The Lancet*, vol. 365, no. 9453, pp. 43–52, 2005.

[90] H. Peltola, "Worldwide *Haemophilus influenzae* type b disease at the beginning of the 21st century: Global analysis of the disease burden 25 years after the use of the polysaccharide vaccine and a decade after the advent of conjugates," *Clinical Microbiology Reviews*, vol. 13, no. 2, pp. 302–317, 2000.

[91] O. S. Levine, B. Schwartz, N. Pierce, and M. Kane, "Development, evaluation and implementation of *Haemophilus influenzae* type b vaccines for young children in developing countries: current status and priority actions," *The Pediatric Infectious Disease Journal*, vol. 17, no. 9, supplement, pp. S95–S113, 1998.

[92] Lessons learned: new procurement strategies for vaccines. Final report to the GAVI board, GAVI Alliance: Mercer Management Consulting, 2002, http://www.gavi.org/library/gavi-documents/supply-procurement/mercer-report-on-vaccine-procurement.

[93] M. C. Danovaro-Holliday, S. Garcia, C. de Quadros, G. Tambini, and J. K. Andrus, "Progress in vaccination against *Haemophilus influenzae* type b in the Americas," *PLoS Medicine*, vol. 5, no. 4, article e87, 2008.

[94] M. Landaverde, J. L. Di Fabio, G. Ruocco, I. Leal, and C. de Quadros, "Introduction of a conjugate vaccine against Hib in Chile and Uruguay," *Revista Panamericana de Salud Pública*, vol. 5, no. 3, pp. 200–206, 1999.

[95] J. D. Wenger, J.-L. DiFabio, J. M. Landaverde, O. S. Levine, and T. Gaafar, "Introduction of Hib conjugate vaccines in the non-industrialized world: experience in four 'newly adopting' countries," *Vaccine*, vol. 18, no. 7-8, pp. 736–742, 1999.

[96] A. Hamidi, C. Boog, S. Jadhav, and H. Kreeftenberg, "Lessons learned during the development and transfer of technology related to a new Hib conjugate vaccine to emerging vaccine manufacturers," *Vaccine*, vol. 32, no. 33, pp. 4124–4130, 2014.

[97] J. B. Milstien, P. Gaulé, and M. Kaddar, "Access to vaccine technologies in developing countries: Brazil and India," *Vaccine*, vol. 25, no. 44, pp. 7610–7619, 2007.

[98] M. Beurret, A. Hamidi, and H. Kreeftenberg, "Development and technology transfer of *Haemophilus influenzae* type b conjugate vaccines for developing countries," *Vaccine*, vol. 30, no. 33, pp. 4897–4906, 2012.

[99] F. Mawas, G. Newman, S. Burns, and M. J. Corbel, "Suppression and modulation of cellular and humoral immune responses to *Haemophilus influenzae* type B (Hib) conjugate vaccine in Hib-diphtheria-tetanus toxoids-acellular pertussis combination vaccines: a study in a rat model," *Journal of Infectious Diseases*, vol. 191, no. 1, pp. 58–64, 2005.

[100] Arabio Company, 2006, http://www.arabio.com/index.html.

[101] S. A. Plotkin, "Vaccines: the fourth century," *Clinical and Vaccine Immunology*, vol. 16, no. 12, pp. 1709–1719, 2009.

[102] G. M. Glenn, D. N. Taylor, X. Li, S. Frankel, A. Montemarano, and C. R. Alving, "Transcutaneous immunization: a human vaccine delivery strategy using a patch," *Nature Medicine*, vol. 6, no. 12, pp. 1403–1406, 2000.

[103] A.-S. Beignon, J.-P. Briand, S. Muller, and C. D. Partidos, "Immunization onto bare skin with heat-labile enterotoxin of *Escherichia coli* enhances immune responses to coadministered protein and peptide antigens and protects mice against lethal toxin challenge," *Immunology*, vol. 102, no. 3, pp. 344–351, 2001.

[104] A.-S. Beignon, J.-P. Briand, R. Rappuoli, S. Muller, and C. D. Partidos, "The LTR72 mutant of heat-labile enterotoxin of *Escherichia coli* enhances the ability of peptide antigens to elicit CD4⁺ T cells and secrete gamma interferon after coapplication onto bare skin," *Infection and Immunity*, vol. 70, no. 6, pp. 3012–3019, 2002.

[105] G. M. Glenn, T. Scharton-Kersten, R. Vassell, C. P. Mallett, T. L. Hale, and C. R. Alving, "Transcutaneous immunization with cholera toxin protects mice against lethal mucosal toxin challenge," *The Journal of Immunology*, vol. 161, no. 7, pp. 3211–3214, 1998.

[106] C. M. Gockel, S. Bao, and K. W. Beagley, "Transcutaneous immunization induces mucosal and systemic immunity: a potent method for targeting immunity to the female reproductive tract," *Molecular Immunology*, vol. 37, no. 9, pp. 537–544, 2000.

[107] S. Godefroy, L. Goestch, H. Plotnicky-Gilquin et al., "Immunization onto shaved skin with a bacterial enterotoxin adjuvant protects mice against Respiratory Syncytial Virus (RSV)," *Vaccine*, vol. 21, no. 15, pp. 1665–1671, 2003.

[108] R. Tierney, A.-S. Beignon, R. Rappuoli, S. Muller, D. Sesardic, and C. Partidos, "Transcutaneous immunization with tetanus toxoid and mutants of *Escherichia coli* heat-labile enterotoxin as adjuvants elicits strong protective antibody responses," *Journal of Infectious Diseases*, vol. 188, no. 5, pp. 753–758, 2003.

[109] B. Quiambao, O. Van Der Meeren, D. Kolhe, and S. Gatchalian, "A randomized, dose-ranging assessment of the immunogenicity and safety of a booster dose of a combined diphtheria-tetanus-whole cell pertussis-hepatitis B-inactivated poliovirus-*Hemophilus influenzae* type b (DTPw-HBV-IPV/Hib) vaccine vs. co-administration of DTPw-HBV/Hib and IPV vaccines in 12 to 24 months old Filipino toddlers," *Human Vaccines & Immunotherapeutics*, vol. 8, no. 3, pp. 347–354, 2012.

[110] H. Kalies, V. Grote, T. Verstraeten, L. Hessel, H.-J. Schmitt, and R. Von Kries, "The use of combination vaccines has improved timeliness of vaccination in children," *Pediatric Infectious Disease Journal*, vol. 25, no. 6, pp. 507–512, 2006.

[111] L. E. Happe, O. E. Lunacsek, D. T. Kruzikas, and G. S. Marshall, "Impact of a pentavalent combination vaccine on immunization timeliness in a state medicaid population," *Pediatric Infectious Disease Journal*, vol. 28, no. 2, pp. 98–101, 2009.

[112] V. Baldo, P. Bonanni, M. Castro et al., "Combined hexavalent diphtheria-tetanus-acellular pertussis-hepatitis B-inactivated poliovirus-*Hemophilus influenzae* type b vaccine; Infanrix hexa: twelve years of experience in Italy," *Human Vaccines and Immunotherapeutics*, vol. 10, no. 1, pp. 129–137, 2014.

[113] H. Kalies, V. Grote, A. Siedler, B. Gröndahl, H.-J. Schmitt, and R. von Kries, "Effectiveness of hexavalent vaccines against invasive *Haemophilus influenzae* type b disease: Germany's experience after 5 years of licensure," *Vaccine*, vol. 26, no. 20, pp. 2545–2552, 2008.

[114] H. O. Hallander, T. Lepp, M. Ljungman, E. Netterlid, and M. Andersson, "Do we need a booster of Hib vaccine after primary vaccination? A study on anti-Hib seroprevalence in Sweden 5 and 15 years after the introduction of universal Hib vaccination related to notifications of invasive disease," *APMIS*, vol. 118, no. 11, pp. 878–887, 2010.

[115] M. S. Amstey, R. Insel, J. Munoz, and M. Pichichero, "Fetal-neonatal passive immunization against *Hemophilus influenzae*, type b," *American Journal of Obstetrics and Gynecology*, vol. 153, no. 6, pp. 607–611, 1985.

[116] J. A. Englund, W. P. Glezen, C. Turner, J. Harvey, C. Thompson, and G. R. Siber, "Transplacental antibody transfer following maternal immunization with polysaccharide and conjugate *Haemophilus influenzae* type b vaccines," *Journal of Infectious Diseases*, vol. 171, no. 1, pp. 99–105, 1995.

[117] M. S. Einhorn, D. M. Granoff, M. H. Nahm, A. Quinn, and P. G. Shackelford, "Concentrations of antibodies in paired maternal and infant sera: relationship to IgG subclass," *The Journal of Pediatrics*, vol. 111, no. 5, pp. 783–788, 1987.

[118] M. K. Park, J. A. Englund, W. P. Glezen, G. R. Siber, and M. H. Nahm, "Association of placental transfer of anti-*Haemophilus influenzae* type b polysaccharide antibodies with their V regions," *Vaccine*, vol. 14, no. 13, pp. 1219–1222, 1996.

[119] A. M. Krieg, "Lymphocyte activation by CpG dinucleotide motifs in prokaryotic DNA," *Trends in Microbiology*, vol. 4, no. 2, pp. 73–77, 1996.

[120] V. E. Schijns, "Immunological concepts of vaccine adjuvant activity," *Current Opinion in Immunology*, vol. 12, no. 4, pp. 456–463, 2000.

[121] C. A. Janeway Jr. and R. Medzhitov, "Introduction: the role of innate immunity in the adaptive immune response," *Seminars in Immunology*, vol. 10, no. 5, pp. 349–350, 1998.

[122] M. Roman, E. Martin-Orozco, J. S. Goodman et al., "Immunostimulatory DNA sequences function as T helper-1-promoting adjuvants," *Nature Medicine*, vol. 3, no. 8, pp. 849–854, 1997.

[123] N. S. Greenspan and L. J. N. Cooper, "Intermolecular cooperativity: a clue to why mice have IgG3?" *Immunology Today*, vol. 13, no. 5, pp. 164–168, 1992.

[124] F. D. Finkelman, J. Holmes, I. M. Katona et al., "Lymphokine control of in vivo immunoglobulin isotype selection," *Annual Review of Immunology*, vol. 8, pp. 303–333, 1990.

[125] A. R. Foxwell, J. M. Kyd, and A. W. Cripps, "Nontypeable *Haemophilus influenzae*: pathogenesis and prevention," *Microbiology and Molecular Biology Reviews*, vol. 62, no. 2, pp. 294–308, 1998.

[126] M. R. Loeb and D. H. Smith, "Outer membrane protein composition in disease isolates of *Haemophilus influenzae*: pathogenic and epidemiological implications," *Infection and Immunity*, vol. 30, no. 3, pp. 709–717, 1980.

[127] S. J. Barenkamp, R. S. Munson Jr., and D. M. Granoff, "Subtyping isolates of *Haemophilus influenzae* type b by outer-membrane protein profiles," *The Journal of Infectious Diseases*, vol. 143, no. 5, pp. 668–676, 1981.

[128] M. Comanducci, S. Bambini, B. Brunelli et al., "NadA, a novel vaccine candidate of *Neisseria meningitidis*," *Journal of Experimental Medicine*, vol. 195, no. 11, pp. 1445–1454, 2002.

[129] C. A. Janeway, P. Travers, M. Walport, and M. Chlomchik, *Immunobiology*, Garland Science Publishing, New York, NY, USA, 6th edition, 2005.

[130] N. A. Mitchison, "T-cell-B-cell cooperation," *Nature Reviews Immunology*, vol. 4, no. 4, pp. 308–312, 2004.

[131] F. Y. Avci and D. L. Kasper, "How bacterial carbohydrates influence the adaptive immune system," *Annual Review of Immunology*, vol. 28, pp. 107–130, 2010.

[132] B. A. Cobb, Q. Wang, A. O. Tzianabos, and D. L. Kasper, "Polysaccharide processing and presentation by the MHCII pathway," *Cell*, vol. 117, no. 5, pp. 677–687, 2004.

[133] Á. G. Barrientos, J. M. de la Fuente, T. C. Rojas, A. Fernández, and S. Penadés, "Gold glyconanoparticles: synthetic polyvalent ligands mimicking glycocalyx-like surfaces as tools for glycobiological studies," *Chemistry—A European Journal*, vol. 9, no. 9, pp. 1909–1921, 2003.

[134] F. Y. Avci, X. Li, M. Tsuji, and D. L. Kasper, "A mechanism for glycoconjugate vaccine activation of the adaptive immune system and its implications for vaccine design," *Nature Medicine*, vol. 17, no. 12, pp. 1602–1609, 2011.

[135] H. Amir-Kroll, L. Riveron, M. E. Sarmiento, G. Sierra, A. Acosta, and I. R. Cohen, "A conjugate vaccine composed of a heat shock protein 60 T-cell epitope peptide (p458) and *Neisseria meningitidis* type B capsular polysaccharide," *Vaccine*, vol. 24, no. 42-43, pp. 6555–6563, 2006.

[136] N. Cohen, M. Stolarsky-Bennun, H. Amir-Kroll et al., "Pneumococcal capsular polysaccharide is immunogenic when present on the surface of macrophages and dendritic cells: TLR4 signaling induced by a conjugate vaccine or by lipopolysaccharide is conducive," *The Journal of Immunology*, vol. 180, no. 4, pp. 2409–2418, 2008.

[137] S. Könen-Waisman, A. Cohen, M. Fridkin, and I. R. Cohen, "Self heat-shock protein (hsp60) peptide serves in a conjugate vaccine against a lethal pneumococcal infection," *Journal of Infectious Diseases*, vol. 179, no. 2, pp. 403–413, 1999.

[138] F. Falugi, R. Petracca, M. Mariani et al., "Rationally designed strings of promiscuous CD4$^+$ T cell epitopes provide help to *Haemophilus influenzae* type b oligosaccharide: a model for new conjugate vaccines," *European Journal of Immunology*, vol. 31, no. 12, pp. 3816–3824, 2001.

[139] K. Baraldo, E. Mori, A. Bartoloni et al., "Combined conjugate vaccines: enhanced immunogenicity with the N19 polyepitope as a carrier protein," *Infection and Immunity*, vol. 73, no. 9, pp. 5835–5841, 2005.

[140] R. Rana, J. Dalal, D. Singh et al., "Development and characterization of *Haemophilus influenzae* type b conjugate vaccine prepared using different polysaccharide chain lengths," *Vaccine*, vol. 33, no. 23, pp. 2646–2654, 2015.

[141] A. Bardotti, G. Averani, F. Berti et al., "Physicochemical characterisation of glycoconjugate vaccines for prevention of meningococcal diseases," *Vaccine*, vol. 26, no. 18, pp. 2284–2296, 2008.

[142] M. Bröker, P. M. Dull, R. Rappuoli, and P. Costantino, "Chemistry of a new investigational quadrivalent meningococcal conjugate vaccine that is immunogenic at all ages," *Vaccine*, vol. 27, no. 41, pp. 5574–5580, 2009.

[143] P. Costantino, R. Rappuoli, and F. Berti, "The design of semisynthetic and synthetic glycoconjugate vaccines," *Expert Opinion on Drug Discovery*, vol. 6, no. 10, pp. 1045–1066, 2011.

[144] E. Altindis, "Antibacterial vaccine research in 21st century: from inoculation to genomics approaches," *Current Topics in Medicinal Chemistry*, vol. 13, no. 20, pp. 2638–2646, 2013.

[145] M. N. Baeshen, A. M. Al-Hejin, R. S. Bora et al., "Production of biopharmaceuticals in *E. coli*: current scenario and future perspectives," *Journal of Microbiology and Biotechnology*, vol. 25, no. 7, pp. 953–962, 2015.

[146] N. A. Baeshen, M. N. Baeshen, A. Sheikh et al., "Cell factories for insulin production," *Microbial Cell Factories*, vol. 13, article 141, 2014.

[147] N. A. El-Baky and E. M. Redwan, "Therapeutic alpha-interferons protein: structure, production, and biosimilar," *Preparative Biochemistry & Biotechnology*, vol. 45, no. 2, pp. 109–127, 2015.

[148] N. A. El-Baky, V. N. Uversky, and E. M. Redwan, "Human consensus interferons: bridging the natural and artificial cytokines with intrinsic disorder," *Cytokine & Growth Factor Reviews*, vol. 26, no. 6, pp. 637–645, 2015.

[149] E.-R. M. Redwan, "Cumulative updating of approved biopharmaceuticals," *Human Antibodies*, vol. 16, no. 3-4, pp. 137–158, 2007.

[150] E.-R. M. Redwan, "Animal-derived pharmaceutical proteins," *Journal of Immunoassay and Immunochemistry*, vol. 30, no. 3, pp. 262–290, 2009.

[151] Y. Liao, E. M. El-Fakkarany, B. Lönnerdal, and E. M. Redwan, "Inhibitory effects of native/recombinant full-length camel lactoferrin and its N/C lobes on hepatitis C virus infection of Huh7.5 cells," *Journal of Medical Microbiology*, vol. 61, part 3, pp. 375–383, 2012.

[152] E.-R. M. Redwan, A. Fahmy, A. E. Hanafy, N. A. EL-Baky, and S. M. A. Sallam, "Ovine anti-rabies antibody production and evaluation," *Comparative Immunology, Microbiology and Infectious Diseases*, vol. 32, no. 1, pp. 9–19, 2009.

[153] E.-R. M. Redwan, S. M. Matar, G. A. El-Aziz, and E. A. Serour, "Synthesis of the human insulin gene: protein expression, scaling up and bioactivity," *Preparative Biochemistry and Biotechnology*, vol. 38, no. 1, pp. 24–39, 2008.

[154] N. Jenkins, "Modifications of therapeutic proteins: challenges and prospects," *Cytotechnology*, vol. 53, no. 1–3, pp. 121–125, 2007.

[155] G. Walsh and R. Jefferis, "Post-translational modifications in the context of therapeutic proteins," *Nature Biotechnology*, vol. 24, no. 10, pp. 1241–1252, 2006.

[156] J. Ihssen, M. Kowarik, S. Dilettoso, C. Tanner, M. Wacker, and L. Thöny-Meyer, "Production of glycoprotein vaccines in *Escherichia coli*," *Microbial Cell Factories*, vol. 9, article 61, 2010.

[157] M. Kowarik, S. Numao, M. F. Feldman et al., "N-linked glycosylation of folded proteins by the bacterial oligosaccharyltransferase," *Science*, vol. 314, no. 5802, pp. 1148–1150, 2006.

[158] V. S. Terra, D. C. Mills, L. E. Yates, S. Abouelhadid, J. Cuccui, and B. W. Wren, "Recent developments in bacterial protein glycan coupling technology and glycoconjugate vaccine design," *Journal of Medical Microbiology*, vol. 61, no. 7, pp. 919–926, 2012.

[159] M. Wacker, D. Linton, P. G. Hitchen et al., "N-linked glycosylation in *Campylobacter jejuni* and its functional transfer into *E. coli*," *Science*, vol. 298, no. 5599, pp. 1790–1793, 2002.

[160] A. A. Ollis, S. Zhang, A. C. Fisher, and M. P. DeLisa, "Engineered oligosaccharyltransferases with greatly relaxed acceptor-site specificity," *Nature Chemical Biology*, vol. 10, no. 10, pp. 816–822, 2014.

[161] J. D. Valderrama-Rincon, A. C. Fisher, J. H. Merritt et al., "An engineered eukaryotic protein glycosylation pathway in *Escherichia coli*," *Nature Chemical Biology*, vol. 8, no. 5, pp. 434–436, 2012.

[162] J. Cuccui and B. Wren, "Hijacking bacterial glycosylation for the production of glycoconjugates, from vaccines to humanised glycoproteins," *The Journal of Pharmacy and Pharmacology*, vol. 67, no. 3, pp. 338–350, 2015.

[163] J. H. Merritt, A. A. Ollis, A. C. Fisher, and M. P. Delisa, "Glycans-by-design: engineering bacteria for the biosynthesis of complex glycans and glycoconjugates," *Biotechnology and Bioengineering*, vol. 110, no. 6, pp. 1550–1564, 2013.

[164] M. Wetter, M. Kowarik, M. Steffen, P. Carranza, G. Corradin, and M. Wacker, "Engineering, conjugation, and immunogenicity assessment of *Escherichia coli* O121 O antigen for its potential use as a typhoid vaccine component," *Glycoconjugate Journal*, vol. 30, no. 5, pp. 511–522, 2013.

[165] A. C. Fisher, C. H. Haitjema, C. Guarino et al., "Production of secretory and extracellular N-linked glycoproteins in *Escherichia coli*," *Applied and Environmental Microbiology*, vol. 77, no. 3, pp. 871–881, 2011.

Permissions

The contributors of this book come from diverse backgrounds, making this book a truly international effort. This book will bring forth new frontiers with its revolutionizing research information and detailed analysis of the nascent developments around the world.

We would like to thank all the contributing authors for lending their expertise to make the book truly unique. They have played a crucial role in the development of this book. Without their invaluable contributions this book wouldn't have been possible. They have made vital efforts to compile up to date information on the varied aspects of this subject to make this book a valuable addition to the collection of many professionals and students.

This book was conceptualized with the vision of imparting up-to-date information and advanced data in this field. To ensure the same, a matchless editorial board was set up. Every individual on the board went through rigorous rounds of assessment to prove their worth. After which they invested a large part of their time researching and compiling the most relevant data for our readers.

The editorial board has been involved in producing this book since its inception. They have spent rigorous hours researching and exploring the diverse topics which have resulted in the successful publishing of this book. They have passed on their knowledge of decades through this book. To expedite this challenging task, the publisher supported the team at every step. A small team of assistant editors was also appointed to further simplify the editing procedure and attain best results for the readers.

Apart from the editorial board, the designing team has also invested a significant amount of their time in understanding the subject and creating the most relevant covers. They scrutinized every image to scout for the most suitable representation of the subject and create an appropriate cover for the book.

The publishing team has been an ardent support to the editorial, designing and production team. Their endless efforts to recruit the best for this project, has resulted in the accomplishment of this book. They are a veteran in the field of academics and their pool of knowledge is as vast as their experience in printing. Their expertise and guidance has proved useful at every step. Their uncompromising quality standards have made this book an exceptional effort. Their encouragement from time to time has been an inspiration for everyone.

The publisher and the editorial board hope that this book will prove to be a valuable piece of knowledge for researchers, students, practitioners and scholars across the globe.

List of Contributors

María A. Hidalgo, María D. Carretta, Stefanie E. Teuber, Cristian Zárate, Leonardo Cárcamo and Rafael A. Burgos
Laboratory of Molecular Pharmacology, Institute of Pharmacology and Morphophysiology, Faculty of Veterinary Sciences, Universidad Austral de Chile, Independencia 631, 5110566 Valdivia, Chile

Ilona I. Concha
Institute of Biochemistry and Microbiology, Faculty of Sciences, Universidad Austral de Chile, Independencia 631, 5110566 Valdivia, Chile

Carlos F. M. Morris, Muhammad Tahir, Mariana S. Castro and Wagner Fontes
Laboratory of Biochemistry and Protein Chemistry, Department of Cell Biology, Institute of Biology, University of Brasilia, 70910-900 Brasilia, DF, Brazil

Samina Arshid
Laboratory of Biochemistry and Protein Chemistry, Department of Cell Biology, Institute of Biology, University of Brasilia, 70910-900 Brasilia, DF, Brazil
Laboratory of Surgical Physiopathology (LIM-62), Faculty of Medicine, University of Sao Paulo, 01246-904 Sao Paulo, SP, Brazil

Roberta Fedele, Massimo Martino and Giuseppe Irrera
Hematology and Stem Cell Transplant Unit, Azienda Ospedaliera BMM, 89100 Reggio Calabria, Italy

Anna Grazia Recchia
Biotechnology Research Unit, Azienda Sanitaria Provinciale di Cosenza, 87051 Aprigliano, Italy

Massimo Gentile
Hematology Unit, Azienda Ospedaliera di Cosenza, 87100 Cosenza, Italy

Fortunato Morabito
Biotechnology Research Unit, Azienda Sanitaria Provinciale di Cosenza, 87051 Aprigliano, Italy
Hematology Unit, Azienda Ospedaliera di Cosenza, 87100 Cosenza, Italy

Léa Campos de Oliveira
Laboratório de Medicina Laboratorial (LIM03), Hospital das Clínicas, Faculdade de Medicina, Universidade de São Paulo, 05403-000 São Paulo, SP, Brazil

Anna Carla Goldberg
Hospital Israelita Albert Einstein, 05652-900 São Paulo, SP, Brazil
Instituto de Investigação em Imunologia, Instituto Nacional de Ciência e Tecnologia, 05403-000 São Paulo, SP, Brazil

Maria Lucia CarnevaleMarin
Laboratório de Imunologia, Instituto do Coração (InCor), Hospital das Clínicas, Faculdade de Medicina, Universidade de São Paulo, 05403-000 São Paulo, SP, Brazil
Laboratório de Histocompatibilidade e Imunidade Celular (LIM19), Hospital das Clínicas, Faculdade de Medicina, Universidade de São Paulo, 05403-000 São Paulo, SP, Brazil

Karina Rosa Schneidwind
Departamento de Hepatologia, Instituto da Crianç̧a, Hospital das Clínicas, Faculdade de Medicina, Universidade de São Paulo, 05403-000 São Paulo, SP, Brazil

Amanda Farage Frade
Divisão de Alergia e Imunologia Clínica, Faculdade de Medicina, Universidade de São Paulo, 05403-000 São Paulo, SP, Brazil

Jorge Kalil
Instituto de Investigação em Imunologia, Instituto Nacional de Ciência e Tecnologia, 05403-000 São Paulo, SP, Brazil
Laboratório de Imunologia, Instituto do Coração (InCor), Hospital das Clínicas, Faculdade de Medicina, Universidade de São Paulo, 05403-000 São Paulo, SP, Brazil
Laboratório de Histocompatibilidade e Imunidade Celular (LIM19), Hospital das Clínicas, Faculdade de Medicina, Universidade de São Paulo, 05403-000 São Paulo, SP, Brazil
Divisão de Alergia e Imunologia Clínica, Faculdade de Medicina, Universidade de São Paulo, 05403-000 São Paulo, SP, Brazil

Irene Kasue Miura, Renata Pereira Sustovich Pugliese, Vera Lucia Baggio Danesi and Gilda Porta
Departamento de Hepatologia, Instituto da Criança, Hospital das Clínicas, Faculdade de Medicina, Universidade de São Paulo, 05403-000 São Paulo, SP, Brazil

Eileen S. Kim, Jennifer E. Kim, Mira A. Patel, Antonella Mangraviti and Jacob Ruzevick
Department of Neurosurgery, Johns Hopkins University School of Medicine, Baltimore, MD 21205, USA

Michael Lim
Department of Neurosurgery, Johns Hopkins University School of Medicine, Baltimore, MD 21205, USA
Department of Oncology, Johns Hopkins University School of Medicine, Baltimore, MD 21205, USA

Daniel Feijó and Natalia Tavares
Centro de Pesquisas Gonçalo Moniz (CPqGM), 40296-710
Salvador, BA, Brazil

Rafael Tibúrcio and Mariana Ampuero
Centro de Pesquisas Gonçalo Moniz (CPqGM), 40296-710
Salvador, BA, Brazil
Universidade Federal da Bahia (UFBA), 40170-115
Salvador, BA, Brazil

Cláudia Brodskyn
Centro de Pesquisas Gonçalo Moniz (CPqGM), 40296-710
Salvador, BA, Brazil
Universidade Federal da Bahia (UFBA), 40170-115
Salvador, BA, Brazil
Instituto de Investigação em Imunologia (iii), 01246-903
São Paulo, SP, Brazil

Dragana Odobasic
Centre for Inflammatory Diseases, Monash University,
Department of Medicine, Monash Medical Centre,
Clayton, VIC 3168, Australia

A. Richard Kitching and Stephen R. Holdsworth
Centre for Inflammatory Diseases, Monash University,
Department of Medicine, Monash Medical Centre,
Clayton, VIC 3168, Australia
Department of Nephrology, Monash Health, Clayton,
VIC 3168, Australia

Mingming Wei, Suli Zhang and Huirong Liu
Department of Physiology and Pathophysiology, School
of Basic Medical Sciences, Capital Medical University,
Beijing 100069, China
Beijing Key Laboratory of Metabolic Disorders Related
Cardiovascular Diseases, Capital Medical University,
Beijing 100069, China

Chengrui Zhao
Department of Physiology, Basic Medical Department,
Fenyang College of Shanxi Medical University, Fenyang,
Shanxi 032200, China

Li Wang
Department of Pathology, Shanxi Medical University,
Taiyuan, Shanxi 030001, China

XinliangMa
Department of Physiology and Pathophysiology, School
of Basic Medical Sciences, Capital Medical University,
Beijing 100069, China
Beijing Key Laboratory of Metabolic Disorders Related
Cardiovascular Diseases, Capital Medical University,
Beijing 100069, China
Department of Emergency Medicine, Thomas Jefferson
University, 1025Walnut Street, College Building, Suite
808, Philadelphia, PA 19107, USA

Ekaterina A. Ivanova
Department of Development and Regeneration, KU
Leuven, 3000 Leuven, Belgium

Alexander N. Orekhov
Institute of General Pathology and Pathophysiology,
Moscow 125315, Russia
Institute for Atherosclerosis Research, Skolkovo
Innovation Center, Moscow 121609, Russia
Department of Biophysics, Biological Faculty, Moscow
State University, Moscow 119991, Russia

Lu Zhang
Department of Nephrology, The First Affiliated Hospital
of Xiamen University, Xiamen 361003, China

Guixiu Shi
Department of Rheumatology and Clinical Immunology,
The First Affiliated Hospital of Xiamen University,
Xiamen 361003, China

**Stefanie Hoyer, Isabell A. Pfeiffer, Tanushree Jaitly,
Gerold Schuler, Julio Vera, Niels Schaft and Jan Dörrie**
Department of Dermatology, Universitätsklinikum
Erlangen, Erlangen, Germany

**Kerstin F. Gerer, Sabrina Prommersberger and Sandra
Höfflin**
Department of Dermatology, Universitätsklinikum
Erlangen, Erlangen, Germany
Department of Genetics, Friedrich-Alexander-Universität
Erlangen-Nürnberg, Erlangen, Germany

Luca Beltrame
Department of Oncology, Istituto di Ricerche
Farmacologiche Mario Negri, Milan, Italy

Duccio Cavalieri
Department of Neurosciences, Psychology, Drug Research
and Child Health, University of Florence, Florence, Italy

Tana A. Omokoko, Andrea Breitkreuz and Petra Simon
Division of Translational and Experimental Oncology,
Department of Medicine III, Johannes Gutenberg
University, Freiligrathstrasse 12, 55131 Mainz, Germany
BioNTech Cell & Gene Therapies GmbH, An der
Goldgrube 12, 55131 Mainz, Germany

Uli Luxemburger and Ugur Sahin
Division of Translational and Experimental Oncology,
Department of Medicine III, Johannes Gutenberg
University, Freiligrathstrasse 12, 55131 Mainz, Germany
BioNTech AG, An der Goldgrube 12, 55131 Mainz,
Germany

Shaheer Bardissi
BioNTech Cell & Gene Therapies GmbH, An der
Goldgrube 12, 55131 Mainz, Germany

Magdalena Utsch
Ganymed Pharmaceuticals AG, An der Goldgrube 12,
55131 Mainz, Germany

Özlem Türeci
Division of Translational and Experimental Oncology, Department of Medicine III, Johannes Gutenberg University, Freiligrathstrasse 12, 55131 Mainz, Germany Ganymed Pharmaceuticals AG, An der Goldgrube 12, 55131 Mainz, Germany

Clara Mônica Lima
Postgraduate Program in Health Sciences, Federal University of Bahia School of Medicine, 40025-010 Salvador, BA, Brazil
Immunology Service, Professor Edgard Santos University Hospital, Federal University of Bahia, 40110-060 Salvador, BA, Brazil
Department of Otolaryngology, Federal University of Bahia, 40110-060 Salvador, BA, Brazil

Silvane Santos
Immunology Service, Professor Edgard Santos University Hospital, Federal University of Bahia, 40110-060 Salvador, BA, Brazil
National Institute of Science and Technology of Tropical Diseases (CNPq/MCT), 40110-060 Salvador, BA, Brazil
Department of Biological Sciences, State University of Feira de Santana (UEFS), 44036-900 Feira de Santana, BA, Brazil

Adriana Dourado, Natália B. Carvalho and Valéria Bittencourt
Immunology Service, Professor Edgard Santos University Hospital, Federal University of Bahia, 40110-060 Salvador, BA, Brazil

Marcus Miranda Lessa
Postgraduate Program in Health Sciences, Federal University of Bahia School of Medicine, 40025-010 Salvador, BA, Brazil
Department of Otolaryngology, Federal University of Bahia, 40110-060 Salvador, BA, Brazil

Isadora Siqueira
Immunology Service, Professor Edgard Santos University Hospital, Federal University of Bahia, 40110-060 Salvador, BA, Brazil
Gonçalo Moniz Research Center, Oswaldo Cruz Foundation (FIOCRUZ), 40296-710 Salvador, BA, Brazil

Edgar M. Carvalho
Postgraduate Program in Health Sciences, Federal University of Bahia School ofMedicine, 40025-010 Salvador, BA, Brazil
Immunology Service, Professor Edgard Santos University Hospital, Federal University of Bahia, 40110-060 Salvador, BA, Brazil
National Institute of Science and Technology of Tropical Diseases (CNPq/MCT), 40110-060 Salvador, BA, Brazil
Gonçalo Moniz Research Center, Oswaldo Cruz Foundation (FIOCRUZ), 40296-710 Salvador, BA, Brazil

Michelle Amantéa Sugimoto
Programa de Pós-Graduação em Ciências Farmacêuticas, Faculdade de Farmácia, Universidade Federal de Minas Gerais, 31270-901 Belo Horizonte, MG, Brazil
Departamento de Análises Clínicas e Toxicológicas, Faculdade de Farmácia, Universidade Federal de Minas Gerais, 31270-901 Belo Horizonte, MG, Brazil
Laboratório de Imunofarmacologia, Departamento de Bioquímica e Imunologia, Instituto de Ciências Biológicas, Universidade Federal de Minas Gerais, 31270-901 Belo Horizonte, MG, Brazil

Juliana Priscila Vago
Departamento de Análises Clínicas e Toxicológicas, Faculdade de Farmácia, Universidade Federal de Minas Gerais, 31270-901 Belo Horizonte, MG, Brazil
Laboratório de Imunofarmacologia, Departamento de Bioquímica e Imunologia, Instituto de Ciências Biológicas, Universidade Federal de Minas Gerais, 31270-901 Belo Horizonte, MG, Brazil
Programa de Pós-Graduação em Biologia Celular, Departamento de Morfologia, Instituto de Ciências Biológicas, Universidade Federal de Minas Gerais, 31270-901 Belo Horizonte, MG, Brazil

MauroMartins Teixeira
Laboratório de Imunofarmacologia, Departamento de Bioquímica e Imunologia, Instituto de Ciências Biológicas, Universidade Federal de Minas Gerais, 31270-901 Belo Horizonte, MG, Brazil

Lirlândia Pires Sousa
Programa de Pós-Graduação em Ciências Farmacêuticas, Faculdade de Farmácia, Universidade Federal de Minas Gerais, 31270-901 Belo Horizonte, MG, Brazil
Departamento de Análises Clínicas e Toxicológicas, Faculdade de Farmácia, Universidade Federal de Minas Gerais, 31270-901 Belo Horizonte, MG, Brazil
Laboratório de Imunofarmacologia, Departamento de Bioquímica e Imunologia, Instituto de Ciências Biológicas, Universidade Federal de Minas Gerais, 31270-901 Belo Horizonte, MG, Brazil
Programa de Pós-Graduação em Biologia Celular, Departamento de Morfologia, Instituto de Ciências Biológicas, Universidade Federal de Minas Gerais, 31270-901 Belo Horizonte, MG, Brazil

Ekua W. Brenu, Sandra Ramos and Don Staines
The National Centre for Neuroimmunology and Emerging Diseases, Griffith Health Institute, Griffith University, Gold Coast, Australia

Simon Broadley
School of Medicine, Griffith University, Gold Coast, Australia

Thao Nguyen, Samantha Johnston and Sonya Marshall-Gradisnik
The National Centre for Neuroimmunology and Emerging Diseases, Griffith Health Institute, Griffith University, Gold Coast, Australia
School of Medical Science, Griffith University, Gold Coast, Australia

Liusong Yin and Timothy P. Hickling
Pharmacokinetics, Dynamics and Metabolism-New Biological Entities, Pfizer, Andover, MA 01810, USA

Xiaoying Chen and Abhinav Tiwari
Pharmacokinetics, Dynamics and Metabolism-New Biological Entities, Pfizer, Cambridge, MA 02138, USA

Paolo Vicini
Pharmacokinetics, Dynamics and Metabolism-New Biological Entities, Pfizer, San Diego, CA 92121, USA

Fulvia Ceccarelli, Carlo Perricone, Enrica Cipriano, Cristiano Alessandri, Francesca Romana Spinelli, Antonio Sili Scavalli, Guido Valesini and Fabrizio Conti
Reumatologia, Dipartimento di Medicina Interna e Specialitá Mediche, Sapienza Universitá di Roma, 00161 Rome, Italy

Paola Borgiani, Cinzia Ciccacci, Sara Rufini and Giuseppe Novelli
Department of Biomedicine and Prevention, Section of Genetics, School of Medicine, University of Rome "Tor Vergata", 00133 Rome, Italy

Robert C. Allen
Department of Pathology, Creighton University School of Medicine, Omaha, NE 68131, USA

Omar Rafael Alemán, NancyMora, Ricarda Cortes-Vieyra and Carlos Rosales
Departamento de Inmunología, Instituto de Investigaciones Biomédicas, Universidad Nacional Autónoma de México, 04510 México, DF, Mexico

Eileen Uribe-Querol
División de Estudios de Posgrado e Investigación, Facultad de Odontología, Universidad Nacional Autónoma de México, 04510 México, DF, Mexico

Meital Cohen-Mazor, Rafi Mazor, Inbal Ziv and Shifra Sela
Eliachar Research Laboratory, Western Galilee Hospital, 22100 Nahariya, Israel
Technion Faculty of Medicine, 3525433 Haifa, Israel

Batya Kristal
Technion Faculty of Medicine, 3525433 Haifa, Israel
Department of Nephrology and Hypertension, Western Galilee Hospital, 22100 Nahariya, Israel

Erik B. Kistler
Department of Anesthesiology & Critical Care, VA San Diego Healthcare System, San Diego, CA 92161, USA

Judith Chezar
Hematology Laboratory, Western Galilee Hospital, 22100 Nahariya, Israel

Vidula T. Vachharajani
Department of Anesthesiology, Wake Forest School of Medicine, Winston-Salem, NC 27157, USA
Department of Internal Medicine, Wake Forest School of Medicine, Winston-Salem, NC 27157, USA

Tiefu Liu
Department of Internal Medicine, Wake Forest School of Medicine, Winston-Salem, NC 27157, USA
Fudan University, Shanghai Public Health Clinical Center, Shanghai 201508, China

Xianfeng Wang and Charles E. McCall
Department of Anesthesiology, Wake Forest School of Medicine, Winston-Salem, NC 27157, USA

Jason J. Hoth and Barbara K. Yoza
Department of Surgery, Wake Forest School of Medicine, Winston-Salem, NC 27157, USA

Adi Essam Zarei
Biological Sciences Department, Faculty of Science, King Abdulaziz University, P.O. Box 80203, Jeddah 21589, Saudi Arabia
Main Medical Laboratory, Medical Services, Saudi Airlines, P.O. Box 167, Cost Center 507, Jeddah 21231, Saudi Arabia

Hussein A. Almehdar
Biological Sciences Department, Faculty of Science, King Abdulaziz University, P.O. Box 80203, Jeddah 21589, Saudi Arabia

Elrashdy M. Redwan
Therapeutic and Protective Proteins Laboratory, Protein Research Department, Genetic Engineering and Biotechnology Research Institute, City for Scientific Research and Technology Applications, New Borg EL-Arab, Alexandria 21934, Egypt